Orthopedic/Neurology Words and Phrases

Second Edition

Orthopedics
Neurology
Neurosurgery
Neuroradiology
Podiatry
Rehabilitation
Rheumatology/Genetics
Chiropractic

Health Professions Institute • Modesto, California • 2000

Orthopedic/Neurology Words and Phrases
Second Edition

Orthopedics, Neurology, Neurosurgery, Neuroradiology, Podiatry, Rehabilitation, Rheumatology/Genetics, Chiropractic

Sally C. Pitman
Editor & Publisher
Health Professions Institute
P. O. Box 801
Modesto, CA 95353-0801
Phone 209-551-2112
Fax 209-551-0404
Web site: http://www.hpisum.com
E-mail: hpi@hpisum.com

Printed by
Parks Printing & Lithograph
Modesto, California

ISBN 0-934385-03-3
Last digit is the print number: 9 8 7 6 5 4 3 2 1

Preface

When the first edition of *Orthopedic/Neurology Words and Phrases* was introduced in 1994, it represented a landmark in quick-reference word books. Here at last was a reference that combined two very different yet interrelated medical specialties—orthopedics and neurology—with subspecialties such as chiropractic, podiatry, and rehabilitation medicine. It was enthusiastically received and lauded by its readers.

But the practice of medicine is dynamic, and so is its terminology. Healthcare documentation requires knowledge of and access to a broad spectrum of new words and phrases. Hundreds of new drugs, many of them developed through recombinant technology for orthopedic and neurology patients, have appeared since 1994.

In that vein, *Orthopedic/Neurology Words and Phrases*, second edition, sets another milestone in excellence and value. Its 870 pages and over 70,000 entries make word-researching easier and more accurate for the production-oriented healthcare professional. In addition to the standard medical specialties of orthopedics, neurology, neurosurgery, podiatry, rehabilitation, and chiropractic, this new edition includes terms from neuroradiology, rheumatology, genetics, alternative medicine, complementary medicine, Chinese medicine, and recombinant technology. Hundreds of drugs, both prescription and over-the-counter, have been added.

We are also pleased to present a special feature in this edition: in the Appendix are three tables of bones, muscles, and nerves. Medical transcriptionists especially will appreciate listings of these common anatomic structures in both English and their Latin equivalents.

As always, *Orthopedic/Neurology Words and Phrases* is extensively cross-referenced to assure greater success in finding a desired word or phrase. Terms were gathered from thousands of actual orthopedic and neurology transcripts, from medical journals and textbooks, and through extensive research on the Internet. Invaluable assistance in verifying the accuracy of entries and reconciling discrepancies from various authoritative references was provided by John H. Dirckx, M.D., medical editorial consultant.

We are grateful to Bron Taylor and Susan Turley, the main contributors of terminology to the first edition. Research for this second edition was done primarily by Linda C. Campbell and Diane S. Heath, with editorial assistance from Georgia Green. We thank Arleen McGovern and Toni Mercadante for sharing their terminology research. Our warmest gratitude is also extended to those readers who called or wrote with comments and suggestions on the first edition; this book is better because of their feedback.

Sally C. Pitman, MA
Editor & Publisher

How to Use This Book

The words and phrases in this book are alphabetized letter by letter of all words in the entry, ignoring punctuation marks and words or letters in parentheses. The possessive form ('s) is omitted from eponyms for ease in alphabetizing. Numbers are alphabetized as if written out, with the exception of subscripts and superscripts which are ignored.

Eponyms appear alphabetically as well as under the nouns they modify. For example, *Ogden epiphyseal fracture classification* is found alphabetically under the O's as well as under the main entries *classification* and *fracture*. *Magnevist* is found in the M's as well as under *imaging agent*.

The main entry *drugs* includes descriptive terms related to drugs, not the names of pharmaceuticals. The names of hundreds of medications used in orthopedics and neurology as well as the various subspecialties included in this book appear under the entry *medications*. Names of various radiology imaging studies have been combined under the broad category *imaging,* while names of various kinds of technology are listed under the broad terms *device* and *system*.

In medical dictation physicians may arbitrarily refer to an operative procedure as an *approach*, *method*, *operation*, *procedure*, *repair*, or *technique*, or by the type of procedure, such as *arthroplasty* and *osteotomy*. Thus, all procedures are listed alphabetically by the eponym as well as under the type of procedure and under the main entry *operations*.

Many anatomical terms are found in the book, but no attempt was made to be comprehensive. The appendix includes tables of bones, muscles, and nerves, with both English and Latin forms in tabular form for quick reference.

Main entries with a lengthy list of subentries include the following:

activity on EEG	fracture	reflex
bone	graft	retractor
brace	imaging	scale
cast	joint	score
cerebrospinal fluid	lesion	screw
classification	ligament	sign
deformity	medications	splint
device	MRI	support
disease	muscle	suture
electrode	nerve	syndrome
electroencephalogram	operations	system
electromyogram	orthosis	test
epilepsy	plate	tumor
forceps	prosthesis	view

A, a

AA (acetabular anteversion)
AAA (diagnostic arthroscopy, operative arthroscopy, and possible operative arthrotomy)
AAA bone
AAASPS (African-American Antiplatelet Stroke Prevention Study)
AACPDM (American Academy for Cerebral Palsy and Developmental Medicine)
AAHKS (American Association of Hip and Knee Surgeons)
AAHS (American Association for Hand Surgery)
AAI (axial acetabular index)
AAMI (age-associated memory impairment)
AAN (American Academy of Neurology)
AANA (Arthroscopy Association of North America)
AANS (American Association of Neurological Surgeons)
AAOFAS (American Association of Orthopaedic Foot and Ankle Surgeons)
AAO (awake, alert, and oriented)

AAOP (American Association of Orthotists and Prosthetists)
AAOS (American Academy of Orthopaedic Surgeons)
AAOS classification of acetabular abnormalities
AAOS/HKOD Questionnaire
AAOS Knee Society Clinical Rating Score
AAOS POI (American Academy of Orthopedic Surgeons Pediatrics Outcomes Instrument)
AAOx3 (awake, alert, and oriented x 3 [person, place, and time])
AAPMR (American Academy of Physical Medicine and Rehabilitation)
AAPSM (American Academy of Podiatric Sports Medicine)
AAROM (active ankle joint complex range of motion)
AAROM (active assisted range of motion)
AARP (American Association of Retired Persons)
AAS (American Autonomic Society)
abarticular gout
abasia

abate, abated
abatement
Abbe operation
Abbott brace
Abbott-Fisher-Lucas arthrodesis
Abbott-Gill epiphyseal plate exposure
Abbott-Lucas shoulder operation
Abbreviated Injury Scale (AIS)
ABC (aneurysmal bone cyst)
ABD (abdominal) dressing
ABD pad
abdominal brace position
abdominal bracing
abdominal epilepsy
abdominal internal oblique muscle
abdominal migraine
abdominal muscles
abdominal reflex
abdominopelvic splanchnic nerves
abdominis rectus muscle
abducens (or abducent) nerve (sixth
    cranial nerve)
abducens (or abducent) nucleus
abducens nerve palsy
abducens nerve paresis
abduct, abductor
"a-b-duction" (as dictated)
abduction fracture
abduction stress test
abductor digiti minimi muscle
abductor digiti quinti (ADQ) muscle
abductor digiti quinti (ADQ) tendon
abductor hallucis muscle
abductor lurch (gluteus medius gait)
abductor pollicis brevis (APB) muscle
abductor pollicis brevis (APB) tendon
abductor pollicis longus (APL) muscle
abductor pollicis longus (APL) tendon
abductovalgus, hallux
Abercrombie neuronal cell count
    formula
aberrant patterns (of sweating, hair
    distribution, color)
aberrations, intersegmental
abet, abetted, abetting
ABGs (arterial blood gases)
ABG (autogeneous bone graft)

ABGd imaging agent
ABI (ankle/brachial index)
ABI (auditory brain stem implant)
ability (pl. abilities)
    bathing and dressing
    abstracting
    conceptual
    constructional
    following (of the eyes)
    positive
ability to abstract
ability to attend
ABJS (Association of Bone and Joint
    Surgeons)
ablation
    nerve
    radical nail bed
    stereotactic or stereotaxic
    surgical
    total pituitary
    Zadik total nail bed
ablator, Concept
ablative arthroplasty
ablative laser therapy
ablative surgery
ABLB (alternate binaural loudness
    balance) test
Abnormal Involuntary Movement
    Scale (AIMS)
abnormality
    acral
    bony
    bulbar
    cranial nerve
    cytoarchitectonic
    focal
    frontal plane growth
    functional
    gray matter
    neuroendocrine
    perfusion
    restrictive
    soft tissue
    torsional
    tracer
    ultrastructural
    vasculature

abnormality *(continued)*
  vessel wall
  white matter
aboral direction
ABOS (American Board of
  Orthopaedic Surgery)
above-elbow prosthesis
above-knee prosthesis
ABR (auditory brain stem response)
  threshold
abrader, cartilage
Abramson catheter
abrasion arthroplasty
abrasions and contusions
Abrikosov tumor
abrupt vessel closure
abscess (pl. abscesses)
  actinomycotic brain
  acute
  arthrifluent
  Aspergillus cerebral
  bone
  brain
  Brodie metaphyseal
  cerebral
  collar button
  daughter
  encapsulated brain
  epidural
  extradural
  frontal
  growth plate
  horseshoe
  intradural
  intraosseous
  lumbar epidural
  metaphyseal
  midpalmar
  Paget
  postoperative
  Pott
  psoas
  serous
  spinal epidural (SEA)
  subaponeurotic
  subdural
  subgaleal

abscess *(continued)*
  subperiosteal
  subungual
  suture
  thecal
  thenar space
absence attack
absence seizure (see *seizure*)
absence status (seizure)
absent ataxia
absent bow-tie sign
absent consensual constriction (pupil)
absent thumb
Absolute absorbable screw
absolute latency
absolute neck diameter of aneurysm
absolute perfusion value
absolute scotomata
absorbable polyparadioxanone pin
absorbent cover dressing (ACD)
absorptiometry
  double-photon (DPA)
  dual x-ray
  fan-beam x-ray
  single-photon (SPA)
  single-energy x-ray (SXA)
absorption
  bony
  impaired
  linear
  lysosomal
absorption cavity
absorption of radionuclide
abstraction
abstract thinking
abulia
abulic mental changes
abut, abutted, abutting
abutment splint
AC (acromioclavicular) joint
  separation
AC (anterior commissure)
ACA (American Chiropractic
  Association)
ACA (anterior cerebral artery)
ACA (anterior choroidal artery)

ACAD (atherosclerotic carotid artery disease)
academy (see also *association; committee; society*)
    American Academy of Neurology
    American Academy of Orthopedic Surgeons (AAOS)
acalculia
    aphasic
    visual-spatial
Acanthamoeba meningitis
acanthopelvis
ACAT (automated computed axial tomography)
ACB (asymptomatic carotid bruit)
accelerated chondral wear
accelerated hyperfractionated radiotherapy
accelerometer device
accelerator
    Bevatron
    linear
    Philips linear
accelerator nerves
acceptance, weight (of gait)
accessory atlantoaxial ligament
accessory bones (sesamoid bones of foot or hand)
accessory flexor muscle of foot
accessory ligament
accessory nerve, vagal
accessory oculomotor nucleus
accessory ossicle
accessory phrenic nerves
accessory plantar ligament
accessory recess
accessory volar ligament
accident
    ATV (all-terrain vehicle)
    cardiovascular
    cerebrovascular (CVA) (stroke)
    compensable
    horseback riding
    motorcycle (MCA)
    motor vehicle (MVA)
    rollerblading
    skateboarding

accident *(continued)*
    snowboarding
    vascular
    vehicular
acclivity
accommodation reflex
Accommodator arch support
ACCR (American Chiropractic College of Radiology)
Accucore II core biopsy needle
Accuflate tourniquet
accuDEXA bone densitometer
Accu-Flo CSF reservoir
Accu-Flo dura film
Accu-Flo polyethylene bur hole cover
Accu-Flo silicone rubber bur hole cover
Accu-Flo ventricular catheter
AccuLength arthroplasty measuring system
Accu-Line dual pivot
Accu-Line femoral resector
Accu-Line guide
Accu-Line knee instrumentation
Accu-Line tibial resector
accumulation, abnormal tracer
accumulation, p53
accuracy, spatial
AccuSharp carpal tunnel release instrument
Accuson 128XP ultrasound
Accuson Sequoia ultrasound device
AccuSway balance measurement system
Accutom low-speed diamond saw
Accu-Tron microcurrent machine
Accuzyme enzymatic debriding agent
ACD (absorbent cover dressing)
Ace bandage
Ace-Colles fixator
Ace-Colles frame technique
Ace-Colles half ring
Ace-Fischer external fixator
acellular dermal allograft
    AlloDerm
    XenoDerm
Ace screw

acetabular angle of Sharp
acetabular anteversion (AA)
acetabular bone
acetabular cup (see *cup*)
acetabular depth to femoral head
   diameter (AD/FHD)
acetabular dysplasia
acetabular fossa
acetabular head index (AHI)
acetabular labrum
acetabular notch
acetabular osteolysis   — petrusio
acetabular recess
acetabular roof
acetabulectomy
acetabuloplastic round chisel
acetabuloplasty
acetabulum (pl. acetabula)
   deep-shelled
   dysplastic
   true
acetazolamide challenge test
Ace Unifix fixation device
Ace wrap
acetic acid iontophoresis
acetylcholine esterase
acetylcholine receptor antibody
   (AChRab)
ACF (anterior cervical fusion)
ACG knee replacement system
ACh (acetylcholine) receptor
achalasia, cricopharyngeal
acheiria
ache, achy, aching
aches and pains
ache, weather-
Achilles bulge sign
Achilles bursa
Achilles jerk
Achilles paratendinitis
Achilles squeeze test
Achilles tendon (tendo Achillis)
Achilles tendon autograft
Achilles tendon lengthening
Achilles tendon reflex
Achilles tendon rupture
Achilles tendon shortening

Achilles + ultrasound bone
   densitometer
Achillis, tendo
achillodynia
achillorrhaphy
achillotenotomy
Achillotrain tendon support
aching pain
achondroplasia
achondroplastic dwarfism
AChR (acetylcholine receptor) antibody
AChRab (acetylcholine receptor
   antibody)
achromatopsia
achy feeling
ACI (autologous chondrocyte
   implantation)
ACI (Autologous Chondrocyte
   Implantation) Register
acid
   arachidonic
   bichloroacetic
   phytanic
acid class, pyranocarboxylic
acidophilic pituitary tumor
acidosis, ischemic lactic
aciduria
   argininosuccinic
   methylmalonic
Ackerman criteria for osteomyelitis
ACL (anterior cruciate ligament)
ACL-Ab (anticardiolipin antibodies)
ACL drill guide
ACL graft
ACL guide set
AC Lite functional knee brace
ACL repair
Acland clamp or clip
Acland clamp-applying forceps
Acland double-clamp approximator
Acland microvascular clamp
aclasia, diaphyseal
ACLR (anterior capsulolabral
   reconstruction)
ACM (acute confusional migraine)
ACoA (anterior communicating artery)
Acoma scanner

Acor Quikform I or II shoe
acorn, Midas Rex
acoustical shadowing on ultrasound
acoustic impedance
acoustic nerve
acoustic nerve tumor
acoustic neurinoma
acoustic neuroma
acoustic reflex threshold
AC-PC (anterior commissure-
    posterior commissure) line
AC-PC plane
acquired post-traumatic syringomyelia
acquired flatfoot
acquired myopathy
acquired nystagmus
acquired toxoplasmosis
acquisition time (MRI)
ACR (American College of
    Rheumatology)
ACR classification of arthritis
Acra-Cut cranial perforator
Acra-Cut cranioblade
Acra-Cut Spiral craniotome blade
Acra-Cut wire pass drill
acral abnormality
Acrel ganglion
ACRM (American Congress of
    Rehabilitation Medicine)
acrocallosal syndrome
acrocephalosyndactylism
acrocephalosyndactyly
Acro-Flex artificial disk
acromacria
AcroMed plate
AcroMed screw
AcroMed VSP (variable screw
    placement) fixation system
acromegaly
acrometastasis
acromial angle
acromial bone
acromioclavicular (AC) joint
acromioclavicular meniscus
acromioclavicular osteolysis
acromiocoracoid ligament
acromiohumeral interval (AHI)

acromion
    curved
    flat
    hooked
acromionectomy, Armstrong
acromioplasty
    anterior
    arthroscopic
    decompressive
    McLaughlin
    Neer
    revision
acro-osteosclerosis
acropachy
acroparesthesia of limbs
acropectorovertebral dysplasia
acrosyndactyly, Apert
Acrotorque hand engine
acrylic cement
Acryl-X orthopedic cement removal
    system
ACS acetabular liner
ACSM (American College of Sports
    Medicine)
Act support
ACTH (adrenocorticotropic hormone)
    antibody
ACTH-producing pituitary adenoma
ACTH-producing pituitary tumor
Actinomadura madurae
Actinomyces
actinomycetoma
actinomycosis with epidural granuloma
actinomycotic brain abscess
action
    scotomata of
    tenodesis
    viscoelastic
action myoclonus
action potential
Action Research Arm (ARA) Test
Activa tremor control therapy system
activating procedures on EEG
activating techniques
    hyperventilation
    photic stimulation

activating techniques *(continued)*
  stroboscopic light
  sleep
activator
  recombinant tissue-type
    plasminogen
  tissue-type plasminogen
activator table
active assisted range of motion
  (AAROM)
active biplanar MR imaging guidance
active core cooling
active deformers (muscle action in
  arthritis)
active dorsiflexion
active extension against gravity
active range of motion (AROM)
  exercise
Active supports and braces
activities
  high-impact
  instrumental activities of daily
    living (IADL)
activities of daily living (ADLs)
activity (pl. activities)
  aerobic
  dynamic
  neuronal
  overhead
  striatal
  telomerase
  tremor-related
activity on EEG
  alpha
  asymmetrical epileptiform
  asymmetrical generalized
    epileptiform
  background
  barbiturate-induced spindle-like
  beta
  bilateral
  burst of
  burst of delta
  burst of slow wave
  burst of theta
  cerebral
  delta

activity on EEG *(continued)*
  desynchronization
  diffuse distribution of
  discontinuous
  distribution of
  electrocerebral
  electrographic seizure
  epileptiform
  excessive diffuse low and medium
    wave beta
  extracerebral
  focal delta slow wave
  focal epileptiform
  focal interictal epileptiform
  frontal intermittent rhythmic delta
    (FIRDA)
  frontal rhythmic theta
  generalized delta
  generalized distribution
  generalized epileptiform
  generalized paroxysmal fast
  high-voltage slow and sharp
  ictal epileptiform
  interictal epileptiform
  interictal localized
  intermittent rhythmical delta
    activity (IRDA)
  lateralized
  lateralized epileptiform
  level of
  localized delta
  localized epileptiform
  low-amplitude
  low-voltage
  medium-voltage beta
  monomorphic
  monorhythmic frontal delta (MFD)
  monorhythmic sinusoidal delta
  noncerebral
  nonepileptiform
  occipital dominant intermittent
    rhythmic delta
  occipital intermittent rhythmical
    delta (OIRDA)
  paroxysmal alpha
  paroxysmal beta
  paroxysmal delta

activity on EEG *(continued)*
  paroxysmal theta
  polymorphic delta
  polyrhythmic
  posterior dominant
  post-traumatic epileptiform
  propagation of
  pseudoepileptiform
  reflex neurologic
  rhythmic
  rhythmical spindle-shaped
  runs of
  scattered dysrhythmic slow
  serotonergic
  sleep
  slow-wave
  spectral peak frequency of
  spiking
  spindle-like
  theta
  triphasic slow-wave
  unilateral epileptiform
  unilateral focus of
  widespread distribution
activity level
Activity-Lite knee brace
Activity Losses Assessment (ALA)
activity restriction
activity status
Actonel (risedronate)
actual leg length test
ACU-derm wound dressing
ACU-dyne antiseptic
Acufex ankle distractor
Acufex arthroscopic instruments
Acufex bioabsorbable fixation device
Acufex bioabsorbable Suretac suture
Acufex bioabsorbable suture anchor
Acufex biting forceps
Acufex curet
Acufex distractor pin
Acufex gouge
Acufex knee laxity arthrometer
Acufex mallet
Acufex meniscal basket
Acufex meniscal stitcher
Acufex osteotome

Acufex probe
Acufex rasp
Acufex TAG rod
Acufex T-fix suture anchor
Acufex tibial guide
Acumed instruments and devices
acuity, central visual
Acumeter
acupoint
AcuPressor myotherapy tool
acupressure ear-probe reflexology
  device
acupressure without needles
acupuncture
  electro-acupuncture
  Korean hand
acupuncture laser
Acuson imaging system
AcuSpark piezoelectrical device
Acustar surgical navigation system
acutance, image edge profile
acute acquired hemiplegia
acute aphonia
acute ascending motor paralysis
acute avulsion fracture
acute brain syndrome
acute cerebellar hemispheric lesion
acute chorea
acute compartment syndrome
acute confusional state
acute exertional compartment
  syndrome (AECS)
acute exogenous reaction
acute foot strain
acute gout
acute hematogenous arthritis
acute hematogenous osteomyelitis
  (AHO)
acute infective gangrene
acute inflammatory demyelinating
  polyradiculoneuropathy (AIDP)
acute inflammatory polyradiculopathy
acute labyrinthine disorder
acute meningitis
acute phase reactant
acute purulent meningitis
acute repetitive seizure (ARS) disorder

acute spinal arthritis
acute stretch injury
acute stroke
acute transverse myelitis (ATM)
acute whiplash
ACUTENS transcutaneous nerve
    stimulator
Acutrak fusion system
Acu-Treat electro-acupuncture
AD (Alzheimer disease)
ADA (American Dietetic Association)
    diets for athletes
adactyly (adactylia)
Adam and Eve splint
adamantinoma
Adamkiewicz (also Adamkiewitz)
    artery of
    syndrome of the great radicular
        artery of
Adams forward-bending test for
    scoliosis
Adams position test
Adams procedure
Adams saw
Adams splint
Adapta physical therapy table
adapter
    Christmas tree
    chuck
    collet screwdriver
    French
    Hudson chuck
    Jacobs chuck
    Lloyd
    Mayfield
    Trinkle chuck
    VCS clip
Adaptic dressing
Adaptic gauze
Adaptic packing
Adaptic sponge
adaptive equipment
ADAS (Alzheimer's Disease
    Assessment Scale)
ADAS noncognitive subscale
ADC (AIDS dementia complex)

ADC (analog-to-digital) conversion
    quantization error (MRI)
ADCA (autosomal-dominant cerebellar
    ataxia), type II
Adcon-L anti-adhesion barrier
ADD (attention deficit disorder)
addiction medicine
addiction therapy
addictive disease
Addis test
Add-On Bucky digital x-ray image
    acquisition system
adduct
"a-d-duction" (as dictated)
adduction, Edgarton-Grand thumb
adduction fracture
adduction stress to fingers
adduction to neutral
adductor canal
adductor hiatus
adductor magnus
adductor minimus muscle
adductor muscle
    great
    long
    short
adductor muscle of great toe
adductor pollicis muscle (thumb)
adductor sweep of thumb
adductor tendon
adductor tendon and lateral capsular
    release
adductor tenotomy and obturator
    neurectomy (ATON)
adductor tubercle
adductus
    metatarsus (MTA)
    true metatarsus (TMA)
adenocarcinoma, metastatic
adenohypophysectomy
adenohypophysial
adenohypophysis
adenoma
    acidophilic
    acinous
    ACTH-producing pituitary

adenoma *(continued)*
  basophilic
  chromophobic
  cutaneous
  eosinophilic
  glycoprotein-secreting
  gonadotropin-secreting
  intraspinal
  nonsecreting pituitary
  null-cell
  pituitary
  prolactin-secreting
  sebaceum
  suprasellar
adenopathy
Adenoscan contrast medium
adenosine diphosphate pathway
AD/FHD (ratio of acetabular depth to
  femoral head diameter)
ADH (antidiuretic hormone) secretion,
  inappropriate
ADHD (attention deficit/hyperactivity
  disorder)
adherent tape, benzoin
adhesed
adhesion
  capsular
  fibrous
  intra-articular
  leukocyte-endothelial
  subacromial bursal
  subdeltoid bursal
adhesion molecule
adhesive (see also *cement; glue*)
  APR cement fixation
  Aron Alpha
  benzoin
  Biobrane
  Coe-pak paste
  Cover-Roll gauze
  Coverlet
  cyanoacrylate
  Fibrijet
  fibrin glue
  Histoacryl glue
  hydroxyapatite

adhesive *(continued)*
  Implast bone cement
  ligand
  LPPS hydroxyapatite
  medical
  methyl methacrylate
  Palacos cement
  Simplex
  Superglue (cyanoacrylate)
  Surfit
  Surgical Simplex P
  Zimmer low viscosity
adhesive arachnoiditis
adhesive capsulitis (frozen shoulder)
ADI (atlantodens interval)
adiabatic fast passage (MRI)
adiadochokinesia
Adie-Holmes pupil
Adie pupils
Adie syndrome
Adie tonic pupil
adipose graft
adipose ligament
adipose tissue
adiposogenital dystrophy
aditus pelvis
adjunctive glucocorticoid therapy
Adjustable Leg and Ankle
  Repositioning Mechanism
  (ALARM)
adjusting table
adjustive treatment (chiropractic)
adjustment
  atlas
  chiropractic spinal
  vectored
adjustment of the articulations and
  adjacent tissues
adjuvant-induced arthritis (AIA)
adjuvant radiation therapy
Adkins arthrodesis
Adkins spinal fusion
ADL (adrenoleukodystrophy)
ADL indices
ADLs (activities of daily living)
  extended
  hierarchical scales of

ADLs *(continued)*
  indices of
  instrumental
Adolescent and Pediatric Pain Tool
  (APPT)
adolescent hallux valgus
adolescent idiopathic scoliosis (AIS)
adolescent tibia vara
Adorno Rogers wheelchair
ADQ (abductor digiti quinti) muscle
ADRDA (Alzheimer's Disease and
  Related Disorders Association)
adrenal medullary tissue, autologous
adrenaline
adrenergic neurotransmission
adrenocortical coma
adrenoleukodystrophy (ADL),
  X-linked recessive
Adriamycin (doxorubicin)
ADROM (ankle dorsiflexion range of
  motion)
ADR Ultramark 4 ultrasound
ADS (anterior dynamized system)
  orthosis
AD7C cerebrospinal fluid test for
  Alzheimer disease
Adson-Anderson cerebellar retractor
Adson aneurysm needle
Adson bayonet dressing forceps
Adson bipolar forceps
Adson brain-exploring cannula
Adson brain retractor
Adson brain suction tip
Adson brain suction tube
Adson-Brown tissue forceps
Adson bur
Adson cerebellar retractor
Adson chisel
Adson clip-introducing forceps
Adson conductor
Adson cranial rongeur
Adson dissecting hook
Adson dressing forceps
Adson drill
Adson drill guide
Adson dural hook
Adson dural knife

Adson dural needle holder
Adson dural protector
Adson elevator
Adson enlarging bur
Adson exploring cannula
Adson forceps
Adson ganglion scissors
Adson hemilaminectomy retractor
Adson hemostatic forceps
Adson hypophyseal forceps
Adson knife
Adson knot tier
Adson laminectomy chisel
Adson maneuver
Adson micro dressing forceps
Adson micro tissue forceps
Adson-Mixter neurosurgical forceps
Adson modified maneuver
Adson needle
Adson needle holder
Adson nerve hook
Adson perforating bur
Adson periosteal elevator
Adson retractor
Adson right-angle knife
Adson-Rogers cranial bur
Adson rongeur
Adson saw
Adson saw guide
Adson scalp clip
Adson scalp needle
Adson scissors
Adson sign
Adson suction tube
Adson test
Adson tissue forceps
Adson-Toennis scissors
Adson twist drill
Adson wire saw
ADT (anterior drawer test)
AdTech electrode grid
AdTech electrode strip
ADTRA composite external fixator
  ring
adult-onset ankylosing spondylitis
  (AOAS)
advanced cortical disease

Advanced mobile-bearing knee implant
Advanced NMR Systems scanner
advanced practice nurse (APN)
advancement
    fronto-orbital
    heel-cord
    tendon
    transcranial frontofacial
    VMO (vastus medialis obliquus)
Advance PS total knee system
advancer
Advanta Orthopaedics instruments
    and devices
Advantage electromyography system
AdvanTeq II TENS unit
Advantim revision knee system
adventitia
adventitial forceps
adventitious bursa
adventitious movements
adversive attack
adversive fields (visual)
adversive motor seizure
AE (above-elbow) amputation
AECS (acute exertional compartment
    syndrome)
aEEG (amplitude-integrated EEG)
AE1, AE3 antibody
AER (apical ectodermal ridge)
aerate, aerated, aeration
aerobe
aerobic dance
    high-impact (HIAD)
    low-impact (LIAD)
aerobic exercise
Aeroplast dressing
aerosolized Tc-DTPA
aerosolized Tc-PYP
AERx pain management system
Aesculap ABC cervical plating system
Aesculap bipolar cautery forceps
Aesculap forceps
Aesculap head holder
Aesculap-PM noncemented femoral
    prosthesis
Aesculap screw
aesthetic, aesthetically

aesthetic surgery
AF (anterior frontal) electrode
    (AF_3, AF_4, AF_7, AF_8, AF_z)
AF (arcuate fasciculus)
affect
    blunted
    flat
    inappropriate
    infantile
    labile
    normal
    pseudobulbar
    shallow
affective behavior
affective changes
affective prodrome of epilepsy
affective prodrome of migraine
affective symptoms of seizures
afferent digital lesion
afferent digital nerves
afferent nerve lesion
afferent neuron
afferent proprioception
afferent pupillary defect
AFI total hip replacement prosthesis
A5 pulley
AFO (ankle-foot orthosis)
    articulated
    molded
    posterior leaf-spring
    standard shell
AFO brace
AFP (alpha-fetoprotein) test
A-frame electrode
after-discharge on EEG
after-nystagmus, cycles of
AG (angular gyrus)
AGC (anatomically graduated
    component)
AGC Biomet total knee system
AGC femoral prosthesis
AGC knee prosthesis
AGC tibial prosthesis
age
    biologic
    bone
    chronologic

...r cavernous

...ory

...sock

...nflammatory

...ating polyradiculopathy)

...nal memory

...ual

...alking

...DS (acquired immunodeficiency
syndrome)

AIDS-defining illness

AIDS dementia complex (ADC)

AIDS encephalopathy

AIDS myelopathy

AI 5200 diagnostic ultrasound system

Aiken osteotomy

AIM CPM (continuous passive
motion) for hand and legs

aimer
femoral
tibial

AIMS (Abnormal Involuntary
Movement Scale)

AIMS (Arthritis Impact Measurement
Scale)

AIMS2 (Arthritis Impact Measurement
Scales–Symptoms [Pain])

AIMS2 Hand Subscale

Ainsworth modification of Massie nail

AIOD (aortoiliac obstructive disease)

AIOSM (American Institute of
Orthopaedic and Sports Medicine)

air-bone gap

Aircast Air-Stirrup brace

Aircast Cryo-Cuffs

Aircast pneumatic air stirrup

Aircast pneumatic walker

Aircast Rolimeter

Aircast Swivel-Strap brace

Aircast walking brace

air cisternography

AirCom compression-molded polyethylene

air-conduction threshold

air-contrast studies

air cuff

air DonJoy patellofemoral brace

Air-Dyne bicycle

air embolism of the brain

AirFlex carpal tunnel splint

air hunger

Airis II open MRI system

air myelogram

AIROM (active integral range of
motion)

airplane brace

airplane cast

airplane splint shoulder brace

air plethysmography

Airprene Action knee brace

Airprene hinged knee prosthesis

air pressure splint

air splint

Air-Stirrup Ankle Training Brace

Airtrac ambulatory cervical/lumbar
traction system

AIS (Abbreviated Injury Scale)

AIS (adolescent idiopathic scoliosis)

Aitken classification of epiphyseal
fracture

Aitken femoral deficiency

AIT-082 (Neotrofin)

AJ (ankle jerk)

AJC (ankle-joint complex)

AJCC (American Joint Commision
on Cancer)

AKA (above-knee amputation)

akathisia, tardive

A-K diamond knife

Akin bunionectomy

akinesia

akinesthesia

akinetic drop attack

akinetic drop spell

akinetic mutism
alert
apathetic

akinetic seizure

akinetic spell

Akin osteotomy

Akros extended-care mattress

Akros pressure mattress
AKS (American Knee Society)
ala (pl. alae), sacral
ALA (Activity Losses Assessment)
ALAAD (aromatic L-amino acid
    decarboxylase)
alalia
Alanson amputation
alar bone
alar ligament
alarm clock headache
ALARM (Adjustable Leg and Ankle
    Repositioning Mechanism)
Albee bone graft
Albee-Compere fracture table
Albee-Delbert operation
Albee hip arthrodesis
Albee lumbar spinal fusion
Albee olive-shaped bur
Albee shelf procedure
Albers-Schönberg disease
    (Schoenberg)
Albert Grass Heritage digital EEG
    system
Albert knee operation
Alberts Famous Faces Test
albicans, Candida
Albinus muscle
Albright-Chase arthroplasty
Albright-McCune-Sternberg syndrome
albumin, radioiodinated serum (RISA)
albuminocytologic dissociation in
    Guillain-Barré disease
Albunex ultrasound imaging agent
Alcock canal
alcohol, blood levels of
alcoholic blackout
alcoholic amnesia
alcoholic epilepsy
alcoholic hallucinosis
alcoholic intoxication
alcoholic myopathy
alcoholic paraplegia
alcoholic stupor
alcohol-precipitated epilepsy
alcohol-related seizure

alcohol withdrawal
alcohol withdrawal seizures
alcohol withdrawal syndrome
alcohol withdrawal tremor
Alden CDI orthotic
aldosteronoma
alendronate (Fosamax)
alert and oriented x 3 (to person,
    place, and time)
alert and oriented x 4 (to person,
    place, time, and future plans)
alerting maneuver on EEG
alerting stimulus on EEG
alertness
    level of
    state of
Alexander chisel
Alexander costal periosteotome
Alexander disease
Alexander-Farabeuf periosteotome
Alexander-Farabeuf rasp
alexandrite (solid-state) laser
alexia
    anterior
    central
    posterior
    tactile
alexia with agraphia
alexia without agraphia
Alexian Brothers overhead frame
alfacalcidol (One-Alpha)
algesimeter
    Aly
    Björnström
alginate-collagen gel
algodystrophy
AlgoMed infusion system
algometer
algorithm, alignment-correction
aliasing on EEG
aliasing, temporal
Alice 4 diagnostic sleep system
alien hand sign
align, aligned
aligner
    Charnley femoral inlay
    femoral

aligner *(continued)*
  patellar
  tibial
alignment
  anatomic
  angular
  fracture fragment
  integrity and
  lower extremity
  poor
  rotational
  three-plane
  torsional
  transverse-plane
  two-plane
  vertebral body
alignment-correction algorithm
alignment of fracture fragments
alignment of vertebral bodies
alignment rod
Alimed insert
Alimed wrist/thumb support
alimentary seizure
Aliplast insoles
aliquorrhea (low CSF production)
Alivium implant metal
Alkphase-B
ALL (anterior longitudinal ligament)
all-median-nerve hand
all-terrain vehicle (ATV)
all-ulnar-nerve hand
allachesthesia
allele (pl. alleles)
  APOE-e4
  unmethylated
Allen arm/hand surgery table
Allen arthroscopic elbow positioner
Allen arthroscopic knee positioner
Allen arthroscopic wrist positioner
Allen maneuver
Allen open reduction of calcaneus
  fracture
Allen shoulder/wrist arthroscopy
  traction system
Allen sign
Allen stirrups
Allen test

Allen wrench
Allender vertical laminar flow room
Allevyn dressing
Allis clamp
Allis forceps
Allis sign
Allis tissue forceps
Allman classification of acromioclavicular injury
Allman modification of Evans ankle
  reconstruction
allochiria (allocheiria)
allocortex
AlloDerm acellular dermal autograft
alloesthesia
allodynia
Allofix freeze-dried cortical bone pin
allogeneic bone graft
allogeneic cytokine-secreting cellular
  vaccine
allogenic chondrocyte
allogenic marrow transplantation
allogenic transplantation
allogenous bone graft
allograft
  acellular dermal
  block
  bone
  bone-tendon-bone
  fresh frozen
  frozen radiated wedge
  lyophilized spinal dural
  osteochondral
  Red Cross freeze-dried
  structural anterior column
  wedgeAllport retractor
allograft transplantation
AlloGrip bone vise
allopurinol (Zyloprim)
alloy
  cobalt-chromium
  stainless steel
  Ti-Nidium
  Ti6A14V
  Wood
All-Tronics scanner
Alm wound retractor

Aloka SSD ultrasound system
Alouette amputation
ALP (ankle ligament protector)
Alpers disease
Alpers syndrome
alpha activity
alpha angle (on x-ray)
alpha band on EEG
alpha blocking on EEG
alpha-BSM bone repair material
alpha-fetoprotein
alpha frequency band on EEG
alpha frequency coma
alpha frequency range
alpha index
alpha motor neuron
alpha pattern on EEG
alpha rhythm on EEG
alpha spindles on EEG
AlphaStar table
Alphatec mini lag-screw system
    (MLS)
alpha tocopherol
alpha wave on EEG
ALP Plus ankle brace
ALPS (anterior locking plate system),
    Amset
ALS (Amyotrophic Lateral Sclerosis)
    Association
ALS (amyotrophic lateral sclerosis)
    bulbar-onset
    carcinomatous
    limb-onset
    spinal form of
ALS Functional Rating Scale (ALS-
    FRS)
alta, patella
Alta tibial/humeral reconstruction rod
alteplase (recombinant tissue plasmino-
    gen activator) (Activase)
alteration in blood-brain barrier
alteration in consciousness
altered mechanical strength of allograft
altered mental status
altered metabolism
alternans, hemiplegia

alternate binaural loudness balance
    (ABLB) test
alternate hemiplegia
alternating motion rate (AMR)
alternating oculomotor hemiplegia
alternating single-leg support (running
    gait)
altitudinal anopsia
altitudinal hemianopsia
Alumafoam splint
alumina bioceramic joint replacement
    material
aluminum oxide ceramic coating
Alu 1 insertion
Alu 1 sequence
Alvar condylar bolt
Alvarado collateral ligament protector
Alvarado knee holder
Alvarado leg holder
alveolar bone fracture
alveolar nerve
    inferior
    superior
alveolar rhabdomyosarcoma
alveolodental ligament
Aly algesimeter
ALZ-50 protein marker for Alzheimer
    disease
Alzheimer disease (presenile dementia)
Alzheimer Disease Asssessment Scale
    (ADAS)
Alzheimer neurofibrillary degeneration
Alzheimer-type, senile dementia
    (SDAT)
AMA Guide to Evaluation of
    Permanent Impairment
amalgam
amaurosis
    central
    cerebral
    uremic
amaurosis centralis
amaurosis fugax
ambidexterity
ambidextrous
ambient cistern

ambifixation
AMBI hip screw
ambilevosity
ambilevous
AMBI wrist brace
amblyaphia
amblyopia ex anopsia (lazy eye)
amblyopia, toxic (toxic retinoneuropathy)
ambon
ambulant
ambulate with assistance
ambulate with support
ambulate without assistance
ambulate without support
ambulation
   brace-free
   toe-touch
ambulation skills
Ambulators shoe
ambulatory EEG recording
ambulatory patient
ambulatory status
ambulatory with a cane
ambulatory with assistance
AMC total wrist prosthesis
AMD (arthroscopic microdiskectomy)
AMD (articular motion device)
AME (American Medical Electronics)
AME (Austin Medical Equipment)
AME bone growth stimulator
AME microcurrent TENS unit
AME PinSite Shield
amebiasis (see *amoebiasis*)
amelia
amenorrhea, exercise-induced
amentia
American Academy for Cerebral Palsy
   and Developmental Medicine
   (AACPDM)
American Academy of Neurology
   (AAN)
American Academy of Orthopaedic
   Surgeons (AAOS)
American Academy of Orthopedic
   Surgeons Pediatrics Outcomes
   Instrument (AAOS POI)

American Academy of Physical
   Medicine and Rehabilitation
   (AAPMR)
American Academy of Podiatric
   Sports Medicine (AAPSM)
American Association for Hand
   Surgery (AAHS)
American Association of Hip and
   Knee Surgeons (AAHKS)
American Association of Homes for
   the Aging
American Association of Mental
   Deficiency
American Association of Neurological
   Surgeons (AANS)
American Association of Orthopaedic
   Foot and Ankle Surgeons (AAO-
   FAS)
American Association of Orthotists
   and Prosthetists (AAOP)
American Association of Retired
   Persons (AARP)
American Autonomic Society (AAS)
American Board of Orthopaedic
   Surgery (ABOS)
American Chiropractic Association
   (ACA)
American Chiropractic College of
   Radiology (ACCR)
American College of Rheumatology
   (ACR)
American College of Sports Medicine
   (ACSM)
American Congress of Rehabilitation
   Medicine (ACRM)
American Diabetes Association (ADA)
   Foot Council
American Dietetic (*not* Diabetic)
   Association diets for athletes
American EEG Society
American Foundation for the Blind
American Geriatrics Society
American Institute of Orthopaedic and
   Sports Medicine (AIOSM)
American Joint Commision on Cancer
   (AJCC) staging system for soft-
   tissue sarcoma

American Knee Society (AKS) score
American Musculoskeletal Tumor
    Society rating scale
American Nursing Home Association
American Orthopaedic Foot and Ankle
    Society (AOFAS) ankle-hindfoot
    score
American Orthotic and Prosthetic
    Association (AOPA)
American Parkinson's Disease
    Association
American Physical Therapy
    Association (APTA)
American Podiatric Medical
    Association (APMA)
American Rheumatism Association
    (ARA)
American Seating Access-O-Matic bed
American Shoulder and Elbow
    Surgeons (ASES) shoulder score
American Society for Surgery of the
    Hand (ASSH)
American Society for Testing and
    Materials (ASTM)
American Spinal Cord Injury
    Association classification
American Sports Medicine Institute
    (ASMI)
Americans with Disabilities Act
    (ADA)
americium (Am) radioactive source
A-Methapred (methylprednisolone
    sodium succinate)
Amfit orthotic system
AMI contrast medium
Amigo mechanical wheelchair
aminoaciduria
    arginase deficiency
    argininosuccinic
    Baló
    carnosinemia
    citrullinemia
    cystathioninuria
    Devic
    Hartnup disease
    histidinemia
    homocystinuria

aminoaciduria *(continued)*
    hydroxyisovaleric
    hyper-ß-alaninemia
    hyperlysinemia
    hyperprolinemia
    hypersarcosinemia
    hypervalinemia
    isovaleric acidemia
    maple-syrup urine disease
    Marchiafava-Bignami
    methylmalonic
    neonatal tyrosinemia
    oasthouse urine disease
    Pelizaeus-Merzbacher
    phenylketonuria (PKU)
    primary
    saccharopinuria
    Schilder
    sulfite oxidase deficiency
    tyrosinemia
aminocaproic acid
Amipaque contrast medium
amiprilose hydrochloride (Therafectin)
amitriptyline (Elavil)
AMK (Anatomic Modular Knee) total
    knee system
AML (amyotrophic lateral sclerosis)
AML (anatomic medullary locking)
AML hip prosthesis
AML Tang femoral prosthesis
AM-MI orthopedic table
Ammon horn (mesial temporal)
    sclerosis
ammonia toxicity
amnesia
    alcoholic
    amnesic
    antegrade
    anterograde
    auditory
    Broca
    circumscribed
    concussion
    continuous
    dissociative
    emotional
    episodic

amnesia *(continued)*
   generalized
   global
   hippocampal
   hysterical
   infantile
   ictal
   Korsakoff
   lacunar
   localized
   olfactory
   organic
   partial
   patchy retrograde
   postconcussive
   posthypnotic
   post-traumatic
   psychogenic
   retroactive
   retrograde
   selective
   shrinking retrograde
   tactile
   transient
   transient global (TGA)
   traumatic
   verbal
   visual
amnesiac
amnesic aphasia
amnestic state
amnestic syndrome
amobarbital sodium test
A-mode ultrasound
amoebiasis, cerebral (or amebiasis)
   Entamoeba histolytica
   Iodamoeba buetschlii
amorphosynthesis
amorphous silicon filmless digital
   x-ray detection technology
Amoss sign
amoxicillin
ampakine CX-516
Ampalex (CX516)
amphiarthrosis
amphiregulin, human
amplifier drift on EEG

amplitude (on EEG)
   absolute band
   absolute EP (evoked potential)
   asymmetry
   local reduction in
   peak-to-peak
   reduction of
   relative band
   SNAP (sensory nerve action
     potential)
   very low
   waveform
amplitude-integrated EEG (aEEG)
ampullar nerve
   anterior
   inferior
   lateral
   superior
amputation
   above-elbow (AE)
   above-knee (AK) (AKA)
   Alanson
   Alouette
   Beclard
   below-knee (BK) (BKA)
   Berger interscapular
   Bier
   Boyd ankle
   Bunge
   Burgess below-knee
   button toe
   Callander
   Carden
   chop
   Chopart hindfoot
   circular supracondylar
   closed flap
   complete
   congenital
   digital
   femoral head
   fingertip
   fish-mouth
   forearm
   forefoot digital
   forequarter
   Gritti-Stokes distal thigh

21   **amputation • anal**

amputation *(continued)*
  guillotine
  Hey
  incomplete
  index ray
  interinnominoabdominal
  interphalangeal
  interscapular
  interscapulothoracic
  Jaboulay
  Kirk distal thigh
  Le Fort
  Lisfranc
  midthigh
  nonreplantable
  one-stage
  Pirogoff
  ray
  replantable
  supramalleolar open
  Syme
  Syme ankle disarticulation
  Teale
  toe
  transcarpal
  transcondylar
  translumbar
  transmetatarsal (TMA)
  traumatic
  two-stage
  Vladimiroff-Mikulicz
amputation neuroma
amputation stump
amputee
AMR (alternating motion rate)
Amrex muscle stimulator
Amrex SynchroSonic muscle
  stimulation-ultrasound
AMS (accelerator mass spectrometry)
Amset ALPS (anterior locking plate
  system)
Amset R-F fixation system
Amset R-F rod
Amset R-F screw
Amsler grid visual test
Amspacher-Messenbaugh technique

Amstutz resurfacing procedure
Amstutz total hip replacement
Amstutz-Wilson osteotomy
AMTR (anteromedial temporal lobe
  resection)
amusia
AMX knee brace
amyelination
amygdala of cerebellum
amygdalofugal pathway
amygdalohippocampectomy
amygdaloid nuclear complex
amygdalotomy
amyloidoma
amyloidosis, skeletal
amyloid precursor protein gene
amyostatic syndrome
amyotrophic lateral sclerosis (ALS)
Amyotrophic Lateral Sclerosis
  Association (ALSA)
amyotrophic type of spongiform
  encephalopathy
amyotrophy
  Aran-Duchenne
  asthmatic
  brachial
  diabetic
  dystonic
  neuralgic
  neuritic
  primary progressive
  progressive nuclear
  syphilitic
amytal provocation test
ANA (antinuclear antibody) test
anabolic steroids, nandrolene
  decanoate
anabolism
anachronism on EEG
anaerobe, anaerobic
analgesia, patient controlled (PCA)
anal nerves, inferior
analog-to-digital converter
analogous
anal reflex
anal wink

anal wink reflex
analysis
  aggrecan
  biomechanical
  cephalometric
  chi-square
  computer-assisted EEG signal
  computerized EEG signal
  DeLee radiographic
  EEG autoregressive model for
    signal
  EEG digital signal
  EEG spectral
  electro-oculographic
  EVa HiRES Motion Analysis
  footprint
  force-plate-foot
  F-Scan foot pressure
  Fuscger
  gait
  hydrophobic cluster
  kinematic
  kinetic gait
  Kruskal-Wallis one-way analysis
  linear regression
  Mann-Whitney U
  multilinear regression
  Pearson correlation coefficients
  power spectral (PSA)
  quantitative EEG
  Rasch
  Sassouni
  segregation
  short EEG epoch FFT
  signal
  single-strand conformation
    polymorphism
  Spearman rank correlation
    coefficient
  total body neutron activation
    (TBNAA)
analysis of variance (ANOVA)
analyzer
  Arthrodial Protractor range-of-
    motion
  Sam Jr. posture
Anametric total knee system

anaplastic astrocytoma
anaplastic glioma
anarithmetria
anarthria
anastomosis
  extradural
  intradural
  Ma-Griffith end-to-end
  Ma-Griffith tendon
  Martin-Gruber
  Riche-Canieu
anastomotic pseudoaneurysm
anatomic alignment
anatomic graduated components
  (AGC) in joint replacement
anatomic landmarks
anatomic medullary locking (AML)
anatomic neck
anatomic position
anatomic snuffbox
anatomic variant
ANB cephalometric measurement
anchor (also *suture anchor*)
  Acufex T-fix suture
  Anchorlok soft-tissue
  Anspach suture
  Bio-Anchor suture
  Bio-Phase suture
  Biologically Quiet Mini-Screw
    suture
  Catera suture
  Corkscrew suture
  FASTak suture
  FASTIN
  G2 or GII
  GII EasyAnchor
  GII Snap-Pak
  GLS suture
  Harpoon suture
  In-Tac bone-anchoring system
  intraosseous suture
  knotless suture
  Micro QuickAnchor
  MicroMite suture
  Mini GLS
  Mini QuickAnchor
  Mini-Revo Screw suture

anchor *(continued)*
  Mitek bone
  Mitek GII suture
  Mitek knotless suture
  Mitek Superanchor
  Multitak SS suture
  OBL RC5 soft tissue
  Ogden
  Panalok RC absorbable soft tissue
  Parachute corkscrew suture
  PeBA suture
  Radial Osteo Compression (ROC)
    soft-tissue
  Sherlock threaded suture
  Stryker wedge suture
  SuperAnchor suture
  suture
  Tacit threaded
  TAG suture
  T-fix suture
  traction
  UltraFix MicroMite suture
anchor hole
Anchorlok soft-tissue anchor
anchor plate
anchor splint
anchorage-dependent growth
anchoring fibers of hand
anchoring system, bone
anchovy
  interposition
  tendon interposition
  tensor fasciae latae
anchovy spacer
anconeal fossa (also anconal fossa)
anconeus muscle flap
anconoid
Andersch tympanic nerve
Anderson acetabular prosthesis
Anderson-Adson scalp retractor
Anderson classification of tibial
  pseudoarthrosis
Anderson-D'Alonzo classification
Anderson distractor
Anderson fixation apparatus
Anderson fixation device
Anderson-Fowler procedure

Anderson-Green growth prediction
Anderson-Hutchins tibial fracture
Anderson-Neivert osteotome
Anderson screw placement technique
Anderson splint
Anderson tendon tunneller
Anderson traction
Andersson hip status system
André hook
Andrews iliotibial band reconstruction
Andrews osteotome
Andrews spinal surgery frame
Andrews SST-3000 spinal surgery
  table
androgen
android pelvis
anechoic area
anemic hypoxia
anencephaly
AnervaX vaccine
anesthesia
  ankle block
  axillary block
  Bier block
  bulbar
  compression
  continuous intravenous regional
    (CIVRA)
  crash induction of
  doll's head
  dolorosa
  epidural block
  femoral nerve block
  gauntlet
  general
  general endotracheal
  general orotracheal
  glove
  glove and stocking
  hysterical
  infraclavicular block
  inhalation, inhalant
  intercostal nerve block (ICNB)
  interscalene block (ISB)
  interscalene catheter
  intrathecal
  intravenous regional (IVRA)

anesthesia *(continued)*
   lateral femoral cutaneous nerve
     block
   local standby
   Mayo block
   peripheral nerve block
   popliteal nerve block
   regional ankle block
   ring block
   saddle
   scalene block
   sciatic nerve block
   segmental
   short-acting block (SAB)
   spinal
   supraclavicular brachial block
   tactile
   thalamic hyperesthetic
   thermal
   transthecal digital block
   traumatic
anesthesic region
anesthetic block
aneurysm
   arteriovenous
   aspergillotic
   basilar artery
   basilar trunk
   berry intracranial
   brain
   carotid
   cavernous carotid
   cavernous sinus
   cerebral
   Charcot-Bouchard intracerebral
   circle of Willis
   clinoid
   clip ligation of
   clipping of
   coating of
   congenital arteriosclerotic
   cranial
   de novo
   dissecting
   dissecting intracranial
   dolichoectatic dissecting
   dome of

aneurysm *(continued)*
   extracerebral
   extracranial
   false
   feeding artery of
   fundus of
   fusiform
   giant
   great cerebral vein of Galen
   hunterian ligation of
   internal carotid artery
   intracerebral
   intracranial
   M1 segment
   miliary
   mirror-image
   mycotic intracranial
   neck of
   neoplastic
   nonatherosclerotic
   PICA (posterior inferior cerebellar
     artery)
   posterior circulation
   posterior communicating artery
   precursor sign to rupture of
   prerupture of
   racemose
   rebleeding of
   rerupture of
   ruptured intracranial
   sacciform
   saccular
   serpentine
   spindle-shaped
   thrombosed
   thrombotic
   trapping of
   traumatic intracranial (TICA)
   true
   tubular
   unruptured
   wide-necked intracranial artery
   wrapping of
aneurysmal bone cyst (ABC)
aneurysmal bruit
aneurysmal bulging
aneurysmal dilatation

aneurysmal hemorrhage
aneurysmal rebleed
aneurysmal trapping
aneurysmal vein
aneurysm clip applicator
aneurysmectomy
aneurysm needle
aneurysmoplasty
aneurysmorrhaphy
aneurysmotomy
Angelchik antireflux prosthesis
Angell James dissector
Angell James hypophysectomy forceps
angel-wing sign
Anghelescu sign
angiitis, granulomatous giant cell
angiofibroblastic proliferation
angiogram, angiograph, angiography
　carotid
　catheter
　cerebral
　cine
　computed tomographic (CTA)
　digital subtraction (DSA)
　digital subtraction cerebral
　digital subtraction rotational
　directional color (DCA)
　dobutamine thallium
　DSA (digital subtraction)
　dynamic tagging MR
　elastic subtraction spiral CT
　Epistar subtraction
　equilibrium radionuclide
　four-vessel cerebral
　gated blood pool
　gated equilibrium radionuclide
　gated nuclear
　gated radionuclear
　gated radionuclide
　IDIS (intraoperative digital
　　subtraction)
　innominate
　intercostal artery
　internal carotid
　intra-arterial digital subtraction
　　(IADSA)

angiogram *(continued)*
　intra-arterial DSA (digital
　　subtraction)
　intravenous DSA (digital
　　subtraction)
　magnetic resonance (MRA)
　postembolization
　postoperative
　preoperative
　radionuclide (RNA)
　Seldinger
　small-angle double-incidence
　　(SADIA)
　spinal
　STAR
　stereotactic cerebral
　stereotaxic cerebral
　superselective
　3D (three-dimensional)
　3D gadolinium-enhanced MR
　3DFT magnetic resonance
　3D helical CT
　3D inflow MR
　3D phase-contrast MR (3D-PCA)
　time-of-flight (TOF)
　transvenous digital subtraction
　tumor blush on
　velocity encoding on brain MR
　vertebral
angiographically confirmed
angiographically occult intracranial
　vascular malformation (AOIVM)
angiographic catheter
angiographic finding
angiographic recanalization
angiographic targeting
angiographic vessel occlusion
angiography (see *angiogram*)
angiolipoma, spinal
angioma
　arteriovenous
　cavernous
　cutaneous
　intracranial cavernous
　intradermal
　venous

Angiomat contrast delivery system
angiomatosis
  bacillary
  cerebroretinal
  corticomeningeal
  Divry-van Bogaert familial
  encephalotrigeminal
  leptomeningeal
  retinocerebral
angiomatosis of retina
angiomyolipoma, multifocal
angioparalytic blockade
angiopathy, cerebral amyloid
angioplastic meningioma
angioplasty
  stent-assisted
  transluminal
angiopneumography
angiosarcoma
angiotomomyelography
AngioVista angiographic system
Angiovist contrast medium
angle
  acetabular
  acromial (of scapula)
  alpha (on x-ray)
  antegonial
  anteroposterior talocalcaneal
    (APTC)
  arch
  Bauman
  Beatson combined ankle
  bimalleolar
  Boehler (Böhler) calcaneal
  Boehler lumbosacral
  Bragg
  C
  calcaneal inclination
  calcaneal pitch
  calcaneoplantar
  carrying
  CE (capital epiphysis)
  center-edge (C-E)
  central collodiaphyseal (CCD)
  cephalic
  cephalometric
  cerebellopontile (CPA)

angle *(continued)*
  cerebellopontine (CPA)
  Citelli
  Clarke arch
  Cobb lumbar
  Cobb scoliosis
  Codman
  condylar
  costal
  costolumbar
  costophrenic (CP)
  costosternal
  costovertebral (CVA)
  craniofacial
  distal articular
  dorsoplantar talometatarsal
  dorsoplantar talonavicular
  Drennan metaphyseal-epiphyseal
  Euler
  fan
  femorotibial (FTA)
  first-fifth intermetatarsal
  first metatarsal
  first-second intermetatarsal
  flip
  foot-progression (FPA)
  Garden
  Gissane
  gonial
  hallux dorsiflexion (DFA)
  hallux interphalangeus
  hallux valgus (HVA)
  hallux valgus interphalangeus
  Hibbs metatarsocalcaneal
  Hilgenreiner
  IM (intermetatarsal)
  increased carrying
  intermetatarsal (IMA) I or II
  infrasternal
  interlaminal
  intersegmental
  Kite
  Konstram
  lateral plantar metatarsal
  lateral talocalcaneal (LATC)
  lateral tarsometatarsal
  Laurin

angle *(continued)*
 Laurin lateral patellofemoral
 Louis
 Lovibond angle
 Ludovici
 Ludwig
 lumbosacral joint
 mandibular
 Meary metatarsotalar
 mediolateral radiocarpal
 Merchant congruence
 metaphyseal-epiphyseal
 metatarsocalcaneal
 metatarsotalar
 metatarsus adductus
 metatarsus primus
 Mikulicz
 navicular-to-first metatarsal
 neck-shaft
 nu
 nutation
 occipitocervical
 Pauwel
 pelvic femoral
 Pirogoff
 pitch
 plantar metatarsal
 pontine
 proximal articular set (PASA)
 Q
 radiocarpal
 Ranke
 resting forefoot supination
 sacrohorizontal
 sacrovertebral
 scapular
 set
 Sharp
 slip
 spinographic
 sulcus
 talar-tilt
 talocalcaneal (subtalar)
 talocrural
 talometatarsal
 talonavicular
 tarsometatarsal

angle *(continued)*
 TC
 thigh-foot (TFA)
 tibiofemoral (TFA)
 tibiotalar
 tilting
 TMA-thigh (transmalleolar axis)
 trajectory
 transmetatarsal (TMA)
 valgus
 valgus carrying
 varus
 varus metatarsophalangeal (MTP)
 vertebrophrenic
 Wiberg
 Wiltze
 xiphoid
 angled tomographic slice
 angle from horizontal plane
 angle from vertical plane
 angle of anteversion
 angle of declination of metatarsal
 angle of greatest extension (AGE)
 angle of greatest flexion (AGF)
 angle of incongruity
 Angle splint
 angular frequency
 angular gyrus (AG)
 angular hinge clamp
 angular momentum
 angular process of orbit
 angulated fracture
 angulation
  cephalic
  degrees of valgus
  degrees of varus
  forefoot
  post-traumatic
  spinal
 anhidrosis
 animation, suspended
 anisocoria
 anisotrophy, curvature
 ankle
  autologous reverse graft to
  disk of
  eversion sprain of

ankle *(continued)*
 footballer's
 fractured
 fused
 fusion of
 giving way of
 instability of
 inversion injury of
 mortise of
 neuropathic
 snowboarder's
 sprained
 swelling of
 syndesmosis sprain of
 synthetic graft bypass to
 tailor's
 transmalleolar
 twisted
 Wiltse osteotomy of
ankle Air-Stirrup
ankle/arm blood pressure index
ankle/arm index
ankle block
ankle bone
ankle brace
ankle/brachial blood pressure index
ankle/brachial pressure ratio
ankle disk
ankle dorsiflexion range of motion
 (ADROM)
ankle dressing, Cryo/Cuff
ankle eversion
ankle-foot orthosis (AFO)
ankle fracture
ankle fusion
ankle instability
ankle inversion-eversion range of motion
ankle jerk (AJ)
ankle jerk reflex
ankle joint
ankle joint complex (AJC)
ankle-level arteriotomy
ankle ligament protector (ALP)
ankle mortise
ankle mortise widening
ankle orthosis, Malleoloc anatomic
ankle pump

Ankle Score
ankle sprain
Ankle Stabilizing Orthosis (ASO)
 support
ankle systolic pressure
anklet, elastic
ankylodactyly
ankylosing spondylitis
ankylosis (pl. ankyloses)
 bony
 extracapsular
 false
 fibrous
 intracapsular
 joint
 ligamentous
 shoulder
 spurious
 vertebral
anlage (pl. anlagen)
 cartilaginous
 radial head
 ulnar
anlage à priori
ANMR Insta-scan MR scanner
anneal, annealed
annexin I
ANNs (artificial neural networks)
annular calcification
annular cartilage
annular fibrosis
annular foreshortening
annular fracture
annular hypoplasia
annular ligament of finger
annular pulley
annuli (pl. of annulus)
annuloplasty, IDET (intradiscal
 electrothermal)
annulospiral fibers
annulotomy
annulus (also anulus)
annulus fibrosus
annulus fibrosus disci intervertebralis
annulus, fissure of
annulus of Vieussens
anococcygeal ligament

anococcygeal nerve
anomalous vertebral artery
anode
anoia
anomalous insertion
anomalous movement
anomaly, anomalies
  congenital
  cranial
  multiple congenital (MCA)
  vascular
anomia
  color
  finger
  tactile
anomic aphasia
anomie
anopsia, altitudinal
anosmia, anosmic
anosodiaphoria
anosognosia
anosognosis
anosteoplasia
anostosis
ANOVA (analysis of variance)
anoxemia
anoxia
  acute
  birth
  cerebral
  consumptive
  perinatal
anoxic damage
anoxic encephalopathy
anoxic hypoxia
anoxic ischemia
ansa (pl. ansae)
ansa of Vieussens
anserine bursitis syndrome
anserinus, pes
Anspach Cement Eater
Anspach craniotome
Anspach power drill
Anspach reamer
Anspach suture anchor
antagonist muscle groups
antagonists, cytokine

antalgic gait
antalgic limp
anteater sign
antebrachial fascia
antebrachium
antecubital fossa
antecubital vein
anteflexion
antegonial angle
antegonial notch
antegrade amnesia
antegrade femoral nailing
Antegren monoclonal antibody
antenna
anterior ampullar nerve
anterior antebrachial nerve
anterior apprehension test
anterior auricular muscle
anterior auricular nerves
anterior calcaneoastragaloid ligament
anterior cardiac vein
anterior cerebellar artery syndrome
anterior cervical fusion (ACF)
anterior cervical intertransverse
  muscles
anterior cingulate gyrus tumor
anterior circulation ischemia
anterior circulation stroke
anterior colliculus
anterior column of spine
anterior communicating artery
  distribution infarction
anterior compartment syndrome
anterior corpus
anterior corticospinal tract
anterior costotransverse ligament
anterior costovertebral ligament
anterior costoxiphoid ligament
anterior cruciate instability with pivot
  shift
anterior cruciate ligament (ACL) drill
  guide
anterior cruciate ligament repair
anterior crural nerve
anterior cutaneous nerves of abdomen
anterior descending artery
anterior dynamized system (ADS)

anterior ethmoidal nerve
anterior feet view
anterior femoral cutaneous nerves
anterior fibular ligament
anterior foot draw sign
anterior gray column of cord
anterior head region
anterior horn-cell disease
anterior horn-cell motor impairment
anterior horns of spinal cord
anterior hypothalamus
anterior inferior cerebellar artery
    (AICA)
anterior inferior cerebral artery
    (AICA)
anterior inferior communicating artery
    (AICA)
anterior inferior iliac spine
anterior inferior tibiofibular ligament
anterior innominate test
anterior instability
anterior intercostal artery
anterior interhemispheric cistern
anterior interhemispheric fissure
anterior interosseous nerve
anterior labial nerves
anterior lobe, midline tumor of
anterior longitudinal ligament
anterior maxillary spine
anterior medial ankle ligament
anterior median fissure of cord
anterior mediastinum
anterior metatarsal arch
anterior oblique ligament
anterior posterior intercommissural
    line
anterior posterior laxity of knee
anterior radioulnar ligament
anterior rectus muscle of head
anterior scalene muscle
anterior scrotal nerves
anterior serratus muscle
anterior shear
anterior shin splints
anterior spinal artery syndrome
anterior spinal fusion (ASF)
anterior spinal line

anterior spinocerebellar tract
anterior spinothalamic tract
anterior superior iliac spine (ASIS)
anterior supraclavicular nerve
anterior talar dome
anterior talofibular ligament
anterior talotibial ligament
anterior tibial artery
anterior tibial compartment syndrome
anterior tibial muscle
anterior tibial nerve
anterior tibiofibular ligament
anterior tibiotalar ligament
anterocollis
anterograde amnesia
anterolateral white matter of cord
anterolisthesis
anteromedial humeral head defect
    (reverse Hill-Sachs)
anteromesial temporal discharge on
    EEG
anteroposterior (AP) (also anterior-
    posterior)
antetorsion, femoral
anteversion
    angle of
    femoral
    Magilligan technique for measuring
    neutral
anteversion determination,
    Budin-Chandler
anteverted
anthropoid pelvis
anthropometric measurement
anti-AChR (antiacetylcholine receptor)
    antibody
anti-aggregant, platelet
antiangiogenesis
anti-annexin I monoclonal antibody
antibiotic and saline solution
antibiotic-impregnated beads
antibiotic-impregnated polymethyl
    methacrylate (PMMA)
antibody
    acetylcholine receptor antibody
        (AchRab)
    AChR (acetylcholine receptor)

antibody *(continued)*
ACL-Ab (anticardiolipin antibody)
ACTH
AE1
AE3
anti-ACh receptor
anti-AChR (antiacetylcholine
   receptor)
anti-annexin I monoclonal
anticardiolipin (ACL-Ab)
anticitrullinated peptide
anti-C1q
antiendothelial
antiglioma monoclonal antibody
   kinase C
anti-Hu
antineutrophil cytoplasmic
antiphosphatidylethanolamine
antiphospholipid
antiproteasome autoantibody
anti-Ri
antiribonucleoprotein
anti-RNA polymerase
antistriated muscle
antivascular endothelial growth
   factor
anti-VGCC
beta-endorphin
Borrelia burgdorferi
CAM 5.2
cytokeratins
EMA (epithelial membrane antigen)
GFAP (glial fibrillary acidic protein)
glutinin 1
growth hormone
kinase C antiglioma monoclonal
lectins
luteinizing hormone
MG (myasthenia gravis)
monoclonal
neuron-specific enolase (NSE)
neutralization
neutralizing
NSE (neuron-specific enolase)
prealbumin
prolactin hormone
RCA (*Ricinus communis* agglutinin 1)

antibody *(continued)*
S-100 protein
St. Louis encephalitis
thyrotropin hormone
UE (Ulex europaeus)
vimentin
VZ (varicella-zoster)
anticardiolipin antibodies (ACL-Ab)
anticitrullinated peptide antibodies
anti-C1q autoantibodies
anticoagulant-induced hemorrhage
anticonvulsant drugs
anticoagulant, lupus
anticonvulsant intoxication, hypersensitivity reaction
anticonvulsants
   blood levels of
   hypersensitivity reaction to
antidepressants, tricyclic
antidromic (sensory) conduction studies
antidromic vasodilator mechanism
antiembolism hose
antiembolism stockings, Orthawear
antiendothelial antibodies
antiepilepsirine
antiepileptic effect of drug
antigen
   antiproliferating cell nuclear
   carcinoembryonic (CEA)
   epithelial membrane (EMA)
   von Willebrand factor
antigravity muscles
anti-Hu antibody
anti-inflammatory drug
anti-Ki-67
antimalarial
antimyoclonic effect of drug
antineurofilament
antineutrophil cytoplasmic antibodies
antinuclear antibody (ANA) test
antioxidant therapy
antiparkinsonism
antiphosphatidylethanolamine
   antibodies
antiphospholipid antibody syndrome
   (APS)
antipronation taping

antiproteasome autoantibodies
antiprotrusio cage
antiresorptive medication
anti-RI antibody
antiribonucleoprotein antibody
anti-RNA polymerase antibodies
antirotation device
anti-sense oligonucleotide
antiseptic, ACU-dyne
Anti-Shox foot cushion
anti-siphon device
antistreptolysin O (ASO) titer
antithrombin III
antithrombotic therapy
anti-TNF therapy
antitragus muscle
antivascular endothelial growth factor
     antibody
antivibratory gloves
anti-VGCC antibodyAnton syndrome
Antoni A cell
Antoni-A classification of neurinoma
Antoni B cell
Antoni-A classification of neurinoma
antrum, Malacarne
anulus (see *annulus*)
anvil
     Bunnell
     Hurteau skull plate
anvil bone
anvil sign
anvil test
AO (Arbeitsgemeinschaft für Osteo-
     synthesefragen) surgical technique
AOA halo traction cervical collar or
     support
AOAS (adult-onset ankylosing
     spondylitis)
AO-ASIF compression technique
AO-ASIF implant
AO-ASIF screw
AO blade plate
AO classification of ankle fracture
AO cortical screw
AO-Danis-Weber classification of
     ankle fractures
AO drill bit

AOFAS (American Orthopaedic Foot
     and Ankle Society) hindfoot scor-
     ing system
AO fracture pattern
AOIVM (angiographically occult
     intracranial vascular malformation)
AO minifragment set
AO nail
AOPA (American Orthotic and
     Prosthetic Association)
AO plate
AO pseudoisochromatic color plate test
AO reconstruction plate
AO reduction forceps
aortic arch injection of contrast
aortic nerve
aortic valve prosthesis
aortoplasty, SFA (subclavian flap
     aortoplasty)
AO semitubular plate
AO spongiosa screw
AO spoon plate
AO technique
AO tension band technique
AOVM (angiographically occult
     vascular malformation)
AP (anteroposterior or anterior-
     posterior)
     AP film
     AP projection
     AP supine portable view
     AP view
APACHE II measure of disease
     severity
apallic patient
apallic state
apallic syndrome
apathy
apatite and wallstonite-containing
     glass-ceramic (AW-GC)
APB (abductor pollicis brevis) muscle
A-P cutter
ape hand (simian griffe)
ape hand of syringomyelia
ape-like hand
aperiodic complex
aperiodic wave

Apert acrosyndactyly
Apert disease
Apert syndrome
aperture
apex
  orbital
  petrous
apex of head of femur
apex of head of fibula
apex of head of patella
apex of horn of spinal cord
apex of petrous portion of temporal
  bone
Apfelbaum mirror
aphagia
aphalangia
aphasia
  acoustic
  acquired epileptic
  acquired fluent
  ageusic
  amnemonic
  amnesic
  amnestic
  anomic
  associative
  ataxic
  auditory
  Benson-Geschwind classification of
  Broca
  combined
  commissural
  complete
  conduction
  cortical
  dynamic
  expressive
  expressive-receptive
  fluent
  frontocortical
  frontolenticular
  functional
  gibberish
  global
  graphomotor

aphasia *(continued)*
  Grashey
  hypophonic
  impressive
  intellectual
  jargon
  Kussmaul
  lenticular
  Lichtheim
  major motor
  mixed
  motor
  nominal
  nonfluent
  optic
  parieto-occipital
  partial nominal
  pathematic
  pictorial
  psychosensory
  receptive
  semantic
  sensory
  subcortical
  syntactical
  tactile
  temporoparietal
  total
  transcortical (motor)
  transcortical (sensory)
  transcortical mixed
  true
  verbal
  visual form of Wernicke
  Wernicke
Aphasia Screening Test, Halstead-
  Wepman
aphasic error
aphasic patient
aphasic seizure
aphasic speech
  fluent
  nonfluent
aphasiology
aphemia

aphonia
  acute
  functional (hysterical)
  hysterical (functional)
aphthous
API (arterial pressure index)
apical corn
apical ligament of dens ligament
apical posterior artery
apices (pl. of apex)
apiculate waveform
APL (abductor pollicis longus) muscle
APL (abductor pollicis longus) tendon
aplasia, cerebellar
APLD (automated percutaneous
  lumbar diskectomy)
Apley grinding test
Apley scratch test
Apley sign
Apley test, two-part
APM (anterior papillary muscle)
APMA (American Podiatric Medical
  Association)
APN (advanced practice nurse)
apnea
  central
  central sleep
  mixed sleep
  obstructive
  obstructive sleep
  sleep
apneic seizures
apneustic breathing
apneustic period
apodia
apo E (apolipoprotein E) genotype
APOE polymorphism
APOE-e4 allele
Apogee ultrasound device
apogeotropic nystagmus
A point
apolipoprotein E (apo E) genotype
Apollo DXA bone densitometry
  system
Apollo prosthesis
Apollo triple-lumen papillotome
aponeurectomy

aponeurorrhaphy
aponeurosis
  bicipital
  digital
  epicranial
  palmar
  plantar
  tendon
aponeurosis of tendon
aponeurotic band
aponeurotic triangle
aponeurotic troika
aponeurotomy
apophyseal fracture
apophyseal joint
apophysis of Rau
apophysis, apophyseal
apophysitis
  calcaneal
  iliac
  traction
apoplectic
apoplexy
  Broadbent
  cerebellar
  delayed
  pineal
  pituitary
  postpartum
  post-traumatic (of Bollinger)
  Raymond
apoptosis, neuronal
apoptotic cell
apotentiality, cerebral
APP (platelet amyloid precursor
  protein)
apparatus (see *device*; *orthosis*)
appearance
  beaten-silver (of the skull)
  disheveled
  isodense
  onion peel (on x-ray)
  unkempt
appendicular ataxia
appendicular bone mass measurement
appendicular skeletal muscle (ASM)
appendicular skeleton

apperceptive disorder
appliance (see *device*; *orthosis*)
application of traction device
applicator
    aneurysm clip
    scalp clip
applier
    bayonet clip
    clip
    Ligaclip
    Mayfield miniature clip
    Mayfield temporary aneurysm clip
    mini
    vari-angle clip
apposing articular surfaces
apposition
    bone-to-bone
    fracture in close
apprehension shoulder
apprehension test
approach (see *incision*; *operation*)
    CW subpectoralis
    endoscopic retroperitoneal thoraco-
      abdominal
    holistic
    interforniceal
    ipsilateral
    keyhole
    Kocher-Langenbach
    lateral
    median parapatellar
    orbitozygomatic
    posterolateral
    pterional
    subchoroidal
    subforniceal
    transforaminal
    translabyrinthine
    transsylvian
    transventricular
    vastus-splitting
    veterinary
approximator (see also *contractor*)
    Acland double-clamp
    double-clamp
    Lalonde tendon
    Lemmon sternal

approximator *(continued)*
    Neuromeet universal soft tissue
    sternal
    Van Beck nerve
APPT (Adolescent and Pediatric Pain
    Tool)
APR (anatomic porous replacement)
APR acetabular prosthesis
APR cement fixation
APR femoral prosthesis
APR II hip prosthesis
APR total hip system
apractognosia
apractic (or *apraxic*)
apraxia
    akinetic
    amnestic
    Bruns gait
    buccofacial
    callosal
    cerebral mapping of
    classic
    constructional
    cortical
    disconnection
    dressing
    ideational
    ideokinetic
    ideomotor
    innervation
    Liepmann
    limb-kinetic
    magnetic
    motor
    ocular
    oculomotor
    oral
    pure limb
    sensory
    transcortical
apraxic disorder (or apractic)
apraxic dysarthria (or apractic)
APRL (Army Prosthetics Research
    Laboratory) prosthesis
apron, quadriceps
aprotinin
APS (air plasma spray) hydroxyapatite

APTA (American Physical Therapy
  Association)
APTC (anteroposterior talocalcaneal)
  angle
Aquaphor gauze dressing
Aquaplast splint
AquaShield orthopedic cast cover
Aquasorb hydrogel dressing
Aquatech cast padding
aquatic exercise program
aquatic rehabilitation
aqueduct
  cerebral
  forking of sylvian
  gliosis of
  mesencephalon
  midbrain
  Monro
  sylvian
  ventricular
aqueduct compression
aqueduct occlusion
aqueduct stenosis
Aquilion CT scanner
ARA (Action Research Arm Test)
ARA (American Rheumatism
  Association)
arachidonic acid
arachidonic acid metabolite
arachnodactyly
  congenital
  contracture
arachnodactyly
arachnoid canal
arachnoid cyst
arachnoid granulation
arachnoid of uncus
arachnoid-shape Beaver blade
arachnoid villi
arachnoiditis
  adhesive
  basilar
  fibrosing
  perimedullary
  spinal
arachnoiditis of opticochiasmatic
  cistern

Arafiles elbow arthrodesis
Arafiles prosthesis
Arana-Iniquez intracranial cyst
  removal technique
Aran-Duchenne amyotrophy
Arantius ligament
Arava (leflunomide)
arborization
arborize
arbovirus (arthropod-borne)
arbovirus meningo-encephalitis
arboviruses, group b (causing
  encephalitis)
arc
  carpal
  Leksell stereotactic
  monosynaptic reflex
  stereotactic
arc of motion
arcade
  Frohse ligamentous
  Struthers
  superficialis
Arcelin view
arch
  anterior atlas
  anterior metatarsal
  articular
  atlas
  carpal
  cervical aortic
  coracoacromial
  deep
  flat
  flattened longitudinal
  Hapad metatarsal
  Hapad scaphoid
  hemal
  high
  Hillock
  hypoplastic
  longitudinal plantar
  metal
  neural
  neural vertebral
  palmar arterial
  plantar

arch *(continued)*
  plantar arterial
  posterior atlas (C1)
  posterior metatarsal
  pubic
  subpubic
  superciliary
  superficial palmar arterial
  tarsal
  transverse
  vertebral
  zygomatic
arch-height index
arch-height ratio
archicortex
arch index
archimedean hand drill
architectural alterations of bone
architecture
  bony
  brain
  foot
arch of atlas
archplasty
arch support
  plantar
  Plastizote
  Whitman
arcuate artery
arcuate complex
arcuate fasciculus (AF)
arcuate ligament
arcuate movement
arcuate nucleus
arcuate popliteal ligament
arcuate pubic ligament
arcus atlantis
arcus palmaris profundus
arcus palmaris superficialis
arcus parieto-occipitalis
arcus pedis transversalis
arcus plantaris
arcus plantaris profundus
arcus pubicus
arcus vertebrae
arcus vertebralis
arcus volaris profundus

Arduan (pipecuronium)
area (see also *region*)
  Broca
  Brodmann
  callosal (parolfactory nerve)
  language
  olfactory
  parietal association
  parietotemporal
  premotor
  sclerotic
  sclerotome
  septal
  watershed
  Wernicke
Aredia (pamidronate disodium)
areflexia, pupillary
areflexic dystasia, Roussy-Levy
  hereditary
areolar plane
areolar tissue, dorsum of hand
arginase deficiency
argininosuccinic aciduria
argon beam coagulator
argon laser
Argyll Robertson pupils of tabetic
  neurosyphilis
argyrophil plaque
arhinencephaly
Aricept (donepezil Hcl)
Ariel computerized exercise system
Arisotospan (triamcinolone)
arithmetical epilepsy
Arizona ankle brace
Arizona Health Science Center-Volz
  elbow prosthesis
Arizona leg support
arm
  abductor lever
  flail
  Leyla
  linebacker's
  outrigger
  Popeye
  tackler's
  3 Degree of Freedom robotic
  manipulator

arm *(continued)*
  4 Degree of Freedom robotic
    manipulator
  5 Degree of Freedom robotic
    manipulator
  6 Degree of Freedom robotic
    manipulator
  Utah artificial
  Yasargil Leyla retractor
arm abduction test
armboard, Flexisplint flexed
armchair splint
arm cuff
arm drift
arm roll testing
Armistead technique
arm sling
Armstrong acromionectomy
Armstrong plate
arm swing, synkinetic
arm swing with gait
Army bone gouge
Army-Navy retractor
Army osteotome
Arnold-Chiari deformity
Arnold-Chiari malformation
Arnold-Chiari syndrome
Arnold lumbar brace
Arnold nerve
AROM (active range of motion)
  exercises
aromatic L-amino acid decarboxylase
  (ALAAD)
Aron Alpha adhesive
arousal-attentional fatigue
arousable patient
arousal from sleep
array
  compressed spectral (on EEG)
  linear electrode
  reduced EEG electrode
array of electrodes
array processor
arrector pili muscles
arrest
  epiphyseal
  growth

arrest of speech
arrest reaction
arrested derotation of foot position
Arrow absorbable meniscal repair
  device
arrow, meniscal (or meniscus)
arrow pin clasp
ARS (acute repetitive seizure) disorder
Artane (trihexyphenidyl)
arterial blood gases (ABGs)
arterial ligament
arterial line
arterial pressure index (API)
arterial tonus
arteriogram, arteriography
  arch and carotid
  cerebral
  contrast
  selective cerebral
  vertebral
  vertebrobasilar
arteriography (see *arteriogram*)
arteriolar muscle tone
arteriosclerosis, cerebral
arteriosclerotic intracranial aneurysm
arteriotomy, ankle-level
arteriovenous angioma
arteriovenous fistula (AVF)
arteriovenous interhemispheric
  angioma
arteriovenous malformation (AVM)
arteriovenous oxygen difference
  (AVDO$_2$)
arteritis
  cranial
  Horton giant cell
  spinal cord
  Takayasu
  temporal
  viral intracerebral
artery (pl. arteries)
  A1-A5 segments of anterior cerebral
  aberrant
  Adamkiewicz (Adamkiewitz)
  aneurysm of internal carotid
  aneurysm of posterior communicating
  angular MCA (middle cerebral a.)

artery *(continued)*
    anomalous vertebral
    anterior cerebral (ACA)
    anterior choroidal (ACA or AChA)
    anterior communicating (ACoA)
    anterior inferior cerebellar (AICA)
    anterior inferior cerebral (AICA)
    anterior inferior communicating
       (AICA)
    anterior spinal
    anterior spinal canal
    anterior temporal branch of
       posterior cerebral
    ascending frontoparietal (ASFP)
    basal perforating
    basilar
    bifurcation of anterior communicating
    bifurcation of common carotid
    bifurcation of internal carotid artery
    bifurcation of middle cerebral
    brachiocephalic
    branch of
    calcarine
    callosomarginal
    carotid
    cerebral
    cervical
    choroidal
    choroidal branch of internal carotid
       artery
    choroidal pericallosal
    circumflex
    common carotid (CCA)
    compression of
    C1-C5 segments of internal carotid
    cortical branch of middle cerebral
    costocervical
    course of
    deltoid branch of posterior tibial
    dissection of
    dorsal spinal
    dural
    dynamic entrapment of vertebral
    embryonic
    en passage feeder
    external carotid (ECA)
    extracranial vertebral

artery *(continued)*
    extradural
    familial fibromuscular dysplasia of
    feeder
    feeding
    friable
    frontopolar (FPA)
    genicular
    internal carotid (ICA)
    intracavernous internal carotid
    intracranial vertebral
    lateral posterior choroidal (LPCh)
    lenticulostriate
    leptomeningeal
    MCA (middle cerebral)
    medial posterior choroidal (MPCh)
    median sacral
    meningeal
    meningohypophyseal trunk (MHT)
    mesencephalic
    mesenteric
    middle cerebral (MCA)
    middle meningeal
    M1-M5 segments of middle cerebral
    nodular induration of temporal
    nutrient
    occipital branch of external carotid
    occlusion of
    ophthalmic
    pachymeningeal feeding
    paramalleolar
    paramedian thalamopeduncular
    parietal MCA
    parieto-occipital branch of posterior
       cerebellar
    peduncular segment of superior
       cerebellar
    perforating
    persistent trigeminal
    pericallosal
    petrous segment of carotid
    plantar metatarsal
    plaque-containing
    P1-P4 segments of posterior cerebral
    pontine
    post-temporal MCA
    posterior cerebral (PCA)

artery *(continued)*
   posterior choroidal
   posterior communicating (PCA)
   posterior inferior cerebellar (PICA)
   posterior parietal
   posterior spinal
   posterior temporal
   posterolateral spinal (PLSA)
   precommunicating segment of
     anterior cerebral
   primitive trigeminal (PTA)
   proximal digital
   radial digital
   radicular
   radiculomedullary
   radiculospinal
   recurrent (of Heubner)
   retinal
   scalp branch of external carotid
   segmental branch of vertebral
   splenial branch of posterior
     cerebral artery
   subclavian
   superficial temporal (STA)
   superior cerebellar (SCA)
   supraclinoid carotid
   thalamocaudate
   thalamogeniculate
   thalamoperforating
   thyrocervical trunk of subclavian
   transverse cervical
   trifurcation of middle cerebral
   twig of
   ulnar anesthetic
   ulnar digital
   vertebral basilar
artery island flap
artery-vein-nerve bundle
Arth-Aid (capsaicin/aloe)
Arthopor acetabular cup
Arthopor cup prosthesis
Arthopor pad
Arthopor II acetabular prosthesis
arthralgia
   migratory
   subtalar
   temporomandibular joint

arthrectomy
arthrempyesis
Arthrex arthroscopy instruments
Arthrex coring reamer
Arthrex femoral guide
Arthrex instruments and systems
Arthrex tibial guide
arthrifluent abscess
arthritic talonavicular changes
arthritis (pl. arthritides)
   acute hematogenous
   acute spinal
   adjuvant-induced
   AIA (adjuvant-induced arthritis)
   allergenic
   assignment criteria for rheumatoid
   Bekhterev
   Brucella
   cervical
   Charcot
   degenerative
   Fries score for rheumatoid
   gold therapy for rheumatoid
   gonococcal
   gouty
   inflammatory
   juvenile rheumatoid (JRA)
   Lyme
   Marie-Strümpell
   migratory
   monarthritis
   neuropathic
   New York diagnostic criteria
     for rheumatoid
   oligoarthritis
   osteoarthritis
   Outerbridge staging of degenerative
   pantalocrural
   pantrapezial
   pauciarticular
   polyarticular juvenile rheumatoid
   post-traumatic
   psoriatic
   pyogenic
   rheumatoid (RA)
   Rome criteria for rheumatoid
   Salmonella

arthritis *(continued)*
  sarcoid
  septic
  seronegative
  seropositive rheumatoid
  spinal
  staphylococcus
  Steinbrocker classification of
    rheumatoid
  suppurative
  traumatic
  tuberculous
  ulnar deviation of hand in
    rheumatoid
  undifferentiated oligoarthritis
arthritis deformans
Arthritis Foundation
Arthritis Helplessness Index (AHI)
Arthritis Impact Measurement Scales
  (AIMS)
Arthritis Impact Measurement Scales–
  Symptoms (Pain) (AIMS2)
Arthritis Quality of Life Scale
Arthrobot-Zimmer
ArthroCare electrosurgical systems
  and instruments
ArthroCare Wand thermal probe
arthrocele
arthrocentesis
arthrochalasis
arthrochondritis
arthroclasia
arthrodesed digit
arthrodesis (see also *operation*)
  Albee hip
  anterior slot graft arthrodesis
  arthroscopic subtalar
  atlantoaxial
  Baciu-Filibiu dowel ankle
  Badgley
  Benyi modification of Lambrinudi
    triple
  bimalleolar approach to ankle
  Blair tibiotalar
  Brett
  Brockman-Nissen
  Brooks atlantoaxial

arthrodesis *(continued)*
  calcaneocuboid
  Campbell
  Carroll
  Chandler
  Chapchal knee
  Charcot hip
  Charnley ankle
  Charnley-Houston
  Chuinard-Petersen ankle
  closing wedge
  Compere-Thompson
  compression screw
  cone
  distraction-compression bone graft
  double
  dowel
  extra-articular subtalar
  fused
  Gallie ankle
  Gallie atlantoaxial
  Gant hip
  Gill-Stein
  Grice extra-articular subtalar
  Grice-Green extra-articular subtalar
  Grice-Green subtalar
  Guttmann subtalar
  hallux interphalangeal (IP) joint
  hindfoot
  Ilizarov ankle
  interbody
  internal fixation compression
  intertransverse process
  intra-articular
  Lambrinudi triple
  Lapidus modified
  lesser tarsal
  Mann-Coughlin
  Mann-Thompson-Coughlin
  McKeever
  metatarsocuneiform
  metatarsophalangeal joint
  midfoot
  Moberg
  Müller (Mueller)
  Nalebuff
  naviculocuneiform joint

arthrodesis *(continued)*
  nonfused
  occipitocervical
  pantalar
  Potenza
  Potter
  scapulothoracic
  Schneider
  sliding
  spinal
  Stone
  subtalar
  talonavicular
  tibiocalcaneal
  tibiotalar
  transfibular
  transmalleolar ankle
  triple
  Uematsu shoulder
  ulnocarpal
arthrodial articulation
Arthrodial Protractor range-of-motion
  analyzer
arthrodiastasis
arthrodynia
arthrodysplasia
arthroempyesis
arthroendoscopy
arthroereisis, staple
arthrofibrosis
Arthro-Flo arthroscopic irrigation system
Arthro-Flo irrigator
Arthro-Flo system
arthrogram, arthrography
  Brostrom-Gordon
  coronal computed tomographic
    (CCTA)
  CT (computed tomography)
  double-contrast
  gadolinium-enhanced magnetic
    resonance imaging
  Gordon-Brostrom single-contrast
  indirect magnetic resonance
  indirect MR
  joint
  MR

arthrogram *(continued)*
  saline-enhanced MR (of shoulder)
  single-contrast
arthrogryposis multiplex congenita
arthrokatadysis
arthrokleisis
arthrolith
Arthro-Lok blade
Arthro-Lok system
arthrolysis
arthromeningitis
arthrometer
  Acufex knee laxity
  Genucom
  joint
  KT-1000 joint
  KT-1000/Jr
  KT-1000 knee ligament
  KT-1000/S
  KT-2000
  Medmetric KT-1000 knee laxity
  Robinson
  stress-testing
  Stryker knee laxity
arthroncus
arthroneuralgia
Arthron hip and shoulder impact
  protectors
arthronosos
arthro-onychodysplasia
arthro-ophthalmology, hereditary
  progressive
arthropathology
arthropathy
  Charcot
  crystal-related
  inflammatory
  Jaccoud
  midfoot
  neuropathic (NA)
  neuropathic spinal
  post-traumatic
  systemic lupus erythematosus (SLE)
  tabetic
arthrophyma
arthrophyte

arthroplasty (see also *operation*)
    ablative
    abrasion
    Albright-Chase
    ankle
    Aufranc-Turner
    Bowers radial
    capitellocondylar total elbow
    Carroll and Taber
    cemented total hip
    cementless surface replacement
    cementless total hip
    Clayton resection
    constrained ankle
    Cracchiolo-Sculco implant
    Crawford-Adams acetabular cup
    cuff-tear
    cup
    ELP stem for hip
    excision
    extensor brevis
    failed implant
    fascial
    forefoot
    four-in-one
    Girdlestone
    Global total shoulder
    Gore-Tex interpositional
    Gustilo-Kyle cementless total hip
    Hamus wrist
    hemijoint
    hip (cup on cup)
    implant
    interpositional elbow
    irradiated chondral graft
        implantation
    Irvine ankle
    Johnson resection
    laser image custom (LICA)
    Kates forefoot
    Keller
    Keller resection
    Kocher-McFarland hip
    Koenig metatarsophalangeal joint
    Koenig MPJ implant and
    LICA (laser image custom)
    Mann resection

arthroplasty *(continued)*
    Mark II Sorrells hip
    Mayo ankle
    Mayo resection
    McAtee-Tharias-Blazina
    McKee-Farrar total hip
    Meuli
    modified mold and surface
        replacement
    monospherical total shoulder
    mosaic
    Mumford-Gurd
    Neer hemiarthroplasty
    New England Baptist
    primary
    Putti-Platt
    resection
    revision
    Schlein elbow
    silicone implant
    Stanmore shoulder
    surface replacement
    Sutter silicone metacarpophalangeal
        joint
    Swanson interpositional wrist
    Swanson metatarsophalangeal joint
    Swanson PIP joint
    tendon interposition
    Thackray low-friction
    total ankle
    total articular resurfacing (TARA)
    total hip (THA)
    total knee (TKA)
    triaxial total elbow
    Tupper
    UCLA anatomic shoulder
    unicompartmental joint
    Vainio
    Valenti
    Volz total wrist
arthroplasty implant technique, great
    toe (GAIT)
arthropod bite
ArthroProbe arthroscopic laser
ArthroProbe laser system
arthropyosis
arthrorheumatism

arthroscintigraphy
arthroscope
  angled
  Baxter angled
  Dyonics
  Eagle straight-ahead
  GoldenEye
  panoview
  Storz oblique
  Stryker viewing
  Trio
  Wolf
arthroscopically assisted autogenous
  patellar tendon reconstruction
arthroscopically assisted mini-open
  rotator cuff repair
arthroscopic bioabsorbable tack repair
  of shoulder
arthroscopic capsular shift
arthroscopic debridement
arthroscopic examination
arthroscopic glenohumeral release
arthroscopic inferior capsular split
  technique
arthroscopic knot
arthroscopic labrectomy
arthroscopic microdiskectomy (AMD)
arthroscopic mosiacplasty
arthroscopic open-staple capsulorrhaphy
arthroscopic outside-in technique
arthroscopic pump
arthroscopic resection, screw fixation
arthroscopic sheath
arthroscopic subacromial decompression
arthroscopic subtalar arthrodesis
arthroscopic suture anchor repair of
  shoulder
arthroscopic synovectomy
arthroscopic system, McCain TMJ
arthroscopic transacromial repair of
  coracoacromial ligament
arthroscopic transglenoid suture repair
  of shoulder
arthroscopic transhumeral reconstruction of rotator cuff tear

arthroscopic wafer procedure
arthroscopy
  Allen shoulder
  ankle
  diagnostic and operative
  electrothermal
  extraarticular
  Gillquist
  knee
  metacarpophalangeal
  second-look
  wrist
arthroscopy-assisted patellar tendon
  substitution
Arthroscopy Association of North
  America (AANA)
arthroscopy entry portal, stab wound
arthrosis
  crystal-induced
  degenerative
  IRM spiral
  post-traumatic
  trapeziometacarpal
arthrosis deformans
ArthroSorb solidifier material
arthrosynovitis
Arthrotek RC needle
arthrotome
arthrotomography of shoulder, double
  contrast
arthrotomy
  Magnuson-Stack shoulder
  medial parapatellar
  subtalar
ArthroWand
arthroxerosis
arthroxesis
articular capsule
articular cartilage autograft
articular cartilage degeneration
articular cartilage volume
articular cortex
articular disk
articular facet
articular fracture
articular fragment
articular gout

articular muscle
articular nerve
articular process
articular rheumatism
articular surfaces
  apposing
  contiguous
articular wear
articulate
articulating bone ends
articulation (see also *joint*)
  acromioclavicular
  arthrodial
  atlantoaxial
  atlanto-occipital
  bicondylar
  body contour orbit
  calcaneocuboid
  carpal
  carpometacarpal
  carporadial
  cartilaginous
  compound
  condylar
  costovertebral
  cuneonavicular
  DIP (distal interphalangeal)
  distal radioulnar
  disturbance of
  foot
  glenohumeral
  humeral
  humeroradial
  humeroulnar
  incudomalleolar
  intercarpal
  interchondral
  intermetacarpal
  intermetatarsal
  interphalangeal
  intertarsal
  metacarpophalangeal
  metatarsophalangeal
  occipitocervical
  patellofemoral
  PIP (proximal interphalangeal)

articulation *(continued)*
  proximal radioulnar
  radiocarpal
  radiohumeral
  radioulnar
  sacroiliac
  scapuloclavicular
  spheroid
  sternocostal
  subtalar
  superior tibial
  talocalcaneal
  talocalcaneonavicular
  talocrural
  talonavicular
  tarsometatarsal
  temporomandibular
  thorax
  tibiofibular
  transverse tarsal
  trochoid
  ulnoligamentous
  zygapophyseal
articulation disturbance
articulation of pisiform bone
articulatory skills
articulatory tics
artifact, asymmetric
artifact-free EEG
artifact on EEG
  asymmetric
  blink
  cardiac pacemaker
  electrode-popping
  eye-blink
  glossokinetic
  lateralized
  movement
  muscle
  nonbiological
  nonphysiologic
  paper stop
  perspiration
  physiologic
  pikelike
  pulse wave

artifact on EEG *(continued)*
  spikelike
  rhythmic
  stimulus
artifact on x-ray
artificial limb, Utah
artificial neural networks (ANNs)
artificial pneumothorax
Artoscan M (MRI system)
ARUM pin for fixation of Colles
  fracture
aryepiglottic muscle
arytenoid cartilage
ASBAH (Association for Spina Bifida
  and Hydrocephalus)
A-scan ultrasound
ascending activating system
ascending hemiplegia
ascending reticular activating system
ascending septae from the deltoid
  tuberosity
ascending tract
Asch forceps
Asch splint
ASCT (autologous stem cell transplantation)
ASD (antisiphon device), Heyer-Schulte
ASE (axilla, shoulder, elbow) bandage
aseptic fashion
aseptic felon (herpetic whitlow)
aseptic loosening
aseptic meningitis
aseptic necrosis
aseptic uremic meningitis
ASES (American Shoulder and Elbow
  Surgeons) shoulder score
ASF (anterior spine fusion)
ASFP (ascending frontoparietal) artery
Asher physical build assessment
  technique
Ashhurst fracture classification
Ashhurst sign
Ashhurst splint
Ashworth implant arthroplasty
Ashworth scale
Ashworth score of muscle spasticity

ASIA (American Spinal Injury
  Association)
ASIA impairment scale for classifica-
  tion of spinal cord injury
ASIF (Swiss Association for the Study
  of Internal Fixation)
ASIF blade plate
ASIF chisel
ASIF plate
ASIF screw
ASIS (anterior superior iliac spine)
A68 protein marker
ASM (appendicular skeletal muscle)
ASMI (American Sports Medicine
  Institute)
Asnis cannulated screw
Asnis 2 guided screw
ASO (Ankle Stabilizing Orthosis)
  support or brace
ASO (antistreptolysin O) titer
Aspen electrocautery
Aspen laparoscopy electrode
aspergillosis, intracranial
aspergillosis of the central nervous
  system
aspergillotic aneurysm
Aspergillus fumigatus
Aspergillus invasion of the nervous
  system
Aspergillus niger
asphyxia
  neonatal
  perinatal
aspiration
  bone marrow
  joint
  joint fluid
  stereotactic
  therapeutic
aspirator
  Cavitron ultrasonic surgical (CUSA)
  Sharplan ultrasonic
  Sonocut ultrasonic
assay
  Bayer Immuno 1 Dpd
  boron

assay *(continued)*
  clonality
  coagulate
  Immuno 1 Dpd
  immunoprecipitation
  kinase
  PreVue *B. burgdorferi* antibody
    detection
  Pyrilinks-D
  radioisotope clearance
assessment (see also *index, scale,
    score*)
  Activity Losses (ALA)
  BASC (Behavioral Assessment
    System for Children)
  Behavioral Assessment System for
    Children (BASC)
  BFM (Brunnstrom-Fugl-Meyer)
    impairment
  Brunnstrom-Fugl-Meyer (BFM)
    arm impairment
  CFQ-for-others
  closed-chain functional
  environmental
  functional
  Glasgow Assessment Scale
  global assessment of sensory
    disturbance
  home
  immunohistochemical
  isokinetic strength
  JAFAR (Juvenile Arthritis Func-
    tional Assessment Report)
  Juvenile Arthritis Functional
    Assessment Report (JAFAR)
  Moire topographic scoliosis
    screening assessment
  Musculoskeletal Function
    Assessment
  quality of life
  RADAR (Rapid Assessment of
    Disease Activity in Rheuma-
    tology)
  rehabilitation
  Rivermead Motor Assessment

assessment *(continued)*
  SANE (Single Assessment Numeric
    Evaluation)
  Stone and Neale Daily Coping
  ASSH (American Society for Surgery
    of the Hand)
  ASSI (Accurate Surgical and Scientific
    Instruments Corp.)
  ASSI coagulator
  ASSI bipolar coagulating forceps
  ASSI cranio blade
  ASSI wire pass drill
  assignment criteria for rheumatoid
    arthritis
  assist
    handheld
    maximal assist of one or more
    minimal
    standby
  assistant, chiropractic (C.A.)
  Assistant Free calibrated femoral-tibial
    spreader
  association (also *academy, college,
    committee, society*)
    American Association of Hip and
      Knee Surgeons (AAHKS)
    American College of Rheumatology
      (ACR)
    American Diabetes Association
      (ADA) Foot Council
    American Dietetic Association
    American Association of Mental
      Deficiency
    American Podiatric Medical
      Association (APMA)
    American Rheumatism (ARA)
    Amyotrophic Lateral Sclerosis (ALS)
      Association
    Consortium to Establish a Registry
      for Alzheimer's Disease
      (CERAD)
    French Alzheimer Collaborative
      Group
    National Collegiate Athletic (NCAA)
    National Association for Mental
      Health

association *(continued)*
    National Association for the Deaf
    National Association for the
        Visually Handicapped
    National Institute of Neurological
        Communicative Disease and
        Stroke, Alzheimer's Disease and
        Related Disorders Association
    Orthopedic Trauma Association
        (OTA)
    Pediatric Rheumatology Disease
        Registry
    Visiting Nurse
    World Federation of Neurology
associational thalamic nuclei
association cortex of parietal lobes
Association for Spina Bifida and
    Hydrocephalus (ASBAH)
Association of Bone and Joint
    Surgeons (ABJS)
associations
    clang
    loose
associative visual agnosia
astasia
astasia-abasia
astatic seizures
astereognosis (tactile agnosia)
asterion
asterixis (hepatic encephalopathy
    tremor)
asthenia, asthenic
ASTM (American Society for Testing
    and Materials)
ASTM designation of Biophase
Aston cartilage reduction
astragalar bone
astragalocalcaneal
astragalocrural
astragaloscaphoid bone
astragalotibial
astragalectomy
astragalus (talus), aviator's
astroblast
astroblastoma

astrocyte
    fibrous
    gemistocytic
    plasmatofibrous
    protoplasmic
astrocytic gliosis
astrocytic tumor
astrocytoma
    anaplastic
    fibrillary
    gemistocytic
    glioblastoma multiforme
    grades 1-4
    high-grade
    intracranial
    low-grade (LGA)
    pilocytic
    protoplasmic
    supratentorial
astrocytoma tumor
astrocytosis
astroglial tumor
astrogliosis
Astro-Med Albert Grass Heritage
    digital EEG system
asymmetric hyperreflexia
asymmetric tonic neck reflex (ATNR)
asymmetrical loading of lower
    extremity
asymmetry
    amplitude
    cranial growth
    facial
    interhemispheric
    limb length
    skull
    thermal
asyndesis
asyndetic communication
asynergia, asynergic
Atak knee brace
Atasoy-Kleinert flap
Atasoy palmar flap
Atasoy triangular advancement flap
Atasoy V-Y technique

ataxia
  absent
  appendicular
  atactic
  Bruns
  cerebellar
  crural
  equilibratory
  familial paroxysmal kinesigenic
  familial spastic
  Friedreich
  frontal
  gait
  Greenfield classification of
    spinocerebellar
  hereditary spastic
  ipsilateral cerebellar
  kinesigenic
  limb
  limb-gait
  locomotor
  Marie hereditary spastic
  mild
  moderate
  sensory
  severe
  spinocerebellar
  sporadic
  truncal
ataxia of cerebellar origin
ataxia of posterior column origin
ataxia-telangiectasia
ataxic breathing
ataxic dysarthria
ataxic gait
ataxic hemiparesis (AH)
ataxic paraplegia
ataxic respiration
ataxic speech
ATD (assistive technology devices)
atelocollagen gel
Aten olecranon screw
ATF (anterior talofibular ligament)
atheroma, carotid bifurcation
atherosclerosis, extracranial carotid
  artery

atherostenosis
atherothrombotic brain infarction
athetoid palsy, pure
athetosis, double congenital
athetotic
athlete
  differently abled
  high-power
athlete's diet, American Dietetic
  Association
athlete's foot
athlete's pseudonephritis
Athlete's Shoulder Scoring System
athletic caloric requirements
Ativan (lorazepam)
Atkin epiphyseal fracture
Atkinson endoprosthesis
ATL (anterior temporal lobectomy)
ATL real-time Neurosector scanner
Atlanta brace orthosis
atlantoaxial arthrodesis
atlantoaxial articulation
atlantoaxial interval
atlantoaxial joint
atlantoaxial rotary subluxation
atlantoaxial separation
atlantoaxial stabilization
atlantomastoid
atlanto-occipital articulation
atlanto-occipital dissociation
atlanto-occipital fusion
atlanto-occipital junction
atlanto-occipital membrane
atlanto-odontoid
atlas adjustment
atlas of neck (C1, first cervical
    vertebra)
  arch of
  burst fracture of the
  compression fracture of the
  transverse ligaments of the
AtlasPlan neurosurgery software
atlas vertebral subluxation complex
ATM (acute transverse myelitis)
ATNR (asymmetric tonic neck reflex)
ATODC (atraumatic osteolysis of
    distal clavicle)

ATON (adductor tenotomy and
  obturator neurectomy)
atonic bladder
atonic seizure
atony (atonia)
atopognosia
atracurium besylate
atraumatic
atraumatic osteolysis of distal clavicle
  (ATODC)
atretic
atrium of ventricle
Atromid (clofibrate)
atrophic dementia
  Alzheimer
  Pick
  senile
atrophic lesion of brain
atrophic neuroarthropathy
atrophied muscle
atrophy
  brachial muscular
  brain
  cerebellar
  cerebral
  cerebral surface
  cortical
  dentatorubral
  dentatorubropallidoluysian
  disuse
  dorsum sellae
  Duchenne-Aran spinal muscular
  eccentric
  frontotemporal
  Gudden
  hemisphere
  hippocampal
  Kugelberg-Welander juvenile spinal
    muscle
  Leber optic
  lesser (of disuse)
  lobar (of Pick)
  localized muscular
  Marie-Foix-Alajouanine cerebellar
  Menzel olivopontocerebellar
  multiple system (MSA)
  muscle

atrophy (continued)
  neurogenic
  olivopontocerebellar
  parenchymatous
  peroneal muscular
  postneuritic
  primary optic
  progressive neuropathic muscle
  progressive post-polio muscle
    (PPPMA)
  quadriceps
  scapuloperoneal muscular
  spinal cord
  spinal muscular (SMA)
  subacute denervation
  subcortical
  Sudeck osteoporotic
  sulcal
  temporal horn
  Vulpian-Bernhardt spinal muscular
  Welander distal muscular
  Werdnig-Hoffmann spinal muscular
attachment
  capsular
  cerebellar
  commissural
  dural
  fibrous
  Hudson cerebellar
  ligamentous
  Pearson
  tendon-bone
  tendinous
attack
  adversive
  akinetic drop
  brain
  cataleptic
  cephalalgic
  cephalgic
  cryptogenic drop
  decerebrate
  drop
  epileptic drop
  factitious
  falling
  jackknife

attack *(continued)*
   kinesigenic
   masticatory
   motor jacksonian
   psychomotor
   salaam
   sensory jacksonian
   sleep
   Stokes-Adams
   transient hemisphere (THA)
   transient ischemic (TIA)
   vagal
   vasospastic
   waking
attack absence
Attenborough knee prosthesis
attend, ability to
attention
   fix and focus
   heightened
   raptus of
attention deficit disorder (ADD)
attention deficit/hyperactivity disorder
   (ADHD)
attention span
attenuate, attenuated
attenuating
attenuation, broadband ultrasound
attenuation coefficient on MRI scan
attenuation of alpha rhythm on EEG
attenuation of tendons
attenuation value on MRI scan
attitude, over-dependent
Atton disease
attrition rupture of tendon
ATV (all-terrain vehicle) accident
ATV (anterior terminal vein)
a2-macroglobulin (a2M)
A2 pulley
A-2000 BIS (Bispectral Index) monitor
atypical absence seizure (petit mal
   variant)
atypical giant cell tumor
atypical neuroleptic
auditory agnosia
auditory brain stem implant (ABI)

auditory brain stem response (ABR)
   threshold
auditory cortex, primary
auditory division of eighth cranial nerve
auditory evoked potential
auditory evoked response
auditory localization
auditory nerve (cochlear)
auditory ossicles, muscles of
auditory radiation
auditory seizure
auditory symptoms
Aufranc cobra hip prosthesis
Aufranc cobra retractor
Aufranc modification of Smith-
   Petersen cup
Aufranc osteotome
Aufranc retractor
Aufranc-Turner acetabular cup
Aufranc-Turner arthroplasty
Aufranc-Turner hip prosthesis
Aufricht glabellar rasp
auger
augmenting response on EEG
augmentor nerves (cervical splanchnic
   nerves)
Augustine boat nail
aula
auliplexus
aulix
aura
   auditory
   déjà vu
   epigastric
   epileptic
   gustatory
   hysterical
   intellectual
   jamais vu
   kinesthetic
   migraine
   migrainous
   motor
   olfactory
   reminiscent
   sensory

aura *(continued)*
    shimmering light with
    status
    tactile pricklings with
    tingling with
    uncinate
    visual shimmering with
    visual shining with
    visual sparkling with
    wavering light with
AuRA cemented total hip system
aura of migraine
aura symptoms in migraine
auricular fissure
auricular ligament
auricular nerve
    anterior
    great
    internal
    posterior
    vagus nerve
auriculo-osteodystrophy
auriculotemporal nerve
auriculotherapy
Aurum
Aussies-Isseis unstable scoliosis
Austin-Akin bunionectomy
Austin bunionectomy
Austin Moore chisel
Austin Moore hemiarthroplasty
Austin Moore hip prosthesis
Austin Moore hook
Austin Moore impactor
Austin osteotomy
Australian X viral encephalitis
autism
    akinetic
    infantile
autistic thinking
autoantibody, antiproteasome
autoantigen
autochthonous graft
autoecholalia
Autoflex II CPM (continuous passive
    motion) unit
autofusion

Autogenesis automator for Ilizarov
    screws
autogenous bone graft
autogenous cartilage transplantation
autogenous osteocartilage transfer
autogenous peroneus longus free graft
    technique
autogenous replantation of meniscal
    cartilage
autograft
    Achilles tendon
    bone-patellar tendon-bone (BPB)
    bone-retinaculum-bone
    bridge
    bulk
    free revascularized
    iliac crest
    ipsilateral
    osteochondral shell
    semitendinosus/gracilis
    tendon-bone
autograft hamstring augmentation
autograft replacement with
    nonmeniscal tissue
autoimmune response
Auto-Implant procedure
autologous adrenal medullary tissue
autologous blood
autologous bone strut
autologous chondrocyte implantation
    (ACI)
autologous cultured chondrocytes
autologous graft
autologous growth factor (AGF)
autologous pericranium
autologous reverse graft to ankle
autologous stem cell transplantation
    (ASCT)
autologous vein-covered stent
automated cerebral blood flow
    analyzer
automated computerized axial
    tomography (ACAT)
automated percutaneous lumbar
    diskectomy (APLD)
automatic dysreflexia

automatic behavior
automatic bladder, in spinal cord
  syndromes
automatic bladder reflex
automatic phrase level
automatism
  chewing
  epileptic
  facial expression
  gestural
  ictal
  lip smacking
  mumbling
  patting
  scratching
  swallowing
Automator device
autonomic denervation
autonomic dysfunction
autonomic failure
autonomic hyperactivity
autonomic hyperreflexia
autonomic hyperventilation
autonomic nerve
autonomic nervous system
autonomic neuropathy
autonomic or accessory oculomotor or
  Edinger-Westphal nucleus
autonomous nodule
Autophor ceramic hip prosthesis
Autophor femoral prosthesis
autoregulation of cerebral blood flow
auto-reinforced polyglycolide rods
autosomal dominant disorder
autosomal dominant inheritance
autosomal dominant myoclonic
  dystonia
Auto Suture vascular clip applier
  system
autosympathectomization, spontaneous
autosympathectomy secondary to
  diabetic neuropathy
autotenodesis
autotopagnosia
Avanta soft skeletal implants
avascular chondroepiphyseal trans-
  plants

avascular necrosis (AVN)
AVDO$_2$ (arteriovenous oxygen difference)
AVEEG (audiovisual electroencephalogram)
Avellis syndrome
averaging, spike
Averett hip prosthesis
Averill total hip replacement
aviator's astragalus
Avila technique
A-V Impulse System
Avitene "flour"
Avitene microfibrillar collagen
  hemostat
AVM (arteriovenous malformation)
AVN (avascular necrosis)
avoidance gait
avulse
avulsed fracture fragment
avulsion
  bony
  coracoid tip
  epiphyseal
  iatrogenic
  ligament
  nail plate
  patellar tendon
  spinal nerve root
  traumatic
avulsion chip fracture
avulsion fracture
avulsion fragment
AVVM (angiographically visualized
  vascular malformation)
A wave form on ICP monitor
awareness
  heightened
  lapse of
  postural
AW-GC (apatite- and wallstonite-
  containing glass-ceramic)
awl
  angled
  Aufranc
  bone
  curved

awl *(continued)*
  DePuy
  Ender
  Küntscher
  pointed
  reaming
  rectangular
  Rush
  square-shaped
  Swanson lunate
  Swanson scaphoid
  T-handled
  Zuelzer
Axer-Clark procedure
Axer varus derotational osteotomy
axial acetabular index (AAI)
axial compression forces
axial compression fracture
axial compression of foot
axial flag flap
axillary arch muscle
axillary block anesthesia
axillary nerve
axial load and torque
axial loading, spinal
axial malrotation
axial manual traction test
axial musculature
axial neuritis
axial pattern flap
axial percutaneous pinning
axial plane
axial scan
axial section
axial skeleton
axial slice
axial spinal system
axial spin density
axial traction
Axiom total knee system
axis (neck) (C2, second cervical
  vertebra)
axis (pl. axes)
  anatomic
  ankle mortise
  basibregmatic
  basicranial

axis *(continued)*
  bimalleolar foot
  cortical hinge
  craniospinal
  distal reference (DRA)
  eccentric axis of ankle rotation
  femoral shaft
  flexion-extension
  hypothalamic-pituitary
  hypothalamic-pituitary-adrenal
  hypothalamoneurohypophyseal
    (HNA)
  leg
  long
  longitudinal
  mechanical
  metatarsal
  proximal reference (PRA)
  rotation
  single
  spinal
  subtalar
  transcondylar (TCA)
  vertical
  weightbearing
  Z-axis
Axis ankle brace
axis length
axis ligament
axle lock and bumper
axodendritic synapse
axoid
axon
  centrally directed
  distally directed
axonal neuropathy
axonal sprouting
axon degeneration
axon flare
axon hillock
axon loss
axon regeneration
axon regrowth
axon sprouting
axon terminal
axon transection
axon transport

axonapraxia
axonopathic neurogenic thoracic outlet
 syndrome
axonopathy
axonotmesis
axoplasm
axoplasmic flow and papilledema

Axostim nerve stimulator
Ayers needle holder
Ayres tactile discrimination stereognosis test
azathioprine (Imuran)
Azorean disease
azotemic osteodystrophy

B, b

Baastrupi syndrome
Babcock scissors
Babcock sentences
Babcock stainless steel wire
Babcock wire-cutting scissors
"babies" the injured part
Babinski-Fröhlich syndrome
Babinski-Nageotte syndrome
Babinski percussion hammer
Babinski reflex
Babinski sign
BA (bioactive) bone cement
BacFix system
bacillary angiomatosis
bacitracin solution
Baciu-Filibiu dowel ankle arthrodesis
back
    arching of
    industrial
backache
Backbiter
Back Bubble gravity traction unit
back crease
back exercise techniques
    bilateral arm raise
    bridge
    calf raise
    functional squats

back exercise techniques *(continued)*
    gluteal/hamstring raise
    hip hinge
    kneeling reciprocal
    partial sit-ups
    quadruped
    reciprocal arm raise
    reverse lunge
    side lunge
    side-lying
    superman
    Williams flexion
backfire fracture
background activity on EEG
background disorganization on EEG
background subtraction technique
Back Hammer muscle stimulator
Backhaus towel clamp
Backhaus towel forceps
Back-Huggar lumbar support cushion
Backlund biopsy needle
back manipulation
backpack palsy
backpack paralysis
Back Revolution Stick
Back Revolution traction/exercise unit
back-scatter, optical
back school

Back Specialist chiropractic table
BackStrong lumbar extension machine
BackTracker
Back Trainer spinal exercise system
baclofen (Lioresal)
Bacon bone rongeur
Bacon cranial rongeur
Bacon raspatory
Bacon rongeur
Bacon thoracic shears
bacterial cerebritis
bacterial meningitis
Bacterium anitratum meningitis
bactogen (slang for bacterial antigen in CSF)
Badgley arthrodesis
Badgley laminectomy retractor
Badgley resection of iliac wing
Badgley retractor
Badgley rib spreader
Bad Wildungen Metz (BWM) spine system
BAEP (brain stem auditory evoked potential)
Baer bone-cutting forceps
Baer bone rongeur
Baer rib shears
BAER (brain stem auditory evoked response)
bag balm
bag, stereotactic
Bagby angled compression plate
Bahler hinge
BAI (Barthel ADL Index)
bail-lock knee joint
Bailey-Badgley cervical spine fusion
Bailey conductor
Bailey-Dubow technique
Bailey-Gibbon rib contractor
Bailey-Gigli saw guide
Bailey rib contractor
Bailey rib spreader
Bailey saw guide
Bailey wire saw
Baillinger, inner stripe of
BAK/C (cervical) interbody fusion system

baked-brain phenomenon
Baker cyst
Baker-Hill osteotomy
Baker lateral semitendinosus transfer
baker's leg (genu valgum)
BAK fusion cage
BAK interbody fusion system
BAK laparoscopic procedure
BAK/Proximity interbody fusion implant
BAK/T (thoracic) interbody fusion system
Balacescu-Golden technique
balance
    coronal
    dopaminergic-cholinergic
    dynamic ambulatory
    dynamic standing balance
    homeostatic
    sagittal
    sitting
    standing
    static and dynamic sitting
    static and dynamic standing
Balance Master rehabilitation evaluation
balance padding
balanced suspension
balancing, tendon
Baldwin Bowers radioulnar joint repair
Balint syndrome
Balkan fracture frame
Balkan splint
ball
    cold-weld femoral
    ExerFlex
    Gymnic
    Jurgan pin
    Silastic
    Thera-Band exercise
    therapy
ball-and-socket giant pseudarthrosis
ball-and-socket joint
ball-and-socket synovial joint
Ballantine hemilaminectomy retractor
ball-bearing eye sign
ball bearing, Steinmann pin with

Ballenger-Hajek chisel
Ballenger knife
Ballenger periosteotome
Ballenger swivel knife
ballism
ballistic injury
ballistic wound
ball of foot
balloon
  occlusion
  Spiegelberg epidural
ballooned floor of ventricle
ballooning of the sella
ballooning of vertebral interspace
ballottement
  distal ulna
  patella
ball skill performance
ball valve tumor
balm, bag
balmoral laced shoe
balneotherapy
Baló disease
Baló sclerosis
balsa wood filler block
Baltic myoclonus syndrome
Baltimore Therapeutic Equipment
  Work Simulator
Bamberger-Marie disease
Bamberger sign
banana Beaver blade
banana sign
Bancaud phenomenon on EEG
Bancroft sign
band
  alpha
  alpha frequency
  AO tension
  aponeurotic
  arm
  beta
  beta frequency
  Broca diagonal
  calf
  constriction
  delta frequency
  deossification

band *(continued)*
  external
  fascial
  frequency band on EEG
  Gennari
  iliotibial (IT)
  internal
  lateral
  lucent
  oligoclonal band in CSF
  Parham
  Parham-Martin
  Partridge
  pretendinous band of hand
  scar
  subsurface white
  tennis elbow arm
  theta frequency
bandage (see also *dressing*)
  Ace adherent
  adhesive
  ASE (axilla, shoulder, elbow)
  Barton
  capeline
  Champ elastic
  Comperm tubular elastic
  Fabco gauze
  gum rubber Martin
  Hamilton
  Helenca
  Heliodorus
  Hippocrates
  Hueter
  Hydron Burn Bandage
  compression
  Conco elastic
  cotton elastic
  cravat
  crepe
  demigauntlet
  Desault
  Dressinet netting
  E Cotton
  elastic
  elastic wrap
  Elastic Foam
  Elastomull

bandage *(continued)*
- Elastoplast
- Esmarch
- Fabco gauze
- figure of 8 interscapular
- Flex-Foam
- Flex-Master
- Flexilite conforming elastic
- Fractura Flex
- gauntlet
- Gibney
- Gibson
- immobilizing
- Kerlix
- Kling elastic
- malleable metal finger splints
- Martin sheet rubber
- nonadhesive
- Nu Gauze sterile gauze
- Ortho-Trac adhesive
- Ortho-Vent nonadhesive
- Pavlik
- plaster of Paris (POP)
- PRN
- Redigrip pressure
- replantation
- restrictive
- Ribble
- Richet
- Sayre
- scultetus
- self-adhering
- sling and swathe
- spica
- spiral
- starch
- stockinette
- Tricodur compression support
- Tricodur Epi (elbow) compression
- Tricodur Omos (shoulder) compression
- Tricodur Talus (ankle) compression
- Tru-Support
- Tru-Support EW (elastic wrap)
- Tru-Support SA (self-adhering)
- Tubigrip
- tubular elastic

bandage *(continued)*
- two-inch gauze
- Velpeau
- Webril
- Bandage Gard cast protector
- band around head, feeling of
- B&L pinch gauge
- Bandi patellofemoral score
- Band-It magnetic elbow support
- band of Gennari
- Bandi procedure
- band tenodesis
- Bane bone rongeur
- Bane-Hartmann bone rongeur
- Bane mastoid rongeur
- Bane rongeur forceps
- Bangerter muscle forceps
- banjo cast
- banjo splint
- Bankart procedure for shoulder dislocation
- Bankart-Putti-Platt operation
- Bankart retractor
- Bankart shoulder prosthesis
- Bankart tack
- Banks-Laufman approach
- Bantam wire-cutting scissors
- bantenadesis

bar
- bony
- cartilaginous
- congenital
- Denis Browne (DB)
- distraction
- fibrous
- Fillauer
- Gerster traction
- intramedullary
- L
- Leyla
- Livingston
- lumbrical
- metatarsal flatfoot
- opponens
- parallel
- patellar
- quad

bar *(continued)*
  rigid
  spacer
  spondylitic
  spondylotic
  spreader
  Stephen spreader
  supraorbital
  tarsal
  Thornton
  Tommy trapeze
  torsion
  traction
  trapeze
  unsegmented vertebral
barber's chair sign
barbiturate coma
barbiturate poisoning
barbiturates, blood screen for
barbotage
Bardeen disk
bar defect
Bardeleben bone-holding forceps
Bardeleben rasp
Bardinet ligament
Bard-Parker blade
Bard-Parker knife
Bard-Parker scalpel
Bareskin knee positioner
baresthesia
barked
Barkow ligament
bar-like ventral defect on myelography
Barlow hip instability test
Barlow maneuver
Barlow sign
Barlow splint
Barlow test
barognosis
Baron suction tube
baroreceptor nerve (pressoreceptor
  nerve)
baroreceptors in the carotid bulb
Barouk button space for hallux valgus
  deformity
Barouk cannulated bone screw

Barouk microscrew with shortening
  osteotomy
Barouk microstaple
Barouk spacer
Barraquer needle holder
Barrasso-Wile-Gage arthrodesis
barrel chest
Barré-Lieou syndrome
barrier
  blood-brain (BBB)
  blood-spinal cord
  Capset (calcium sulfate) bone graft
Barr-Record ankle arthrodesis
Barsky procedure
Barthel ADL Index (BAI)
Bartlett nail fold excision
Barton-Cone tong traction
Barton fracture
Barton skull traction tongs
basal caloric requirements
basal cistern
basal chordae
basal endothelium-derived relaxing
  factor
basal ganglia
basal ganglia calcifications
basal ganglia of cerebellum
basal joint of thumb
basal layer
basally
basal movements
basal neck fracture
basal part of brain
basal part of temporal lobe
basal short axis slice
basal skull fracture
basal vein of Rosenthal
basal zone
BASC (Behavioral Assessment System
  for Children)
base
  cranial
  dorsal spinal cord horn
  Dycal
  posterior spinal cord horn
  skull

baseball elbow
baseball finger
baseball shoulder
baseball splint
baseball stitch or suture
Baseline Bubble inclinometer
baseline distortion on EEG
Baseline hand dynamometer
base of brain
base wedge osteotomy
basiarachnitis
basiarachnoiditis
basibregmatic axis
basicranial
basicranial axis
basilar artery insufficiency syndrome
basilar artery migraine headache
basilar bone
basilar cavernous fistula
basilar cistern
basilar ectasia
basilar fracture
basilar insufficiency
basilar intracerebral hemorrhage
basilar invagination
basilar occlusion
basilar skull fracture
basilar suture
basilar syndrome
basilar trunk aneurysm
basilar vertebral artery disease
Basile screw
basilic vein
basioccipital bone
basiocciput tumor
basion
basis pontis
basistyloid fovea
basket
   Acufex meniscal
   forward-biting
   shovel-nose Schutte
basket-weave ankle taping
BASMI (Bath Ankylosing Spondylitis
   Metrology Index)
basocervical fracture

basophilic adenoma
basophilic pituitary tumor
basophilism
   Cushing
   pituitary
Bassen-Kornzweig syndrome
Basser syndrome
Bassett electrical stimulation device
basswood splint
Batchelor-Brown arthrodesis
Batchelor modified procedure to
   correct hindfoot valgus deformity
Batch-Spittler-McFaddin knee
   disarticulation
Bateman shoulder procedure
Bateman UPF (universal proximal
   femur)
Bateman UPF II bipolar endoprosthesis
Bateman UPF II bipolar hip prosthesis
Bateman UPF II shoulder prosthesis
bath (pl. baths)
   contrast
   hot and cold contrast
   hot sulfur
   mud pack
   paraffin (PB)
   paraffin oil
   sitz
   whirlpool
Bath Ankylosing Spondylitis Disease
   Activity Index (BASDAI)
Bath Ankylosing Spondylitis
   Functional Index (BASFI)
Bath Ankylosing Spondylitis
   Metrology Index (BASMI)
bathing and dressing ability
batrachian (frog) gait or posture
Batson plexus
Batson vertebral brain system
Battelle Developmental Inventory
   (BDI)
Batten disease
Battery
   Cambridge Test
   Halstead-Reitan
   Memory Efficiency subtest

Battery *(continued)*
   neuropsychological
   Rand Functional Limitations
   Rand Physical Capacities
   Rand Social Health
   Rivermead Perceptual Assessment
      (RPAB)
battery of tests, neuropsychologic
Battery of Memory Efficiency subtest
Battle sign
battledore incision
bat-wing appearance
Batzdorf cervical wire passer
Batzdorf cervical wire twister
Bauerfeind orthopedic products
Bauer-Tondra-Trusler technique
Bauman angle
Baumgard-Schwartz tennis elbow
   technique
Bavarian splint
Baxter angled arthroscope
Bayer Immuno 1 Dpd assay
Baylor splint
Bayne classification for ulnar ray defi-
   ciency (types I through IV)
Bayne classification of radial agenesis
bayonet dislocation
bayonet fracture dislocation
bayonet leg
bayonet-point wire
bayonet position of fracture
BBB (blood-brain barrier)
BBC (biceps, brachialis, coraco-
   brachialis) muscles
BB shot
B-cell surface marker of CNS
   neoplasm
BDD (blistering distal dactylitis)
BDD (body dysmorphic disorder)
BDH (biologically designed hip)
   prosthesis
BDI (Battelle Development Inventory)
BDNF (brain-derived neurotrophic
   factor)
BDRS (Blessed Dementia Rating
   Scales)

BDRS information-memory-
   concentration test
B–D (Becton-Dickinson) spinal needle
beach chair position
beads
   antibiotic-impregnated
   gentamicin
   methylmethacrylate
   PMMA (polymethylmethacrylate)
   targeting
bead-blasted prosthesis
beaked cervicomedullary junction
beaking of head of talus
beaking, talonavicular
beak-like osteophyte formation
Beall-Webel-Bailey technique
BEAM (brain electrical activity map
   or mapping)
beam-hardening artifact
beanbag
bearing
   ceramic-on-ceramic
   metal-on-metal
   polar
bear's paw hand
beaten silver appearance of skull
beat-knee syndrome
Beath needle
Beath pin
Beath view
Beatson combined ankle angle
Beau line
Beauvais disease
Beaver blade
   arachnoid shape
   banana
   cataract knife
   discission knife
   keratome
   retrograde
   rosette
   sickle shape
Beaver cataract knife
Beaver DeBakey blade
Beaver keratome blade
Bebax shoe for forefoot deformity

Bechtol acetabular component
Bechtol hip prosthesis
Bechtol shoulder prosthesis
Beck Cognitive subscore
Beck Depression Inventory
Beckenbaugh technique
Becker external drain
Becker-Kiener dystrophy
Becker muscular dystrophy (BMD)
Becker suture
Becker tendon repair
Becker-type muscular dystrophy
Becker variant of Duchenne dystrophy
Beckman-Adson laminectomy blade
Beckman-Eaton laminectomy retractor
Beckman EEG instrument, 20-channel
Beckman laminectomy retractor
Beckman-Weitlaner laminectomy
   retractor
Beck Questionnaire
Beck-Steffee total ankle prosthesis
Beclard amputation
Becton technique
bed
   American Seating Access-O-Matic
   BioDyne
   Borg-Warner orthopedic
   Burke Bariatric
   Cardiopulmonary Paragon 8500
   Carrom orthopedic
   Chick-Foster orthopedic
   circle
   CircOlectric
   Clinitron air
   DMI orthopedic
   Flexicair
   FluidAir
   Foster
   fracture
   Gatch
   gatched
   Goodman orthopedic
   Hausted orthopedic
   high air loss
   high muscular resistance
   Hill-Rom orthopedic
   Hollywood

bed *(continued)*
   Inland Super Multi-Hite orthopedic
   Inter-Royal frame orthopedic
   Joerns orthopedic
   Keane Mobility
   KinAir
   Lapidus
   low air loss
   Magnum 800
   Medicus
   Mega-Air
   Mega Tilt and Turn
   nail
   orthopedic
   primary tumor
   Pulmonair 40
   Restcue
   RotoRest
   Simmons Multi-Matic orthopedic
   Simmons Vari-Hite orthopedic
   skeletal
   Skytron
   SMI 3000
   SMI 5000
   Smith-Davis Converta-Hite
      orthopedic
   Stryker
   Superior Sleeprite Hi-Lo orthopedic
   TheraPulse
   Tilt and Turn Paragon
   tumor
   Ultra-Flex orthopedic
bed cradle
bedfast
bed mobility skills
bed of nail
bed of rib
bedrest
bedridden
bed wedge, Duo-Cline (by Bodyline)
Beebe wire-cutting scissors
beefy tongue
Beere Precision Medical
   instruments/devices
bees' nest
Beeson cast spreader
Beeson plaster spreader

Beevor sign
behavior
 affective
 aggressive
 automatic
 cognitive
 drug-seeking
 explosive
 hyperactive
 illness
 impulsive
 inappropriate
 infantile
 interictal
 pain
 rehabilitation
 repetitive
 sequential
 semipurposeful
 stereotypical
 tic-like
Behavioral Assessment System for
 Children (BASC)
behavioral changes
Behavioral Inattention Test (BIT)
behavioral mapping
Behavioral Pathology in Alzheimer's
 Disease rating scale
Behavioral Risk Factor Surveillance
 System (BRFSS)
Behavior Rating for Dementia Scale
 (BRDS)
Behr syndrome
Beighton criteria for hypermobility
 syndrome
Bekhterev arthritis
Bekhterev layer
Bekhterev-Mendel reflex
Bekhterev spondylitis
Bekhterev sitting test
Belfast regime
Bell-Dally cervical dislocation
Bellemore-Barrett-Middleton-Scougall-
 Whiteway technique
Bellini ligament
Bell long thoracic nerve
Bell-Magendie law

Bell muscle
Bell palsy
Bell phenomenon
bellringer category
Bell suture
Bell-Tawse open reduction technique
Bellucci alligator scissors
belly of muscle
belly press test
Belos compression pin
below-elbow prosthesis
below-knee prosthesis
belt
 cast
 Meek pelvic traction
 MicroTeq portable
 obesity
 pelvic traction
 Posey
 Reed cast
 rib
 Silesian
 test
 tub
 waist suspension
 Zim-Zap rib
Benadryl (diphenhydramine)
Bence Jones protein
bench examination
bench, tub
bender
 BendMeister rod
 French rod
 rod
 Rush
bendable metallic rod
bending fracture
Bendixen-Kirschner traction
BendMeister rod bender
bends, the (caisson disease)
benediction posture
Benedikt ipsilateral oculomotor paralysis
Benedikt syndrome
Benefen (ibuprofen topical gel)
BeneJoint (capsaicin, glucosamine,
 chondroitin sulfate)
Benemid (probenecid)

benign capillary hemangioblastoma
benign essential tremor
benign familial neonatal convulsions
(BFNC)
benign functional vertigo
benign hypermobile joint syndrome
benign lymphocytic choriomeningitis
benign pain syndrome
benign paroxysmal positional vertigo
(BPPV)
benign raised intracranial pressure
benign senescent forgetfulness
benign X-linked recessive muscular
dystrophy
Benink tarsal index
Bennett basic hand dislocation
Bennett basic hand fracture
Bennett basic hand splint
Bennett bone elevator
Bennett bone retractor
Bennett fracture
Bennett lesion
Bennett posterior shoulder approach
Bennett quadriceps plastic procedure
Bennett tibial retractor
Benson-Geschwind classification of
aphasia
bent-knee pelvic tilts
bent malleable retractor
Benton Visual Retention Test
bentonite flocculation test (BFT)
Benyi modification of Lambrinudi
triple arthrodesis
benzoin adherent tape
BeOK hand exercise putty
Berens muscle clamp
Berens muscle forceps
Berger interscapular amputation
Berger rhythm (on EEG)
Bergeron chorea
BERG (balloon-assisted, endoscopic,
retroperitoneal, gasless) lumbar
interbody fusion
Bergman mallet
Bergstrom cannula
Berliner percussion hammer
Berman-Gartland metatarsal osteotomy

Berman-Moorhead metal locator
Bermuda spica cast
Bernard-Horner syndrome
Berndt-Hardy classification of
transchondral fracture
Berndt-Hardy talar lesion staging
Berndt hip ruler
Bernese periacetabular osteotomy
berry aneurysm
Berry ligament
Berstein cast table
Bertillon cephalometer
Bertin bone
Bertin ligament
besipirdine hydrochloride
beta activity
beta adrenergic receptor blocker
beta amyloid
beta frequency band
beta index
beta pattern
beta rhythm
Betaseron (interferon beta-1b)
Betaseron needle-free delivery system
beta spindles
beta wave
Betadine Helafoam solution
Betadine scrub solution
Betadine soak
Bethesda bone
Bethune-Coryllos rib shears
Bethune periosteal elevator
Bethune rib shears
BETS (benign epileptiform transients
of sleep)
Betz giant pyramidal cell
Bevatron accelerator
bevel, beveled, beveling
Bevin shoe
Beyer rongeur forceps
Beyer-Stille bone rongeur
BFM arm assessment (Brunnstrom-
Fugl-Meyer)
BFNC (benign familial neonatal
convulsions)
BFT (bentonite flocculation test)
B.H. Moore procedure

BHT (blunt head trauma)
Biad SPECT imaging system
Bi-Angular shoulder prosthesis
biarthrodial muscles
biarticular bone-cutting forceps
biarticular bone shears
bias, flexion
bias potential
Bias hip prosthesis
biaxial synovial joint
Biaxial Weave composite prosthesis
BICAP (bipolar cautery probe) unit
biceps
    long head of (LHB)
    short head of (SHB)
biceps brachii muscle
biceps femoris muscle
biceps jerk (BJ), stretch reflex
biceps-labral complex
biceps stretch reflex
biceps tendon tenodesis
bicerebral infarction
Bichat canal
Bichat ligament
bichloroacetic acid
bicipital groove tenderness test
bicipital tendinitis
bicipital tuberosity
Bickel intramedullary rod
Bickel leg holder
Bickel-Moe procedure
Bickerstaff migraine
bicondylar articulation
bicondylar fracture
bicoronal synostosis
bicorrectional Austin osteotomy
bicortical iliac bone graft
bicortical screw
Bicro-Lyte ankle stirrup
bicycle
    Air-Dyne
    FES exercise
    Pedlar portable stationary
bidirectional traction
Bielschowsky head tilt test
Bielschowsky-Jansky disease
Biemer-Clip aneurysm clip

Bier amputating saw
Bier block anesthesia
Bier lumbar puncture needle
Bier saw
bifida, spina
bifocal manipulation with distraction
bifrontal headache
bifurcated ligament
bifurcation
    basilar artery
    carotid
    common carotid artery
    middle cerebral artery
Bigelow calvarium clamp
Bigelow ligament
Bigelow maneuver, reverse
big toe
BIH (benign intracranial hypertension)
bihemispheral insult
bihemispheric lesion
bi-ischial diameter
Bike ankle brace
bikini skin incision
bilateral Babinksi sign
bilateral carotid artery occlusion
bilateral carotid stenosis
bilateral cerebral dysfunction
    metabolic
    structural
bilateral corticobulbar disease
bilateral decortication
bilateral frontal lobe disease
bilateral hallux valgus (HV)
bilateral hemisphere dysfunction
bilateral hyperreflexia
bilateral interfacet dislocation
bilateral orbital frontal cortex
bilateral paralysis
bilateral pyramidal sign
bilateral simultaneous stimulation
bilateral synchrony on EEG
bilateral theta slowing (on EEG)
bilateral upper motor neuron
    (supranuclear) dysfunction
Bilhaut-Cloquet procedure
Bill bar (bone)
Bilos pin

bimalleolar ankle fracture
Bi-Metric hip prosthesis
binder (see also *bandage*; *dressing*)
    Dale abdominal
    Helenca
    scultetus
binding, biological
bind wire
Bing-Horton syndrome
binocular acuity change
Binswanger dementia
Binswanger disease
Binswanger encephalopathy
bioabsorbable interference screw
bioabsorbable suture
Bio-Anchor suture anchor
Bio-Boot
Biobrane adhesive
Biobrane glove
biocalibration
bioceramic joint replacement material
Bio-Chromatic hand prosthesis
Bioclad acetabular prosthesis
Bioclusive transparent dressing
biocompartmental replacement of knee
Biocoral
biodegradable calcium phosphate
    cement
biodegradable fixation device
biodegradable implant
biodegradable synthetic polymer
Biodel
Biodex dynamometer
Biodex isokinetic exercise system
BioDyne bed
bioelectrical repair of delayed union or
    nonunion
biofeedback, EMG
Biofit acetabular prosthesis
Biofix absorbable fixation
Biofix biodegradable implant
Biofix Meniscus Arrow
Biofix system pin
BioFlex medical magnets
Bio-Form gloves
Biofreeze with ILEX pain-relieving
    gel

Bioglass (calcium salts, phosphorus,
    sodium salts, silicon)
Bio-Groove acetabular prosthesis
Bio-Groove Macrobond HA femoral
    prosthesis
BioHy high molecular weight sodium
Bio-Interference screwdriver
Bio-Interference tibial screw
Biojector
Biokinetics pedobarograph
Biolectron bone growth stimulator
biologic age
Biologically Quiet mini-screw suture
    anchor
Biologically Quiet screw
Biologically Quiet stapler
biological osteosynthesis
Biolox ball head for hip replacement
Biolox ceramic coating
biomechanical extensometry testing
biomechanical imbalance
biomechanical integrity of joint
biomechanical stress
biomechanics, gait
biomechanics of limb length
    discrepancy
Biomet acetabular cup
Biomet AGC knee prosthesis
Biomet button
Biomet hip prosthesis
Biomet instruments or devices
Biomet Ultra-Drive cement remover
Bio-Modular shoulder prosthesis
Bio-Moore endoprosthesis
Bionicare 1000 stimulator system
Bionix absorbable cannulated screw
Bio-Oss synthetic bone material
Biophase, ASTM designation of
Biophase implant metal
Bio-Phase suture anchor
BioPolyMeric graft
BioPro instruments or devices
bioprosthesis
biopsy (pl. biopsies)
    bone
    bone marrow
    brain

biopsy *(continued)*
   channel and core
   cone
   CT (computed tomography) guided
   Dunn
   forage core
   freehand CT guided
   Michele vertebral
   muscle
   nerve
   onion bulb changes on
   open brain
   point-in-space stereotactic
   punch
   stereotactic brain
   StereoGuide stereotactic needle
     core
   stereotactic aspiration
   stereotactic core needle (SCNB)
   sural nerve
   synovial
   targeted brain
   temporal artery
   transnasal
   Tru-Cut needle (TCNB)
   ultrasound-guided echo
   ultrasound-guided stereotactic
biopsy specimen
biopsy trephine
BioScrew absorbable interference
   screw
Biosensor biomechanical testing
   system
bioskills
Bio Skin braces and supports
Bio Skin DP wrist support
Bio Skin Q (quadrant) knee brace
BioSorbFX SR self-reinforced plate
   and screw
BioSorb suture
Biosound AU (Advanced Ultrasonography) system
Biospec Bruker spectroscopy
Biospec imaging system
BioStinger low profile fixation device
BioStop G bone cement restrictor
Biosyn synthetic monofilament suture

Biotex implant metal
Bio-Thesiometer
Biothotic foot orthosis
BIOWARE software
biparietal bossing
biparietal diameter (BPD)
biparietal hump wave
biparietal suture
biparietotemporal hypometabolism
bipartite patella
bipartite sesamoid
bipennate muscle
biphasic wave
biplanar angular correction
biplane roadmapping
biplaning of osteotomy
BIPLED (bilateral independent periodic
   lateralizing epileptiform discharge)
bipolar affective illness
bipolar EEG recording
bipolar hip replacement
bipolar montage
Bircher bone/cartilage clamp
Bircher-Ganske cartilage forceps
Bircher meniscotome
Bircher meniscus knife
Bircher-Weber technique
Bird & Cronin wrist brace
birdcage splint
birdlike facies
birefringent lipid crystals
birth fracture
birth paralysis
bisection, AP malleolar
Bis-Gd-mesoporphyrine (Bis-Gd-MP)
   imaging agent
Bishop-Black tendon tucker
Bishop chisel
Bishop clamp
Bishop-DeWitt tendon tucker
Bishop-Harmon forceps
bishop's nod
Bishop-Peter tendon tucker
bispinous diameter
bit (see *drill bit*)
BIT (Behavioral Inattention Test)
bitemporal hemianopsia

bite, arthropod
biter, Stille bone
bituberous diameter
bivalved cylinder cast
bivalved pancake plaster hand cast
BJ (biceps jerk)
Björnström algesimeter
BKA (below-knee amputation)
Black and Decker drill
Black-Broström staple technique
Blackburn traction
black dot heel
black eye
blackout, alcoholic
Black rasp
bladder
  atonic
  automatic bladder in spinal cord
    syndromes
  centrally uninhibited
  motor paralytic
  neurogenic
  refluxing spastic neurogenic
  sensory paralytic
  spastic neurogenic
  uninhibited
bladder knock in distance runners
blade (see also *knife*)
  arachnoid shape
  arthroscopic
  banana
  Bard-Parker
  Beaver cataract
  Beaver-DeBakey
  Beaver discission
  Beaver keratome
  Beckman-Adson laminectomy
  Beckman-Eaton laminectomy
  carotid
  cartilage shaver
  Caspar
  cataract
  chisel
  chondroplasty
  copper
  craniotome
  crescentic

blade *(continued)*
  Curdy
  deep
  discission
  double-edged razor
  drill
  Dyonics arthroscopic
  Feild (*not* Field)
  full curve
  Gigli saw
  Hebra
  Hibbs
  Incisor arthroscopic
  K
  keratome
  knife
  laminectomy
  malleable
  meniscal trimmer
  meniscectomy
  Meyerding laminectomy
  Meyerding-Scoville
  Micro-Aire
  mini-meniscus
  MVR
  notchplasty
  oscillating
  partial curve
  Paufique
  PowerCut drill
  razor
  retractor
  retrograde
  rosette
  Scoville
  sickle shape
  skin
  spinal retractor
  Superblade
  Swann-Morton surgical
  Synovator arthroscopic
  synovectomy
  Taylor spinal retractor
  Temperlite saw
  3 M Maxi Driver
  tracheal
  tri-radial resector

blade bone
bladeless scalpel handle
blade plate (see also *plate*)
   ASIF
   Giebel
   10-hole
Blair ankle fusion
Blair-Brown skin graft
Blair chisel
Blair elevator
Blair-Morris-Dunn-Hand arthrodesis
Blair palate hook
Blair talar body fusion
Blair tibiotalar arthrodesis
blanch
Blanchard traction device
blanching
Blatt capsulodesis
Blazina prosthesis
bleb, myelin
Bleck classification of metatarsus
   adductus
Bleck recession technique
Bledsoe fracture brace
bleed (noun) (see *hemorrhage*)
bleeders, persistent
blennorrhagic swelling
blepharospasm
Blessed Behavior Scale
Blessed Dementia Rating Scales
   (BDRS)
Blessed Information Memory
   Concentration (BIMC) Test
Blessed-Roth Dementia Scale (BRDS)
blind headache (preceded by visual
   phenomena)
blindness
   cortical
   hysterical
   ipsilateral monocular
   monocular
   total cortical
   transient cortical
   transient monocular (TMB)
   word
blind spot in visual field

blind spots (from multiple sclerosis)
blind spots, migrainous
blind tibial outflow tracts
blink artifact
blink reflex to corneal stimulation
blinking, reflex
Bliskunov implantable femoral distractor
blister
   bone
   fracture
blistering distal dactylitis (BDD)
Bloch equation
block (see also *anesthesia*)
   anesthetic
   axillary
   axillary anesthetic
   balsa wood filler
   Bier anesthetic
   bone
   Campbell posterior bone
   cutting
   digital nerve
   epidural steroid
   filler
   frequency-dependent conduction
   Gill posterior bone
   Howard bone
   Inclan posterior bone
   intercostal nerve (ICNB)
   interscalene (ISB)
   Kohs
   median nerve anesthetic
   Mikhail bone
   nerve
   patellar tendon bone
   peripheral nerve
   phenol nerve
   radial nerve anesthetic
   regional
   scalene
   sphenopalatine ganglion
   spinal (by cord compression)
   stellate sympathetic ganglion
   Styrofoam filler
   subarachnoid
   supraclavicular anesthetic

block *(continued)*
   sympathetic ganglion
   ulnar nerve anesthetic
   ventricular
blockade
   depolarization
   regional sympathetic
block allograft
block design test
blocker's exostosis
blocking, alpha
Block-Sulzberger syndrome
Blom-Singer tracheoesophageal fistula
blood (see *hemorrhage*)
   autologous
   intraparenchymal
   intraventricular
   new
   old
   subdural
blood behind tympanic membrane
blood-brain barrier (BBB)
blood deficiency (Chinese medicine term)
blood flow (see *flow*)
blood flow analyzer, automated cerebral
blood flow, supratentorial cerebral
blood gases, arterial (ABGs)
blood patch for post-LP headache
blood pool imaging
blood-spinal cord barrier
blood stagnation (Chinese medicine term)
blood supply, longitudinal
blood vessel tumor
bloody cerebrospinal fluid (CSF)
bloody tap
Bloomberg sign
Bloom-Raney modification of Smith-Robinson technique
Bloom splint
Bloom syndrome
blotting, Western
Blount disease
Blount displacement osteotomy
Blount fracture

Blount lamina spreader
Blount retractor
Blount-Schmidt Milwaukee brace
blow-in fracture
blowout fracture
blucher laced shoe
blue reticulated chondroid
blue spells (intermittent autonomic dysfunction)
blue toe syndrome
Blumenbach clivus
Blumensaat line
Blumenthal bone rongeur
Blumer shelf
Blundell Jones hip osteotomy
blunt carotid injury
blunt head trauma (BHT)
blunt spike and wave complex
blur, saccadic
blurring of disk margins
blurring of vision in multiple sclerosis
blush
   tumor
   vascular
B lymphocyte
BMC (bone mineral content)
BMD (Becker muscular dystrophy)
BMD (bone mineral density)
BMI (body mass indices)
BMIPP SPECT scan
BMP (bone marrow pressure)
BMP (bone morphogenic protein)
BMP-2 (recombinant human bone morphogenetic protein-2 [rhBMP-2])
BNMSE (Brief Neuropsychological Mental Status Examination)
BOA (British Orthopaedic Association)
board
   arm
   Euroglide MKII slide
   Flexisplint flexed arm
   Hadfield hand
   hand
   slide
   spine
   Spri Xercise

board *(continued)*
  Tegtmeier hand
  vertical foot
  wobble
  Yucca
BoarderAnkle brace
boathead
bobbing
  head
  ocular
Bobechko hook
Bobechko spreader
Bobrath technique
Bochdalek muscle
Bock knee prosthesis
Bock nerve
Bodenstab tourniquet
BODI knee extension orthosis
Bodnar retractor
body (pl. bodies)
  alignment of vertebral
  carotid
  coccygeal
  Cowdry-type intranuclear inclusion
  foreign (retained)
  geniculate
  Hirano
  height of vertebral
  inclusion
  intra-articular
  juxtarestiform
  Lafora
  Lewy
  loose
  Luys
  mamillary
  navicular
  Negri
  nemaline
  ossified
  osteochondritic loose
  pacchionian
  Pick
  pineal
  psammoma
  restiform
  retained foreign

body *(continued)*
  rhinencephalic mamillary
  rice joint
  scapular
  Schwann cell
  trapezoid
  Vater-Pacini
  Verocay
  vertebral
body dysmorphic disorder (BDD)
body dystonia
body exhaust system
body fat calipers
Body Gard neoprene support
Body Glove orthopedic products
body jacket cast
body jacket, halo
body mass index (BMI)
body mechanics
body of scapula
body of vertebra
Body Sticks massager
Boeck sarcoid
Boehler (Böhler)
Boehler angle
Boehler-Braun leg frame
Boehler-Braun splint
Boehler extension bow
Boehler guidelines
Boehler-Steinmann pin holder
boggy synovitis
boggy synovium
Bohlman cervical vertebrectomy
Bohlman triple-wire fusion
Boies forceps
Bollinger, posttraumatic apoplexy of
bolster
  abduction
  padded
  rubber
  Telfa
bolt (see also *pin*)
  Alvar condylar
  Barr
  bone lock
  Camino microventricular
  Camino ventricular

bolt *(continued)*
cannulated
condylar
Fenton
fixation
Harris
Holt
Moreira
slotted
subarachnoid
tibial
tibiofibular
trochanteric
Webb-Andreesen condylar
Webb stove
wire fixation
Zimmer tibia
bolt cutter
Boltzmann distribution
bolus, cotton
Bombelli-Mathys-Morscher hip
prosthesis
Bondek absorbable suture
bond, heat labile hydrogen
Bond splint
bone (see Table of Bones in
Appendix)
AAA
accessory
accessory navicular
acetabular
acromial
alar
Albers-Schönberg (Schoenberg)
marble
Albrecht
Allofix freeze-dried
alveolar supporting
ankle
anvil
arch of
areolae of
articular lamella of
articular tubercle of
astragalar
astragalocalcaneal
astragalocrural

bone *(continued)*
astragaloscaphoid
astragalotibial
astragalus
atlas
autogenous
axis
basal
basilar
basioccipital
basisphenoid
Bertin
Bethesda
bicortical iliac
blade
bleeding
Bonfiglio
breast
bregmatic
Breschet
brittle
bundle
calcaneal, calcaneus
Calcitite
calvarial
cancellated
cancellous
cannon
capitate
carpal
cartilage
cavalry
central
cervical vertebral
chalky
cheek
chevron (V-shaped)
clavicle
clavicula
coccygeal vertebral
coccyx
coffin
collar
compact
continuity of
convoluted
coronary

bone *(continued)*
cortical
cortical cancellous
costal
coxal
cranial
crest of iliac
cribriform
cubital, cubitus
cuboid
cuneiform
dead
dense
depression of nasal
dermal
destruction of
devitalized portion of
diastasis of cranial
digits of hand
distal phalanx
dorsal talonavicular
Durapatite
eburnated
elbow (olecranon process of ulna)
electrical stimulation of
endochondral
enetral
epactal
epihyal
epihyoid
epiphysis
epipteric (Flower)
episternal
erosion of epiphyseal
ethmoid
exercise
exoccipital
fabella
facial
femoral
femur
fibula
first cuneiform
flank
flat
Flower (epipteric)
fourth turbinated

bone *(continued)*
fracture running length of
fragile
fragment of
fragmental
freeze-dried
freshening of
frontal (skull)
Goethe (preinterparietal)
greater multangular (trapezium)
hallucal sesamoids
hamate
heel
heterotopic
highest turbinated
hip
hollow (pneumatic)
hooked (hamate)
humerus
hydroxyapatite
hyoid
hyperplastic
iliac
iliac cancellous
ilium
immature
incarial
incisive
incomplete fracture of
incus
infected
inferior nasal concha
inferior turbinate
inflammation of
innominate
intermaxillary
intermediate cuneiform
interparietal
Interpore
intracartilaginous
interchondral
intramembranous
irregular
ischial
ischium
ivory
ivorylike

bone *(continued)*
  jaw
  jugal (zygomatic)
  knuckle
  Krause
  lacrimal
  lamellar
  lamellated
  lateral cuneiform
  lenticular
  lentiform
  lesser multangular
  lingual
  long (pipe)
  long axis of
  lunate
  lunocapitate
  luxated
  malar
  malleolus
  malleus
  mandible
  mandibula
  marble
  mastoid
  mature
  maxilla, maxillary
  maxilloturbinal
  medial cuneiform
  medullary
  membrane of
  metacarpal
  metastasis to
  metatarsal
  middle cuneiform
  middle phalanx
  middle turbinate
  morcellized
  mortise of
  multangular
  nasal
  navicular
  necrotic
  neoplasm of
  newly woven
  Nicoll
  nonlamellar (woven)

bone *(continued)*
  nonlamellated
  occipital
  odontoid
  orbicular
  orbitosphenoidal
  osteonal
  osteopenic
  osteoporosis of
  osteoporotic
  pagetoid
  palatine
  parietal
  patella
  pedal
  pelvic
  perichondral (periosteal)
  perilesional
  periosteal
  periotic
  peroneal
  petrosal
  petrous temporal
  phalangeal
  ping-pong
  pipe (long)
  Pirie (dorsal talonavicular)
  pisiform
  pneumatic
  porous
  post-traumatic atrophy of
  postsphenoid
  preinterparietal (Goethe)
  premaxillary
  presphenoid
  primitive
  proliferation of
  prominence of
  proximal phalanx
  pterygoid
  pubic
  pyramidal (triquetral)
  quadrilateral
  radius
  raw
  refractured
  replacement (endochondral)

bone *(continued)*
- resurrection
- reticulated (woven)
- rib
- rider's
- Riolan
- rudimentary
- sacral vertebra
- sacrum
- scaphoid
- scapula
- sclerotic
- scroll
- second cuneiform
- semilunar
- septal
- sesamoid
- shank (cannon)
- shin
- short
- sieve
- sphenoid
- sphenoidal turbinated
- sphenoturbinal
- splint
- splintered
- spoke
- spongy
- squamo-occipital
- squamous-type
- stapes
- sternum
- stirrup
- subchondral
- subperiosteal new
- substitution
- superior turbinated
- supernumerary sesamoid
- supracollicular spike of cortical
- suprainterparietal
- supraoccipital
- suprapharyngeal
- suprasternal
- supreme turbinate
- sutural
- tail
- talus

bone *(continued)*
- tarsal
- temporal
- thick
- thigh
- thoracic vertebrae
- three-cornered
- tibia
- tongue (hyoid)
- trabecular
- trapezium
- trapezoid of Henle
- trapezoid of Lyser
- triangular wrist
- triquetral
- triquetrum
- tuberculosis of
- tubular
- tumor-bearing
- turbinate, turbinated
- tympanic
- tympanohyal
- ulna
- unciform
- Unilab Surgibone
- upper jaw
- vascular
- vesalian
- Vesalius
- vomer
- wedge
- weightbearing
- wing
- wormian
- woven
- wrist
- xiphoid
- yoke
- zygomatic

bone absorption
bone age according to Greulich and Pyle
bone age ratio
bone allograft
bone and limb growth velocity ratios
bone atrophy
bone bank
bone biopsy

bone block
bone-blocking procedure
bone borer
bone cement, Surgical Simplex P
    radiopaque
bone chip
bone conduction threshold
bone core
bone cutter, Horsley
bone-cutting forceps
bone debris
bone demineralization
bone densitometer, QDR-1500 or
    QDR-2000
bone density
bone density study
bone deposits, endochondral
bone destruction, localized
bone destructive process
bone dowel
bone dysplasia
bone ends
bone erosion
bone fixation surface coating
bone formation, subperiosteal new
bone-forming sarcoma
bone-forming tumor
Bonefos (disodium clodronate tetra-
    hydrate)
bone fracture (see *fracture*)
bone fragment
bone graft (see *graft*)
Bone Grafter instrument
bone graft incorporation
bone graft punch
bone graft ratcheting T-handle
bone graft substitute material, CHAG
    (coralline hydroxyapatite Goniopora)
bone growth stimulator, Orthofix
    Cervical-Stim
bone harvesting
bone-healing cascade
bone holder, three-paw
bone imaging
bone implant
bone infarct
bone infection

bone island
bone length study
bonelet
bone lock bolt
bone loss, periprosthetic
bone marrow
bone marrow edema pattern
bone marrow pressure (BMP)
bone marrow stimulating technique
bone mass, loss of
bone maturation
bonemeal tablet
bone metastases, occult
bone "mets" (slang for *metastases*)
bone mineral content (BMC)
bone mineral density (BMD)
bone mineralization
bone morphogenic protein (BMP)
bone mulch screw
bone or joint pathology
bone paste
bone-patellar tendon-bone (BPB) auto-
    graft
bone phase image
bone pinhole
Bone Plast bone replacement material
bone plate
bone plug
bone plug extractor
bone powder
bone rasp
bone remodeling
Bone Plast Healos Hedrocel
bone resorption
bone resurfacing
bone-retinaculum-bone autograft
bone rongeur
bone round needle
bone scaffold
bone scan (see also *imaging*)
    isotope
    triple phase
    TSPP rectilinear
bone scintigraphy
bone screw
bone sequestrum
bone shaft

bone shears, biarticular
bone sialoprotein
bone skid
bone sliver
bones of digits
BoneSource hydroxyapatite cement
bone spicule
bone spike
bone spreader
bone spur
bone stock
bone substance
bone surface lesion
bone survey
bone-tendon exposure
bone-tendon graft
bone ultrasound attenuation (BUA)
bone wax
bone wedge resection
bone window
bone wire guide
Bonfiglio bone graft
Bonfiglio bone replacement material
Bonfiglio modification of Phemister
   technique
Bonney hallux valgus outcome scale
Bonney-Kessel dorsiflexionary tilt-up
   osteotomy
bony (see also *bone*)
bony abnormality
bony ankylosis
bony apposition
bony architecture
bony avulsion
bony bridging
bony callus
bony callus formation
bony change
bony decompression
bony defect (acoustic window)
bony deformity
bony deposit
bony destruction
bony disruption
bony eburnation
bony encroachment
bony enlargement

bony erosion
bony excrescence
bony exostosis
bony fragment
bony fusion
bony healing
bony ingrowth
bony island
bony landmark
bony lysis
bony necrosis and destruction
bony osteophyte
bony overgrowth
bony pelvis
bony proliferation
bony prominence
bony protuberance
bony rarefaction
bony reabsorption
bony resorption
bony ridge
bony sclerosis
bony skeleton
bony spicule
bony spur
bony spurring
bony stability
bony structures, demineralized
bony tenderness
bony thorax
bony tufts of fingers
bony union, solid
Book Butler book-grip device
"boomerang" ovoid-shaped tendon
boomerang wrist support
boom, overhead
boot
   Bunny
   cast
   fluid barrier
   gelatin compression
   Gibney
   Hang Ups gravity
   Moon snowboard
   Multi Podus
   rocker
   Sorrel-type snowboard

boot *(continued)*
    Unna
    Unna paste
    Venodyne
    Wilke
Booth test
Booth wire osteotomy
boot-top fracture
boot wrap, Unna
Boplant Surgibone
Bora operation
Borchardt olive-shaped bur
Borden-Spencer-Herman osteotomy
border
    corticated
    crescentic
    interosseous
    sternal
borer
    bone
    cork
Borg-Warner orthopedic bed
Borggreve-Hall technique
Bornholm disease
boron assay
boron delivery agent
boron neutron capture therapy
Borrelia burgdorferi antibody
BOS (base of skull)
Bose nail fold excision
boss, bossing
bosselated, bosselation
bossing
Boston Children's Hospital grading
    system
Boston Classification System
Boston Diagnostic Aphasia Exami-
    nation
Boston LINAC (linear accelerator)
Boston Naming Test
Boston neurosurgical couch
Boston scoliosis brace
Boston soft body jacket
Boston thoracic brace
Boston thoracic splint
Bosworth femoroischial arthrodesis

Bosworth fracture
Bosworth lumbar spinal fusion
Bosworth procedure
Bosworth screw
Bosworth screwdriver
Bosworth shelf procedure
Botallo foramen
Botallo ligament
both-bone forearm fracture
Botox (botulinum A toxin)
bottle sign
botulinum A toxin (Botox)
botulinum toxin (BTX)
botulinum toxin type B (Neurobloc)
bottoming out of prosthetic component
Bouchard node
bouche de tapir (tapir's mouth)
Bouge needle
bouncing, ligamentous
bound, stimulus
boundary lubrication
boundary, tumor
Bourgery ligament
Bourneville disease
Bourneville-Pringle disease
boutonnière deformity of finger
boutonnière staging
Bovero muscle ("sucking muscle")
Bovie electrocautery apparatus
bovine bone substitute
    Boplant Surgibone
    Lubboc
bovine calf knee capsule
bovine collagen graft
bovine cough
bovine myelin (Myloral)
bovine spongiform encephalopathy
    ("mad cow disease") (BSE)
bow
    aiming
    Boehler extension
    extension
    finger extension
    Framer finger extension
    Kirschner wire traction
    posterior

bow *(continued)*
    Schwarz finger extension
    traction
    wire traction
bow boring rack
Bowden cable suspension system
bowed legs
bowel and bladder dysfunction
Bowen-Grover meniscotome
Bowers radial arthroplasty
bowing deformity
bowing of forearm
bowing of tendons in arthritis
bowl, cement mixing
Bowlby splint
bowleg (genu varum)
bowler's thumb
Bowman angle
Bowman muscle (ciliary muscle)
bowstringing
bowstring sign
bowstring splint
bowstring tear
bow-tie sign
box
    anatomic snuffbox
    fiducial
    high-toe
    ligamentous
    snuffbox
    toe
box and block test of arm disability
boxcar effect
boxer's elbow
boxer's fracture of metacarpal
boxer's nose
boxer's punch fracture
boxwood mallet
Boyd amputation
Boyd-Anderson biceps tendon repair
Boyd bone graft
Boyd-Bosworth procedure
Boyd formula
Boyd fracture
Boyd-Griffin classification
Boyd-McLeod procedure
Boyd-Sisk posterior capsulorrhaphy

Boyes brachioradialis transfer
Boyes-Goodfellow hook
Bozzini light conductor
BPA (burst-promoting activity)
BPA (p-boronophenylalanine)
BPA-fructose
BPB (bone-patellar ligament-bone)
    autologous graft
BPB (bone-patellar tendon-bone) graft
BPPV (benign paroxysmal positional
    vertigo)
BPS spinal angiographic catheter
BPTB (bone-patellar tendon-bone)
Bq (becquerel)
brace, bracing (see also *bar; orthosis;*
        splint; strap; support)
    Abbott
    accommodative
    AC Lite functional
    Active ankle
    Activity-Lite knee
    adjustable
    AFO
    Aircast Air-Stirrup
    Aircast Cryo/Cuff
    Aircast pneumatic air stirrup
    Aircast Swivel-Strap
    Aircast walking
    air DonJoy patellofemoral
    airplane
    Airprene Action knee
    Air-Stirrup Ankle Training Brace
    AMBI wrist
    AMX knee
    ankle
    Ankle Ligament Protector (ALP)
    APL Plus ankle
    Arizona ankle
    Arnold lumbar
    ASO ankle
    Atak knee
    athletic
    Axis ankle
    back
    Bike ankle
    Bio Skin ankle
    Bio Skin Q (quadrant) knee

brace *(continued)*
    bipivotal hinge knee
    Bird & Cronin wrist
    Bledsoe
    Blount-Schmidt Milwaukee
    BoarderAnkle
    Body Sport ankle
    Boehler
    boot
    Boston scoliosis
    Boston thoracic
    bowleg
    Brite-Life wrist
    cable twister
    caliper
    Callender derotational
    Cam Walker ankle (or leg)
    Can Am
    Carpal Lock CTS
    carpenter's
    CASH spinal
    cast
    Castaway leg
    Cast Boot polypropylene hip abduction brace
    Castiglia ankle
    Centec Formfit ankle
    cervical
    cervical collar
    chairback
    Charleston nighttime bending
    Charleston scoliosis
    Charnley
    Cheetah ankle
    CHH cervical
    Chopart
    CI (Combined Instabilities) functional knee
    Cinch Lock CTS wrist
    clam-shell
    Cole hyperextension
    contraflexion
    controlled-motion
    Cook walking
    cool CPB
    Cooper ankle
    cowhorn

brace *(continued)*
    CPB (Controlled Position Brace)
    CRS (Counter Rotation System)
    Cruiser hip abduction
    Cryo/Cuff
    CTi (or C.Ti.)
    CTi2 knee
    custom-fitted
    cutout patellar
    D.A.C.O.
    Dalco Astro ankle
    Darco back
    DarcoGel ankle
    Dennyson cervical
    derotational
    dial-lock
    DonJoy
    DonJoy Gold Point knee
    DonJoy Quadrant shoulder
    DonJoy Universal ankle
    donut support
    dorsiflexion stop
    drop-foot
    drop-lock knee
    Drytex RocketeSoc ankle
    Dura-Flex back
    dynamic abduction
    eclipse ankle
    economy ROM
    EconoSoc ankle
    elastic knee sleeve
    Elite knee
    English
    felt
    Flagg fiberglass knee
    FlexTech knee
    Florida cervical
    Florida J-24; J-35; J-45; J-55
    foot-ankle
    footdrop
    49er knee
    four-point cervical
    4-point SuperSport functional knee
    four-poster cervical
    Frazer wrist
    Futuro
    Friedman

brace *(continued)*
- functional
- gait lock splint (GLS)
- Galveston metacarpal
- Genutrain knee
- GLS (gait lock splint)
- Gold Point knee
- Goldthwait
- GII (Generation II) Unloader ADJ knee
- Generation II Unloader Select knee
- GoldPoint ACL functional knee
- GoldPoint hinged knee
- GoldPoint PCL functional knee
- Guilford cervical
- H buttress support patellofemoral
- Hennessy knee
- high-tide walking
- Hi-Top foot/ankle
- hinged knee
- horseshoe patellofemoral
- Hudson
- hyperextension
- I-Plus humeral
- Ilfield
- InCare ankle
- Industrial Work
- internal tibial torsion
- Intrepid functional knee
- ischial weightbearing
- IsoDyn knee
- J-55 postfusion
- Jewett
- Jewett-Benjamin cervical
- Jewett contraflexion
- Jewett hyperextension
- Jewett postfusion
- Juzo
- Kalassy ankle
- Key wrist
- Kicker Pavlik harness
- King cervical
- Klengall
- Klenzak spring
- knee
- knee cage
- knee MD

brace *(continued)*
- KneeRanger hinged knee
- Knight back
- Knight-Taylor thoracic
- knock-knee
- Korn Cage knee
- KS 5 ACL
- Kydex
- kyphosis
- lace-on
- lace-up ankle
- lacing
- lacing ankle
- lateral buttress support J patellofemoral
- Legend ACL functional knee
- Legend PCL functional knee
- Lerman cervical halo
- Lenox Hill derotational knee
- Liberty CMC thumb
- limb
- long arm
- long leg
- long leg hinged
- low tide walking
- LSU reciprocation-gait orthosis
- lumbar
- lumbosacral
- Lyman-Smith
- MacCausland lumbar
- Magnetic Support
- M-Brace knee
- McClintoch
- McCollough internal tibial torsion
- McDavid ankle
- MCL (medial collateral ligament)
- MC walker
- MD (Medical Design)
- Medipedic Multicentric knee
- Miami TLSO scoliosis
- Milwaukee scoliosis
- Minerva cervical
- Monarch knee
- Moon Boot
- Mooney
- Mueller ATF
- Mueller Lite ankle

brace *(continued)*
  Multi-Lig knee
  Multi-Lock knee
  Murphy
  neoprene RocketSoc
  Nevin ankle
  Newington
  Newport MC hip orthosis
  Nextep knee
  night
  no-stretch RocketSoc
  nonweightbearing
  OAsys knee
  offloading knee
  OPAL knee
  Oppenheim
  Orthotech Controller knee
  OS-5/Plus 2 knee
  osteoarthritis padded night sleeve
  out-of-cast ankle
  oyster-shell
  P.C. Williams
  Palumbo stabilizing knee
  pantaloon
  Parachutist ankle
  patellar stabilization
  patellar tendon-bearing (PTB)
  patellofemoral
  pelvic
  performer ultralight knee
  PFT (postop flexor tendon) traction
  Phelps
  Philadelphia Plastizote cervical
  piano-wire dorsiflexion
  Playmaker functional knee
  PlayTuf knee
  PMT halo system
  Pneu Knee air support
  postfusion
  Procare Ankle-Lock
  Pro-8 ankle
  Proline Stomatex shoulder
  PTS knee
  Quadrant shoulder
  range of motion
  reamer

brace *(continued)*
  Rhino Triangle polypropylene hip
    abduction
  rigid postoperative
  RocketSoc ankle
  Rolyan tibial fracture
  ROM walker
  Saltiel
  SAS II (shoulder arm system)
  SAWA shoulder
  Schanz
  SCOI shoulder
  scoliosis
  Scottish Rite
  Selectively Lockable knee
  Seton hip
  short arm
  short leg caliper (single or double
    bar)
  short leg double upright
  six-point knee
  SmartBrace
  SmartWrap elbow
  snap-lock
  SOMI (sternal occipital mandibular
    immobilizer)
  Sports
  Sports-Caster I and II knee
  Stardox wrist
  Stealth knee
  stirrup
  stop action
  Stromgren ankle
  Stubbs 4-way clavicle
  ST walker
  Sully shoulder stabilizer
  Sure Step ankle
  Swede-O Ankle Lok
  Swede-O-Universal
  Swivel-Strap
  Taylor-Knight
  Teufel
  Thermoskin
  Thomas
  thoracolumbosacral (TLSO)
  3-D fracture walker

brace *(continued)*
   TLSO (thoracolumbosacral orthosis)
   toe-drop
   Toronto
   total anatomical hinge knee
   Townsend knee
   Tracker knee
   Trinkle
   Tru-Fit
   Tuli's Cheetah ankle
   UBC (University of British
     Columbia)
   Ultrabrace
   unilateral calcaneal (UCB)
   unloader
   Varney acromioclavicular
   Victorian
   walking
   Warm Springs
   Watco
   weightbearing
   Wheaton Pavlik Harness
   Williams
   Wilmington scoliosis
   Yale
   Zimmer reamer
   Zinco CAM Walker
   Zinco Minerva cervical
   Zinco Multi-Lig
brace/corset, Hoke lumbar
bracelet test
brachial-basilar insufficiency
brachial muscle (brachialis)
brachial plexopathy
brachial plexus neuropathy
brachialgia
brachiocephalic lymph nodes
brachiocephalic muscle
brachiocephalic trunk of aorta
brachiocephalic vein
brachioradialis muscle
brachioradialis reflex
brachioradialis tendon
brachioradial muscle (brachioradialis)
brachium (pl. brachia)
brachium conjunctivum
brachium of colliculus

brachycephalic head shape
brachycephaly
brachydactyly
brachymetatarsia
brachytherapy
   ^{125}I or I-125
   ^{192}I or I-192
   interstitial
   remote afterloading (RAB)
   volumetric interstitial
bracing, abdominal
bracket, longitudinal epiphyseal
Brackett-Osgood-Putti-Abbott
   technique
Brackett osteotomy
Brackmann facial nerve monitor
Brackmann II EMG system
Braden flushing reservoir
Bradford fracture frame
Bradycor
Brady-Jewett technique
bradykinesia
bradykinin
Brady leg splint
bradyphemic
bradyphrenia
Bragard sign
Bragg ionization peak
Bragg peak, helium ion
Bragg peak photon beam therapy
Bragg peak radiosurgery
Brahms procedure
Braille TeleCaption system
brain
   architecture of
   base of
   edematous
   inflammation of
   metastasis to
   split
   unicameral
   Virchow-Robin spaces of
   water on the
   wet
brain abscess (see *abscess*)
brain activity
brain and spinal cord

brain anoxia
"brain attack"
brain biopsy
brain concussion
brain contusion
brain cyst
brain dead patient
brain death syndrome
brain deformation
brain-derived neurotrophic factor
(BDNF)
brain disease, organic (OBD)
brain dysfunction
   diffuse
   minimal
brain edema
brain electrical activity map
(or mapping) (BEAM)
brain function
brain-impaired person
brain ischemia
brain laceration
brain lesion
brain mantle
brain map (or mapping)
brain mass, posterior fossa
brain parenchyma, bleeding into
brain perfusion scintigraphy
brain perfusion SPECT
brain plasticity
brain proteins 130 and 131
brain scan (see *imaging*)
brain spatula
   Children's Hospital
   D'Errico
   Payton
   Scoville
brain spatula spoon, Ray
brain stem (or brainstem)
brain stem auditory evoked potential
(BAEP)
brain stem auditory evoked response
(BAER)
brain stem compression
brain stem damage (Widowitz sign)
brain stem demyelination

brain stem disease
brain stem displacement
brain stem dysfunction
brain stem encephalitis
brain stem evoked potential
brain stem function
brain stem gaze mechanism
brain stem glioma tumor
brain stem hemorrhage
brain stem herniation
brain stem infarct (or infarction)
brain stem lesion
brain stem, motor nuclei in the lower
brain stem pyramidal tract
brain stem reflex
brain stem reticular formation
brain stem signs
brain stem stimulation
brain stem stroke
brain stem symptom
brain stem syndrome
brain surface matching technique
brain swelling
brain syndrome, organic (OBS)
brain temperature monitoring
brain tests
   BAEP (brain stem auditory evoked
     potential)
   BAER (brain stem auditory evoked
     response)
   EP (evoked potential)
   ER (evoked response)
   MEP (multimodality evoked
     potential)
   noninvasive
   SEP (somatosensory evoked
     potential)
   SER (somatosensory evoked
     response)
   VEP (visual evoked potential)
   VER (visual evoked response)
brain-to-background ratio
brain tumor (see *tumor*)
brain tumor forceps
Brain variation, hip arthroplasty
brain wave activity

brain window
branch
  digital
  distal
  feeding
  motor
  phalangeal
  proper digital nerve
branched calculus
branch of artery
Brand forceps
Brand palmaris tendon stripper
Brand plantaris stripper
Brandt-Daroff vertigo exercises
Brand tendon-holding forceps
Brand tendon-passing forceps
Brand tendon transfer technique
Brand tendon-tunneling forceps
Brannock foot measuring device
Brannon-Wickstrom technique
Brant aluminum splint
Brantigan-Voshell procedure
brassiere, Jobst
Braune muscle
Braun shoulder tenotomy
Braun skin graft
Braun-Yasargil right-ankle clip
Bravais-jacksonian epilepsy
Bray score
BRDS (Behavior Rating for Dementia
  Scale)
bread-crumbling movement
breakable screw
breaker (see *cast breaker*)
break screw extractor
break screw trephine
breastbone
breast stroker's knee
breathholding spells
breathing
  apneustic
  ataxic
  diaphragmatic
  labored
Breck pin
bregma
bregmatic bone

bregmatic space
bregmatomastoid suture
Breg orthopedic products
Bremer AirFlo halo vest
Bremer Halo Crown cervical collar
Breschet bone
Breschet sinus
Brett arthrodesis
Brett-Campbell tibial osteotomy
Breuerton x-ray view of hand
BRFSS (Behavioral Risk Factor
  Surveillance System) questionnaire
bridegroom's palsy
bridge
  bony
  interthalamic
  osseous
  osteophytic
  skin
  suture
bridge autograft
Bridge hip system
bridge of meniscus
bridging, bony
bridging osteophytes
bridging syndesmophytes
bridging veins
bridle suture
Brief Cognitive Rating Scale (BCRS)
Brief Neuropsychological Mental
  Status Examination (BNMSE)
Brief Test of Attention
Brigham brain tumor forceps
Brigham prosthesis
Brighton electrical stimulation system
brim sign
Brink-Yesavage Geriatric Depression
  Scale
brisement therapy
Brissaud scoliosis
Brissaud syndrome
Bristow coracoid process transfer
Bristow-Helfet procedure
Bristow-May procedure
Bristow periosteal elevator
Bristow rasp
Bristow shoulder reconstruction

Brite-Life wrist brace
British Orthopaedic Association (BOA)
British test
Brittain ischiofemoral arthrodesis
brittle bone disease (osteogenesis
  imperfecta)
brittle bones failure
broach
  barbed
  Charnley femoral
  drilling
  femoral
  femoral prosthesis
  Harris
  intramedullary
  Mittlemeir
  root canal
  smooth
  Swanson intramedullary
  Zimmer femoral canal
broached
broadband ultrasound attenuation
broadest muscle of back
broad maxillary ridge
Brobdingnagian disorder of visual
  perception
Broberg score
Broca aphasia
Broca area
Broca convolution
Broca diagonal band
Broca gyrus
Broca motor speech area of brain
Broca region
Broca syndrome
Brockman-Nissen arthrodesis
Brockman procedure of foot
Broden view
Brodie abscess
Brodie bursa
Brodie disease
Brodie knee
Brodie ligament
Brodie metaphyseal abscess
Brodmann area
Brodmann cytoarchitectonic fields
broken bone

bromhidrosis
bronchoesophageal muscle
Bronstrom thermal procedure
Brooke Army Hospital tendon repair
  splint
Brooker classification of heterotopic
  ossification
Brooker femoral nail
Brooker-Wills nail
Brookes-Jones tendon transfer
Brooks atlantoaxial arthrodesis
Brooks cervical fusion operation
Brooks-Gallie cervical fusion
Brooks-Jenkins atlantoaxial fusion
Brooks-Seddon tendon transfer
Brook wire
Broomhead approach
broom-stick cast
Brophy periosteal elevator
Broström-Gordon arthrography
Broström-Gould ankle instability
  operation
Browlift bone bridge system
Brown-Adson tissue forceps
Brown-Cushing forceps
Brown knee joint reconstruction
Brown rasp
Brown-Roberts-Wells (BRW) head
  ring halo
Brown-Roberts-Wells stereotactic head
  frame
Brown-Séquard paralysis
Brown-Séquard syndrome
Brown tendon sheath syndrome
Brown tissue forceps
brown tumor (osteoclastoma)
Brown two-portal carpal tunnel release
Broxine (broxuridine) radiation sensi-
  tizer
Bruce protocol
Brucella arthritis
Brucella osteomyelitis
brucellosis, cerebral
Bruck disease
Brücke muscle (Crampton muscle)
Brudzinski sign
Brudzinski test

Bruel-Kjaer ultrasound scanner
Bruening chisel
Bruening-Citelli rongeur
Bruininks-Oseretsky Test of Motor
    Proficiency
bruisability
bruise, MRI bone
bruit (pl. bruits)
    aneurysmal
    asymptomatic carotid (ACB)
    carotid
    cranial
    high-pitched
    loud
    subclavian
Brunhilde strain (type I poliomyelitis
    virus)
Brunner modified incision
Brunner palmar incision
Brunner rib shears
Brunnstrom-Fugl-Meyer (BFM) arm
    impairment assessment
Bruno-Helfand physical therapy
Bruns ataxia
Bruns bone curet
Bruns gait apraxia
Bruns nystagmus
Bruns plaster shears
Bruns syndrome
Bruser skin incision (knee surgery)
brush
    delta
    Dr. Joseph's Original Footbrush
bruxism
BRW (Brown-Roberts-Wells) stereo-
    tactic head ring
BRW-Mayfield head adapter
Bryan-Morrey elbow approach
Bryant sign
Bryant traction
BSE (bovine spongiform encepha-
    lopathy)
BSSS (benign small sharp spike)
BTE (Baltimore Therapeutic
    Equipment)
BTE Assembly Tree
BTE Bolt Box

BTE Dynamic Lift
BTE Work Simulator
BTS (Back Therapy System),
    NordiCare
BTX (botulinum toxin)
BUA (bone ultrasound attenuation)
bubble ventriculography
bubbly bone lesion
buccal midazolam
buccal nerve
buccinator nerve (buccal nerve)
buccofacial apraxia
buccopharyngeal muscles
Buch-Gramcko gouge
Buchholz acetabular cup
Buchholz ankle prosthesis
Buchholz hip prosthesis
Buck bone curet
Buck cement restrictor insertor
Buck convoluted traction apparatus
Buck elevator
bucket, Denis Browne
bucket-handle tear
bucket-handle fracture
bucket-handle tear of knee meniscus
Buck-Gramcko pollicization
buckle fracture
buckle, wire-fixation
Buckley chisel
Buck neurological hammer
Buck percussion hammer
Buck periosteal elevator
Buck plug
Buck Redi-Traction apparatus
Buck restrictor
Buck splint
Buck traction stockinette
Bucky view
Bucky x-ray tray
Bucy cordotomy knife
Bucy-Frazier coagulation cannula
Bucy-Frazier suction cannula
Bucy laminectomy rongeur
Budde-Greenberg-Sugita stereotactic
    head frame
Budde halo retractor system
Budde retractor

buddy splint
buddy taping of fingers
Budge, ciliospinal center of
Budin-Chandler anteversion
  determination
Budin hammertoe splint
Budin toe splint
Buechel-Pappas total ankle prosthesis
Buerger Allen exercise
Buerger disease
Buerger symptom
BUE strength
buffalo hump
buffy coat of blood
Bugg-Boyd technique
buildup of seizure discharges
bulb
  baroreceptor in the carotid
  carotid
  high jugular (HJB)
  irrigation
  jugular
  olfactory
bulbar abnormality
bulbar form of ALS (amyotrophic
  lateral sclerosis)
bulbar intracerebral hemorrhage
bulbar-onset ALS (amyotrophic lateral
  sclerosis)
bulbar palsy
bulbar reflex
bulb dynamometer
bulbocavernous muscle
bulb of internal jugular vein
bulb of occipital horn of lateral ventricle
bulb of posterior horn of lateral
  ventricle
bulb syringe
bulbo cavernous reflex
bulbous stump
bulbus (n.), bulbous (adj.)
bulge of disk
bulging disk
bulk autograft
bulk, muscle
bulla (pl. bullae)
bulldog response (chewing reflex)

bull's eye deformity
bull's eye images
bull's eye map (mapping)
bull's eye polar map
bull's eye sign
bullet
  hollow-point
  stabilizing
  tri-point
bull-neck appearance
bullosa, recessive dystrophic
  epidermolysis
bullous
bump
  hip
  inion
  runner's
bumper fracture
Buncke technique
bundle
  Flechsig
  Gowers
  maculoneural
  neurovascular
  Schultze
bundle bone
bundle function
bundle-nailing method of treating bone
  shaft fracture
bundle of Vicq d'Azyr
Bunge amputation
bunion complex
bunionectomy
  Akin
  Austin
  Austin-Akin
  base wedge osteotomy
  chevron
  closing wedge osteotomy
  crescentic base wedge osteotomy
  DuVries-Mann modified
  Hauser
  Joplin
  juvenile
  Kelikian modified Z osteotomy
  Keller
  Kreuscher

bunionectomy *(continued)*
  Lapidus
  Mayo
  McBride
  Mitchell
  Mitchell osteotomy
  modified Mau
  modified McBride
  open base wedge osteotomy
  rotational scarf osteotomy
  scarf osteotomy
  Silver
  Stone
  supratubercular wedge osteotomy
  tailor's
  tricorrectional
  Wu
  Z
bunionette
  excision of
  tailor's
bunionette-hallux valgus-splay foot
  complex
bunion last
bunion, tailor's
bunk bed fracture
Bunker foot-piece
Bunnell active hand and finger splints
Bunnell anvil
Bunnell crisscross suture
Bunnell digital exertion measurer
Bunnell dissecting probe
Bunnell drill
Bunnell finger extension splint
Bunnell finger loop
Bunnell forwarding probe
Bunnell hand drill
Bunnell knuckle-bender splint
Bunnell-Littler test
Bunnell modification of Steindler
  flexorplasty
Bunnell posterior tibial tendon transfer
  operation
Bunnell reverse knuckle bender splint
Bunnell safety-pin splint
Bunnell splint
Bunnell stitch

Bunnell suture
Bunnell technique of pulley recon-
  struction
Bunnell tendon needle
Bunnell tendon passer
Bunnell tendon slippers
Bunnell tendon stripper
Bunnell tendon suturing technique
Bunnell tendon transfer
Bunnell wire pull-out suture
Bunny Boot orthopedic brace
Bunny Boot splint
bunting hitch
bur (also burr)
  Adson enlarging
  Adson perforating
  Adson-Rogers cranial
  air-driven
  Albee olive-shaped
  arthroplasty
  Bailey
  barrel
  bone
  Borchardt olive-shaped
  Burwell
  Caparosa
  carbide
  cone
  conical
  cranial
  craniotomy
  crosscut
  Cushing cranial
  cutting
  cylindrical
  D'Errico enlarging drill
  D'Errico perforating drill
  dental
  diamond
  Doyen cylindrical
  Doyen spherical
  Dyonics arthroplasty
  enlarging
  finish
  flame tip
  high speed
  high torque

bur *(continued)*
    Hudson bone
    Lindermann
    McKenzie enlarging
    Midas Rex craniotomy
    motorized
    MTM 2
    olive-shaped
    Ossotome
    pear
    perforating
    power
    right-angle
    Rosen
    Rotablator rotating
    round
    Shannon
    spherical
    Stille
    water-cooled power
    Zimmer rotary
Burch-Greenwood tendon tucker
burden of disease
Burford-Finochietto rib spreader
Burford rib spreader
Burgess below-knee amputation
bur hole
bur hole cover
    Accu-Flo polyethylene
    Accu-Flo silicone rubber
buried-knot suture
Burke Bariatric bed
Burkhalter modification of Stiles-
    Bunnell technique
burned-out tabes
Burner phenomenon
Burnham thumb and finger splint
burning-feet syndrome
Burns bench test
Burns ligament
Burns plate
Burow skin flap operation
burr (see *bur*)
bursa (pl. *bursae*)
    Achilles
    adventitious
    anserine

bursa *(continued)*
    bicipitoradial
    Brodie
    calcaneal
    Fleischmann
    flexor
    intermediate
    intermetatarsophalangeal
    ischiogluteal
    Luschka
    Monro
    "no-name, no-fame"
    olecranon
    omental
    plantar
    popliteal
    prepatellar
    radial
    retrocalcaneal
    subacromial
    subdeltoid
    suprapatellar
    trochanteric
    ulnar
bursal adhesion
    subacromial
    subdeltoid
bursal flap
bursal fluid
bursal inflammation
bursal sac
bursectomy
bursitis (pl. *bursitides*)
    anserine
    bicipital
    calcaneal
    chronic retrocalcaneal
    infracalcaneal
    intermetatarsophalangeal
    intertubercular
    ischiogluteal
    olecranon
    patellar
    pes anserine
    pigmented villonodular (PVB)
    postcalcaneal
    posterior calcaneal

bursitis *(continued)*
    prepatellar
    radiohumeral
    retrocalcaneal
    scapulothoracic
    septic
    subacromial
    subdeltoid
    Tornwaldt
    trochanteric
bursocentesis
bursography
bursolith
bursopathy
bursotomy
burst
    asynchronous
    bilaterally synchronous
    bisynchronous
    epileptogenic
    onset
    positive
    rhythmic theta
    spindle
    synchronous
    synchronous paroxysmal
    theta wave
    unilateral
burst compression fracture of atlas
burst fracture of spiral column
bursting fracture
bursting, synchronous paroxysmal
burst of activity
burst of delta activity
burst of muscle potentials
burst of REM
burst of slow wave activity
burst of theta activity
burst phase
burst-promoting activity (BPA)
burst suppression
bursts between hemispheres
bur surgery
Burton sign
Burwell bur
Burwell-Charnley classification of
    fracture reduction

bushing, guide
Busquet disease
Butler fifth toe operation
butterfly flap
butterfly fracture fragment
butterfly-type glioma
buttock sign
button
    Biomet
    Charnley suture
    collared
    Drummond
    Endobutton FM
    Hewson ligament
    padded
    patellar
    periosteal
    polyethylene
    Silastic
    subdural
    suture
    Wisconsin
buttonhole rupture
Button Spacer
button toe amputation
buttress
    Rotator Cuff Buttress (RCB)
    screws used to
buttressing
buttress plate
buzz bleeders
buzzing sensation
BVR (basal vein of Rosenthal)
B wave form on ICP monitor
B wave of cerebrospinal fluid (CSF)
BWM (Bad Wildungen Metz) spine
    system
bypass
    dorsal pedal
    EC-IC (extracranial-intracranial)
    extended tibial in situ
    femorodistal
    femoropopliteal
    intracranial arterial
    short vessel graft
    synthetic graft bypass to ankle

C, c

C.A. (chiropractic assistant)
cable
  braided
  chrome-cobalt
  Dall-Miles cerclage
  Dwyer scoliosis
  Gallie fusion-using
  Howmedica cerclage
  Songer spinal
  twister
cable and screws
cable bar
cable grip system
Cable-Ready cable grip system
cable telemetry EEG
cable twisters as treatment for internal
  tibial torsion
Cabot splint
Cacchione syndrome
cachexia, pituitary
cadaveric biomechanical study
CAD/CAM revision femoral implant
CAD (computer-assisted design)
  femoral prosthesis
cadence locomotion
cadence of gait
Cadenza panty girdle
Cadwell 5200A somatosensory evoked
  potential unit

café au lait spot
Caffey disease
Caffey hyperostosis
Caffinière prosthesis
cage
  antiprotrusio
  BAK fusion
  bony thoracic
  Interfix threaded spinal fusion
  Novus LC threaded interbody
    fusion
  Novus LT titanium threaded
    interbody fusion
  osseocartilaginous thoracic
  Ray TFC threaded fusion
  VariLift spinal
Cairns hemostatic forceps
caisson worker's disease (decompression
  sickness) (the bends)
Cajal interstitial nucleus
calamus scriptorius
Calandriello hip reduction
Calandruccio compression apparatus
Calandruccio fixation device
Calandruccio triangular compression
  fixation device
calcaneal apophysitis
calcaneal bone
calcaneal fracture, intra-articular

calcaneal gait
calcaneal inclination angle
calcaneal osteotomy
calcaneal pain
calcaneal pitch
calcaneal spur
calcaneal spur cookie orthosis
calcaneal spur pad in shoe
calcaneal stance position
calcanectomy
calcaneocavus (clubfoot)
    talipes calcaneus
    talipes cavus
calcaneoclavicular ligament
calcaneocuboid arthrodesis
calcaneocuboid joint
calcaneocuboid ligament
calcaneofibular ligament (CFL)
calcaneonavicular coalition
calcaneoplantar angle
calcaneotibial fusion
calcaneotibial ligament
calcaneovalgocavus
calcaneovalgus flatfoot
calcaneovalgus, pes
calcaneus (foot)
    excursion of the
    paralytic
    pes
    subtalar posterior displacement
    osteotomy of the
    sulcus
    talipes
    thalamic fracture of the
calcaneus altus
calcaneus deformity
calcar avis
calcareous deposits
calcarine cortex
calcarine fissure
calcarine sulcus
calcar pedis
calcar, pivot of
calcar planer
calcar reamer

calcification
    basal ganglia
    cerebral
    costal cartilage
    curvilinear
    dural
    dystrophic
    eggshell
    falx
    fine
    focal
    foci of
    free body
    glial tumor
    gyriform
    intervertebral cartilage
    intervertebral disk
    intracranial
    irregular
    laminated
    ligamentous
    linear
    medial collateral ligament
    metastatic
    periarticular
    periventricular
    pineal body
    pineal gland
    plaque
    plaquing
    sella turcica
    soft tissue
    tramline cortex
calcification of basal ganglia
calcification of dentate nuclei
calcification of falx
calcification of pineal gland
calcific spur
calcific tendinitis
calcific tendinopathy
calcified cartilage
calcified glial tumor
calcified pineal body, shift of
calcify
calcifying

Calcimar (calcitonin salmon)
calcinosis, tumoral
calcis, os
Calcitite bone replacement material
calcitonin salmon
calcium alginate dressing
calcium deposit
calcium deposition
calcium, elemental
calcium gout
calcium hydroxyapatite
calcium pyrophosphate dihydrate
   crystal deposition disease
calculus
   branched
   staghorn
Caldani ligament
Caldwell-Coleman flatfoot technique
Caldwell-Durham tendon transfer
Caldwell hanging cast
Caldwell occipitofrontal view
calf circumference
calf cramps
calf muscle pump (anatomical)
calf squeeze test
calibrated tensiometer
calibration
   biological
   square wave
calibration pulse
calibration voltage
California Verbal Learning Test
California viral encephalitis
Caligamed ankle orthosis
caliper orthosis
calipers
   blunt
   body fat
   Harpenden
   Mitutoyo digital
   Thomas walking
   Townley femur
   vernier
   weight-relieving
Callahan extension of cervical injury
Callahan fusion technique
Callander amputation

Callaway test
Calleja exercises
Callender derotation brace
callosal area
callosal commissurotomy
callosal dysgenesis
callosal formation
callosal gyrus
callosal lesion
callosal sulcus
callosities of the palms
callosity (pl. callosities), plantar
callosomarginal artery
callostomy, corpus
callosum, corpus
callous (adj.), callus (n.)
callus
   bony
   bridging
   central
   definitive
   ensheathing
   external
   florid
   fracture
   intermediate
   permanent
   provisional
callus distraction
callus formation
callus weld
Calman carotid clamp
Calnan-Nicolle metatarsophalangeal
   prosthesis
Calnan-Nicolle synthetic joint prosthesis
caloric requirements
   athletic
   basal
caloric stimulation test
calorics
   cold water
   ice water
calprotectin
calvarial bone
calvarial free bone graft
calvarium (pl. calvaria)
Caltagirone chisel

calvarial bone
calvarium (pl. calvaria)
Calvé-Perthes disease
Cam (controlled ankle motion)
Cam Walker ankle walker
Cam Walker leg brace
Cam Walker leg walker
cambium layer of periosteum
Cambridge test battery
camelback sign
camera
  DyoCam arthroscopic video
  Endius spinal endoscopic
  Enview
  gamma
  Olympus digital
Cameron-Haight periosteal elevator
CAM 5.2 antibody
Camino ICP monitor
Camino intracranial catheter
Camino microventricular bolt
Camino subdural transducer
Camino ventricular bolt
CAMIS (computer-assisted minimally
  invasive surgery)
Camitz opponensplasty
Camitz palmaris longus abductorplasty
Camitz tendon transfer
Campanacci grading system for giant
  cell tumor
Campbell-Akbarnia procedure
Campbell ankle operation
Campbell arthrodesis
Campbell-Goldthwait procedure
Campbell ligament
Campbell nerve root retractor
Campbell periosteal elevator
Campbell posterior bone block
Campbell questionnaire
Campbell root retractor
Campbell tibial osteotomy
Camp corset
Camp Diversity (arthritis program)
Camper chiasma
Camper ligament
camptocormia
camptodactyly

Camurati-Engelmann disease
Canadian Association of Physical
  Medicine and Rehabilitation
  (CAPMR)
Canadian crutches
Canadian Neurological Scale
Canadian Occupational Performance
  Measure
Canakis pin
canal
  Alcock
  arachnoid
  Bichat
  bony semicircular
  carotid
  carpal
  central spinal
  cerebrospinal
  cervical
  condylar
  condyloid
  craniopharyngeal
  Dorello
  Dupuytren
  ethmoidal
  facial nerve
  femoral medullary
  Guyon
  haversian
  Hunter
  hydrops
  iliac
  infraorbital
  intersacral
  intramedullary
  lumbar
  mandibular
  marrow
  mastoid
  maxillary
  medullary
  mental
  musculotubal
  narrowing of spinal
  neural
  orbital
  Richet tibioastragalocalcaneal

canal *(continued)*
  sacral
  semicircular
  spinal
  spinal cord
  supraorbital
  tarsal
  temporal
  tibial medullary
  tibioastragalocalcaneal of Richet
  tight spinal
  trefoil
  vertebral
  Volkmann
  zygomaticofacial
  zygomaticotemporal
canal decompression
Canale-Kelly classification of talar
  neck fracture
Canale osteotomy
canaliculus (pl. canaliculi), bone
canalithiasis of posterior semicircular
  canal
canalith repositioning procedure (CRP)
canal paresis
Can Am brace
Canavan disease
Canavan leukodystrophy
Canavan-van Bogaert-Bertrand disease
cancellated bone
cancellectomy
cancellous bone carrier
cancellous versus cortical bone
cancellus (noun)
candelabra, sylvian
Candella SPTL laser
Candida albicans fungus
Candida albicans meningitis
Candida albicans invasion of
  nervous system
candle-wax appearance of bone
cane
  quad
  single-point
  small-base quad
  tripod
C angle

canine muscle
cannula
  Acufex double-lumen
  Adson brain-exploring
  arthroscopic
  Bergstrom
  biopsy
  brain-exploring
  Bucy-Frazier suction
  coagulating suction
  biopsy
  Deroyal surgical
  Dohrmann-Rubin
  Dorsey ventricular
  Dyonics
  Elsberg brain
  Elsberg ventricular
  Endotrac
  Eriksson muscle biopsy
  exploring
  Fischer ventricular
  Ford Hospital ventricular
  Frazier brain-exploring
  Frazier ventricular
  Haynes brain
  high flow
  inflow
  intraventricular
  Kanavel brain-exploring
  large bore inflow
  large egress
  McCain TMJ
  microirrigating
  outflow
  Portnoy ventricular
  Ray ventricular
  Scott ventricular
  Sedan-Vallicioni
  slotted
  small egress
  suction
  suprapatellar
  ventricular
cannulated guided hip screw system
Cannulated Plus screw system
cantilever external fixator
Cantelli sign

CAOS (computer-assisted orthopedic surgery)
CAP (carotid Amytal procedure)
capability
    energy-absorbing
    load-transmitting
capacitor plate for electrical stimulation
Caparosa bur
Caparosa wire crimper
CAPE (Clifton Assessment Procedures for the Elderly)
CAPE (continuous anatomical passive exerciser)
Capello total hip replacement
Capener lateral rachitomy
Capener splint
capillary endothelium
capillary filling time
capillary hemangioma
capillary microscopy
CAPIT (Core Assessment Program for Intracerebral Transplantation)
capital epiphysis (CE) angle
capital extension
capital flexor
capital fragment
capital mover
capitate bone
capitate fracture
capitate, volar
capitellocondylar total elbow arthroplasty
capitellum
capitolunate joint
capitular epiphysis
capitulocondylar elbow arthroplasty
capitulum
Caplan syndrome
CAPMR (Canadian Association of Physical Medicine and Rehabilitation)
Capner gouge
Capner splint
CaPPi (calcium pyrophosphate)
CAPRIE (clopidogrel versus aspirin in patients at risk of ischemic events) clinical study

CAPS ArthroWand
Capset (calcium sulfate) bone graft barrier
capsular hemiplegia
capsular imbrication
capsular incision
capsular ligament rupture
capsular plane
capsular reefing
capsular release forceps
capsular shrinkage procedure
capsule
    articular
    cartilage
    dorsal
    external
    facet
    Gerota
    internal
    joint
    limb of anterior
    metatarsophalangeal (MTP) joint
    plantar
    posterolateral
    redundant
    rim of
    suprasellar
    talonavicular
    wrist
capsulectomy
    anterior
    circumferential
    silhouette
capsulitis
    adhesive (frozen shoulder)
    dorsal carpal
capsulocaudate infarction
capsulodesis
    Blatt
    dorsal
    intercarpal ligament
    Zancolli
capsulolabral complex
capsuloperiosteal envelope
capsuloplasty, Zancolli
capsuloputaminal infarction
capsuloputaminocaudate infarction

capsulorrhaphy (see *operation*)
   laser-assisted
   medial
   open staple
   pants-over-vest
   staple
   thermal
capsulotomy (see *operation*)
   Curtis PIP joint
   dorsal transverse
   dorsolateral and medial
   L-shaped
   medial V-Y
   stereotaxic anterior
   subtalar
   talonavicular
   transmetatarsal
   V
   vertical
capuloligamentous
caput medusae
carbamazepine (Tegretol)
carbide bur
carbohydrate loading
CarboJet lavage system
carbon dioxide intoxication
carbon fiber resurfacing
carbon monoxide intoxication
carbon tetrachloride poisoning
Carborundum grinding wheel
Carcassonne ligament
Carceau-Brahms ankle arthrodesis
carcinoma
   eccrine
   medullary
carcinomatosis
carcinomatous meningitis
Cardan screwdriver
cardiac ganglion, Wrisberg
cardiac muscle
cardiac nerve
   cervical
   inferior
   middle
   superior
   supreme
   thoracic

cardinal directions of gaze
cardinal ligament
cardioembolic stroke
Cardiopulmonary Paragon 8500 bed
cardiopulmonary splanchnic nerves
cardiovascular seizure
Caregiver Strain Index (CSI)
CareStair half-height step device
car hand controls
Carl P. Jones traction splint
C-arm portable x-ray unit
Carnation corn caps
carnosinemia
Carolina rocker
caroticocavernous fistula
caroticoclinoid ligament
caroticotympanic nerve
carotid angiography
carotid artery endarterectomy
carotid bruit
carotid bulb baroreceptor
carotid cavernous fistula occlusion
carotid collar
carotid distribution TIA (transient
   ischemic attack)
carotid endarterectomy
carotid occlusive disease
carotid plexus
carotid pulses
carotid sheath
carotid sinus nerve (Hering sinus)
carotid siphon
carotid stenosis
   bilateral
   unilateral
carpal arch
carpal articulation
carpal bone fracture
Carpal Care carpal tunnel exerciser
carpal coalition
carpal deviation
carpal dislocation
carpal height index
carpal instability
carpal interval ratio
Carpal Lock cock-up splint
Carpal Lock CTS brace

carpal-metacarpal (see *carpometa-carpal*)
carpal navicular
carpal row
carpal scaphoid bone
carpal stretch test
Carpal Trac traction device
carpal tunnel gloves
carpal tunnel release (CTR)
Carpal Tunnel Stretch exerciser
carpal tunnel syndrome (CTS)
carpal tunnel view
carpal tunnel wrist syndrome
carpectomy, proximal row (PRC)
Carpenter syndrome
carphology
carpometacarpal (CMC)
carpometacarpal articulation
carpometacarpal joint
carpometacarpal ligament
carpometacarpal synovitis
carpopedal spasm
carpophalangeal joint
carporadial articulation
carpus
Carrell fibular substitution technique
Carrell-Girard screw
carrier
    cancellous bone
    Cave-Rowe ligature
    double-headed stereotactic
    ligature
    Yasargil ligature
Carroll and Taber arthroplasty
Carroll arthrodesis
Carroll-Bennett retractor
Carroll bone-holding forceps
Carroll dressing forceps
Carroll hand retractor
Carroll-Legg periosteal elevator
Carroll periosteal elevator
Carroll skin hook
Carroll-Smith-Petersen osteotome
Carroll tendon-pulling forceps
Carroll tendon retriever
Carroll test
Carroll tissue forceps

Carrom orthopedic bed
Carr-Purcell-Meiboom-Gill sequence
carrying angle
car-sickness
Carter foam pillow
Carter immobilization cushion
Carter-Rowe shoulder score
Carter-Rowe view
Carter splint
Carter-Wilkinson criteria for hyper-mobility syndrome
Cartesian coordinate system for neurosurgery
Carticel ACI (autologous chondrocyte implantation)
cartilage
    accessory
    accessory nasal
    alar
    annular
    arthrodial
    articular
    arytenoid
    auditory
    auricular
    basilar
    branchial
    calcified
    cariniform
    ciliary
    circumferential
    conchal
    connecting
    corniculate
    costal
    cricoid
    cryopreserved
    cuneiform
    degenerated
    elastic
    ensiform
    epiglottic
    epiphyseal
    falciform
    fibrocartilage
    fibroelastic
    fibrous

cartilage *(continued)*
  floating
  free flap of
  hyaline
  hyaline articular
  interarticular
  nonossified tarsal navicular
  patellofemoral groove
  physeal
  pitted
  quadrangle
  quadrangular
  roughened
  scored
  semilunar
  shelling off of
  thinned
  thyroid
  tracheal
  triangular fibrocartilage
  triradial
  triradiate
  yellow
cartilage articulation
cartilage bone
cartilage degeneration, articular
cartilage joint
  primary
  secondary
cartilage joint space
cartilage joint symphysis
cartilage oligomeric matrix protein
  (COMP)
cartilage reduction, Aston
cartilage shaver blade
cartilage spaces
cartilaginous anlage
cartilaginous articulation of coccyx
  with sacrum
cartilaginous cap of phalangeal head
cartilaginous glenoid labrum
cartilaginous lesion
cartilaginous navicular
cartilaginous ring
cartwheel fracture

cascade
  diagnostic
  excitotoxic
CASH (cruciform anterior spinal
  hyperextension)
CASH spinal brace
CASH thoracolumbosacral orthosis
CASP (contoured anterior spinal plate)
Caspar alligator forceps
Caspar anterior cervical plating
  technique
Caspar blade
Caspar cervical plate
Caspar cervical screw
Caspar craniotome
Caspari arthroscopic portal
Caspari repair
Caspari suture punch
Caspari transglenoid multiple suture
  technique
casserian ligament
Casser ligament
Casser perforated muscle (casserian
  muscle)
cast, casting
  airplane
  arm cylinder
  banjo
  below-knee walking
  below-the-knee
  bent-knee
  Bermuda spica
  bivalved cylinder
  bivalved pancake plaster hand
  body
  body jacket
  Boston bivalve
  broom-stick
  Caldwell hanging
  corrective
  Cotrel scoliosis
  cotton
  Cotton-Loader position
  cylinder walking
  Dehne

cast *(continued)*
- double hip spica
- double spica
- EDF scoliosis
- Equilizer short leg walking
- extension body
- fiberglass
- figure 8 (figure of 8)
- flexion body
- Fractura Flex
- Frejka
- full thumb spica
- Gaiter
- gauntlet
- gel
- Gelocast
- groin-to-ankle
- Gypsona
- halo
- hanging arm
- Hexcelite
- hinged cylinder
- hip spica
- inhibitive
- intermediate
- Kite clubfoot
- Kite metatarsal
- light
- long arm (LAC)
- long arm thumb spica
- long leg (LLC)
- long leg bent-knee
- long leg walking (LLWC)
- long leg weightbearing (LLWBC)
- Lorenz
- Lovell clubfoot
- MaxCast
- Minerva
- Moe modified Cotrel
- Mooney
- negative impression
- Neufeld
- nonwalking
- O'Donoghue cotton
- one and one-half spica
- one-half spica
- Orfizip wrist

cast *(continued)*
- pantaloon
- patellar tendon-bearing (PTB)
- patellar tendon weightbearing
- petaling edges of
- Petrie spica
- plantar flexion
- plaster of Paris (POP)
- polyurethane
- Quengel
- Risser localizer scoliosis
- Risser turnbuckle
- Sarmiento short leg patellar tendon-bearing
- Sbarbaro spica
- Schmeisser spica
- scoliosis
- serial
- serial wedge
- short arm (SAC)
- short arm fiberglass
- short leg (SLC)
- short leg walking (SLWC)
- shoulder spica
- shroud
- slipper
- spica
- sugar tong
- three-finger spica
- 3M fiberglass
- thumb spica
- toe spica
- toe-to-groin
- toe-to-midthigh
- tone-inhibiting leg
- total contact
- turnbuckle
- univalve
- Unna boot
- Velpeau
- walking
- walking boot
- warm and form
- wedging
- well leg
- windowed

cast application

Castaway ankle walker
Castaway leg brace
Castaway leg walker
castbelt, Posey below-the-knee
cast bender
Cast Boot polypropylene hip abduction
    brace
cast brace
cast breaker
cast cover
    AquaShield orthopedic
    Dryspell
cast cushion
cast cutter
Cast Gard cast protector
Castiglia ankle brace
cast immobilization
Castle procedure
cast padding, cotton
Castroviejo bladebreaker knife
Castroviejo needle holder
cast sock
cast spreader
    Beeson
    Henning
    Hoffer-Daimler
cast syndrome
cast table
cast tape
    Scotchcast 2
    TufStuf II
cast walker
    rubber sole
    Sabel
cast wedge
cast with dorsal (or volar) toe plate
    extension
CAT-CAM conversion
CAT (CT) scan
CAT (CT) scan cradle
CAT (CT) scan gantry
catabolism
cataclysmic headache
Cataflam (diclofenac potassium)
CATCH (Chedoke-McMaster
    Attitudes Toward Children with
    Handicaps) scale

catalepsy
cataleptic attack
catamenial migraine
cataplexy
cataract knife
cataract knife Beaver blade
catastrophic reaction
catatonia
catecholamines
Categories, Functional Ambulation
    (FAC)
category
    bellringer
    ding
    Westin-Turco
Catera suture anchor
Cateye Ergociser
catgut suture
Cathcart Orthocentric hip prosthesis
"cath'd" or "cathed" (slang for
    catheterized)
catheter
    Abramson
    Accu-Flo ventricular
    angiographic
    BPS spinal angiographic
    Camino ICP (intracranial pressure)
    cardiac
    dummy seed
    epidural
    FasTracker
    Fogarty embolectomy
    Foltz
    guide
    guiding
    Heplock
    high pressure
    HNB angiographic
    hyperthermia
    ICP (intracranial pressure)
    indwelling
    interstitial
    intratumoral
    intraventricular
    ITC radiopaque balloon
    kinking of CNS
    low pressure

catheter *(continued)*
    medium pressure
    peritoneal
    Phoenix ventriculostomy
    Portnoy ventricular
    Pudenz peritoneal
    Raimondi peritoneal
    Raimondi spring
    Raimondi ventricular
    Scott silicone ventricular
    Seletz nonrigid ventricular
    Shaw
    Simpson
    SpineCATH intradiscal
    subarachnoid
    subcutaneous ventricular reservoir
    subdural drainage
    toposcopic
    Tracker-10
    Tracker-18
    UltraLite flow-directed micro-
        catheter
    ventricular
catheter angiography
catheterization, superselective
catheter probe, polarographic $P(ti)O_2$
Catlin amputating knife
Catterall classification
caudad
cauda equina compression syndrome
caudal-cranial angulation
caudal ligament
caudally
caudalward
caudate nucleus
caudothalamic groove
cauliflower ear
causalgia
    major
    minor
    trauma-related
causalgic pain
cautery
    Aesculap bipolar
    BICAP
    bipolar

cautery *(continued)*
    Bovie
    Concept handheld
    Mira
    monopolar
    unipolar
cautery probe, McCain TMJ
Cavanaugh-Rogers classification of
    footprints
cave, Meckel
Cave-Rowe ligature carrier
Cave-Rowe shoulder dislocation
    technique
cavernoma
cavernous hemangioma
cavernous malformation
cavernous sinus lesion
cavernous sinus syndrome
cavernous sinus thrombosis
Cavin osteotome
cavitas medullaris
cavitation
Cavitron dissector
Cavitron ultrasonic aspirator (CUSA)
cavity
    absorption
    cotyloid
    epidural
    glenoid
    joint
    marrow
    Meckel
    popliteal
    saclike
    sigmoid cavity of radius
    sigmoid cavity of ulna
    subarachnoid
    subdural
    synovial
    syringomyelic
    syrinx
    trigeminal
cavity of septum pellucidum
cavovalgus
    pes
    talipes

cavovarus
  pes
  talipes
cavovarus foot deformity
cavus
  anterior
  forefoot
  global
  local
  midfoot
  pes
  posterior
  posttraumatic
  talipes
cavus foot deformity
CAWO (closing abductor wedge
  osteotomy)
C-bar web-spacer
CBF (cerebral blood flow)
CBI (convergent beam irradiation)
CBI stereotactic head holder
CBI stereotactic ring
CBS (chronic brain syndrome)
CBT (corticobulbar tract)
CBV (cerebral blood volume)
CBV/CBF ratio
CBVH (Commission for the Blind and
  Visually Handicapped)
CBWO (closed base wedge osteotomy)
CCA (common carotid artery)
CCD (central collodiaphyseal) angle
CCD 1042 (ganaxolone)
CCF (carotid cavernous fistula)
CCMI (custom contour measuring
  instrument), Mark II
CCS (Children's Coma Score)
CCTA (coronal computed tomographic
  arthrography)
CCTV/EEG (closed circuit TV and
  EEG recording)
CD (color Doppler)
CDC (Centers for Disease Control and
  Prevention)
CD (Cotrel-Dubousset) instruments
CD fixation device
CDH (congenital dislocation [or
  dysplasia] of hip)

CD3 (T cell)
CD4 (T cell)
CD43 (leukosialin)
CD68 (macrophage)
CD8 (T cell)
CDI (Cotrel-Dubousset instrumenta-
  tion)
CDP (computerized dynamic posturog-
  raphy)
CE (capital epiphysis) angle of Wiberg
C-E (center-edge) angle
CEA (carcinoembryonic antigen)
CEA (carotid endarterectomy)
Cebotome bone cement drill
Cebotome osteotome
cecocentral scotoma (central cecal)
CECS (chronic exertional compart-
  ment syndrome)
CECT (contrast enhancement of com-
  puted tomographic) head and body
  imaging
Cedell fracture of posterior process of
  the talus
Cedell-Magnusson classification of
  arthritis on x-ray
C-EEG (computerized electroencephalogram)
Ceegraph 128 electroencephalogram
  system
cefotaxime (Claforan)
ceftriaxone (Rocephin)
ceiling-mounted robotic platform
C electrode (central) (C_1-C_6)
Celebrex (celecoxib)
Celestone Soluspan (betamethasone)
celiac nerves
cell (pl. cells)
  agranular chromophobe cell in
    adenohypophysis
  anterior horn
  Antoni A and B
  apoptotic
  B
  Betz
  Betz giant pyramidal
  clonal tumor
  cortical pyramidal

cell *(continued)*
 degeneration of ganglion
 embryonic stem
 ependymal
 excitable
 fibronectin-positive mesenchymal
 foam
 germ
 giant pyramidal Betz
 gitter (microglia) *(not* glitter)
 glial
 globose
 granular cerebellar
 granular chromophil
 hemosiderin-laden
 injured
 intermediolateral horn
 lactotrophic
 motor horn
 multipotential
 myxomatous
 nests of tumor
 neural progenitor
 neural stem
 nigral
 null
 oligodendrocyte
 oligodendroglial
 osteoclastic giant
 osteogenic
 peripheral blood mononuclear
 plasma
 primitive stem
 progenitor skin
 proliferation of
 Purkinje cerebellar
 Renshaw
 Sayk preparation of CSF
 Schwann
 shrinkage of ganglion
 specialized
 spindle
 stromal
 synovial lining
 thalamic pacemaker
CellCept (mycophenolate, mofetil)
cell death, programmed

cell leukodystrophy, globoid
cell-mediated reaction
cell sarcoma, reticulum
cell saver
cellular fibronectin
cellular neurothekeoma
cellulitis
CEM (central extensor mechanism)
cement (see also *adhesive*)
 acrylic bone
 biodegradable calcium phosphate
 bone
 BoneSource hydroxyapatite
 centrifugation of
 CMW bone
 DePuy 1 bone
 Endurance bone
 hydroxyapatite (HA) bone
 Implast bone
 Ketac
 low viscosity
 methylmethacrylate
 Orthocomp
 orthopedic
 Orthoset radiopaque bone
 Osteobond
 Palacos bone
 PMMA bone
 polymerized
 pressurization of
 pressurized
 Protoplast
 radiopaque bone
 removal of excess
 residual
 Simplex
 SRS injectable
 surface
 Surgical Simplex P radiopaque
 Zimmer low viscosity
cementation
cement compactor, acetabular
Cement Eater, Anspach
cemented total hip arthroplasty
cement gun
cementifying fibroma
cementless prosthesis

Cementless Sportorno (CLS) hip arthroplasty stem
cementless surface replacement arthroplasty
cementless technique
cementless total hip replacement
cement line
cement mantle
cementome, Anspach
cemento-ossifying fibroma
cementophyte
cement pump
cement removal
cement restrictor inserter
cement spacer inserter
cement spatula
cement technique
Cemex system
Centec Formfit ankle brace
center
   ciliospinal center of Budge
   cortical
   diaphyseal
   emetic
   growth
   hearing
   motor
   ossification
   pontine lateral gaze
   speech
   visual
   vomiting
center-edge (C-E) angle
center of gravity (CG)
center of joint
center of mass momentum
center of pressure pattern integral
Centers for Disease Control and Prevention (CDC)
centimeter (cm)
central bone (wrist)
central cervical cord syndrome
central collodiaphyseal angle (CCD)
central core disease
central diencephalic herniation syndrome
Central European encephalitis

central facial paresis
central gray matter
Centralign Precoat hip prosthesis
centralizer device
central language deficit
central lesion
central motor pathways disease
central nervous system (CNS)
central nervous system hemorrhage
central nervous system infection
central nervous system toxoplasmosis
central neurogenic hyperventilation
central neuronal hyperexcitability
central nystagmus
central origin weakness
central quadriceps tendon (CQT)
central rays
central recess
central retinal vein thrombosis
central scotoma (pl. scotomata)
central sensory deficit
central sensory loss
central slip of tendon
central stenosis
central sulcus
central tegmental tract
central thrombosis
central venous thrombosis
central visual field
centralization procedure
centrally caused nystagmus
centrally uninhibited bladder
centrencephalic epilepsy
centrencephalic seizure
centrifugal nerve (efferent)
centrifugation of cement
centripetal nerve (afferent)
centripetal wrapping, compressive
centroid
centronuclear myopathy
centroparietal head region
centrotemporal discharges
centrotemporal epilepsy
centrum retractor
cephalad
cephalalgia (cephalgia)
cephalalgic (or cephalgic) attack

cephalgia (cephalalgia)
 cervical
 histamine
cephalgic attack
cephalgic seizure
cephalhematocele
cephalhematoma
cephalic angulation
cephalic index
cephalofacial proportionality
cephalohematocele
cephalohematoma, parietal
cephalometer, Bertillon
cephalometric analysis
cephalometrics
cephalometry
cephalopelvic disproportion (CPD)
cephalopelvimetry
cephalostat
ceramic-on-ceramic bearing surfaces
Ceramion prosthesis
ceratocricoid ligament
CerAxon (citicoline sodium)
cerclage
 cable
 Dall-Miles cable
 Howmedica
cerclage suture
cerclaged component
cerebellar agenesis
cerebellar ataxia
cerebellar cognitive affective syndrome
cerebellar cortical atrophy
cerebellar degeneration
cerebellar dysarthria
cerebellar extension, Hudson
cerebellar fibers
cerebellar fits (seizure)
cerebellar flocculus
cerebellar hemisphere
cerebellar hemorrhage
cerebellar herniation
cerebellar infarction
cerebellar malaria
cerebellar mass
cerebellar notch
cerebellar nystagmus

cerebellar pathway
cerebellar peduncle
cerebellar retractor
cerebellar signs
cerebellar syndrome
cerebellar tonsillar herniation
cerebellar tract
cerebellar tremor
cerebellar vermis
cerebellitis
cerebellopontile (or cerebellopontine)
 angle (CP angle) tumor
cerebellum
 basal ganglia of
 dentate nucleus of
 midline
 petrosal
 Purkinje cells of
 stimulation of the
 unilateral lesion of the
cerebellum tumor
cerebral abscess
cerebral ammonia toxicity
cerebral amoebiasis (amebiasis)
cerebral aneurysm
cerebral angiography
cerebral anoxia
cerebral apotentiality
cerebral aqueduct
cerebral arteries
cerebral arteriography
cerebral arteriovenous fistula
cerebral *Aspergillus* abscess
cerebral atrophy
cerebral autoregulation
cerebral blood flow (CBF)
cerebral blood volume (CBV)
cerebral blood volume/cerebral blood
 flow (CBV:CSF)) ratio
cerebral brain death
cerebral brain flow
cerebral brucellosis
cerebral commissure
cerebral contusion (bruise)
cerebral cortex
cerebral CT venography
cerebral death

cerebral disorder
cerebral dominance
cerebral dysfunction
cerebral dysrhythmia
cerebral edema
cerebral fat embolism
cerebral functions:
    memory
    mood
    orientation
    thinking capacity
cerebral gigantism
cerebral glucose metabolism
cerebral hemidecortication
cerebral hemiplegia
cerebral hemisphere
cerebral herniation
cerebral hypotension
cerebral infarct (infarction)
cerebral infundibulum
cerebral ischemia
cerebral ischemic event
cerebral lesion
cerebral lipidosis
cerebral malaria, *Plasmodium
    falciparum*
cerebral mantle
cerebral metabolic rate of oxygen
    consumption ($CRMO_2$)
cerebral metabolism
cerebral nerves
cerebral nocardiosis
cerebral operculum
cerebral palsy (CP)
    ataxic
    athetoid
    choreoathetoid
    dyskinetic
    dystonic
    extrapyramidal
    flaccid
    hypotonic
    pyramidal
    spastic
cerebral paralysis
cerebral paraplegia
cerebral parenchyma

cerebral peduncle
cerebral perfusion pressure
cerebral perfusion SPECT scan
cerebral phaeohyphomycosis
cerebral poliodystrophy
cerebral potentials
cerebral revascularization
cerebral salt wasting
cerebral signs
cerebral SPECT
cerebral steal syndrome
cerebral substrate
cerebral teratocarcinoma
cerebral thrombophlebitis
cerebral trauma
cerebral vasculopathy
cerebral vasospasm
cerebral Whipple disease
cerebral white matter
cerebri (pl. of cerebrum)
    commotio
    contusio
    falx
    familial gliomatosis
    gliomatosis
    pseudotumor
cerebriform
cerebritis
    bacterial
    saturnine
Cerebrograph
cerebrohepatorenal syndrome
cerebromacular degeneration (CMD)
cerebromeningeal intracerebral hemor-
    rhage
cerebropontocerebellar pathway
cerebroside lipidosis
cerebroside reticulocytosis
cerebroside sulfatase
cerebrospinal fluid (CSF)
    A wave of
    AFB (acid-fast bacilli) in
    anti-Borrelia antibody in
    antibody to herpes simplex in
    antibody to St. Louis encephalitis in
    antigen to *H. influenzae* in
    antigen to meningococci in

cerebrospinal fluid *(continued)*
    antigen to Mycobacterium in
    antigen to pneumococci in
    B wave of
    blood in
    bloody
    C wave of
    C&S (culture and sensitivity)
    cellular pleocytosis in
    centrifuged sediment of
    clear
    cloudy
    coccidioidal complement fixation of
    counterimmune electrophoresis of
    cryptococcal antigen in
    cryptococcal antigen titer of
    CSF-serum HSV antibody ratio in
    culture and sensitivity (C&S) of
    cytology of
    dammed-up
    decreased absorption of
    elevated protein in
    ELISA test on
    erythrocytes in
    flow of
    fungal culture of
    fungal infection of
    fungal screen
    gamma globulin in
    glucose level of
    Gram stain of
    grossly bloody
    H. influenzae antigen in
    hemorrhagic
    herpes simplex antibody titer in
    herpes virus-specific glycoprotein in
    HSV antibody titer in
    hypoglycorrhachia of
    IgG:albumin index of
    IgG:albumin ratio of
    IgG index
    immunoglobulin index of
    increased production of
    increased volume of
    India ink examination of
    India ink stain of
    lactate level of

cerebrospinal fluid *(continued)*
    lactic acid in
    lactic dehydrogenase (LDH) of
    latex particle agglutination test on
    LDH of
    leak of
    leukocytes in
    limulus lysate assay of
    Lyme antibody test on
    Lyme titer of
    lymphocyte:PMN ratio of
    lymphocytes in
    lymphocytic pleocytosis-depressed
        glucose in
    lymphocytosis of
    manometer to measure opening
        pressure of
    meningococci antigen in
    monocytes in
    mononuclear pleocytosis of
    mycobacterial antigen in
    myelin basic protein of
    neutrophils in
    obstruction of flow of
    oligoclonal bands in
    opening pressure of
    plateau wave of
    pleocytosis of
    pneumococci antigen in
    polymorphonuclear cells in
    pressure of
    production of
    protein electrophoresis of
    protein level of
    PRP capsule of *H. influenzae* in
    purulent
    radioimmunoassay of
    RBCs in
    reabsorption of
    red cells in
    routine studies on
    Sayk preparation of
    serologic testing of
    shunting of
    Sicard test on
    spun-down specimen of
    St. Louis encephalitis antibody in

cerebrospinal fluid *(continued)*
  subgaleal
  sugar in
  total protein in
  Traube-Hering-Mayer waves of
  Tyndall effect seen in
  VDRL (Venereal Disease Research
    Laboratory) of
  volume of
  WBCs in
  white cell count of
  white cells in
  xanthochromia of
cerebrospinal fluid fistula
cerebrospinal fluid flow measurement
cerebrospinal fluid leak study
cerebrospinal fluid pathway
cerebrospinal fluid xanthochromia
cerebrotendinous xanthomatosis
cerebrovascular accident (CVA) (stroke)
cerebrovascular circulation
cerebrovascular disease
cerebrovascular insufficiency
cerebrovascular occlusive disease
cerebrum (pl. cerebri)
  central cavity of
  cortex of
  first ventricle of
  great vein of
  lateral ventricle of
  second ventricle of
  third ventricle of
Cerebyx (fosphenytoin)
Ceresine (CPC-211)
Ceretec (technetium 99m)
certified disability examiner
certified hand therapist
Cerva Crane halter
cervical acceleration/deceleration
  syndrome (whiplash)
cervical AOA halo traction
cervical artery dissection
cervical arthritis
cervical brace (see *brace*)
cervical cephalgia

cervical collar or support
  AOA halo traction
  Bremer Halo Crown
  Georgiade visor
  Houston Halo traction
  Mayo rigid
  Miami Acute
  Miami J
  Philadelphia
  Plastizote
  PMT halo system
cervical cord lesion
cervical corpectomy
cervical CT (computed tomography)
cervical disk disease
cervical dorsal outlet syndrome
cervical extension
cervical fracture
cervical halter traction
cervical iliocostal muscle
cervical interspinal muscles
cervical intervertebral foraminal MR
  phlebography (CMRP)
cervical juxtafacet cyst
cervical ligament
cervical mover ligament
cervical movers
cervical muscles or musculature
cervical myelogram
cervical myelopathy
cervical nerve root
cervical nerves
cervical orthosis (see *orthosis*)
cervical outlet
cervical pillow
cervical radiculitis
cervical range of motion (CROM)
cervical retractor
cervical rib
cervical rongeur
cervical rotator muscles
cervical spine (C1-C7 vertebrae)
cervical spine, dens view of
cervical spine injury
cervical splanchnic nerves (augmentor
  nerves)

cervical spondylosis of the spinal cord
cervical spondylosis, washboard effect
    on myelography in
cervical spondylotic myelopathy
    (CMS)
cervical support
cervical sympathectomy
cervical tension myositis (CTM)
cervical traction
    AOA halo
    Bremer halo
    Georgiade visor
    Houston halo
    Miami acute collar
    Miami J collar
    Philadelphia collar
cervical triangle
cervical vertebral instruments, Xiu
cervical vertigo
cervical wire passer, Batzdorf
cervical wire twister, Batzdorf
cervicocerebral
cervicography
cervico-occipital fusion
cervico-ocular reflex
cervicomedullary junction
cervicothoracic level
cervicothoracic region
cervicothoracolumbosacral orthosis
cervicotrochanter
cervicotrochanteric fracture
CES (cauda equina syndrome)
Céstan-Chenais syndrome
CFL (calcaneofibular ligament)
C4 complement component
CFQ (Cognitive Failures Question-
    naire)
CFQ-for-others assessment
CFS (contoured femoral stem) hip
    prosthesis
CFU (colony-forming unit)
CG (center of gravity)
CGIC (Clinical Global Impression
    of Change)
Chaddock reflex
Chaddock sign

CHAG (coralline hydroxyapatite
    Goniopora) bone graft substitute
    material
Chagas disease
chain of electrodes
chain, sympathetic
chains, wheelchair
chair
    ergonomically correct
    Gardner
chairback brace
chairback orthosis
chalk (or chalky) bones
chalky gout
challenge
    hypoglycemic
    vasodilatory
chamber, Pudenz flushing
Chamberlain line
chamfer cut
chamfer reamer
Champ CTS cold therapy wrap
Champ elastic bandage
champagne-bottle legs in Charcot-
    Marie-Tooth disease
Champion Trauma Score (CTS)
Championnière bone drill
Chance vertebral fracture
Chandler arthrodesis
Chandler bone elevator
Chandler felt collar splint
Chandler procedure
Chandler retractor
Chandler spinal perforating forceps
Chandler tendon transfer
change (pl. changes)
    abulic mental
    age-related EEG
    arthritic talonavicular
    behavioral
    binocular acuity
    chondromalacial
    cystic
    dystrophic
    Fairbanks
    focal degenerative

change *(continued)*
  histological tendon
  mental
  monocular acuity
  osteoarthritic
  paroxysmal
  pre-slip
  pupillary
  spondylitic
  subchondral
  Tapper-Hoover
  trophic
  trophic skin
  ultrastructural
  vasomotor
change in mentation
channel (pl. channels)
  EEG recording
  enlarged vascular
  leptomeningeal venous
Chapchal knee arthrodesis
Chaput tubercle
characteristics, stride
Charcot arthropathy
Charcot-Bouchard intracerebral
  aneurysm
Charcot-Bouchard microaneurysm
Charcot chondroma
Charcot cirrhosis
Charcot foot, diabetic
Charcot gait
Charcot joint
Charcot-Marie-Tooth (CMT) disease
  champagne-bottle legs in
  stork's legs in
Charcot-Marie-Tooth syndrome
Charcot restraint orthotic walker
  (CROW)
Charcot spine
Charcot triad
Charest head frame
Charles Bonnet syndrome
Charleston nighttime bending brace
Charleston scoliosis brace
charley horse
Charlie Chaplin-type gait
Charlson Comorbidity Score

Charnley ankle arthrodesis
Charnley bone curet
Charnley brace
Charnley centering ring
Charnley compression apparatus
Charnley compression clamp
Charnley deepening reamer
Charnley drill
Charnley expanding reamer
Charnley external fixation apparatus
Charnley femoral broach
Charnley femoral condyle drill
Charnley femoral condyle radius
  gauge
Charnley femoral inlay aligner
Charnley femoral inlay guillotine
Charnley femoral prosthesis neck
  punch
Charnley femoral prosthesis pusher
Charnley foam suture pad
Charnley-Hastings prosthesis
Charnley hip arthroplasty
Charnley hip replacement
Charnley horizontal retractor
Charnley-Houston shoulder arthrodesis
Charnley Howorth Exflow system
Charnley initial incision retractor
Charnley introducer
Charnley knee retractor
Charnley-Merle D'Aubigné disability
  grading system
Charnley-Mueller hip prosthesis
Charnley pain and function grading
  scale
Charnley pin retractor
Charnley reamer
Charnley socket gauge
Charnley suction drain
Charnley suture button
Charnley taper reamer
Charnley template
Charnley tibial onlay jig
Charnley total hip system
Charnley trochanter holder
Charnley trochanter reamer
Charnley vertical retractor
Charnley wire-holding forceps

Charnley wire passer
Charnley wire tightener
Charriere amputation saw
Charriere bone saw
Chassaignac axillary muscle
Chassaignac tubercle
Chatfield-Girdlestone splint
Chattanooga balance system
Chattanooga traction device
Chatzidakis hinged Vitallium implant
chauffeur's fracture
Chaves muscle transfer
Chaves-Rapp muscle transfer
    technique
checking
checklist
    McGill pain
    Low Back Pain Symptom
    Ways of Coping Checklist
Checkrein deformity
check socket
Chédiak-Higashi syndrome
Chedoke-McMaster Attitudes Toward
    Children with Handicaps (CATCH)
    scale
cheek bone
cheek puffing, repetitive
cheese reaction headache (tyramine)
cheilectomy
    Garceau
    Mann-Coughlin-DuVries
cheilotomy
cheiralgia paresthetica
cheirarthritis
cheirobrachialgia
cheirognostic
cheiromegaly
cheiroplasty
cheiropodalgia
cheirospasm
chemical, chicken (viscoprosthesis)
chemical dependency
chemical neurectomy
chemical rhizotomy
chemical shift
chemical sympathectomy
chemicals, stellate

chemokine
chemoneurolysis
chemonucleolysis, double-needle
chemoprophylaxis
chemoreceptor trigger zone
chemoreceptors
chemotherapy
    intracavitary
    intrathecal
    intratumoral
    neoadjuvant
chemotic eyes in migraine
Cherf leg holder
cherry-red macula of Tay-Sachs
    disease
Cherry-Austin drill
Cherry brain retractor
Cherry-Kerrison laminectomy forceps
Cherry-Kerrison laminectomy rongeur
Cherry laminectomy retractor
Cherry osteotome
Cherry traction tongs
chest expansion test
chest roll
Chesworth Functional Index question-
    naire
chevaux de frise (migraine aura)
chevron bone
chevron laceration
chevron osteotomy
chewing automatism
chewing reflex (bulldog response)
Cheyne periosteal elevator
Cheyne-Stokes respirations
CHH cervical brace
chi, the
CHI (closed head injury)
Chiari-Foix-Nicolesco syndrome
Chiari formation
Chiari innominate osteotomy
Chiari malformation
chiasm
    optic
    tendinous
chiasma, Camper
chiasmal compression
chiasmal lesion

chiasmatic defect
Chick CLT operating table and frame
chicken breast
chicken chemical (viscoprosthesis)
Chick-Foster orthopedic bed
Chick fracture table
Chiene test
chilblains
child, health-handicapped
Child Health Questionnaire PF-50
Child-Pugh score
Children's Coma Score (CCS)
Children's Hospital brain spatula
Children's Hospital hand drill
Children's Hospital scalp clips
Children's Hospital spatula
Childress ankle fixation technique
Childress duck waddle test
Chinese flap
Chinese medicine terms
  blood
  blood deficiency
  blood stagnation
  cold
  cold in the middle burner
  damp heat
  dampness
  deficiency fire or heat
  dryness
  fire
  foot stagnation
  heart blood deficiency
  heart qi deficiency
  heart yin deficiency
  heat
  heat in the blood
  heat toxin
  jing
  kidney yang deficiency
  kidney yin deficiency
  liver blood deficiency
  liver fire
  liver heat
  liver qi stagnation
  liver wind
  liver yang
  liver yang deficiency

Chinese medicine terms *(continued)*
  liver yin deficiency
  lung heat
  lung yang deficiency
  lung yin deficiency
  painful obstruction
  phlegm
  phlegm damp
  phlegm heat
  qi (chi)
  qi deficiency
  qi stagnation
  shao yang disorder
  shen
  spleen dampness
  spleen phlegm
  spleen qi deficiency
  spleen yang deficiency
  stomach qi deficiency
  spleen yang deficiency
  wei qi
  wind
  wind-cold
  wind-heat
chin muscle
chin-occiput piece
chin-tuck swallowing
chip
    cancellous bone
    corticocancellous bone
chip fracture
Chippaux-Smirak arch index
Chirocaine (levobupivacaine)
Chiro-Manis chiropractic table
chiropodical
chiropodist
chiropody
chiropractic (noun)
    doctor of (D.C.)
    sports
    World Federation of (WFC)
chiropractic adjustment
chiropractic assistant (C.A.)
chiropractic joint manipulation
chiropractic laser nonsurgical face lift
chiropractic manual manipulation
chiropractic mattress

chiropractic spinal adjustments
chiropractic thermography
chiropractic x-ray films
chiropractor
chiropraxis
chisel (see also *gouge*)
  acetabuloplastic round
  Adson
  Adson laminectomy
  Alexander
  ASIF
  Austin Moore
  Ballenger-Hajek
  beveled
  Bishop
  Blair
  bone
  Bowen
  box
  Brittain
  Bruening
  Buckley
  Caltagirone
  Cinelli-McIndoe
  Cloward cervical
  Cloward spinal fusion
  cold
  Converse
  Cottle
  D'Errico lamina
  Dautrey
  Fomon
  Freer
  Hajek
  Hibbs
  hollow
  Lambert-Lowman
  laminectomy
  Lexer
  Lowman-Hoglund
  Lucas
  Martin cartilage
  meniscotomy
  Metzenbaum
  Meyerding
  Miles bone
  mortising

chisel *(continued)*
  neurosurgical
  Partsch
  Passow
  Pick
  Puka
  Schwartze
  seating
  Sheehan
  Simmons
  Smillie cartilage
  Smillie meniscotomy
  Smith-Petersen
  square hollow
  Stille bone
  straight
  swan-neck
  Trautmann
  U.S. Army bone
  West bone
chisel fracture
chisel-tip wire
chi-square analysis or test
chloroma
Cho/Cr (choline/creatine ratio)
Cho cruciate ligament reconstruction
choked disk
cholelithiasis
cholesterol emboli
choline acetyltransferase
choline/creatine (Cho/Cr) ratio
cholinergic crisis
cholinergic enzyme
chondral defect
chondral delamination lesion
chondral fragment
chondralgia
chondrectomy
chondrification
chondritis
chondroblastoma
chondrocalcinosis
chondrocyte (pl. chondrocytes)
  autologous
  harvesting of
chondrocyte death
chondrocyte failure

chondrocyte leakage
chondrocyte transplantation
chondrodiastasis
chondrodysplasia
chondrodystrophia calcificans
chondrodystrophia fetalis
chondrodystrophy, myotonic
chondroepiphysitis
chondrofibroma
chondrogenesis
chondroglossus muscle
chondroid, blue reticulated
chondroitin (in osteoarthritis)
chondrolipoma
chondrolysis
chondroma
   Charcot
   extraskeletal
   juxtacortical
   periosteal
   juxtacortical
chondromalacia of the patella
chondromalacia patellae
chondromalacial changes
chondromalacic changes
chondromatosis
   Henderson-Jones
   synovial
chondromatous hamartoma
chondrometaplasia
chondromyofibroma
chondromyxofibroma
chondromyxoid fibroma (CMF)
chondromyxoma
chondromyxosarcoma
chondronecrosis
chondro-osteodystrophy
chondropathology
chondropharyngeal muscles
chondrophyte
chondroplastic
chondroplastic dwarfism
chondroplastic myotonia
chondroplasty blade
chondroplasty, laser
chondroporosis

chondrosarcoma
   clear cell
   differentiated
   extraskeletal
   mesenchymal
   myxoid
   parosteal
   periosteal
chondrosarcomatosis
chondrosteoma
chondrosternal junction
chondrosternoplasty
chondrotomy
chondroxiphoid ligament
Chopart amputation with tendon
   balancing
Chopart ankle dislocation
Chopart hindfoot amputation
Chopart joint
Chopart partial foot prosthesis
Cho-Pat Achilles strap
Cho-Pat knee strap
Cho tendon technique
choppy sea sign
chorda tympani
chordoblastoma
chordocarcinoma
chordoepithelioma
chordoma
   cavern
   lumbosacral
   sacrococcygeal
chordosarcoma
chordotomy (see *cordotomy*)
chorea
   acute
   benign hereditary
   Bergeron
   chronic progressive hereditary
   dancing
   degenerative
   diaphragmatic
   Dubini
   electric
   fibrillary
   hemilateral

chorea *(continued)*
Henoch
hereditary
Huntington
hysterical
juvenile
kinesigenic
limp
lupus-associated
malleatory
methodic
mimetic
minor
Morvan
nocturnal
one-sided
oral contraceptive-induced
paralytic
phenytoin-induced
posthemiplegic
prehemiplegic
rheumatic
rhythmic
saltatory
Schrötter (Schroetter)
senile
simple
Sydenham
thyrotoxicosis-induced
unilateral
choreic dyskinesia
choreic movement disorder
choreic movements
choreic syndrome
choreiform movement
choreoathetoid movement
choreoathetosis
familial paroxysmal
paroxysmal
paroxysmal kinesigenic
phenytoin-induced
psychotic
thyrotoxicosis-induced
choreoathetotic movements
choreoid
choreomania (dancing mania)
choriocarcinoma, pineal gland

choriomeningitis, benign lymphocytic
chorioretinitis
choristoma
choroidal artery
choroid plexus papilloma tumor
choroidal fissure
choroidal pericallosal artery
choroidectomy
Chow endoscopic carpal tunnel release
Chow transbursal technique of endoscopic carpal tunnel release
CHQ (Child Health Questionnaire)
PF-50
Chrisman-Snook ankle technique
Chrisman-Snook reconstruction of
ankle ligaments
Christensen interlocking nail
Christiansen hip prosthesis
Christmas hemophiliac disease
Christmas tree adapter
Christmas tree photopsias
Christmas tree reamer
chromatolysis
chromic suture
chromogranin, immunoreactive
chromophobe adenoma, pituitary
tumor
chromophobe pituitary tumor
chromosomes, double-minute
chronaxy (on EMG)
chrondroblastoma
chronic Achilles tendinitis
chronic ankle sprain
chronic basal meningitis with cranial
nerve paralysis
chronic exertional compartment
syndrome (CECS)
chronic foot strain
chronic functional instability
chronic joint symptoms
chronic leg ulcer
chronic meningitis
chronic musculoskeletal pain syndrome
(CMPS)
chronic opioid therapy
Chronic Pain Self-Efficacy Scale
chronic pain syndrome

chronic paroxysmal hemicrania
chronic pyogenic osteomyelitis
chronic recurrent dislocation of ankle
    joint
chronic retrocalcaneal bursitis
chronic somatic dysfunction
chronic spinal epidural infection
    brucellosis
    coccidioidomycosis
    cryptococcosis
    syphilis
    tuberculous cold abscess
chronic spinal intradural infection
chronic sprain
chronic subdural hematoma (CSDH)
chronic subtalar joint pain
chronic tic
chronic whiplash
chronologic age
chrysiasis
chuck
    hand
    Jacobs
    pin
    universal
chuck key
Chuinard autogenous bone graft
Chuinard-Petersen ankle arthrodesis
CHUK (conserved helix-loop-helix
    ubiquitous kinase)
Chvostek-Weiss sign
chymonucleolysis
chymopapain injection
CI (Combined Instabilities) functional
    knee brace
cicatricial scoliosis
cicatrix
Cicherelli bone rongeur
CIDP (chronic inflammatory
    demyelinating polyradiculopathy)
CIDPN (chronic inflammatory
    demyelinating polyneuropathy)
ciliary ganglion
ciliary ligament
ciliary migraine
ciliary muscle

ciliary nerves
ciliary neuralgia
ciliospinal center of Budge
ciliospinal or pupillary-skin reflex
CINA (Clinical Institute of Narcotic
    Assessment) Scale
Cinch Lock CTS brace
Cincinnati incision
Cincinnati Knee Scoring System
cinefluoroscopy
Cinelli-McIndoe chisel
Cinelli osteotome
cinematographic vision disorder of
    visual perception in migraine
cinereum, tuber
cinesalgia
cingulate gyrus
cingulate herniation
cingulate sulcus
cingulectomy
cingulotomy
cingulum hemispherii
Cintor bone rongeur
Cintor knee prosthesis
CIP (chronic inflammatory poly-
    radiculoneuropathy)
circadian rhythm
circannual cycle
circannual rhythm
circle bed
circle of Vieussens
circle of Weber
circle of Willis
    arterial
    forks of
CircOlectric bed
CircOlectric frame
circuit
    cognitive
    Papez
circulating immune complexes
circulating intercellular adhesion
    molecule-1 (ICAM-1)
circulating intercellular adhesion
    molecule-3 (ICAM-3)
circulating vascular adhesion molecule
    (VCAM)

circulation
  cerebrovascular
  collateral
  leptomeningeal
  parent
  systemic
  spiderweb
circulation stroke
  anterior
  posterior
circulatory arrest, hypothermic
circulatory compromise
circulatory embarrassment
circumduction with spastic gait
circumference
  calf
  head
  pelvic
circumferential dedicated knee coil
    (MRI)
circumferential fracture
circumferentially
circumflex nerve (axillary)
circumlocution of speech
circumoral paresthesia
circumscript aneurysm
circumstantial migraine
circumstantial speech
cirsoid aneurysm
cisatracurium (Nimbex)
CISS (constructive interference in
    steady state)
cistern
  ambient
  arachnoiditis of the opticochiasmatic
  basal
  basal arachnoid
  basilar
  carotid
  cerebellomedullary
  cerebellopontine
  chiasmatic
  chyle
  crural
  effacement of
  great

cistern (continued)
  interpeduncular
  mesencephalic
  opticochiasmatic
  parasellar
  posterior
  prepontine
  puncture of
  quadrigeminal
  subarachnoidal
  suprasellar
  trigeminal
  widening of crural
cisternal puncture
cistern of chiasma
cistern of fossa of Sylvius
cistern of lateral fossa of cerebrum
cistern of Pecquet
cistern of Sylvius
cisternogram, cisternography
  air
  computed tomographic
  indium
  isotope
  metrizamide CT (MCTC)
  nuclear
  oxygen
  radioisotope
  radionuclide
cisternographic
citalopram
Citelli angle
Citelli punch forceps
citicoline sodium (CerAxon)
citrullinemia
Citscope disposable arthroscope
Civinini ligament
CIVRA (continuous intravenous
    regional anesthesia)
CJD (Creutzfeldt-Jakob disease)
CKS (Continuum knee system)
  prosthesis
CKS knee implant
Clado ligament
Claforan (cefotaxime)
Claiborne external fixator

clamp
- Acland microvascular
- Adair breast
- Allis
- angular hinge
- Böhler (Boehler)
- Backhaus towel
- Berens
- Berens muscle
- Bigelo calvarium
- Bircher bone/cartilage
- Bishop
- bone extension
- bone-holding
- Boyes muscle
- bulldog
- C
- Calman carotid
- calvarium
- carotid artery
- cartilage
- Charnley compression
- Crutchfield carotid artery
- Dandy
- Diethrich bulldog
- Dingman bone and cartilage
- double
- Edna towel
- Fukushima C-clamp
- Gardner neurosurgical skull
- Greenberg
- Halifax interlaminar
- Harrington hook
- Harrington rod
- Hoen
- hook
- infant skull
- interlaminar
- intracranial
- Jackson bone extension
- Jacobson bulldog
- Jacobson-Potts vascular
- Javid carotid
- Johns Hopkins bulldog
- Kartchner carotid
- Kelly
- Kern bone-holding

clamp *(continued)*
- Kindt carotid artery
- Kocher
- Lahey
- Lambert-Lowman bone
- Lamis patella
- Lane bone
- Lane bone-holding
- Lewin bone-holding
- Locke
- Lowman bone-holding
- Lowman-Gerster bone
- Lowman-Hoglund bone-holding
- Martin cartilage
- Martin meniscus
- Martin muscle
- Matthew cross-leg
- Mayfield neurosurgical skull
- Mayfield three-pin skull
- Mayo
- meniscus
- microvascular
- mosquito
- Moynihan towel
- muscle biopsy
- Parham-Martin
- patellar
- Pean
- Pemberton spur-crushing
- pin
- Poppen-Blalock carotid
- Price muscle biopsy
- Rayport muscle biopsy
- rod
- saddle
- Salibi carotid artery
- Schlein
- Schwartz temporary intracranial artery
- self-retaining
- Selverstone carotid artery
- Sevrain cranial
- single
- skull
- Slocum meniscal
- Smith bone
- spur-crushing

clamp *(continued)*
  Steinhauser bone
  swivel
  Thompson carotid
  three-point skull
  towel
  trochanter-holding
  Ulrich bone-holding
  vascular
  Verbrugge
  VSF (Vermont spinal fixator)
  Walton cartilage
  Walton meniscus
  wire fixation
  Yasargil carotid
clam-shell brace
Clancy-Andrews reconstruction
Clancy cruciate ligament reconstruction
clang associations
Clark transfer technique
Clarke arch angle
Clarke column
Clarke patellar compression test
Clarus spinescope
clasp, arrow pin
clasp-knife response
classic amnesic spell
  dissociative state
  fugue state
classical abdominal migraine
classic Kaposi sarcoma
classic migraine headache
classic-type spongiform encephalopathy
classification (see also *fracture*)
  AAOS acetabular abnormalities
  ACR
  acromioclavicular injury
  Aitken epiphyseal fracture
  Allman acromioclavicular injury
  American Rheumatism Association
  American Spinal Cord Injury
    Association
  Anderson-D'Alonzo odontoid
    fracture
  Anderson tibial pseudarthrosis
  Antoni-A neurinoma
  AO ankle fracture

classification *(continued)*
  AO-Danis-Weber ankle fracture
  Arco
  Arthritis Impact Measurement
    Scales
  Bayne radial agenesis
  Bayne ulnar ray deficiency (I–IV)
  Bennett thumb fracture
  Benson-Geschwind aphasia
  Berndt-Harty talar lesion staging
  blast injury
  Bleck metatarsus adductus
  Bosniak
  Boston Classification System
  boutonniére
  Boyd-Griffin trochanteric fracture
  Broders tumor index
  Brooker
  Brooker periarticular heterotopic
    ossification (PHO)
  Burwell-Charnley fracture reduction
  Butcher staging
  Caldwell-Moloy
  Canale-Kelly talar neck fracture
  Carnesale-Stewart-Barnes hip
    dislocation
  Catterall
  Cavanaugh-Rogers footprint
  Cedell-Magnusson arthritis
  Cole and Manske first web
    space/thumb (A–D)
  Colonna hip fracture
  Copeland-Kavat metatarso-
    phalangeal dislocation
  D'Antonio acetabular
  Danis-Weber ankle fracture
  Daseler-Anson plantaris muscle
    anatomy
  Delbet hip fracture
  Denis compression fracture (A-D)
  Denis seat belt injury
  Denis spinal injury
  Dickhaut-DeLee discoid meniscus
  Durie and Salmon
  Dyck-Lambert
  Eckert-Davis peroneal tendon
    subluxation

classification *(continued)*
    Ellis
    Engel postoperative seizure
    Essex-Lopresti calcaneal fracture
    Evans intertrochanteric fracture
    Ficat femoral head osteonecrosis
    Ficat stage of avascular necrosis
    Fielding-Magliato subtrochanteric
        fracture
    Floyd peripheral nerve
    Fränkel spinal cord injury
    Freeman calcaneal fracture
    Fries rheumatoid arthritis
    Frykman hand fracture
    Frykman radial fracture
    Frykman wrist fracture
    Garden femoral neck fracture
    Gartland supracondylar fracture
    Gertzbein seat belt injury
    Graf
    Grantham femur fracture
    Greenfield (spinocerebellar ataxia)
    Gumley seat belt injury
    Gustilo-Anderson tibial plafond
        fracture
    Gustilo puncture wound
    Gustilo tibial fracture
    Hahn-Steinthal capitellum fracture
    Hansen fracture
    Hardy-Clapham sesamoid
    Hardy pituitary tumor
    Hawkins talar neck fracture
    Herbert-Fisher fracture
    Herbert scaphoid bone fracture
    Herring lateral pillar
    Hohl tibial condylar fracture
    Holdsworth spinal fracture
    Holdsworth spinal injury
    House-Brackmann facial nerve
        function
    Hughston Clinic injury
    Hunt-Hess aneurysm
    Hunt-Hess neurological
    Hunt-Kosnik aneurysm
    Hunt-Kosnik nuchal stiffness
    Hyams esthesioneuroblastoma
    Hyams tumor

classification *(continued)*
    ILAR
    Ingram-Bachynski hip fracture
    International Classification of
        Epilepsies and Epileptic
        Syndromes
    International Headache Society
    International OCu tetraplegia
    Jahss ankle dislocation
    Jahss metatarsophalangeal joint
        dislocation
    Jeffery radial fracture
    Johnson-Boseker scale
    Johnson-Jahss posterior tibial
        tendon tear
    Jones congenital tibial deficiency
    Jones diaphyseal fracture
    Judet epiphyseal fracture
    Kalamchi-Dawe congenital tibial
        deficiency
    Kelikian nail deformity
    Kellgren degenerative disk
    Kernohan astrocytoma/glioblastoma
    Kernohan brain tumor
    Key-Conwell pelvic fracture
    Kilfoyle condylar fracture
    King thoracic scoliosis
    Kistler subarachnoid hemorrhage
    Kocher-Lorenz capitellum fracture
    Kolb drug addiction
    Kostuik-Errico spinal stability
    Kummel ulnar ray deficiency
        (I–III)
    Kyle fracture
    Lauge-Hansen ankle fracture
    Leung thumb loss
    load sharing
    LSUMC motor and sensory function
    LSUMC nerve injury
    MacNichol-Voutsinas
    Mangled Extremity Severity Score
        (MESS)
    Mason radial fracture
    Mayo elbow fracture
    Mazur ankle evaluation
    McDermott-Scranton
    McLain-Weinstein spinal tumor

classification *(continued)*
   Medical Research Council (MRC) muscle function
   Merland perimedullary arteriovenous fistula
   Meyers-McKeever tibial fracture
   Milch elbow fracture
   Minaar coalition
   Mirra
   Modic disk abnormality
   MRC muscle strength
   MSTS (Musculoskeletal Tumor Society) staging system
   Mueller humerus fracture
   multiaxial
   Nalebuff
   Neer femur fracture
   Neer-Horowitz humerus fracture
   Neer shoulder fracture (I–III)
   Nevaiser frozen shoulder
   Newman radial fracture
   New York diagnostic criteria
   Nurick spondylosis
   O'Brien radial fracture
   O'Rahilly limb deficiency
   Oden peroneal tendon subluxation
   Ogden epiphyseal fracture
   Olerud and Molander fracture
   osteoarthritis grading
   OTA/AO
   Ovadia-Beals tibial plafond fracture
   Paley complications
   Palmer
   Pauwel femoral neck fracture
   Pipkin femoral fracture
   Poland epiphyseal fracture
   Prosthetic Problem Inventory Scale
   Ratliff avascular necrosis
   Riordan club hand
   Riseborough-Radin intercondylar fracture
   Ritchie index
   Rockwood acromioclavicular injury
   Rome criteria
   Rosser Classification of Illness States
   Rowe calcaneal fracture

classification *(continued)*
   Rowe-Lowell fracture-dislocation
   Ruedi-Allgower tibial plafond fracture
   Russell-Rubinstein cerebrovascular malformation
   Sage-Salvatore acromioclavicular joint injury
   Saha shoulder muscle
   Sakellarides calcaneal fracture
   Salter epiphyseal fracture
   Salter-Harris epiphyseal fracture
   Salter-Harris-Rang epiphyseal fracture
   Salter-Harris tibial-fibular injury
   Sanders computed tomography
   Schatzker fracture
   Scranton-McDermott
   Seddon nerve injury
   Seinsheimer femoral fracture
   Shelton femur fracture
   Smith sesamoid position
   Sorbie calcaneal fracture
   Steinbrocker rheumatoid arthritis
   Steinert epiphyseal fracture
   Steward-Milford fracture
   Sunderland nerve injury
   Sundt carotid ulceration
   Swanson
   Synder labral-biceps detachment
   talocalcaneal index
   Temtamy-McKusick
   Thompson-Epstein femoral fracture
   TNM (tumor size, nodal involvement, metastatic progress)
   Torg
   Tronzo intertrochanteric fracture
   Trunkey fracture
   Vostal radial fracture
   Wagner diabetic foot ulcer
   Waldenstrom staging
   walking footprints
   Warren-Marshall
   Wassel thumb duplication
   Watanabe discoid meniscus
   Watson-Jones navicular fracture
   Watson-Jones spinal fracture

classification *(continued)*
    Watson-Jones tibial fracture
    White and Panjabi cervical spine
        x-ray
    WHO (World Health Organization)
        astrocytoma
    Wiberg patellar type (I–III)
    Wilkins radial fracture
    Winquist-Hansen femoral fracture
    Zickel fracture
    Zlotsky-Ballard acromioclavicular
        injury
Claude syndrome
claudication
    neurogenic
    vascular
claustrum
clavicectomy
clavicle (shoulder)
clavicle, condensing osteitis of
clavicotomy
clavicular head of sternocleidomastoid
clavicular notch
clavipectoral fascia
clavus
    interdigital
    soft
clawfoot deformity
    hollow foot
    pes arcuatus
    pes cavus
claw hand (main en griffe)
clawing of toes
clawtoe deformity
clay shoveler's fracture
Clayton forefoot arthroplasty
Clayton-Fowler technique
Clayton resection arthroplasty
CLBP (chronic low back pain)
CLCS (Comprehensive Level of
    Consciousness Scale)
Cleanwheel neurological pinwheel
clean wound
clearance, diametral
cleavable tumor
cleavage fracture

cleavage plane, subintimal
cleavage tear
Cleeman sign
cleft
    intergluteal
    interinnominoabdominal
    Rathke
    synaptic
    ventricular
cleft foot deformity
clefting of meniscus
C-leg System
cleidocranial dysostosis
Cleland ligament in the hand
clenched fist attitude
clenched fist view
Cleveland bone-cutting forceps
Cleveland bone rongeur
Cleveland-Bosworth-Thompson
    technique
Cleveland rongeur
click, clicking
    hip
    Ortolani
click stimulus rate
Clifton Assessment Procedures for the
    Elderly (CAPE)
climbing up the legs (Gowers sign)
clindamycin-impregnated polymethyl-
    methacrylate (PMMA) beads
Clinical Care in America Managed
    Care database
Clinical Dementia Rating (CDR) Scale
clinical EEG recording
Clinical Global Impression of Change
    (CGIC)
Clinical Institute Narcotic Assessment
    (CINA) Scale
clinical seizure manifestation
clinicoanatomic correlation
Clinisert mattress
Clinitron air bed
clinodactyly
clinoid ligament
clinoid venous plexus
Clinoril (sulindac)

clip (see also *clamp*)
Acland
Adson scalp
aneurysm
aneurysm window
Biemer-Clip aneurysm
brain
Braun-Yasargil right-angle
Children's Hospital scalp
cobalt alloy aneurysm
Codman aneurysm
Cologne pattern scalp
Drake aneurysm
fenestrated Drake
Heifitz
hemoclip
hemostasis or hemostatic
Housepan aneurysm
Ingraham-Fowler tantalum
Khodadad
LeRoy-Raney scalp
Ligaclip hemostatic
ligating
Mayfield aneurysm
McFadden temporary aneurysm
McKenzie brain
McKenzie hemostasis
McKenzie silver
Michel
Olivecrona aneurysm
pin
Raney hemostatic
Raney scalp
ring angled
scalp
Schwartz aneurysm
silver
skin
sponge stopper
Sugita aneurysm
Sundt encircling
Sundt-Kees aneurysm window
supracondylar medial
surgical
temporary vessel
titanium aneurysm
vari-angle aneurysm

clip *(continued)*
VCS clip adapter
vessel
Weck
Yasargil vessel
clip applier (or applicator)
Mayfield miniature
Mayfield temporary aneurysm
clipping of aneurysm
clival dura
clival region
clivus meningioma tumor
clivus tumor
clock, Deaf-Blind Alarm
Clodius dissector
clofibrate
clogs
Markell Mobility Health Clogs
wooden postoperative
clonality assay
methylation-based
transcription-based
clonal tumor cell
clonic movement
clonic phase spike and wave
clonic seizure
clonus
ankle
drawn ankle
patellar
persistent
sustained ankle
three-beat
transient
unsustained
clopidogrel bisulfate (Plavix)
Cloquet ligament
closed break fracture
closed circuit TV (CCTV)
closed disk space infection
closed dislocation
closed fracture
closed head injury (CHI)
closed lip (type I) schizencephaly
closed goggle-type eyeguards
closed reduction and internal fixation
Closer suture-based system

close-up view
closing abductor wedge osteotomy
(CAWO)
closing base wedge osteotomy
(CBWO)
closing pressure (on lumbar puncture)
closing wedge high tibial osteotomy
(CWHTO)
closing wedge manipulation and
reapplication of plaster
closing wedge osteotomy
Clostridium perfringens meningitis
Clostridium tetani
closure (see also *suture*)
  delayed
  epiphyseal
  fascial
  growth center
  incomplete
  myofascial
  partial
  physeal
  primary
  purse-string or pursestring
  secondary
  sutureless
  vein patch
closure tasks, sentence
clot
  blood
  evacuation of blood
  old blood
  subarachnoid
  subdural
clothespin graft
clouding of consciousness
Cloutier unconstrained knee prosthesis
cloverleaf Küntscher nail
cloverleaf sign
cloverleaf skull (kleeblattschädel)
Cloward anterior spinal fusion
Cloward blade retractor
Cloward bone graft impactor
Cloward brain retractor
Cloward cautery hook
Cloward cervical chisel
Cloward cervical retractor

Cloward cervical vertebrae spreader
Cloward-Cone ring curet
Cloward-Cushing vein retractor
Cloward depth gauge
Cloward disk rongeur
Cloward dowel cutter
Cloward dowel ejector
Cloward drill guide
Cloward drill tip
Cloward dural hook
Cloward dural retractor
Cloward elevator
Cloward-English laminectomy rongeur
Cloward hammer
Cloward-Harper laminectomy rongeur
Cloward-Hoen laminectomy retractor
Cloward intervertebral disk rongeur
Cloward lamina spreader
Cloward lumbar lamina retractor
Cloward nerve root retractor
Cloward osteophyte elevator
Cloward periosteal elevator
Cloward pituitary rongeur
Cloward punch forceps
Cloward rongeur forceps
Cloward skin retractor
Cloward spinal fusion chisel
Cloward spinal fusion osteotome
Cloward spots
Cloward tissue retractor
Cloward vertebrae spreader
Clozaril (clozapine)
CLS (Cementless Sportorno) hip
  arthroplasty stem
clubbing, cyanosis, and edema
clubbing of fingers and toes
clubfoot (pl. clubfeet)
clubfoot deformity
clubfoot release
clubfoot splint, Denis Browne
clubhand deformity
clumsy gait
clumsy hand dysarthria
clumsy hand syndrome
cluneal nerve
clunk, spontaneous wrist
cluster headache

Clyburn Colles fracture fixator
CMAP (compound motor action potential)
CMAP (compound muscle action potential)
CMC (carpometacarpal) fusion
CMD (cerebromacular degeneration)
CMF (chondromyxoid fibroma)
CMJ (corticomedullary junction) phase imaging
CMO thigh support
CMPS (chronic musculoskeletal pain syndrome)
CMRglu (regional cerebral glucose metabolism)
$CMRO_2$ (cerebral metabolic rate of oxygen consumption)
CMRP (cervical intervertebral foraminal) (MR phlebography)
CMT (Charcot-Marie-Tooth) disease
CMV (cytomegalovirus)
CMV encephalitis
CMV-induced sensorineural hearing loss
CMV meningitis
CMV myelopathy
CMW bone cement
CMW cement gun
CNAP (compound nerve action potential)
CNS (central nervous system)
CNS pin and wire cutter
CNS tumor
coagulase negative
coagulase positive
coagulate assay
coagulator
   argon beam
   ASSI
   bipolar
   Concept bipolar
   hook tip
   Malis bipolar
   Malis CMC-II bipolar
   paddle
   Polar-Mate
   push-pull tip

coagulopathy
coalition
   bony
   calcaneonavicular
   carpal
   fibrous
   intercarpal
   lunate triquetral
   Minaar classification of
   osseous
   talocalcaneal
   tarsal
coapt, coapted
coaptation, skin
coarse up-beat nystagmus
coated Vicryl Rapide suture
coating of aneurysm
Coballoy implant metal
Coballoy twist drill
cobalt alloy aneurysm clip
cobalt-chromium alloy
cobalt-60 Gamma Knife radiosurgical treatment
Coban elastic dressing
Cobb attachment for Albee-Compere fracture table
Cobb curet
Cobb elevator
Cobb gouge
Cobb method of measuring kyphosis
Cobb periosteal elevator
Cobb scoliosis angle
Cobb scoliosis measuring technique
Cobb spinal elevator
Cobb spinal gouge
Cobb syndrome
coblation (cold ablation) method
cobra retractor
Coccidioides immitis
coccidioidomycosis
coccygeal body
coccygeal bone
coccygeal joint
coccygeal muscle
coccygeal nerve
coccygeal procedures
coccygeal spine (coccyx)

coccygectomy
coccygeopubic diameter
coccygodynia
coccygotomy
coccyx
cochlear nerve
cochlear nucleus
    dorsal
    ventral
cochlear nucleus complex
Cochrane Controlled Trials Registry
cock-up deformity of toe
cock-up hand splint
cock-up wrist splint
Cockayne syndrome
cocking injury
Cocklin toe operation, modified
Co-Cr-Mo (cobalt-chromium-
    molybdenum) alloy implant
Co-Cr-W-Ni (cobalt-chromium-
    tungsten-nickel) alloy implant
code
    CPT (Current Procedural
        Terminology)
    DSM (Diagnostic and Statistical
        Manual [of Mental Disorders])
    ICD (International Classification
        of Diseases [of World Health
        Organization]) 9 (ICD-9)
    ICD (International Classification
        of Diseases [of World Health
        Organization]) 10 (ICD-10)
codfish vertebrae
Codivilla tendon lengthening
Codman angle
Codman cranial blade
Codman curet
Codman drill
Codman exercises
Codman-Harper laminectomy rongeur
Codman-Kerrison laminectomy
    rongeur
Codman-Leksell laminectomy rongeur
Codman-Schlesinger laminectomy
    rongeur
Codman sign
Codman slit valve

Codman spinal curet
Codman spinal frame
Codman surgical patties
    non-x-ray detectable
    x-ray detectable
Codman triangle
Codman tumor
Codman wire pass drill
codon
Coe-pak paste
coefficient
    attenuation
    Pearson correlation
    stiffness
    Spearman rank correlation
coenesthesia
coenzyme Q
Coffin-Lowry syndrome
Cofield shoulder prosthesis
Cogan lid-twitch sign
Cogan syndrome
Cognex (tacrine)
cognition
cognitive behaviors
cognitive circuits
cognitive deficit
cognitive development
cognitive disturbance
cognitive dysfunction
Cognitive Failures Questionnaire
    (CFQ)
cognitive function, higher level
cognitive function
cognitive impairment
cognitive morbidity
cognitive planning deficit
cogwheel gait
cogwheeling
cogwheel rigidity
Cohen periosteal elevator
Cohen rongeur
coherence
Coherent light point stimulator
coil
    circumferential dedicated knee
    crossed
    endosaccular

coil *(continued)*
    endovascular
    Golay
    Guglielmi Detachable Coil (GDC)
    gradient
    Helmholtz
    platinum
    radiofrequency (RF)
    receiver
    RF (radiofrequency)
    saddle
    shim
    solenoid
Coiter muscle
colchicine poisoning
Colclough-Scheicher laminectomy
    rongeur
cold compressive dressing
cold-induced brain injury
cold in the middle burner (Chinese
    medicine)
cold provocation test
Cole and Manske classification of first
    web space/thumb (A–D)
Cole fracture frame
Coleman flatfoot technique
Cole osteotomy
collagen-alginate wound dressing
collagen-coated Vicryl mesh
collagen fibrils within tendon
collagen helical structure
collagen matrix
collagen, microcrystalline
collagen shrinkage
collagen type 2 (Colloral)
Collagraft bone graft matrix
collapse
    ventricular
    vertebral body
collapsing scoliosis
collar
    calcar
    carotid
    cervical
    Cowboy Collar
    dural
    dynamization

collar *(continued)*
    Exo-static cervical
    foam
    Forrester-Brown
    implant
    Lewin
    Mayo Thomas
    Miami Acute Care (MAC) cervical
    Miami J cervical
    myocervical rigid
    Nec Loc cervical
    periosteal bone
    Philadelphia cervical
    Philadelphia rigid
    pillow
    Plastizote cervical
    rigid
    Schanz
    Scott countoured cervical
    Scott serpentine cervical
    Scott universal cervical
    serpentine foam
    soft cervical
    Thomas rigid
    Tuxedo
collar bone
collar button abscess
collateral blood flow
collateral, bridging
collateral circulation
collateral-dependent tissue
collateral ligaments of hand
collateral sprouting of neuron
collateral sulcus
collateral vessels
collection, intratendinous fluid
collectomy, shortening
college (see *academy; association;*
    committee; society)
Colles fascia
Colles fracture
Colles ligament
Colles space
Colles splint
collet screwdriver adapter
Collet-Sicard syndrome
collicular fracture of medial malleolus

colliculus (pl. colliculi)
Collier sign
collimation
collimator helmet
Collimator
  Multileaf
  MCAT (modular coded aperture
    technology)
  Millennium MLC-120
  modular coded aperture technology
    (MCAT)
Collimator plugging pattern
Collin amputating knife
Collin-Beard resection of the levator
  muscle
Collins dynamometer
Collins law of survival after brain
  tumor
Collins rib shears
Collis broken femoral stem technique
Collis-Taylor retractor
Collis TDR instruments
Collison drill
Collison plate
Collison screw
collodion dressing
colloidal gold test (of CSF)
colloid cyst of the third ventricle
colloid cyst tumor
colloid oncotic pressure (COP)
colloid volume expansion
Colloral (collagen type 2)
Collostat
Colonna-Ralston ankle approach
Colonna shelf procedure
Colorado microdissection needle
Colorado tick fever viral encephalitis
color agnosia
color-coded duplex sonography
color-coded flow imaging
color desaturation on vision test
color-flow Doppler
color-flow duplex imaging
Colpac
Coltart fracture technique
Columbia neurologic rating scale

column
  anterior gray
  Clarke
  contrast
  demyelination of posterior
  displacement of spinal
  intermediolateral spinal gray
  lateral
  medial
  posterior
  posterior gray
  Prosorba
  vertebral
column of dye
coma
  adrenocortical
  agrypnodal
  alcoholic
  alpha
  alpha frequency
  apoplectic
  barbiturate
  beta
  deep
  depth of
  diabetic
  evolution of
  hepatic
  hyperosmolar nonketotic
  hypopituitary
  incipient
  irreversible
  Kussmaul
  metabolic
  myxedema
  nonketotic hyperglycemic
    hyperosmolar
  pentobarbital
  postanoxic
  psychogenic
  spindle
  theta
  uremic
coma dépassé
comatose
coma vigil

comeback curette
combretastatin A-4
comb rhythm on EEG
combative, combativeness
combined-flexion phenomenon
Comed post-traumatic and postsurgical
  footgear
Comfeel Ulcus occlusive dressing
Comfort Cast stirrup
Comforfoam splint
Comfy Cradle maternity lumbar
  support
Command joint replacement instrument system
commands
  inability to follow
  responds to verbal
  verbal
  unable to follow simple
commemorative sign
comminuted bursting fracture
comminuted intra-articular fracture
Commission for the Blind and
  Visually Handicapped (CBVH)
commissural myelorrhaphy
commissure
  anterior (AC)
  cerebral
  gray commissure of spinal cord
  hippocampal
  posterior (PC)
  white commissure of spinal cord
commissurotomy
  callosal
  central
committee (see also *academy, association, society*), International Knee
  Documentation Committee (IKDC)
commode, bedside
common carotid artery occlusion
common fibular nerve
common migraine headache
common palmar digital nerve
common peroneal nerve palsy
common plantar digital nerve
communicating hydrocephalus

communication
  asyndetic
  embryonic
communication/cognition treatment
community rehabilitation
Comolli sign
COMP (cartilage oligomeeric matrix
  protein)
compact bone
compacter, acetabular cement
Compaction pliers
comparison view
compartment
  anterior
  anterior mediastinal
  deep posterior
  extensor
  extradural
  fifth
  first
  fourth
  infracolic
  infratentorial
  lateral
  medial
  patellofemoral
  plantar
  posterior
  posterolateral
  posteromedial
  second
  sixth
  superficial posterior
  supracolic
  third
Compartmental II knee prosthesis
compartment lesion, posterior
compartment syndrome
Compass hinge
Compassia (dronabinol)
Compass stereotactic system
compensable accident
compensation filter (x-ray)
compensation
  vestibular
  workers'

"compensationitis"
compensatory wedge
Compere fixation wire
Compere-Thompson arthrodesis
Comperm tubular elastic bandage
competency, collateral ligament
complement component C3 and C4
complement deficiency
complement-fixation studies for herpes
   simplex
complete Achilles tendon rupture
complete elective mutism
complete fracture
complete nerve lesion
complete phocomelia
complete ptosis of third nerve paresis
complete sacrectomy
complete tetraplegia (quadriplegia)
complete ulnar nerve palsy
completed stroke
complex
   AIDS dementia (ADC)
   ankle joint (AJC)
   anterior communicating artery
   aperiodic
   arcuate
   atlas vertebral subluxation
   atypical spike and wave
   biceps-labral
   bunion
   bunion–hallux valgus
   bunionette–hallux valgus–splay foot
   capsulolabral
   circulating immune
   cochlear nucleus
   discoligamentous
   Edinger-Westphal
   fabellofibular
   foot-ankle
   gastrocnemius-soleus
   Ghon-Sachs
   hallux valgus–metatarsus primus
   varus
   hindfoot joint
   hippocampal-amygdala
   K
   ligamentous

complex *(continued)*
   Lyme disease
   morphology
   multiple spike
   OEIS
   parkinsonism-dementia
   periodic
   polyspike
   polyspike and slow wave
   quasi-periodic
   Ranke
   sesamoid
   sharp wave
   slow spike and wave
   spike and dome
   spike and wave
   subluxation
   superior olivary
   symptom
   syndesmotic ligament
   tibiocalcaneal joint
   triangular fibrocartilage
   triphasic wave
   vertebrobasilar
complex craniosynostosis
complex multistep task
complex regional pain syndrome
   (CRPS)
complex voluntary movements
Compliant pre-stress prosthetic bone
   implant device
component (see also *prosthesis*)
   acetabular
   AML trial hip
   Amstutz femoral
   Aufranc-Turner femoral
   Bechtol acetabular
   Bombelli-Morscher femoral
   cerclaged
   Charnley narrow stem
   Charnley standard stem
   cobra-design femoral
   complement component C3 and C4
   DePuy trispiked acetabular
   glenoid
   hallucinatory
   Harris-Galante acetabular

component *(continued)*
 head-neck
 humeral
 internal rotary component of force
 metal-backed acetabular
 Neer II humeral
 Press-Fit
 prosthesis
 S-ROM modular femoral
 straight stem femoral
 Tri-Con
 trial femoral
component trial
composite autologous material
composite graft
composite hamstring graft
composite knee score
compound articulation
compound condylar synovial joint
compound dislocation
compound fracture
compound joint
compound muscle action potential
comprehension deficit
Comprehensive Level of
 Consciousness Scale (CLCS)
compression
 brain stem
 cervical cord
 chiasmal
 extradural spinal cord
 interfragmental
 intermittent pneumatic (IPC)
 long axis
 lower lumbar root
 lumbar root
 mean maximal
 median nerve
 multiplanar
 nerve
 nerve root
 orbital mass
 radicular
 spinal cord
compression apparatus
compression arthrodesis
compression flexion injury

compression fracture
compression fracture of atlas
compression-molded polyethylene
compression paralysis
compression plate and screws
compression plus torque theory of
 cervical injury
compression syndrome, root
compression test
 ulnar nerve
 vasopneumatic
compression therapy
compression ultrasonography
compression wrap dressing
compressive centripetal wrapping
compressive hyperextension injury
compressive neuropathy
compressive optic neuropathy
compressor muscle of naris
Comprifix supports
compromise
 circulatory
 immune system
 neural
 subacromial space
 spinal cord
Compro Plus Knee support
Compton clavicle pin
Compumedics sleep system
computed tomographic cisternogram
computed tomography, Xenon-
 enhanced (Xe-CT)
computed-tomography-guided percutaneous trigeminal tractotomy-
 nucleotomy
computer-assisted arthritis detection
computer-assisted design (CAD)
computer-assisted EEG signal analysis
computer-assisted frameless navigation
 technique
computer-assisted minimally invasive
 surgery (CAMIS)
computer-assisted orthopedic surgery
 (CAOS)
computerized cranial tomography
computerized dynamic posturography
 (CDP)

computerized signal analysis of EEG
Comtan (entacapone)
Conaxial total ankle prosthesis
concave-convex surface
concavity-compression mechanism
concealed straight leg raising test
concentrate, inability to
concentration
    lack of
    poor
concentric hamstring contraction
concentric muscle training
Concept ablator
Concept bipolar coagulator
Concept cannulated screw
Concept handheld cautery
Concept shaver
concepts, time/money/number
conceptual ability
Conceptual Series Completion mental
    status test
concha, inferior nasal (skull)
concha of cranium
conchiolin osteomyelitis
Concise compression hip screw
Conco elastic bandage
concomitant heat
concrete thought processes
concretion of cement
concurrent
concussion amnesia
concussion grades
concussion of brain (grades 1-3)
concussion of spinal cord
condensing osteitis of clavicle
conduction
    ephaptic
    motor nerve
    saltatory nerve
conduction aphasia
conduction studies, nerve
conductive jelly or paste
conductor
    Adson
    Bailey
    Davis

conduit
    detour
    peripheral nerve regeneration
condylar articulation
condylar fracture
condylar hypoplasia
condylar lift-off, fluoroscopy-guided
condyle
    external
    femoral
    flare of
    lateral femoral
    medial femoral
    occipital
    tibial
condylectomy, DuVries phalangeal
condyle resection
condylocephalic nailing
condyloid joint
condylotomy
C1-C7 cervical vertebrae
C1-C5 segments of internal carotid
    artery
cone and socket bone
cone arthrodesis
cone biopsy cannula
cone biopsy needle
cone disk
Cone-Grant technique
Cone laminectomy retractor
Cone ring curet
Cone scalp retractor
Cone skull punch forceps
Cone skull traction tongs
Cone suction biopsy curet
Cone suction tube
Cone ventricular needle
Cone wire-twisting forceps
coned-down x-ray view
confabulation of speech
configuration, horizontal dipole
configuration of wave
configuration, winged
confluent, superior
confocal microscopy
Conform dressing

conforming splint
confrontation naming test
confuse, confused
confusion
  episodic
  nocturnal
  postictal
  right-left
confusional episode
confusional state
congenerous muscle
congenita
  myotonia
  pseudohypertrophic musculature
    in myotonia
congenital absence
congenital anomaly
congenital arteriosclerotic aneurysm
congenital bars
congenital CMV infection
congenital double athetosis
congenital dysplasia of the hip (CDH)
congenital flatfoot
congenital glenoid dysplasia
congenital hemivertebra
congenital hippocampal sclerosis
congenital Horner syndrome
congenital idiopathic nystagmus
congenital immature teratoma
congenital insensitivity to pain
congenital intercalary limb absence
congenital intracranial teratoma
congenital latent nystagmus
congenital laxity of ligament
congenital myopathy
congenital nystagmus
congenital primitive neuroectodermal
  tumor
congenital rubella
congenital spastic paraplegia
congenital spondylolisthesis
congenital syringomyelia
congenital terminal limb absence
congenital toxoplasmosis, Sabin-
  Feldman dye test for
congenital vertical talus
congenitally short limb

congestion, flap
Congo red dye
Congress of Neurological Surgeons
congruence of mood and affect
congruent reduction
congruity, joint
congruous cup-shaped reamer
conical point wire
conjoined lateral band (CLB) rerouting
conjugate deviation of the eyes
conjugate eye movements
conjugate fixed gaze
conjugate gaze
conjugate horizontal gaze deviation
conjugate ligament
conjugately, swing
conjugate overshooting
conjugate paralysis
Conley pin
connection
  corticocerebellar
  dendritic
  dentatorubrothalamic
  rostral
connective tissue disease
conoid ligament
Conrad-Bugg trapping of soft tissue
Conradi-Hünermann syndrome
Conray contrast medium
conscious collaboration of the patient
conscious, fully
consciousness
  change in level of
  clouding of
  crude
  declining
  depression of
  discrimination
  episodic changes of
  impaired
  impairment of
  level of
  loss of
  state of
conscious state, parasomniac
consecutive dislocation
consensual constriction

consensual gaze
consensual light reflex
consensual pupillary response
conservative management
Conserve hip system
consolidation
Consortium to Establish a Registry for
    Alzheimer Disease (CERAD)
constant frequency train
Constant-Murley rating scale
Constant score
constant touch perception
continuous performance test
constitution, migrainous
constitutional white finger (primary
    Raynaud phenomenon)
constraint-induced movement therapy
constriction
    absent consensual
    consensual
    direct (eyes)
    hourglass
    pupillary
constriction band syndrome
constrictor muscle of pharynx
constructional ability
constructional apraxia
constructional impairment
constructional praxis
constructive interference in steady state
    (CISS)
construct validity of rehabilitation testing
consumptive anoxia
contact, electrode
contaminated wound
Contantokin-G (Con-G)
content
    bone mineral (BMC)
    brain water (on MRI scan)
content validity of rehabilitation testing
context-free semantic memories
context-rich episodic memories
contiguous articular surfaces
contiguous images (on CT scan)
contiguous slices
contiguous supramarginal gyrus
continuity of bone

continuous passive motion (CPM)
    device
continuous performance test
continuous running suture
continuous wave Doppler study
Continuum bipolar acetabular head
Continuum elliptical acetabular cup
Continuum hip stem
Continuum knee system (CKS)
Continuum P/S total knee
Continuum polyethylene acetabular
    cup
Continuum total knee base plate
contour
    scalloping
    Wiberg type II patellar
Contour DF-80 total hip replacement
contoured waveform
Contour internal prosthesis
Contour scalp retractor
contract enhancement
contractile fibers
contraction
    agonist-antagonist
    concentric hamstring
    eccentric quadriceps
    nonepileptic myoclonic
    Rossolimo
    synergistic
contraction fasciculations
contractor
    Bailey-Gibbon rib
    Bailey rib
    Lemmon rib
    rib
    Sellors rib
contracture
    Dupuytren
    dynamic equinus
    elbow
    equinus
    fixed flexion
    flexion-adduction
    gastroc/soleus (gastrocnemius/
        soleus)
    hip flexion
    ischemic

contracture *(continued)*
 joint
 knee flexion
 muscle
 myostatic
 postpoliomyelitic muscle
 scar
 secondary
 Skoog release of Dupuytren
 soft tissue
 Volkmann ischemic
 web
contralateral facial paralysis
contralateral foot
contralateral hemiparalysis
contralateral hemiplegia
contralateral homonymous inferior
 quadrantanopsia
contralateral homonymous superior
 quadrantanopsia
contralateral loss
contralateral sign
contrast arteriography
contrast baths (hot and cold)
contrast column
contrast enhancement of computed
 tomography (CECT)
contrast medium (pl. media)
 Amipaque
 Conray
 diatrizoate meglumine
 diatrizoate sodium
 18F-fluorodeoxyglucose
 Ethodian (iophendylate)
 gadolinium
 Hexabrix
 Hypaque-76
 iohexol
 iopamidol
 iothalamate meglumine
 ioversol
 ioxaglate meglumine
 ioxaglate sodium
 Isovue-200, Isovue-300, Isovue-370
 Isovue-M 200, Isovue-M 300
 Magnevist
 MD-60

contrast medium *(continued)*
 metrizamide
 Neurolite
 Neurotrast
 OctreoScan (indium-111
  pentetreotide)
 Omnipaque
 Optiray 320
 radiopaque
 Renografin-60
 Reno-M-Dip
 technetium-99 exametazime
 technetium-99 hexametazime
 Visipaque (iodixanol)
contrast-enhanced ultrasound
contrast myelography
contrast-to-noise ratio (MRI)
contrecoup injury
control
 Dupaco knee
 exsanguination tourniquet
 image
 swing phase
Controlled Oral Word Association
 Test
controls
 car hand
 static reflex
 statokinetic reflex
contusio cerebri
contusion
 brain
 cerebral
 contrecoup
 deep-seated
 frontal lobe
 gliding
 hip
 occipital lobe
 parietal lobe
 pontine
 soft tissue
 spinal cord
 temporal pole
contusion of brain or spinal cord
conus ligament
conus medullaris lesion

convergence
  ocular
  visual axis point of
convergence deficit
convergence of eyes
convergence paralysis
convergence-retraction nystagmus
convergence spasm
Converse chisel
Converse periosteal elevator
conversion, CAT-CAM
conversion disorder
conversion, hemorrhagic
conversion reaction, hysterical
conversion symptom
Convery polyarticular disability index
convex
convexity, frontocentral
convexity sinus
convexobasia
convoluted
convolution
  Broca
  cerebral
  Gratiolet
  Heschl
  occipitotemporal
  Zuckerkandl
convolutional
convulsant
convulsion (see also *epilepsy*; *seizure*)
  central
  clonic
  coordinate
  epileptiform
  essential
  febrile
  generalized tonic/clonic (GTC)
  hysterical
  local
  mimetic
  mimic
  paroxysmal
  puerperal
  salaam
  spontaneous
  tetanic

convulsion *(continued)*
  tonic/clonic
  uremic
convulsive disorder
convulsive episode
Cooksey-Cawthorne exercises
Cook walking brace
cookie (pad)
  arch
  Gelfoam
  navicular shoe
  scaphoid shoe
  shoe
cookie cutter
cool CPB brace
cool extension lock splint
Cooley-Baumgarten wire twisters
Cooley rib retractor
Cooley rib shears
cool IROM splint
cool TROM splint
Coonrad hinge prosthesis
Coonse-Adams technique
Cooper ankle brace
Cooper ligament
Coopernail sign
Coopervision irrigation/aspiration
  handpiece
coordinates
  stereotactic
  target
coordination, interlimb
COP (colloid oncotic pressure)
Copaxone (glatiramer acetate)
Copeland fetal scalp electrode
Copeland-Howard shoulder procedure
Copeland-Kavat classification of
  metatarsophalangeal dislocation
Coping Strategies Questionnaire (CSQ)
coplaning procedure
copolymer ankle-foot orthosis
copper wire effect
coprolalia
copropraxia
coracoacromial arch of scapula
coracoacromial ligament
coracoacromial process

coracobrachial muscle (coraco-
  brachialis)
coracoclavicular fixation device
coracohumeral ligament
coracoid notch
coracoid process
coracoid tip avulsion
coracoid tuberosity
coralline hydroxyapatite
Corbett bone rongeur
cord
  anterior horns of spinal
  anterolateral white matter of
  cervical spinal
  cervical spondylosis of spinal
  compression of spinal
  condyle
  encroachment on spinal
  fasciculi of
  fibrous
  heel cord advancement
  intramedullary spinal
  Lissauer tracts of spinal
  lumbar spinal
  medullary
  neoplasm of spinal
  oblique elbow
  pretendinous
  rostral spinal
  sacral spinal
  severely compromised spinal
  spinal
  substantia gelatinosa of spinal
  tethered
  thoracic spinal
  tight heel
  Weitbrecht
Cordase (injectable collagenase)
cord compression
cord damage
  neoplastic
  traumatic
  vascular
cord embarrassment
Cordis implantable drug reservoir
Cordis multipurpose access port
  (MPAP)

Cordis Orbis Sigma shunt valve
cordlike structure
cordotomy, percutaneous
Cordox (CPC-111)
cord portion
corduroy cloth pattern on myelogram
Core ambidextrous cock-up wrist
  splint
Core Assessment Program for Intracerebral Transplantation (CAPIT)
core, bone
core decompression
Core support
corencephalopathy
Core Reflex wrist support
Core Universal elastic knee support
Core Universal elbow support
Core Universal rib support
CorFit lumbosacral support
Corgard (nadolol)
Corin hip arthroplasty system
corkscrew dural hook
corkscrew esophagus (diffuse
  esophageal spasm)
Corkscrew rotator cuff repair system
Corkscrew suture anchor
corn
  apical
  end
  hard
  neurovascular
  plantar
  soft
  web
corneal reflex
corneal response
Cornelia de Lange syndrome
Cornell Scale for Depression,
  Dementia (CSDD)
corner fracture
corner of knee
corniculopharyngeal ligament
corn-picker's pupil
corn removal plaster
Cornwall hip fracture study
corona radiata

coronal computed tomographic
   arthrography (CCTA)
coronal craniectomy
coronal orientation
coronal plane
coronal projection
coronal scalp incision
coronal section
coronal slab
coronal slice
coronal suture
coronal synostosis
coronal view
coronary ligament
coronoid fossa
coronoid process
corpectomy, decompressive
corporal agnosia (somatagnosia)
corpus callostomy, radiosurgical
corpus callosum
   agenesis of
   central bands of
   splenium of
corpus callosum tumors
correction
   biplanar angular
   degree of
   scoliosis
   subluxation
   V-Y plasty
corrective shoe
correlates, neuroanatomic
correlation
   clinicoanatomic
   Pearson
   Pearson-Spearman
   Spearman rank
corrugator cutis muscle of anus
corset
   Camp
   elastic ankle
   Kampe
   leather ankle
   lumbosacral
Cor-Tech guidance to stereotactic
   head frame
cortectomy, parietal

cortex (pl. cortices)
   articular
   association
   bilateral orbitofrontal
   bone
   calcarine
   cerebellar
   cerebral
   eloquent
   entorhinal
   excitomotor
   femoral
   frontal
   higher-order association
   homotypical
   insular
   limbic
   mesiofrontal
   motor
   nonolfactory
   opercular
   orbitofrontal
   parastriate
   parietal
   perirhinal
   perirolandic parietal
   peristriate
   perisylvian
   postsensory
   premotor
   primary auditory
   primary visual
   pyriform
   rolandic
   sensorimotor
   somatosensory parietal
   striate
   visual
cortical activity
cortical adenoma
cortical atrophy
cortical blindness, total
cortical bone
cortical bone screw
cortical branch of middle cerebral
   artery
cortical cancellous bone

cortical cerebellar degeneration
cortical deafness
cortical defect
cortical deficit
cortical desmoid
cortical disease, advanced
cortical dysfunction, post-traumatic
cortical evoked potential
cortical function
cortical functioning, higher
cortical gray matter
cortical hinge axis
cortical hyperintensity
cortical hyperostosis
cortical infarcts, multiple
cortical intracerebral hemorrhage
cortical ischemia
cortical lesion
cortical mapping
cortical margin
cortical metabolism
cortical motor area
cortical necrosis
cortical neuronal dysfunction
cortical scintigraphy
cortical sensory loss
cortical sign
cortical signet ring shadow
cortical sulci
cortical testing
cortical thumb position
cortical transient ischemia
cortical tuber
cortical-type eye deviation
cortical versus cancellous bone
cortical vision
cortical white matter
corticated border
corticectomy
corticifugal pathway
corticobulbar fibers
corticobulbar pathway
corticobulbar tract
corticocallosal dysgenesis
corticocancellous bone graft
corticocancellous bone strip
corticocancellous strut

corticocerebellar connection
corticogram
corticography
corticopontine-cerebellar fibers
corticopontine projection
corticoreticular theory
corticospinal disease
corticospinal fibers
corticospinal motor pathway
corticospinal motor system dysfunction
corticospinal pathway lesion
corticospinal tract fiber
Cortisporin
corticosteroids
corticotomy
  Ilizarov
  percutaneous
  proximal tibia
  subperiosteal
COR/T implant
Corti organ
Coryllos-Doyen periosteal elevator
Coryllos rasp
Coryllos rib shears
Cosamine DS (glucosamine, chondroitin, manganese)
Cosman ICP Tele-Sensor
Cosman-Roberts-Wells (CRW) arc
Cosman-Roberts-Wells (CRW)
  stereotactic head frame
cosmesis
  poor
  subjective
cosmetically acceptable foot
cosmetically and functionally normal
Cosmolon closure for splint
costal angle
costal bone
costal cartilage
costal groove
costal interarticular cartilage
costal margin syndrome
costal notch
costal pleural reflection
costal process
costal sulcus
costal surface

costal tubercle
costectomy
Costen syndrome
costocervical artery
costocervical trunk
costochondral junction of ribs
costochondral junction separation
costochondritis
costoclavicular ligament
costoclavicular maneuver
costoclavicular syndrome
costoclavicular test
costocolic ligament
costodiaphragmatic recess
costolateral
costomediastinal recess
costophrenic (CP) angle blunting
costophrenic recess
costophrenic septal lines
costophrenic sulcus
costosternal angle
costotransversectomy technique
costotransverse joint
costotransverse ligament
costovertebral angle (CVA) tenderness
costovertebral articulation
costovertebral joint
costoxiphoid ligament
Cotrel cast
Cotrel-Dubousset derotation operation
Cotrel-Dubousset hook-rod
Cotrel-Dubousset instrumentation
   (CDI)
Cotrel-Dubousset spinal instrument
Cotrel scoliosis
Cotrel traction
Cottle chisel
Cottle elevator
Cottle-MacKenty elevator
Cottle-MacKenty rasp
Cottle mallet
Cottle osteotome
Cottle rasp
Cottle saw
Cotton ankle fracture

Cotton ankle instability test
Cotton-Berg syndrome
Cotton Loader position cast
cotton (or cottonoid) patty (or pattie)
   moist
   saline-soaked
CO_2 laser (carbon dioxide)
cotyloid cavity
cotyloid ligament
cotyloid notch
couch, neurosurgical
Couch-Derosa-Throop transfer
   technique
cough fracture of a rib
cough headache
cough-sneeze test
council, Foot Council of the American
   Diabetes Association (ADA)
count
   step
   white blood cell
Count a dose device
counter
   extended medial shoe
   Geiger
   heel
Counter Rotation System (CRS)
counterbore, cloverleaf
countermovement
counterpulsation, intra-aortic balloon
countersink, Synthes minifragment
countersunk
countertraction
counterweight
counting chamber, Fuchs-Rosenthal
counting-money tremor
Cournand-Grino arteriogram needle
course
   relapsing
   remitting
course of artery
course of nerve
Covaderm Plus adhesive barrier
   dressing
Coventry femoral osteotomy

Coventry staple
cover
  Accu-Flo polyethylene bur hole
  Accu-Flo silicone rubber bur hole
  pedicle
Coverlet adhesive
Cover-Roll adhesive gauze
Cover-Roll dressing
Cowdry type A intranuclear inclusion
  bodies in herpes simplex
COWS (cold opposite, warm same)
  caloric testing for vestibular function
coxa vara deformity
coxa vara luxans
coxarthria
coxarthritis
coxarthropathy
coxarthrosis, end-stage
coxitic scoliosis
coxitis
Cox multivariate regression scale
Coxsackie A viral encephalitis
Coxsackie B viral encephalitis
coxsackievirus A16
COX-2 (cyclo-oxygenase-2) inhibitor
Cowboy Collar
Cowper ligament
Cozen-Brockway Z-plasty
Cozen test
CP (cerebral palsy)
CP (costophrenic) angle
CPA (cerebellopontile or cerebello-
  pontine angle)
CPAP (continuous positive airway
  pressure), nasal
CPB (Controlled Position Brace)
CPC-111 (Cordox)
CPC-211 (Ceresine)
CP (centroparietal) electrode
  (CP_1-CP_6, CP_z)
CPM (continuous passive motion)
  device
CPM device for wrist, JACE W550
CPM exerciser machine
CPP (cranial perfusion pressure)
CPS (central pain syndrome)
CPS (complex partial seizure)

CPT (congenital pseudarthrosis of
  tibia)
CPT (Current Procedural Terminology) code
CQT (central quadriceps tendon)
crab gait
crabmeat-like appearance
Cracchiolo forefoot arthroplasty
Cracchiolo-Sculco implant arthroplasty
cracked-pot sound
cracking of joint
cradle
CT (computed tomography) scan
  head
  heel
Crafoord thoracic scissors
Craig biopsy needle
Craig splint
Craig vertebral body biopsy instrument
CRAis cryotherapy unit
Cramer wire splint
Cram test
cramp (pl. cramps)
  benign nocturnal
  calf
  heat
  leg
  muscle
  night
  nocturnal leg
  nocturnal muscle
  writer's
Crampton muscle (Bruecke muscle)
Crane mallet
Crane osteotome
Crane shoulder exercise
cranial and caudal angulations
cranial angled view
cranial anomaly
cranial arteritis
cranial base bone defect
cranial base meningioma
cranial base reconstruction
cranial bone
cranial drill set
  Hudson
  Mira Mark III

cranial growth asymmetry
cranial nerves (I-XII)
   I (first) (olfactory)
   II (second) (optic)
   III (third) (oculomotor)
   IV (fourth) (trochlear)
   V (fifth) (trigeminal)
   VI (sixth) (abducens)
   VII (seventh) (facial)
   VIII (eighth) (auditory)
   IX (ninth) (glossopharyngeal)
   X (tenth) (vagus)
   XI (eleventh) (spinal accessory)
   XII (twelfth) (hypoglossal)
cranial nerve abnormalities
cranial nerve deficit
cranial nerve involvement
cranial nerve palsy
cranial nerve paresis
cranial nerves II-XII intact
cranial neuralgia
cranial neuropathy
cranial rongeur
cranial suture
cranial synostosis surgical repair
cranial vessel
cranial view
craniectomy
   bilateral
   coronal
   decompressive
   metopic
   retromastoid
   suboccipital
cranioblade
   Acra-Cut
   Codman
craniocaudad projection
craniocaudal view
craniocervical decompression
craniocerebral penetrating wound
craniocerebral trauma
craniocervical junction
craniofacial dysjunction fracture
craniofacial microsomia
craniofacial reconstruction
craniofacial region

craniofacial remodeling
craniofacial resection
craniomandibular syndrome
craniometric landmark
cranio-orbital deformity
cranio-orbitotemporal neurofibromatosis
craniopharyngioma tumor
cranioplastic powder
cranioplasty, suboccipital
craniorachischisis
craniosacral therapy (CST)
craniosclerosis
craniospinal axis
craniostomy, twist drill
craniosynostosis
   complex
   primary
   syndromic
craniotome
   Anspach
   B5 Midas Rex
   Caspar
   Freiberg
   Hall neurosurgical
   Mira Mark V
   Smith air
craniotome blade
craniotomy
   CT-assisted stereotactic
     (or stereotaxic)
   decompressive
   emergency
   emergent
   frontal
   frontotemporal
   frontotemporoparietal
   keyhole
   osteoplastic
   parietal
   parieto-occipital
   posterior fossa
   pterional
   retromastoid
   stereotaxic or stereotactic
   subfrontal
   suboccipital transmeatal

craniotomy *(continued)*
    supratentorial
    temporo-occipital
    trephine
craniotomy defect
craniotractor
craniovertebral junction
cranium, vertex of
crank test
crash induction of anesthesia
Crawford-Adams acetabular cup
    arthroplasty
Crawford dural elevator
Crawford low lithotomy crutches
Crawford small parts dexterity test
Crawler, Maddacrawler
CRDs (complex repetitive discharges)
C-reactive protein (CRP)
creaking
    alar
    back
    distal medial
    flexion
    infragluteal
    metatarsal-phalangeal
    palmar
    PIP flexion
    popliteal
    popliteal flexion
    skin
    thenar
    ulnar
    wrist
cream, EMLA
crease
    flexion
    volar flexion
Creed dissector
creep
    cyclic (of graft)
    web
creep test
C_z reference montage
Crego elevator
Crego femoral osteotomy
Crego hip reduction
Crego-McCarroll traction

Crego retractor
Cremascoli Ortho devices
cremasteric reflex
cremaster muscle (Riolan muscle)
crepe bandage
crepitation, patellofemoral
crepitus, bony
crepuscular state
crescent-shaped fibrocartilaginous disk
crescentic base wedge osteotomy
crescentic rupture
crest
    articular
    deltoid
    ethmoidal
    frontal
    ganglionic
    gyral
    iliac
    pubic
    sacral
    tibial
Creutzfeldt-Jakob disease
Creutzfeldt-Jakob syndrome
cribriform bone
cribriform plate, meningioma of
cribriform plate of ethmoid bone
cribriform process
"crick" in the neck
cricoarytenoid joint
cricoarytenoid muscle
cricoid cartilage
cricopharyngeal achalasia
cricopharyngeal diverticulum
cricopharyngeal ligament
cricopharyngeal muscle
cricopharyngeal sphincter
cricosantorinian ligament
cricothyroid joint
cricothyroid ligament
cricothyroid muscle
cricotracheal ligament
Crile artery forceps
Crile dissector
Crile forceps
Crile gasserian ganglion knife and
    dissector

Crile head traction
Crile knife
Crile needle holder
Crile nerve hook and dissector
Crile-Wood needle holder
crimper, washer
C ring
crisis
  cholinergic
  myasthenic
  oculogyric
  parkinsonian
  spondylolisthetic
  tabetic
  Tumarkin
crispation
criteria
  Beighton c. for hypermobility
    syndrome
  Carter-Wilkinson c. for hyper-
    mobility syndrome
  EULAR (European League Against
    Rheumatoid) Response Criteria
    for Rheumatoid Arthritis
  Gage & Winter radiographic
  Garcia wrist laxity
  imaging
  Insall
  Mulholland and Gunn
  New York ankylosing spondylitis
  Salter
  WHO/LAR (World Health Organi-
    zation/International League
    Against Rheumatism) Response
    Criteria for Rheumatoid
    Arthritis
criterion-related validity of rehabilita-
  tion testing
CRN (cerebral radiation necrosis)
CROM (cervical range of motion)
cromakalim
Cronbach alpha scale
Crosby-Insall rating scale
cross-chest adduction test
cross-clamp ischemia
crossed coil
crossed hemiplegia

crossed leg/straight leg raising test
crossed reflex
crossed sciatica sign
crossed signs
crossed straight leg raising
crossfire radiation therapy
cross-irrigation of wounds
cross ligament
cross-linked N-telopeptides (NTx)
cross-linked polyethylene
cross-linked polystyrene (PET scan)
Crosslink, TSRH (Texas Scottish Rite
  Hospital)
cross-modal plasticity
crossover innervation
cross-pin, tensioned
cross-union
Crouzon syndrome
CROW (Charcot restraint orthotic
  walker)
Crowe hip scale
Crowe pilot point
crown
  Adaptic
  halo
  Unitek steel
CRP (C-reactive protein)
CRP (canalith repositioning procedure)
  to measure vertigo
CRP concentration scale
CRPS (complex regional pain
  syndrome)
CRS (Counter Rotation System)
  CRS brace
Cr,TM,Ho:YAG crystal laser
cruciate fashion
cruciate four-strand suture technique
cruciate ligament
cruciate muscle
cruciform ligament
cruciform screwdriver
crude consciousness
Cruiser hip abduction brace
crura (see *crus*)
crural ataxia
crural fascia
crural interosseous nerve

crural monoplegia
crural paresis
cruris, fascia
crus (leg) (pl. crura)
  diaphragmatic
  lateral
  left
  medial
crus phenomenon
crush injury
crushing osteochondritis
crutch paralysis
crutch walking, nonweightbearing
crutches
  Canadian
  Crawford low lithotomy
  Lofstrand
  platform
  weightbearing
Crutchfield carotid artery clamp
Crutchfield drill point
Crutchfield hand drill
Crutchfield-Raney skull traction tongs
Cruveilhier joint
Cruveilhier ligament
Cruveilhier paralysis
Cruz trypanosomiasis
CRW (Cosman-Roberts-Wells)
  stereotactic head frame
Cryo/Cuff ankle dressing
Cryo/Cuff boot
Cryo/Cuff compression support
Cryocup ice massager
cryohypophysectomy, transsphenoidal
cryolesion, brain
cryomagnet
cryoprobe
cryosurgery
cryotherapy unit, CRAis
cryostat
cryotherapy and compression
cryotherapy, liquid nitrogen
cryptococcal meningitis
Cryptococcus neoformans
cryptogenic drop attack
cryptotic medial border
crystal genesis

crystal-induced arthroses
crystal-related arthropathy
crystal-related joint disease
crystalline content of resorbable device
crystalloid
crystals
  birefringent lipid
  hydroxyapatite
  oxalate
  sodium urate
  synovial
  urate
  uric acid
CSC3 cervical support cushion
CSF (cerebrospinal fluid)
CSF absorption and production
CSF cytologic study
CSF dissemination
CSF-induced peritonitis
CSF leak (otorrhea or rhinorrhea)
CSF pathway
CSF pleocytosis
CSF serology for lues
C-shaped incision
CSDH (chronic subdural hematoma)
CSF (cerebrospinal fluid)
CSI (Caregiver Strain Index)
CSL (central sacral line)
CSM (cervical spondylotic myelopathy)
C-spine (cervical spine)
CSQ (Coping Strategies Questionnaire)
CSR (complete subtalar release)
  operation
CSSEP (cortical somatosensory
  evoked potential)
CST (craniosacral therapy)
CST (corticospinal tract)
CSTi (cancellous-structured titanium)
CT (computed tomography)
CT-based CAD/CAM revision
  femoral implant
CT bone densitometry
CT bone window photography
CT cisternogram, metrizamide
  (MCTC)
CT-derived target coordinates
CT-guided stereotactic surgery

CT-guided transsternal core biopsy
CT-guided ultrasound
CT holography (CTH)
CT imaging error
CT myelography
CT reconstruction image of skull
CT scan with contrast
CT/SPECT fusion
CT thin section
CT with slip-ring technology
CTA dosimetry
CTAB extraction
CTD (cumulative trauma disorder)
CTDx electrostimulation system
ctenoid spike (silent *c*)
C3 complement component
CTi or C.Ti. brace
CTi2 knee brace
CTLSO (cervicothoracolumbosacral
   orthosis)
CTLV (cross-table lateral view)
CTM (cervical tension myositis)
CTR (carpal tunnel release)
C-TRAX traction
CTS (carpal tunnel syndrome)
CTS (Champion Trauma Score)
CTT (central tegmental tract)
C-2 OsteoCap hip prosthesis
Cuba osteodensitometer
Cubbins screw
Cubbins shoulder dislocation technique
cubist disorder of visual perception
cubital fossa
cubital joint
cubital nerve (ulnar nerve)
cubital tunnel syndrome
cubitocarpal
cubitoradial
cubitus valgus
cubitus varus
cuboid bone (foot)
cuboideonavicular joint
cuboideonavicular ligament
cuboid squeeze technique
cuboid whip technique
cubonavicular joint
cucullaris muscle

cue, cueing (or cuing)
cuff
   air
   arm
   musculotendinous
   pneumatic tourniquet
   rotator
   side
   thigh
cuff of fascia
cuff of tissue
cul-de-sac, dural
Culler hook
Culley splint
cumulative microtrauma
cumulative trauma disorder (CTD)
cuneatus, fasciculus
cuneiform bone (foot)
cuneiform fracture-dislocation
cuneiform joint
cuneiform mortise
cuneiform osteotomy
cuneocuboid joint
cuneocuboid ligament
cuneometatarsal joint
cuneonavicular articulation
cuneonavicular ligament
cuneus
cup (see also *prosthesis*)
   acetabular
   Arthopor
   Aufranc-Turner acetabular
   Aufranc-Turner hip
   Biomet acetabular
   bipolar acetabular
   bipolar prosthetic
   Buchholz acetabular
   ceramic acetabular
   Charnley acetabular
   Continuum elliptical acetabular
   Continuum polyethylene acetabular
   Crawford-Adams acetabular
   custom-made acetabular
   DePuy bipolar
   Hallister heel
   Harris-Galante acetabular
   Hedrocel

cup *(continued)*
    heel
    hip replacement
    Integrity acetabular
    Interseal acetabular
    jumbo acetabular
    Laing concentric hip
    low profile
    Luck hip
    Mueller-type
    McKee-Farrar acetabular
    metal-backed acetabular
    migration of acetabular
    monolithic A1203
    MultiPolar bipolar
    New England Baptist acetabular
    oblong polyethylene acetabular
    Opti-Fix II acetabular
    Osteonics acetabular
    patella
    plastic heel
    porous-coated acetabular
    Press-Fit
    prosthesis
    retroversion of acetabular
    Smith-Petersen
    Sorbothane II heel
    SROM acetabular
    SROM super
    trial acetabular
    Tuli heel
CUP (cancer of unknown primary)
cup arthroplasty
cup-on-cup arthroplasty of the hip
cupping
cupula of semicircular canal
cupulolithiasis of semicircular canal
Curdy blade
curet, curette
    Acufex
    angle-tipped
    angled Scoville
    bone
    bowl
    box
    Bruns bone
    Buck bone

curet *(continued)*
    cement
    Charnley bone
    Cloward-Cone
    Cobb
    Codman spinal
    comeback
    Cone ring
    Cone suction biopsy
    cup
    cupped
    curved
    Daubenspeck
    Dawson-Yuhl-Cone
    Epstein
    Faulkner
    fine
    fine-angled
    45-degree
    forward-angled
    Halle bone
    Hardy hypophysial
    Hatfield
    hex handle
    Hibbs spinal
    Hibbs-Spratt spinal fusion
    horizontal ring
    Howard spinal
    hypophysial
    Innomed bone
    Jansen bone
    Kerpel bone
    Kerrison
    Kevorkian
    Lempert bone
    long
    loop
    Malis
    Marino transsphenoidal
    Martini bone
    mastoid
    Mayfield spinal
    McCain TMJ
    McElroy
    Meyhoeffer bone
    micro
    Moe bone

curet *(continued)*
  oval curved cup
  pituitary
  Raney stirrup loop
  Ray pituitary
  reverse-angled
  Rhoton loop
  Rhoton micro
  Rhoton pituitary
  Rhoton spoon
  Richards
  ring
  ruptured disk
  Schede bone
  Scoville ruptured disk
  Semmes spinal fusion
  short
  Simon
  spinal fusion
  spoon
  Spratt bone
  Spratt mastoid
  stirrup loop
  T-handle
  transsphenoidal
  vertical ring
  Volkmann bone
  Walker ruptured disk
  Williger bone
  Yasargil micro
curettage, intralesional
curetted
curettement
curettings
curls, towel (postoperative exercises)
current
  alternating
  direct
  pulsing
Current Procedural Terminology
  (CPT) code
Curry hip nail
Curschmann-Steinert disease
curse, Ondine
curtain pulled across visual field
Curtin plantar fibromatosis excision
Curtis-Fisher knee technique

Curtis PIP joint capsulotomy
curtsying pupil
curvature (see also *curve*)
  angular
  anterior
  backward
  cervical
  dorsal kyphotic
  flattening of normal lordotic
  greater
  humpbacked spinal
  kyphotic
  lesser
  lumbar
  normal cervical
  radius of
  stomach
curve (pl. curves)
  cervical spine
  fatigue
  flattening of normal cervical
  flattening of normal lumbar
  flattening of normal thoracic
  Kaplan-Meier survival
  King II scoliosis
  lumbar lordotic
  normal lordotic
  standardized growth
  superincumbent spinal
  thoracic spine
curved acromion
curve pattern of scoliosis
curvilinear distortion
curvilinear incision
CUSA (Cavitron ultrasonic aspirator)
CUSALap ultrasonic accessory for
  fragmentation, irrigation, and
  aspiration
Cushing basophilism
Cushing bipolar forceps
Cushing brain depressor
Cushing brain retractor
Cushing brain spatula spoons
Cushing cranial bur
Cushing cranial perforator
Cushing cranial rongeur
Cushing decompression retractor

Cushing disk rongeur
Cushing dressing forceps
Cushing dural hook knife
Cushing elevator
Cushing flat drill
Cushing gasserian ganglion hook
Cushing-Gigli saw guide
Cushing-Hopkins periosteal elevator
Cushing intervertebral disk rongeur
Cushing-Landolt transsphenoidal
     speculum
Cushing Little Joker elevator
Cushing monopolar forceps
Cushing nerve hook
Cushing nerve retractor
Cushing perforator drill
Cushing periosteal elevator
Cushing pituitary elevator
Cushing pituitary rongeur
Cushing pituitary scoop
Cushing pituitary spoon
Cushing response
Cushing retractor
Cushing rongeur forceps
Cushing saw guide
Cushing spatula spoon
Cushing staphylorrhaphy elevator
Cushing syndrome
Cushing tissue forceps
Cushing vein retractor
Cushing ventricular needle
cushion
     abduction
     Anti-Shox foot
     Back-Huggar lumbar support
     Carter immobilization
     cervical
     CSC3 cervical support
     Dry Flotation wheelchair
     FB cast
     foam
     foot
     immobilization
     Isch-Dish Plus
     lumbar
     lumbar support
     Posture Curve lumbar

cushion *(continued)*
     pressure
     pressure relief
     Roho
     Sat-A-Lite seat
     Satalite
     Sorbothane heel
     Viscoheel K
     Viscoheel N
     Viscoheel SofSpot
     wheelchair
cut
     CT
     homonymous field
     tomographic
     visual field
cutaneomucous muscle
cutaneous adenoma
cutaneous angioma
cutaneous femoral nerve
cutaneous icing
cutaneous larva migrans
cutaneous muscle
cutaneous nerve
cutaneous neural tumor
cutaneous vibration threshold
cutoff, nerve root
cutter
     A-P
     bolt
     bone plug
     cast
     Cloward dowel
     CNS pin and wire
     cookie
     cushion throat wire
     diamond pin and wire
     dowel
     end
     femoral
     Howmedica Microfixation System
          plate
     Kalish Duredge wire
     Kirschner wire
     Kleinert-Kutz bone
     Leibinger Micro System plate
     Luhr Microfixation System plate

cutter *(continued)*
    Martin diamond wire
    meniscal
    milling
    Miltex cannulated pin and wire
    motorized meniscus
    multiple action
    pin
    Questrus leading edge
    Rochester harvest bone
    Rochester recipient bone
    side
    Storz Microsystems plate
    Synthes Microsystem plate
    wire
    Wister wire/pin
Cutter cast
cutter guide
cutting jig for chevron osteotomy
cutting probe
cutting, water jet
CUWD (cold up, warm down) test
CVA (cerebrovascular accident)
    (stroke)
CVA (costovertebral angle)
CVM (cryptic vascular malformation)
C washer
C wave form on ICP monitor
C wave of cerebrospinal fluid
CWHTO (closing wedge high tibial
    osteotomy)
C-wire Serter
CW subpectoralis approach
cyanoacrylate (Superglue) adhesive
cyberphysiology
Cybertech 1000 support
Cybex back rehabilitation equipment
Cybex isokinetic test
Cybex I (and II+) exercise system
Cybex test
Cybex 320 EDI inclinometer
Cybex 340 isokinetic rehabilitation and
    testing system
Cybex Torso Rotation Testing and
    Rehabilitation Unit
Cybex Trunk Extension Flexion unit
Cybex II dynamometer

Cybex II (and II+) isokinetic exerciser
cycle
    circannual
    disordered sleep
    gait
    phase shift of sleep-wake
    sleep
    sleep-wake
    sleep-wakefulness
    sleep-waking
    walking
cycles per second (c/sec)
cyclic creep response (of graft)
cyclic loading
cyclo-oxygenase
cyclophosphamide (Cytoxan)
Cyclops syndrome (holoprosencephaly)
cyclosporine
cyclothymia
cyclothymic disorder
cyclotron
    helium
    proton
Cynosure device
Cyon nerve (aortic)
Cyriax physiotherapy
cyst
    aneurysmal bone
    arachnoid watery
    Baker
    bone
    brain
    central nervous system
    cerebral hydatid
    cervical juxtafacet
    colloid
    Dandy-Walker
    dermoid
    enterogenous
    epidermoid
    foramen magnum
    ganglion
    glial
    inclusion
    interhemispheric
    intracranial
    intramedullary epidermoid

cyst *(continued)*
   intraneural ganglion
   intrasellar Rathke cleft
   joint
   juxtafacet
   meniscal
   mucous
   neurenteric
   paraphyseal
   paraventricular
   pilonidal
   pineal
   pituitary
   popliteal
   porencephalic
   primordial
   Rathke cleft (RCC)
   rheumatoid
   sacral
   scalp inclusion
   solitary bone
   subarticular
   subchondral bone
   supracallosal epidermoid
   supraglenoid
   suprasellar arachnoid
   suprasellar Rathke cleft
   supratentorial epidermoid
   sylvian arachnoid
   synovial
   tarsal
   traumatic
   unicameral bone
   unifocal
   xanthomatous Rathke cleft
cystathioninuria
cystatin B gene
cystic brain tumor

cystic changes
cystic encephalomalacia
cystic hygroma
cystic lysis of bone
cystic osteofibromatosis
cystic sac
cystic tumor
cystic wall
cysticercosis
   cerebral
     parenchymal brain
cysticercosis cerebri
cysto-atrial shunt
cystoduodenal ligament
cystoperitoneal shunt
cyst wall
cytarabine liposomal injection
   (DepoCyt)
cytoarchitectonic abnormality
cytoarchitectonic field, Brodmann
cytochrome
cytokeratin immunostain
cytokeratin, low molecular weight
cytokeratins antibody
cytokine antagonists
cytokine, IL1-b
cytokine inhibitor
cytokine secretion pattern
cytology, spinal fluid
cytomegalic inclusion disease
cytomegalovirus (CMV) viral
   encephalitis
cytometry, flow
cytoplasm, scanty
cytotoxic leukocyte test
Cytoxan (cyclophosphamide)
Czerny suture

D, d

DA (degenerative arthritis)
D.A.C.O. brace
Dacron graft
Dacron-impregnated silicone rod
Dacron suture
Dacron synthetic ligament material
dacryocystic epilepsy
dactylitis, blistering distal (BDD)
DAF (dynamic axial fixator)
Dafilon suture
Dagrofil suture
Dahlgren cranial rongeur
DAI (diffuse axonal injury)
Dakin tubing
Dalco Astro ankle brace
Dale abdominal binder
Dale first rib rongeur
Dallas grading system
Dall-Miles cable cerclage
Dall-Miles cable grip system
DALM (dysplasia with associated
    lesion or mass)
daltons of force (SI units)
DALYs (Disability Adjusted Life
    Years)
dam, rubber
damage
    anoxic
    brain

damage *(continued)*
    cerebral
    epileptogenic cerebral
    focal
    hemisphere
    mesial frontal lobe
    myelin
    neoplastic cord
    physeal
    traumatic cord
    vascular cord
D'Ambrosia test
dammed-up CSF (cerebrospinal fluid)
dampened obstructive pulse
dampened pulsatile flow
dampened wave form
damp heat (Chinese medicine term)
dampness (Chinese medicine term)
D'Antonio classification of acetabular
    abnormalities
DANA (designed after natural anat-
    omy) shoulder prosthesis
dance medicine
dancer's fracture
dance, St. Vitus
dancing bear gait
dancing bear syndrome
dancing eyes (opsoclonus or
    opsoclonia)

157

dancing-eyes dancing-feet syndrome
dancing mania (choreomania)
Dandy clamp
Dandy myocutaneous scalp flap
Dandy nerve hook
Dandy neurosurgical scissors
Dandy probe
Dandy scalp hemostatic forceps
Dandy trigeminal nerve scissors
Dandy ventricular needle
Dandy-Walker cyst
Dandy-Walker deformity
Dandy-Walker syndrome (congenital
  hydrocephalus)
Daniel iliac bone graft
Danis-Weber classification of ankle
  fractures
Danniflex CPM exerciser
D'Antonio classification of acetabular
  abnormalities
Dantrium (dantrolene)
Darco back brace
DarcoGel ankle brace
Darco foot splint
Darco medical-surgical shoe and toe
  alignment splint
Darco moldable insole
Darco surgical shoe
Darier disease
darkfield microscopy
Darkschewitsch, nucleus of
  (also Darkshevich, Darkschevich)
Darrach extensor carpi ulnaris
  tenodesis
Darrach-Hughston-Milch fracture
Darrach-McLaughlin shoulder
  technique
Darrach procedure
dart and dome EEG complexes
DAS (double-armed suture)
DASA (distal articular set angle)
Dasco Pro angle finder
Daseler-Anson classification of
  plantaris muscle anatomy
Das Gupta scapulectomy
DASH (Disabilities of the Arm,
  Shoulder, and Hand) scale

dashboard knee injury
DAS 3 (or 4) index
data
  immunohistochemical
  morphometric
  radiology outcomes
  volumetric image
database, Clinical Care in America
  Managed Care
Daubenspeck bone curet
D'Aubigne-Postel postoperative
  function score
Dautrey chisel
Dautrey osteotome
Davey-Rorabeck-Fowler decompres-
  sion technique
David Letterman sign
Davidson-Sauerbruch-Doyen periosteal
  elevator
Davies-Colley syndrome
Davis brain retractor
Davis brain spatula
Davis coagulating forceps
Davis conductor
Davis dural dissector
Davis dural separator
Davis monopolar forceps
Davis muscle-pedicle graft
Davis nerve separator spatula
Davis percussion hammer
Davis rib spreader
Davis saw guide
Davis scalp retractor
DAVM (dural arteriovenous malfor-
  mation)
Davol drain
Dawbarn sign
Dawson encephalitis
Dawson inclusion body encephalitis
Dawson-Yuhl-Cone curet
Dawson-Yuhl gouge
Dawson-Yuhl impactor
Dawson-Yuhl-Kerrison rongeur forceps
Dawson-Yuhl-Key elevator
Dawson-Yuhl-Leksell rongeur forceps
Dawson-Yuhl osteotome
Dawson-Yuhl periosteal elevator

Dawson-Yuhl rongeur forceps
Dawson-Yuhl suction tube
Day fixation device
Day fixation pin
Day fixation staple
DayTimer carpal tunnel support
daze, patient in a
dazed patient
DB (Denis Browne) bar
DBM (demineralized bone matrix)
D.C. (doctor of chiropractic)
DC (dynamic compression) plate
DCA (directional color angiography)
DC-EEG (direct current electro-
  encephalogram)
DC-101 chiropractic table
D-Core support pillow
DCP (dynamic compression plate)
DCS (dorsal column stimulator)
DDD (degenerative disk disease)
DDFP (dodecafluoropentane) imaging
  agent
DDH (developmental dysplasia of hip)
dead arm syndrome
dead feeling
dead space, anatomical
deaf
  National Association for the Deaf
  National Technical Institute for the
    Deaf (NTID)
  Registry of Interpreters for the
    Deaf (RID)
  TeleCaption TV decoders for the
    Deaf
  telecommunication device for the
    Deaf (TDD)
Deaf-Blind Alarm Clock
deaf-blindness
deafferentation pain
deafferentation, visual
deafness
  cortical
  midbrain
  pure word
de Andrade-MacNab occipitocervical
  arthrodesis
Dean bone rongeur

Dean scissors
Deane unconstrained knee prosthesis
death
  brain
  cerebral
  cerebral brain
  suspected cerebral
Deaver retractor
DeBakey endarterectomy scissors
DeBakey forceps
DeBakey rib spreader
DeBastiani distractor
DeBastiani external fixator
DeBastiani frame
Debeyre-Patte-Elmelik rotator cuff
  technique
debilitation
debonded femoral stem prosthesis
Debré-Sémélaigne pseudomyotonia
debride
debridement
  Ahern trochanteric
  arthroscopic
  cortical
  hemidiaphyseal
  Magnuson
  periodic
debris
  bone
  calcium
  extra-articular
  foreign
  gelatinous
  grumous
  intra-articular
  joint
  necrotic
  particle
  particulate
debulk
debulking of tumor
deburring
Decadron rash
decalcification
decalcified dorsum sellae
decancellation, Ogstron-Verebelyi
decancellation procedure

decannulated
decannulation
decarboxylase inhibitor
decarboxylation of levodopa
decelerative injury
decerebrate attack
decerebrate posturing
decerebrate rigidity
decerebration, furious
dechondrification
deciduous
Decker alligator forceps
Decker alligator scissors
Decker microsurgical forceps
Decker microsurgical rongeurs
Decker microsurgical scissors
declamping
deckplate
declarative memory
decompress
decompression
  balloon
  canal
  core
  craniocervical
  laser-assisted disk (LDD)
  microvascular (MVD)
  peripheral nerve
  posterior fossa
  subacromial
  suboccipiital
  suction
  surgical
  tube
decompression fasciotomy
decompression of tumor
decompression sickness (caisson
  disease; the bends)
decompression technique
decompression tube
decompressive carpectomy
decompressive craniectomy
decompressive craniotomy
decompressive laminectomy
decompressive osteotomy
deconditioned foot
deconditioning, muscular

decorticate and decerebrate
decorticate posturing
decorticate rigidity
decortication
decreased tonus
Decubinex pad/protector
decubitus paralysis
decubitus ulcer
decussation
Dee elbow hinge
DEEG (depth EEG)
deep arch
deep artery
deep blade knife
deep-brain-stimulating electrode
deep Doppler velocity interrogation
deep dorsal sacrococcygeal ligament
deep fibular nerve (deep peroneal)
deep flexor muscle of fingers
deep hyperthermia treatment
de-epithelialized rectus abdominis
  muscle (DRAM) flap
deep lesion
deep massage
deep muscles of back
deep peroneal nerve
deep petrosal nerve
deep posterior sacrococcygeal
  ligament
deep respirations
deep-seated contusion
deep-seated lesion
deep-seated tumor
deep-shelled acetabulum
deep temporal nerves
deep tendon reflexes (DTRs)
  hyperactive
  hypoactive
deep tendon reflexes grading
  0 (no response)
  1+ (low normal, with slight
    diminution in response)
  2+ (normal)
  3+ (more brisk than normal, but
    does not necessarily indicate
    a pathologic process)
  4+ (brisk, hyperactive, clonus)

deep transverse frictions
deep transverse metacarpal ligament
deep transverse metatarsal ligament
deep transverse palmar ligament
deep transverse perineal muscle
deep vein thrombosis
deep venous aplasia
deep venous channel
deep venous incompetence
deep venous insufficiency (DVI)
deep venous occlusion
deep venous thrombosis (DVT)
deep white matter track
defecation
defecogram
defect (see also *deformity*)
    afferent pupillary
    anteroapical
    anteromedial humeral head (reverse
       Hill-Sachs)
    arcuate visual field
    bar
    bar-like ventral (in myelography)
    birth
    blood-brain barrier
    bony
    bridging of
    cauliflower-shaped
    centrocecal visual field
    chain-of-lakes filling
    chiasmatic
    chondral
    concomitant
    congenital
    conoventricular
    cortical
    cranial base bone
    craniotomy
    curvilinear
    developmental
    discoid filling
    extradural
    femoral condylar
    fibrous cortical
    field
    filling
    fixed

defect *(continued)*
    fixed intracavitary filling
    fixed perfusion
    focal plaquelike
    frontal
    fusiform
    global cortical
    hemianopic visual field
    homonymous
    impression
    inferoapical
    intercalary
    intraluminal filling
    ischemic
    linear
    lobulated filling
    lucent
    luminal
    mapping of the
    neural tube
    nonhomonymous field
    nonsubperiosteal cortical
    nonuniform rotational (NURD)
    open neural tube
    optic nerve
    osseous
    osteochondral
    parietal field
    partial homonymous field
    pear-shaped
    perfusion
    plication
    polypoid filling
    posterior-superior humeral head
    posteroapical
    postoperative skull
    proprioceptive
    protrusio
    radial ray
    reverse Hill-Sachs
    reversible
    reversible ischemic
    reversible perfusion
    scan
    scintigraphic perfusion
    segmental bone
    septal

defect *(continued)*
  soft tissue
  spontaneous closure of
  stellar
  subcortical
  subperiosteal cortical
  temporal field
  transient perfusion
  trochlear
  visual field
  wedge-shaped
  wire-related
defective response inhibition
deferential artery
defervesce, defervesced
defervescence
Defiance functional knee brace
deficiency
  Aitken femoral
  aminoaciduria
  alpha-1-antitrypsin
  arginase
  complement
  factor VIII
  factor IX
  hemispheral gaze
  mental
  molybdenum cofactor
  myopathic carnitine
  phosphorylase
  protein S
  proximal femoral focal
  pyruvate dehydrogenase complex
  sulfite oxidase
deficiency disease
deficiency fire or heat (Chinese
  medicine term)
deficit
  attention
  central language
  cognitive
  comprehension
  convergence
  cortical
  cranial nerve
  delayed postoperative neurologic
  fixed neurologic

deficit *(continued)*
  emotional
  focal neurologic
  Fränkel classification of spinal cord
    injury
  gaze
  global cognitive
  gross neurologic
  irreversible neurologic
  language
  lateralizing
  march of sensory
  motor
  neural
  neurologic(al)
  peripheral nerve function
  peripheral neural
  posterior column
  postictal
  radicular neural
  resolving (or reversible) ischemic
    neurologic (RIND)
  saddle distribution of sensory
  sensory
  space
  spinal cord injury
  spinal neural
  thalamic
deficits of ideation and speech in
  migraine
Definition PM (Pre-Mantle) femoral
  component
deflection of EEG pen
defography
deformans
  dystonia musculorum
  osteitis
  osteochondrodystrophia
  Paget osteitis
deformation, brain
deformers, active (in arthritis)
deformity (see also *defect*)
  angular
  Arnold-Chiari
  back-knee
  biconcave
  bifid thumb

deformity *(continued)*
  bone
  bony
  boutonnière
  bowing
  bull's eye
  bunion
  bunionette
  buttonhole
  calcaneus
  cavovarus
  cavus foot
  Charcot
  checkrein
  clawfoot
  clawhand
  clawtoe
  cleft foot
  cloverleaf
  clubhand
  cock-up
  cock-up toe
  codfish
  compensatory
  congenital vertical talus foot
  contracture
  cottage loaf
  coxa vara
  cranio-orbital
  cubitus valgus
  cubitus varus
  curly toe
  Dandy-Walker
  digital
  digitus flexus
  dinner fork
  DISI (dorsal intercalary segment
    instability)
  equinovalgus
  equinovarus
  equinovarus hindfoot
  equinus
  Erlenmeyer flask-like
  eversion-external rotation
  femoral head
  flatback
  flatfoot

deformity *(continued)*
  flexible spastic equinovarus
  flexion
  forefoot abduction
  funnel-like
  genu valgum
  genu varum
  gibbous
  gun stock
  Haglund foot
  hallux abductovalgus
  hallux flexus
  hallux malleus
  hallux rigidus
  hallux valgus
  hammer toe
  hatchet-head
  Hill-Sachs
  hindbrain
  hindfoot
  hourglass
  Ilfeld-Holder
  internal rotation
  intrinsic minus
  intrinsic plus
  J hook
  joint
  J sella
  Kirner
  lobster claw
  Madelung
  mallet finger
  mallet toe
  mermaid
  Michel
  neuropathic midfoot
  nondystrophic spinal
  pannus
  pectus excavatum
  pes cavus
  pes planus
  pigeon breast
  planovalgus
  plantar flexion-inversion
  procurvature
  pseudo-Hurler
  recurvatum

deformity *(continued)*
  reduction
  rockerbottom foot
  rotational
  round shoulder
  sabre shin
  scaphoid humpback
  scimitar
  seal fin
  serpentine
  shepherd's crook
  silver fork
  skeletal
  spastic equinovarus
  spastic hindfoot valgus
  splay foot
  split foot
  split hand
  Sprengel
  static foot
  step-down shoulder
  step-off
  supination
  swan-neck
  swan-neck finger
  talus foot
  thumb-in-palm
  torsional
  trefoil
  trigger-finger
  triphalangeal thumb
  turned-up pulp
  ulnar drift (motor)
  valgus
  valgus heel
  varus
  Velpeau ·
  vertical talus foot
  VISI (volar intercalated segment
    instability)
  Volkmann
  wasp tail
  wedging
  windblown
  windswept
Defourmentel bone rongeur
defunctionalization

degeneration
  Alzheimer neurofibrillary
  articular cartilage
  ascending
  atrophic
  axon, axonal
  bony
  brain
  calcareous
  cartilaginous
  cerebellar
  cerebromacular (CMD)
  cobblestone
  collagen
  combined spinal cord
  cortical cerebellar
  corticobasal ganglionic
  corticostriatospinal
  descending
  dystrophic
  familial cerebellar
  ganglion cells
  Gombault
  granulovacular
  gray matter
  great toe, Regnauld-type
  hepatocerebral
  hepatolenticular
  heterogeneous system
  Holmes cortical cerebellar
  lattice
  malignant
  Menzel olivopontocerebellar
  muscle fiber
  muscular
  myxomatous
  neurofibrillary
  Nissl
  olivopontocerebellar
  pallidal
  paraneoplastic cerebellar
  parenchymatous cerebellar
  paving stone
  photoreceptor
  pigmentary, globus pallidus
  primary progressive cerebellar
  progressive

degeneration *(continued)*
    Ramsey Hunt type of inherited
        dentatorubral
    Regnauld-type great toe
    retrograde
    rim
    sclerotic
    secondary
    senile
    spinal
    spinocerebellar
    spongy white matter
    striatonigral
    subacute
    traumatic
    Türck
    Terrien
    transneuronal
    wallerian
    wear and tear
    Zenker
degenerative arthritic change
degenerative change
degenerative disease
degenerative disk disease (DDD)
degenerative joint disease (DJD)
degenerative spine disease
degenerative spondylolisthesis
degenerative spondylosis
degenerative spur
degenerative spurring
degenerative tendinopathy
DeGimard syndrome
degloving injury
deglutition paralysis
Degos disease
degradable polyglycolide rods
degradation, in vivo
degree of correction
dehiscence
    prosthesis
    wound
Dehne three-finger spica cast
dehydroepiandrosterone (DHEA-S)
Deiter nucleus of cerebellum
déjà entendu (already heard)

déjà éprouvé (already tested)
déjà fait (already done)
déjà pensé (already thought)
déjà raconté (already told)
déjà vécu (already lived)
déjà voulu (already desired)
déjà vu (already seen)
dejection
Dejerine aberrant pyramidal tract
Dejerine anterior bulbar syndrome
Dejerine-Davis percussion hammer
Dejerine disease
Dejerine-Klumpke palsy
Dejerine-Klumpke paralysis
Dejerine onion-peel sensory loss
Dejerine percussion hammer
Dejerine-Roussy syndrome
Dejerine sign
Dejerine-Sottas atrophy
Dejerine-Sottas disease
Dejerine-Sottas syndrome
Deknatel autotransfusion system
Deknatel orthopedic autotransfusion
    system
De La Caffinière trapeziometacarpal
    prosthesis
delamination, graft
de Lange syndrome
delay
    developmental
    motor
    reflex relaxation
    regrowth
    sensory
delayed apoplexy
delayed bone imaging
delayed onset muscle soreness
    (DOMS)
delayed postoperative neurologic
    deficit
delayed transport of tracer
delayed traumatic intracerebral
    hematoma (DTICH)
delayed-type hypersensitivity
delayed union
delayed visualization

delay phenomenon
Delbet fracture classification,
    types I-IV
Delbet sign
Delbet splint for heel fracture
DeLee radiographic analysis
deleterious effect
deletion, genomic
deliberant dizziness therapy
delicate crepitation
deliriant
delirifacient
delirious
delirium
    acute
    alcohol withdrawal
    exhaustion
    febrile
    low
    senile
    toxic
    traumatic
delirium-like state
delirium tremens (DTs)
Delitala T nail
Delmege sign of tuberculosis
delivery, timed bolus
DeLorme exercises
delta activity
delta band
delta brush pattern
delta electrode
delta frequency band
delta index
delta occipital pattern
delta pattern
delta phalanx
delta rhythm
delta slowing
Deltasone (prednisone)
delta wave activity
delta waveform
deltoid branch of posterior tibial artery
deltoid insertion over joint
deltoid ligament
deltoid muscle
deltopectoral groove

deltopectoral interval
delusion, delusional
demagnetization field effect
demarcate, demarcated
demarcation, level of
demarcation line
DeMarneffe meniscotomy knife
DeMartel neurosurgical scissors
DeMartel scalp flap forceps
DeMartel wire saw
De Mayo two-point discrimination
    device
Demel wire-tightening forceps
Demel wire-twisting forceps
demented
dementia
    Alzheimer
    atrophic
    Binswanger
    dialysis
    early
    epileptic
    familial
    frontal lobe
    frontotemporal
    global
    lacunar
    multi-infarct
    paralytic
    Pick
    presenile
    primary degenerative
    senile
    subcortical
    thalamic
    toxic
    vascular
    Wernicke
Dementia Behavior Disturbance
    (DBD) Scale
dementia complex
Dementia Mood Assessment Scale
    (DMAS)
Demianoff sign
demifacets
demilune
demineralization, bony

demineralized bone matrix (DBM)
demodulator
demographic data
Demons-Meigs syndrome
DeMuth screw
demyelinating disease
demyelinating neuropathy
demyelination
  brain stem
  large fiber
  posterior column
  postinfectious
  segmental
demyelination of posterior columns
demyelinative disorder
denatured alcohol
denaturization of protein
Denavit-Hartenberg parameters
dendrite
dendritic connections
dendritic lesion
dendritic spine
denervated area
denervated muscle fiber
denervation
  autonomic
  distal
  level of
  proximal
  somatic
  striatal
  sympathetic
  zone of
denervation atrophy
denervation of muscle
dengue viral encephalitis
Denham external fixation
Denham pin
denial
  organic
  psychiatric
Denis Browne bar
Denis Browne clubfoot splint
Denis Browne talipes hobble splint
Denis Browne neuropathy
Denis Browne syndrome

Denis classification of compression
  fracture (A-D)
Denis classification of seat-belt injury
Denis classification of spinal injury
  (A-E)
Denis score
Dennyson-Fulford arthrodesis
Dennyson-Fulford extra-articular
  subtalar arthrodesis
Denonvilliers ligament
de novo mutation
dens (odontoid process of axis)
dense sensory loss
dens fracture
densitometer
  accuDEXA
  Achilles+
  Apollo DXA bone
  bone
  CT
  Cuba osteodensitometer
  DEXA (dual-energy x-ray
    absorptiometry)
  DPX-IQ
  dual-photon
  Expert-XL
  Hologic 2000
  Norland bone
  OsteoGram 2000
  OsteoView digital bone
  photon
  PIXI peripheral
  Prodigy
  Sahara portable bone
  single-photon
densitometry
  bone
  dual-photon
  photon
  scanning
  video (VD)
density (pl. densities)
  air
  bands of
  bone mineral (BMD)
  calcific

density *(continued)*
  calcified
  capillary
  diffuse reticular
  double
  echo
  fluid
  ground-glass
  hazy
  homogeneous soft tissue
  ill-defined
  increased
  linear
  metallifc
  mottled
  nodular
  patchy
  periventricular
  proton
  radiographic
  radiolucent
  radiopaque
  ropy
  soft tissue
  spicular
  spin
  tissue
  variations in
  water
  wedge-shaped
dens view of cervical spine
dental freer elevator
dental nerve
dentate fracture
dentate ligament
dentate line
dentate nucleus of cerebellum
dentate suture of skull
dentato-olivary pathway
dentatorubral degeneration
dentatorubral-pallidoluysian atrophy
dentatorubrothalamic connections in
  upper brain stem
dentatothalamic
denticulate ligament
dentoskeletal relationship

Denucé quadrate ligament
denudation, areas of
denude, denuded, denuding
Denver Developmental Screening Test
Denver hydrocephalus shunt
Deon hip prosthesis
deossification
Depacon (valproate sodium injection)
DePalma modified patellar technique
Department of Vocational
  Rehabilitation (DVR)
dependence, dependency
  chemical
  economic
  emotional
  physical
dependent extracellular fluid accumulation
depersonalization, transient states of
depiction, magnetic resonance
depiction of vasculature
depigmentation of iris with neonatal
  Horner syndrome
depigmented spots in tuberous
  sclerosis
DepoCyt (cytarabine liposomal injection)
depolarization blockade
depolarization, nerve fiber membrane
depolarization of neuronal membrane
depolarize
deposit, deposition
  calcium
  callus
  iron
  monosodium urate crystal
  spontaneous
deposition rate
depressed and compound skull
  fracture
depressed fracture
depression
  endogenous
  exogenous
  fragment
  postictal

depression *(continued)*
  reciprocal
  sinus node
  spinal cord
depression of fragment
depression of tendon reflexes with
  cervical disk disease
depressor, Cushing brain
depressor superciliary muscle
deprivation, sleep
depth EEG (DEEG)
depth electrode electrophysiologic
  study
depth gauge
depth-inlay shoe
Depth orthopedic shoe
depth-sense esthesiometry
depths of wound
DePuy acetabular liner
DePuy AML Porocoat stem prosthesis
DePuy bone cement
DePuy graft preparation table
DePuy nerve hook
DePuy orthopedic implant
DePuy Tri-Lock interlocking
  acetabular cup
de Quervain disease
de Quervain fracture
de Quervain stenosing tenosynovitis
de Quervain tendinitis
derangement
  internal
  mental
derby hat fracture
Derby nail
dermabrader
Dermacentor andersoni
Dermacentor variabilis
dermal electrodes
dermal interposition splint
dermal neurofibroma
Dermalon suture
dermatoarthritis
dermatofibrosarcoma protuberans
dermatomyosarcoma protuberans
dermatomal area
dermatomal diagram of pain

dermatomal distribution of pain
dermatomal pain
dermatomal pattern
dermatomal rash
dermatome
  Brown
  Reese
  sacral
  sensory
  Stryker
dermatome sensory changes with
  cervical disk disease
dermatomyositis
  heliotrope rash of
  intertriginous
dermatophytosis
dermodesis, resection
dermoid cyst of brain
dermoid tumor
dermometer
derotate, derotated
derotation
DeRoyal instruments/devices
D'Errico-Adson retractor
D'Errico bayonet pituitary forceps
D'Errico brain spatula
D'Errico elevator
D'Errico enlarging bur
D'Errico hypophyseal forceps
D'Errico lamina chisel
D'Errico nerve root retractor
D'Errico perforating drill
D'Errico periosteal elevator
D'Errico pituitary forceps
D'Errico retractor
D'Errico skull trephine
D'Errico tissue forceps
D'Errico ventricular needle
desaturation of color on visual test
Desault fracture
Desault sign
Desault wrist dislocation
descending motor pathway
descending tracts
desflurane
desk, Posture-Rite lap
desmalgia

desmectasis
desmitis
desmocytoma
desmodynia
desmoid, cortical
desmoma
desmopathy
desmoplakin
desmoplasia
desmoplastic
desmorrhexis
desmosis
desmotomy
Desormaux endoscope
destructive lesion
desynchronized pattern
DeTakats-McKenzie brain clip forceps
detector
destruction, bone (or bony)
destructive joint disease
destructive lesion
destructive process
destructive tumor
Desyrel (trazodone)
detachable coils
detachment, Snyder labral-biceps
detail
    exquisite
    suboptimal
detecting, collision
detection
    magnetic resonance (MR)
    occult
    quadrature
    radioactivity
    radwaste radioactivity
detection and quantification
detection zone
detector array
detector collimation
deterioration
    intellectual
    irradiation-induced mental
    mental
    mental status
    neurologic(al)
    progressive

deterioration *(continued)*
    radiation-induced mental
    rostral-caudal
    uniform
    uniformly progressive
determinants of gait
    combined ankle and knee motion
    knee flexion during stance phase
    pelvic rotation
    pelvic shift
    pelvic tilt
Determann syndrome
determination, $TCPO_2$ (transcutaneous
    oxygen)
detour conduit
detritus
Deutschländer disease
development
    cognitive
    delayed
developmental causes of limb length
    discrepancy
developmental delay
developmental dyslexia
developmental dysplasia of the hip
    (DDH)
developmental milestones of infants
developmental pathway
deviation
    angular
    carpal
    conjugate eye
    cortical-type eye
    downward eye
    dysconjugate (or disconjugate) eye
    eye
    fracture
    gait
    ipsilateral tonic
    mediastinal
    radial
    right axis (RAD)
    rotary
    skew eye
    tongue
    tonic eye
    ulnar

deviation of eyes to one side
Devic disease
device (also *apparatus*; *orthosis*;
    system)
  accelerometer
  accuDEXA bone densitometer
  Accuson 128XP ultrasound
  Accuson Sequoia
  Accu-Tron microcurrent machine
  Ace-Fischer external fixator
  Ace Unifix fixation
  ACG knee replacement system
  Achilles+ ultrasonometer
  Acryl-X orthopedic cement
    removal system
  activator table
  Activa tremor control therapy
    system
  Acufex bioabsorbable fixation
  Acufex Meniscal Stitcher
  Acumed
  acupressure ear probe
  AcuSpark piezoelectrical
  adjustable aiming
  Advance PS total knee system
  Advance total knee system
  Advantage electromyography
    system
  Advanta Orthopaedics
  Advantim total knee system
  Aesculap ABC cervical plating
    system
  Airis II open MRI system
  Albert Grass Heritage digital EEG
    system
  Alice 4 diagnostic sleep system
  Anderson fixation
  Anderson leg lengthening
  ankle disk
  anterior fixation
  antirotation
  anti-siphon (ASD)
  AO compression
  AO contouring
  Apollo DXA bone densitometer
  Apollo prosthesis
  Aquilion CT scanner

device *(continued)*
  Arthrex coring reamer
  ArthroCare arthroscopic system
  Arthrotek
  ArthroWand
  articular motion (AMD)
  assistive technology (ATD)
  Astro-Med Albert Grass Heritage
    digital EEG system
  Automator
  Auto Suture
  Axiom total knee system
  Axer compression
  BacFix system
  Back Revolution exercise
  Back Revolution stick exercise
  Back Specialist chiropractic table
  BackStrong lumbar extension
    machine
  Back Trainer spinal exercise
  Bad Wildungen Metz (BWM) spine
    system
  BAK/C cervical interbody fusion
  BAK interbody fusion system
  BAK/Proximity interbody fusion
    implant
  Bassett electrical stimulation
  Beere Precision Medical system
  biodegradable fixation
  Biofix absorbable hardware
  Biojector
  Biolectron bone growth stimulator
  Biologically Quiet stapler
  Biomet
  Bionicare 1000 stimulator system
  BioPro
  BioStinger low profile fixation
  BioStop G bone cement restrictor
  Blanchard traction
  body fat calipers
  body-powered prosthetic
  bone graft ratcheting T-handle
  Book Butler book grip
  Bovie electrocautery
  Brannock foot measuring
  Bridge hip system
  Buck convoluted traction

device *(continued)*

Buck Redi-Traction
BWM (Bad Wildungen Metz) spine
  system
Cadwell 5200A somatosensory
  evoked potential unit
Calandruccio triangular compres-
  sion fixation
Cameron fracture
Candella SPTL laser
CAPS ArthroWand
CarboJet lavage sytem
CareStair half-height step
Carpal Care exercise
carpal tunnel stretch
Carpal Trac traction
Carroll tendon retriever
CD (Cotrel-Dubousset) fixation
Ceegraph 128 electroencephalo-
  gram
centralizer
Charcot restraint orthotic walker
  (CROW)
Charnley centering
Charnley compression
Charnley external fixation
Chiro-Manis chiropractic table
closed goggle-type eyeguards
Coherent light point
collapsible internal fixation
compression screw plate
Concept ablator
Conserve hip system
Copeland fetal scalp electrode
coracoclavicular fixation
Cordis implantable drug reservoir
Cordis MPAP system
Corin
coring
Count a dose
CPM (continuous passive motion)
CRAis cryotherapy unit
cranial
Cremascoli Ortho
CROW (Charcot restraint orthotic
  walker)
CRW stereotactic system

device *(continued)*

Cybex 320 EDI inclinometer
Cybex Trunk Extension Flexion
Cynosure
Dall-Miles cable grip system
Day fixation
DC-101 chiropractic table
Denham external fixation
DePuy Tri-Lock interlocking
  acetabular cup
DeWald spinal
Deyerle fixation
diagnostic ultrasound (DUS)
DIGIT-grip
Dr. Grip
driver tunnel locator
Dunn fracture
Duracon total knee system
Durasul acetabular insert
DUS (diagnostic ultrasound
  of shoulder)
Dwyer-Wickham electrical
Dycem
dynamic external fixator
Easy-Pull sock aide
EBI (Electro Biology, Inc.) bone
  healing system
EBI SpF-2 implantable bone
  stimulator
electro-acuscope
electrocautery
Electrodynogram (EDG)
electrotherapy
Ellman International Surgitron
Encore Orthopedics
Endius spinal endoscopic camera
Endo Stitch suturing
EndoFix absorbable interference
  screw
Endopearl fixation
ENDOtec
Endotrac carpal tunnel release
  system
Enview camera
EVa HiRES motion analysis
Evershears surgical instrument
Exactech

device *(continued)*
ExerFlex ball
Exeter intramedullary bone plug
EX-FI-RE external fixation
Exogen SAFHS (sonic accelerated
　fracture healing system)
Extend total hip system
extensor
external fixation
external skeletal fixation
eyeglass-type eyeguards
E-Z reacher
F.A.S.T. 1 intraosseous infusion
　system
FASTak suture anchor system
Feather-Lite reacher
FemoStop femoral artery
　compression arch
fiberoptic intracranial pressure
　monitor
Finger Blocking Tree
5 Degree of Freedom robotic
　manipulator arm
fixating
fixation
flashlamp pulsed dye laser
FLEX H/A total ossicular
　prosthesis
Flexi-Grip exercise putty
F. L. Fischer microsurgical
　neurectomy bayonet scissors
FluoroScan mini C-arm imaging
　system
foot roller
Foundation total hip system
four-bar external fixation
4 Degree of Freedom robotic
　manipulator arm
Fox internal fixation
fracture
Freehand surgically implanted
　neuroprosthetic system
Fuji FCR9000 computed radiology
　(CR) system
Fukushima retraction system
GAIT (great toe arthroplasty
　implant technique) spacer

device *(continued)*
Gaitmat II
Galileo evoked potential electro-
　encephalograph
Gemini chiropractic table
Georgiade fixation
GIA stapler
Giliberty
Gingrass and Messer pins
GliaSite radiation therapy
GoldenEye arthroscope
Golgi
GoodKnight 318 sleep monitoring
　system
GII EasyAnchor
Gyro-Flex upper extremity
halo fixation
halo vest
halo-pelvic distraction
handgrip ergometer
Hare
Harrington fixation
Harrington outrigger
Harrington-Kostuik distraction
Hemaquet PTCA sheath with
　obturator
Hemi Sling for shoulder
　subluxation
Heyer-Schulte antisiphon
hinged Ilizarov
Hirschhorn compression
Hoffmann external fixation
Hoffmann mini-lengthening fixation
Hoffmann-Vidal external fixation
Hologic DXA
Homer-Wright pseudorosette
Hot/Ice Cold Therapy Cooler
Hough ("huff") hoe
Howmedica Universal compression
　screw
Howmedica-Osteonics
Ho:YAG laser
hybrid Ilizarov halo apparatus
ICLH
iiRAD DR1000 digital x-ray
IMiG-MRI
Imount total knee replacement

device *(continued)*

IMP-Capello arm support
Ikuta fixation
Ilizarov
implantable bone anchor
Implex
Infinity hip system
Innomed
Instron 1000
Instrument Makar
interferential stimulator
Inter Fix threaded spinal fusion
  cage
internal fixation
Interpore
Interseal acetabular cup
intramedullary fixation
INVOS cerebral oximeter
Isometer
JACE-STIM electrotherapy
  stimulation
JACE W550 CPM (continuous
  passive motion) wrist
Jackson spinal surgery and imaging
  table
Jeter lag screws or position screws
J-FX bipolar head
Johnson & Johnson
Kambin-Gellman lumbar diskec-
  tomy instrumentation
Kanavel brain-exploring cannula
Kaneda distraction
Kempf internal screw fixation
Kessler fixation
Kinamed
Kin-Con
kinesiologic testing
KineTec hip CPM
Kinetikos
Kinetron muscle strengthening
Kirschenbaum foot positioner
Kirschner
Kneed-It Kneeguard
knife/sleeve
Knifelight surgical knife and light
knot pusher

device *(continued)*

knot tier
Kronner external fixation
Kuhlman cervical traction
Küntscher traction
Kusch'kin Ace wheelchair
Lasermedic Microlight 830
LaserPen
Laserscope
Leander chiropractic table
leather lacer gauntlet
leg extension power rig
Legasus Sport CPM (continuous
  passive-motion)
leg-holding
Leinbach
Leveron doorknob turner
ligament augmentation
Light Talker computerized
  communication device
linear percussion machine
Linear total hip system and hip
  stem
Link Orthopaedics
Linvatec
lion jaw tenaculum
Lloyd chiropractic table
Luque fixation
MacKinnon-Dellon Diskriminator
  (two-point)
Magnes 2500 WH (whole head)
  imager
magnetically compatible
Mark VII cooling vest
Mark II Kodros radiolucent awl
MCAT (modular coded aperture
  technology) collimator
McLaughlin osteosynthesis
MEDmetric
Medtronic SynchroMed infusion
Meduck anesthesia monitor
Meniscus Arrow fixation
Merry Walker ambulation device
Microlight 830 laser device
Micro-Probe tip
Micro Quick Anchor

device *(continued)*
Microscribe 3DX digitizer
Micro-Z neuromusculator
  stimulator
Millennium MLC-120
Minerva neurosurgical robot
Miya hook ligament carrier
Mobilimb CPM
Modulock posterior spinal fixation
Morse taper stem
MTS servo-hydraulic testing
  machine
Mueller compression (Müller)
MultiBoot
Multifire VersaTack stapler
MultiLock hip prosthesis
Multilok hand operating table
MuscleMax electrical muscle
  stimulator
MuscleSense electrical muscle
  stimulator
nail-bending
nail-plate
Natural-Hip system
Natural-Knee II system
Nauth traction
Nautilus
NC-stat nerve conduction system
NervePace
Neufeld
NeuroCybernetic Prosthesis (NCP)
NeuroLink II EEG data acquisition
  system
NeuroMap system
Neuromeet universal soft tissue
  approximator
NexGen complete knee replacement
  components
NightOwl pocket polygraph
North Coast reacher
Novus LC threaded interbody
  fusion cage
Novus LT titaniuim interbody
  fusion cage
Obwegeser-Dalpont internal screw
  fixation
oculomotor

device *(continued)*
Olympia VACPAC back support
Ommaya reservoir
Omni-Flexor physical therapy
Optical Tracking System (OTS)
Orthion traction
Orthotron
Ortho Dx stimulator for knee
  rehabilitation
Orthofix external fixator
Orthofix intramedullary nail
OrthoLogic 1000 bone growth
  stimulator
OrthoNail intramedullary fixation
OrthoPAT perioperative autotrans-
  fusion system
orthoposer
OSCAR ultrasonic system
OsteoGram 2000 densitometer
Osteomed
Osteonics Omnifit-HA hip stem
Osteonics Scorpio posterior cruciate
  retaining total knee system
OsteoView digital bone
  densitometer
OTI
OTIS (oscillating techniques for
  isometric stabilization)
Oxford unicompartmental
Padgett hydraulic hand
  dynamometer
Parham-Martin fracture
passive traction table
Padgett baseline pinch gauge
Padgett hydraulic hand
  dynamometer
Paratrend 7 and 7+ blood gases
  sensor
Patella Pusher
PCL Pro
PCReflex infrared tracking system
pDEXA bone densitometer
PDN (prosthetic disk nucleus)
Pedlar portable stationary bicycle
Peltier thermode
Perception 5000 PC-based ultra-
  sound scanner

device *(continued)*
  Percuss-O-Matic "jackhammer"
  percutaneous diskoscope
  percutaneous electrical neurostimu-
    lator (PENS)
  percutaneous epidural neurostimu-
    lator (PENS)
  Perfecta hip system
  peripheral nerve regeneration
    conduit
  PGK (Panos G. Koutrouvelis,
    M.D.) stereotactic
  Photon Radiosurgery System (PRS)
  Physio-Stim Lite bone growth
    stimulator
  Picket Fence leg positioner
  piezoelectrical stimulator
  Pivot Pole walking
  PIXI peripheral densitometer
  Pixsys Flashpoint
  plate and screw fixation
  platinum coil
  PMT halo system
  pneumatic compression
  PodoFlex
  Polar Care ice therapy
  polycarbonate eyeguards
  Poly-Dial insert
  Polytechnic foot pressure
    measuring plate
  Poppen Ridge Sensitometer
  Posture Pulley neck exercise
  Posture Pump spine trainer
  Posture S'port
  Posturite writing board
  Power Web Jr. upper extremity
  Preston pinch gauge
  Private Practice vibration reminder
    disk
  Prodigy densitometer
  Profix total knee system
  ProtectaCap
  Pro-Trac measurement
  PSH-25GT transcranial imaging
    transducer
  QDR-1500 or QDR-2000 bone
    densitometer

device *(continued)*
  quadriceps boot
  Questus Leading Edge arthroscopic
    grasper cutter
  QUS-2 calcaneal ultrasonometer
  Quengel
  radiolucent spine frame
  Rancho anklet foot control
  Ray TFC (threaded fusion cage)
  RCB (Rotator Cuff Buttress)
  Redi-Trac traction
  Reflex exercise and rehab
    equipment
  ReflexPro linear percussion
  Reichert-Mundinger stereotactic
  Re-Lax-O chiropractic table
  REMstar Reliance CPAP
  Repose surgical system
  Response rehab and fitness
    equipment
  Rezinian external fixation
  Rezinian interbody
  RFG-3CF radiofrequency generator
  Richards lag screw
  Risser table
  RMC knee replacement
  Rochester bone trephine
  rod-mounted targeting
  Roger Anderson compression
  Roger Anderson external fixation
  Rolyan Firm D-Ring wrist support
  SAFHS (sonic accelerated fracture
    healing system) 2000
  SANS (Stoller afferent nerve
    stimulation) device
  Saunders lumbar traction
  Schiek back support
  screen plate
  screw fixation
  Scully Hip S'port hip
  S*D*sorb meniscal stapler
  Secor I (or II) drug pump
  Secor implantable drug reservoir
  semirigid carbon fiber-reinforced
    plastic plate
  sequential compression
  SergiScope robotic microscope

device *(continued)*
Servox
shock absorbent heel pad
Silverstein facial nerve monitor
Single-Day Baxter infuser
6 Degree of Freedom robotic
manipulator arm
Sleepscan Traveler ambulatory
polysomnography system
Slot distraction
SmartTack fixation
snap fit
Sock-Assist
Sofamor Danek
Sofamor spinal
Sof-Gel palm shield
Somanetics INVOS cerebral
oximeter
SomaSensor
sonic accelerated fracture healing
system (SAFHS) 2000
sonic massager
Sophy programmable pressure
valve
Sorbie-Questor total elbow system
S.O.S. total hip and knee system
SoundScan Compact bone
sonometer
SoundScan 2000 bone sonometer
Southwick pin-holding
Spectrum tissue repair system
SpinaLogic-1000 bone growth
stimulator
Spinal Stim bone growth stimulator
S-ROM modular femoral and hip
prosthesis
Stableloc II external fixator system
Stage-1 single-stage dental implant
StairClimber assist
Staodyn TENS
Sta-Peg subtalar implant
Statak
Steeper Gripper prosthetic
StelKast
Stoller afferent nerve stimulation
Stryker Howmedica Osteonics
Stryker knee joint laxity

device *(continued)*
Stryker Surgilav
Surgilav
STx lumbar traction
Sukhtian-Hughes fixation
Sulzer Orthopedic
SuperQuad assistive
Suretac bioabsorbable shoulder
fixation
Surgitome
Sutter-CPM knee
SwingAlong walker caddie
Synergy rehabilitation
Synergy spine rehab system
Synthes drill
TA-55 Auto Suture stapler
Taylor pinwheel
Tekscan in-shoe monitoring
Telectronics electrical stimulation
Telos SE ankle stress
tensioning
Thera-Band
Thera-P Bar
Therex programmable drug pump
ThermaStim muscle stimulator
ThermaWave warming device
thermocouple-controlled radio
frequency
Thermophore moist heat pads
Thermoskin arthritic knee wrap
3 Degree of Freedom robotic
manipulator arm
3M modular shoulder system
tilt board
toe straight
trampoline
Transcend total hip system
transcranial imaging transducer
triangular compression fixation
True/Lok external fixator system
TS-930 electric-powered foot reflex
stimulator
TSRH pedicle fixation
unconstrained elbow
Ulco
Ultima C femoral component
Ultra-Sling abduction

device *(continued)*
  Unidose drug delivery system
  UniPuls electrostimulation
  universal force-movement sensor
  Vac-Lok immobilization cushion
  Varigrip spine fixation system
  VariLift spinal cage
  VCS clip adapter
  Veley headrest
  Veri-Sketch
  Vernier calipers
  Versalok low back fixation system
  VersaTack stapler
  vibratome
  Vidal-Adrey modified Hoffmann
    external fixation
  Viewing Wand surgical digitizer
  visor halo fixation
  Volkov-Oganesian external fixation
  Wagner distraction
  Wagner external fixation
  Wagner leg lengthening
  Wagner-Schanz screw
  Waldemar Link GmbH
  Warm 'n Form lumbosacral corset
  Wasserstein fixation
  Wehbe arm holder
  Weil-type Swanson-design
    hammertoe implant
  WEST-foot sensory nerve tester
  WinPAD mouse pad
  Winsford self-feeder
  wood probe
  Wrightlock posterior fixation
    system
  Wright Medical
  Wrist Pro wrist support
  Writing Bird
  Xercise Band exercise
  YAG (yttrium-aluminum-garnet)
    laser
  ZD neurosurgical localizing unit
  Zenith chiropractic table
  Zickel medullary
  Zickel supracondylar fixation
  Zielke distraction
  Zimmer electrical stimulation

device *(continued)*
  Zimmer orthopedic
  Zimmer Statak suture
  Zipzoc stocking compression
    dressing and wrap
  ZTT I and ZTT II acetabular cups
device independent (DVI)
DeVilbiss cranial rongeur
DeVilbiss rongeur forceps
DeVilbiss skull trephine
devitalized soft tissue
devoid of circulation
DeWald spinal appliance
Dewar-Barrington clavicular disloca-
  tion technique
Dewar cervical operation
Dewar-Harris shoulder technique
Dewar procedure
DEXA (dual-energy x-ray absorptiom-
  etry) densitometer
dexanabinol (HU-211)
DEXA scan for bone density determi-
  nation
Dexon suture
Dexter hand evaluation
dexterity
  finger
  manual
dextroposed
dextroposition
dextrorotatory
dextrorotoscoliosis
dextroscoliosis
Deyerle II pin
Deyerle plate
Deyerle sciatic tension test
Deyerle sign
Deyerle technique
DF80 (Wilson-Burstein) hip internal
  prosthesis
DFA (hallux dorsiflexion angle)
DFI (dye fluorescence index)
DFS (distraction-flexion stage)
DGR cranial perforator
DH pressure relief walker
diabetes insipidus
diabetes mellitus

diabetic amyotrophy
diabetic Charcot foot
diabetic coma
diabetic encephalopathy
diabetic gangrene
diabetic neuroarthropathy of the foot
  and ankle
diabetic neuropathy
diabetic peripheral neuropathy
diabetic pseudotabes
Diabetic Quality of Life (DQOL)
  score
diabetic sequelae
diabetic third nerve mononeuropathy
diabetic third nerve palsy
Diabetic D-Sole foot orthosis
diacondylar fracture
diadochokinesia
diadochokinesis
diagnosis
  clinical
  differential
  empirical
  gold standard of
  noninvasive
  pathologic
  postoperative
  preoperative
  presumptive
  radiologic
  roentgenographic
  sonographic
  tentative
  ultrasound
  working
Diagnostic and Statistical Manual III—
  Revised (DSM-III-R)
diagnostic arthroscopy and
  debridement
diagnostic cascade
diagnostic procedure
diagnostic radiology
diagnostic radiopharmaceutical
diagnostic range ultrasound
diagnostic ultrasound (DUS) machine
diagonal conjugate diameter
diagram, movement

Dial Away Pain 400 electrotherapy
  unit
dial lock brace
dialysis dementia
diamagnetic shift
diamagnetic susceptibility
diametaphyseal
diametaphysis
diameter (or dimension)
  absolute neck
  anteroposterior (AP)
  artery
  bi-ischial
  biparietal (BPD)
  coil to vessel
  increased AP (anteroposterior)
  intercristal
  intertuberal
  luminal
  maximum AP (anteroposterior)
  midsagittal (MSD)
  minimal luminal
  narrow anteroposterior
  orthonormal
  sacropubic
  spinal cord
  stenosis
  transverse
diametral clearance
diamond bur
Diamond-Gould syndactyly operation
diamond nail
Diamond pin and wire cutter
diamond point wire
diamond rasp
diapering, triple
diaphragm
  muscular crus of
  sella turcica
  styloid
diaphragmatic breathing
diaphragmatic crus (pl. crura)
diaphragmatic ligament
diaphragmatic muscle
diaphragmatic nerve
diaphyseal cortical mortise
diaphyseal aclasia

diaphyseal cortical mortise
diaphyseal dysplasia
diaphyseal fracture
diaphyseal nonunion
diaphysectomy
diaphysis (pl. diaphyses)
diaplasis
diarrhea, weekend
diarthrodial joint
diarthrosis
Dias-Giegerich fracture technique
diaschisis
   cerebral
   crossed cerebellar
Diasonics
diastasis
   fracture
   sutural
   syndesmotic
   tibiofibular
diastasis of sutures
Diastat (diazepam rectal gel)
diastatic fracture
diastatic skull fracture
diastematomyelia
diastrophic dwarfism
diathermy
   Mettler Autotherm
   microwave (MWD)
   shortwave (SWD)
diathesis
   epileptic
   migraine
diatrizoate meglumine imaging agent
diatrizoate sodium imaging agent
diazepam (Valium)
diazepam rectal gel (Diastat)
DiChiara hand tray
Dickhaut-DeLee classification of
   discoid meniscus
Dickinson calcaneal bursitis technique
Dickinson-Coutts-Woodward-Handler
   osteotomy
Dickson-Diveley foot procedure
Dickson osteotomy
Dickson transplant technique
diclofenac (Pennsaid)

diclofenac potassium (Cataflam)
diclofenac sodium (Voltaren)
diclofenac sodium and misoprostol
   (Arthrotec)
DICOM (Digital Imaging and Communications in Medicine) interface
DID (document image decoding)
didactylism
diencephalic autonomic epilepsy
diencephalic herniation
diencephalic seizure
diencephalon
diet
   Evers
   gluten-free
   gouty
   high manganese
   low purine
   MacDougall
   purine-free
   tea and toast
   tyramine
dietary supplements, Phytodolor
diet for athletes, American Dietetic
   Association
diethylenetriaminepentaacetic acid
   (DTPA) imaging agent
Diethrich bulldog clamp
differential diagnosis
differential latency test
differentially abled athlete
differential pressure valve
differential variable reductance transducer (DVRT)
differentiated
differentiation
difficulty
   phrase completion
   word finding
diffraction
   beam
   high resolution
   high temperature
   x-ray
diffraction peak
diffuse axonal injury (DAI)
diffuse axonal tearing in head injury

diffuse brain dysfunction
diffuse cerebral disease
diffuse delta slowing (on EEG)
diffuse encephalopathic process
diffuse encephalopathy
diffuse esophageal spasm (corkscrew
    esophagus)
diffuse idiopathic skeletal (or sclerotic)
    hyperostosis (DISH)
diffuse neurofibroma
diffuse sclerosing osteomyelitis
diffuse sclerosis
diffuse syphilitis meningitis
diffuse thalamic projection system
diffuse tract disease
diffuse uptake
diffusion
    anisotropic
    spectral
    thermal
diffusion and perfusion magnetic reso-
    nance imaging
diffusion coefficient
diffusion magnetic resonance imaging
diffusion pulse sequence
diffusion therapy
diffusion-weighted pulse sequence
diflunisal (Dolobid)
digastric muscle
digastric nerve
DiGeorge syndrome
Digi-Flex finger exerciser
Digikit finger and toe pneumatic
    tourniquet
Digirad gamma camera
digit (pl. digits)
    accessory
    arthrodesed
    flail
    replanted
    supernumerary
    syndactylization of
Digit-Aid fifth toe splint
digital branches
digital color (color of digit)
digital equipment system
digital exertion measurer

digital flexor tendon quartet
digital fluoroscopy
digital frequency analysis
digital grasp method
digital image processing (DIP)
Digital Imaging and Communications
    in Medicine (DICOM) protocol
digital imaging of articular cartilage
digital joint
digitally fused CT and radiolabeled
    monoclonal antibody SPECT
    images
digital microcirculation
digital nerve block
digital nerve repair
digital opposers
Digital OsteoView 2000
digital parabola (toe length)
digital paresthesia
digital plethysmography
digital pressure transducer
digital radiography
digital replantation
digital roadmapping
digital rotational angiography (DRA)
digital runoff
digital signal analysis
digital storage
digital subtraction angiography (DSA)
digital subtraction rotational
    angiography
digital to analog converter
digital unraveling
digital vascular imaging (DVI)
digital videoangiography
DIGIT-grip device
digitized slices
digitized spinography
digitizer (see *scanner*)
digit repetition test
digit reversal test
Digitron digital subtraction imaging
    system
Digitron DVI/DSA computer
digit span test of recall after head
    injury
digit symbol test

digitus annularis (ring finger)
digitus medius (middle finger)
digitus minimus (little finger)
digitus primus (thumb)
digitus secundus (index finger)
digitus valgus
digitus varus
dihydroergotamine mesylate
  (Migranal) nasal spray
Dilantin (phenytoin)
dilantinization
Dilantin loading
Dilantin rash
dilatation (dilation)
  aneurysmal
  annular
  arterial
  balloon
  cavitary
  fusiform
  periportal sinusoidal
  pupillary
  sulcus
  ventricular wall
dilatation and hypertrophy
dilatation of the sulcus
dilatation of the ventricle
dilated and fixed pupils
dilated pupil
dilation (see *dilatation*)
dilator, Eder-Puestow metal olive
dilator muscle
DILE (drug-induced lupus erythematosus)
dilution curve
dilution, isotopic
dimelia, ulnar
dimension
  absolute artery
  arterial
  axial
Dimension/C femoral stem
Dimension hip prosthesis
diminished systemic perfusion
diminutive vessel
Dimon-Hughston fracture fixation
Dimon osteotomy

dimple of bone
dimple, pilonidal
dimple sign
DIMS (disorder of initiating and maintaining sleep)
ding category (mildest category of
  concussion)
Dingman bone and cartilage clamp
Dingman bone-holding forceps
Dingman mouth gag
Dingman osteotome
dinner fork deformity
diode detector
diode, infrared light-emitting
diode laser
Diodrast contrast medium
Dionosil contrast medium
DIP (distal interphalangeal)
DIP articulation
DIP joint
DiPalma shoe lift
diparesis, spastic
diphasic wave
diphenhydramine (Benadryl)
diplegia, spastic
diplopia
  central
  horizontal
  unequivocal
  vertical
diploscope
dipolar broadening
dipolar interaction
dipole
  corneoretinal
  horizontal
diprotrizoate contrast medium
dipyridamole handgrip test
direct constriction
direct current ablation (DCA)
direct current (DC) energy
direct fracture
directional color angiography (DCA)
director, grooved
direct pour of liquid nitrogen
direct visualization
dirty shadowing

Disabilities of Arm, Shoulder, and
Hand (DASH) scale
Disability Adjusted Life Year
(DALYs)
disability benefits
global measures of
learning
mobility
neurologic
partial permanent
pedal
percent of total
permanent
post-traumatic chronic
progressive
tapping tests of arm
total
Viscolas heel pain and
Disability Division of the Social
Services Administration
disabled for work
disarticulate
disarticulation
Batch-Spittler-McFaddin knee
Boyd hip
elbow
hip
knee
shoulder
wrist
disc (see *disk*)
discectomy (see *diskectomy*)
discharge, discharges
anteromesial temporal
bilateral independent periodic
lateralizing
epileptiform (BIPLED)
bilaterally synchronous
biphasic
centrotemporal
complex repetitive (CRD)
contralateral
decrescendo
dive bomber
epileptic
epileptiform burst
focal epileptiform

discharge *(continued)*
generalized epileptiform
ictal focal epileptiform
ictal generalized spike and wave
interictal focal epileptiform
interictal generalized spike and
wave
interictal spike
irregular
lateralizing
local contralateral
midtemporal
multifocal spike
myokymic
myotonic
neuromyotonic
paroxysmal
periodic lateralizing epileptiform
(PLED)
polyspike and wave
regular
rhythmical midtemporal (RMTD)
rolandic epileptiform
sharp and slow wave
spike
spike and wave
subclinical
synchronous bilateral PLED
discernible findings
discharges of adults, subclinical
rhythmical EEG (SREDA)
discission knife
discitis (diskitis)
discogenic
discogram (see *diskogram*)
discography (see *diskography*)
discoid lateral meniscus
discoid rash
discoid shadow
discoligamentous complex
discoligamentous injury
disconjugate (or dysconjugate) gaze
disconjugate eye deviation
disconnection apraxia
disconnection syndrome
discontinuity
discontinuous basement membrane

discopathy
discrepancy
  biomechanics of limb length
  leg length
discrepant intellectual functioning
discrete bleeding source
discrete blood supply
discrete lesion
discrete mass
discrete neurofibroma
discriminant analysis
discriminate
discrimination
  fine tactile
  moving two-point
  sensory
  static two-point
  Sweet two-point
  temperature
  two-point
discrimination consciousness
discriminator
discus (pl. disci)
disease (also *disorder*; *syndrome*)
  advanced cortical
  Albers-Schönberg (Schoenberg)
  albuminocytologic dissociation in
    Guillain-Barré
  Alexander
  Alper
  Alzheimer (presenile dementia)
  amyotrophic lateral sclerosis (ALS)
  anterior horn cell
  Apert
  Atton
  Azorean-Joseph-Machado
  Baló
  basilar vertebral artery
  Bassen-Kornzweig
  Batten
  Bielschowsky-Jansky
  bilateral corticobulbar
  bilateral frontal lobe
  Binswanger
  Blount
  Bornholm
  Bourneville-Pringle

disease *(continued)*
  brain stem
  brancher enzyme deficiency
  brittle bone
  Brodie
  Buerger
  bulky metastatic
  Caffey
  caisson worker's
  calcium pyrophosphate dihydrate
    crystal deposition
  Calvé-Perthes
  Canavan
  Canavan-van Bogaert-Bertrand
  carnitine palmityltransferase (CPT)
    deficiency
  carotid artery
  carotid occlusive
  central core
  central motor pathways
  central nervous system
  cerebellar
  cerebrovascular
  cervical disk
  Chagas
  champagne-bottle legs in Charcot-
    Marie-Tooth
  Charcot joint
  Charcot-Marie-Tooth (CMT)
  cherry-red macula of Tay-Sachs
  Christmas hemophiliac
  congenital disorder (skeletal
    hypoplasia)
  connective tissue
  cortical
  cortical gray matter
  corticospinal
  Creutzfeldt-Jakob (CJD)
  crystal-related joint
  Curschmann-Steinert
  cytomegalic inclusion
  Darier
  Debré-Sémélaigne
  degenerative
  degenerative disk
  degenerative disorder
    (osteoarthritis)

disease *(continued)*
degenerative joint (DJD)
degenerative spinal
Dejerine
Dejerine-Sottas
demyelinating
de Quervain
destructive joint
developmental disorder (scoliosis)
Devic
diffuse cerebral
diffuse tract
disk
distal tandem
diver's
dopa-responsive dystonia (DRD)
Dubini
Duchenne
Duplay
Eales
Ehrenfeld
Emery-Dreifuss
emotional lability following
  infectious neurologic
end organ
Engelmann
Erb-Goldflam
Erb-Landouzy
Erdheim-Chester
Eulenburg
extracranial carotid occlusive
Fabry
facioscapulohumeral muscle
  atrophy
Fahr
familial paroxysmal choreoathetosis
Farber
Fazio-Londe
fibromuscular
flareup of
Flatau-Schilder
focal demyelinating
Foix-Alajouanine
Forbes
Forbes-Cori
Forestier
Freiberg

disease *(continued)*
Freiberg-Kohler
Friedreich
frontal lobe
Fukuyama
Garré
Gaucher
Gerstmann-Straussler-Scheinker
Gilbert
glial
Goldflam
Gorham
Gowers
Greenfield
Haglund
Hallervorden-Spatz
hand, foot, and mouth
Hand-Schüller-Christian
Hartnup
hepatocerebral
hereditary multiple exostoses
hereditary striatopallidal
heterogeneous system
histiocytosis X group
Holmes cerebellar degeneration
Hunt
Huntington
Hurler
Hurst
Iceland (or Icelandic)
intractable
intraneuronal inclusion
intrauterine cytomegalic inclusion
Iselin
Jaffe
Jakob-Creutzfeldt
Jansky-Bielschowsky
jeep driver's
Joseph
Kearns-Sayre
Kienböck (Kienboeck) lunato-
  malacia
Kimura
Kinnier-Wilson
knee knob of Osgood-Schlatter
Köhler (Koehler)
König (Koenig)

disease *(continued)*
   Kümmell (Kuemmell)
   Krabbe
   Kufs
   Kugelberg-Welander
   Lafora body
   Landouzy-Dejerine
   large vessel d. of diabetic foot
   Leber
   Legg
   Legg-Calvé-Perthes
   Legg-Perthes
   Leigh
   leptomeningeal
   Letterer-Siwe
   Lhermitte-Duclos
   Lichtheim
   Lindau-von Hippel
   lipid storage
   Little
   long tract
   Lou Gehrig
   lower motor neuron
   Lyme
   maple syrup urine (MSUD)
   Machado-Joseph
   macrovascular
   "mad cow"
   Marchiafava-Bignami
   Marie-Bamberger
   Marie-Charcot-Tooth
   Marie-Foix-Alajouanine
   Marie-Strümpell (Struempell)
   McArdle
   Menkes
   metabolic bone
   microgeodic
   microvascular
   milk alkali
   milk leg
   Milroy
   mixed connective tissue (MCTD)
   Morquio
   Morvan
   motor neuron (MND)
   moyamoya
   multicore

disease *(continued)*
   multiple system atrophy (MSA)
   multisystem
   neoplastic disorder
   neurodegenerative brain
   neurologic
   neuromuscular
   neurotraumatic evolution of
      Charcot joint
   Niemann-Pick
   oasthouse urine
   obsessive-compulsive disorder
      (OCD)
   oculocraniosomatic
   Ollier
   Oppenheim
   organic brain (OBD)
   Osgood-Schlatter
   Paget (of bone)
   Panner
   parietal lobe
   Parkinson
   Parsonage-Turner
   Pelizaeus-Merzbacher
   Pellegrini-Stieda
   Perthes
   Peyronie
   phytanic acid storage
   Pick
   Pompe
   posterior column
   posterolateral sclerosis
   postherpetic neuralgia (PHN)
   Pott
   Preiser
   prion
   pseudomyotonia
   psoriatic onychopachydermo-
      periostitis
   pulseless
   Quervain (see *de Quervain*)
   Rabot
   Raynaud
   Refsum
   retinal pathways
   rippling muscle
   Roth-Bernhardt

disease *(continued)*
  Roussy-Lévy
  Santavuori-Haltia
  Santavuori-Haltia-Hagberg
  scapuloperoneal muscle atrophy
  Scheuermann
  Schilder
  Schmitt
  Seever
  Seitelberger
  Sever
  Sinding Larsen–Johansson (SLJD)
  small vessel disease of diabetic foot
  Spielmeyer-Vogt
  Spielmeyer-Vogt-Sjögren
  spinocerebellar
  spondylodiskitis
  Steele-Richardson-Olszewski
  steroid-induced bone
  Still
  Strümpell-Lorrain
  Sudeck
  Takayasu
  Tangier
  Tay-Sachs
  Thiemann
  Thomsen
  traumatic disorder
  Trevor
  unilateral supranuclear
  Unverricht
  Unverricht-Lafora
  Unverricht-Lundborg
  upper motor neuron
  vertebrobasilar
  Vogt
  von Economo
  von Eulenberg
  von Gierke
  von Hippel-Lindau
  von Recklinghausen
  Voorhoeve
  VTED (venous thromboembolic)
  wasting
  Welander
  Werdnig-Hoffmann
  Whipple

disease *(continued)*
  white matter
  Wilson
  wing-beating tremor of Wilson
  Wolman
  disease-free vessel wall
  disease-modifying antirheumatic drugs
    (DMARDs)
  disease-modifying therapy
  disease of motor units
  disease of retinal pathways
  disease specific measures of
    impairment
  disequilibrium (or dysequilibrium)
  disequilibrium state
  DISH (diffuse idiopathic sclerosing
    hyperostosis)
  DISH (diffuse idiopathic skeletal
    hyperostosis)
  disheveled appearance
  dishpan fracture
  DISI (dorsal intercalary segment
    instability)
  DISIDA (diisopropyliminodiacetic
    acid) scan
  disimpaction
  disinhibitions of a frontal lobe
    syndrome
  disinsertion of tendon
  disinterest
  disjointing
disk (also *disc*)
  acromioclavicular joint
  articular
  Bardeen primitive
  Bowman
  bulge of
  bulge (or bulging)
  cartilaginous (of epiphysis)
  cervical vertebral
  choked
  contained
  crescent-shaped fibrocartilaginous
  distal radioulnar joint
  epiphyseal
  extruded
  fibrocartilaginous

disk *(continued)*
   fibrous ring of
   fixation
   frayed
   growth
   H
   hard
   Hensen
   herniated
   herniated cervical
   herniated intervertebral (HID)
   herniated lumbar
   herniated sacral
   herniated thoracic intervertebral
   herniation of lumbosacral
     intervertebral
   herniation of thoracic intervertebral
   hydrodynamic potential of
   I
   interarticular
   intervertebral
   intra-articular
   isotropic
   locking
   lumbar vertebral
   lumbosacral vertebral
   mandibular
   massive herniated
   midline herniation of
   pale
   pallid swelling of
   protruding
   ruptured
   Schiefferdecker
   sequestered
   slipped
   soft
   tactile
Diskard head halter
disk bulge
disk bulging
Disk-Criminator sensory tester
disk disease
diskectomy (also *discectomy*)
   automated percutaneous lumbar
     (APLD)
   cervical

diskectomy *(continued)*
   Cloward fusion
   massive herniated
   Merkel tactile
   microendoscopic
   microlumbar
   microsurgical
   midline herniation of
   noncontained
   percutaneous automated
   percutaneous lumbar
   protruded (or protruding)
   ruptured
   sequestered
   sequestrated
   slipped intervertebral
   SMALL (same-day microsurgical
     arthroscopic lateral-approach
     laser-assisted) fluoroscopic
   Smith-Robinson
   soft
   sternoclavicular joint
   tactile
   temporomandibular joint
   thoracic vertebral
   thoracolumbar vertebral
   triangular
   vacuum
   vertebral
   Williams
disk extrusion
disk fragment
disk herniation
diskiform
disk interspace
diskitis
disk margin
disk material
disk matrix proteoglycans
disk maturation
diskogenic pain
diskogram, diskography (discography)
   cervical
   intervertebral
   intranuclear
   provocative
diskovertebral infection

disk plication
disk protrusion
disk rongeur
disk space, height of
disk space infection
disk space narrowing
disk to magnetic field orientation
disk water signal
dislocate, dislocated
dislocation
  anterior hip
  anterior-inferior
  Bankart shoulder
  bayonet
  Bell-Dally cervical
  Bennett basic hand
  boutonnière hand
  bursting
  carpal
  carpometacarpal
  central
  Chopart ankle
  chronic recurrent ankle joint
  closed
  complete
  complicated
  compound
  congenital dislocation of hip (CDH)
  congenital dysplasia of hip (CDH)
  consecutive
  Desault wrist
  divergent elbow
  facet
  fracture
  frank
  gamekeeper's
  habitual
  Hill-Sachs shoulder
  hip
  homolateral fracture-dislocation
  incomplete
  interphalangeal
  irreducible
  isolated
  Jahss classification of ankle
  joint
  Kienböck (Kienboeck)

dislocation (continued)
  knee
  Lisfranc
  lunate
  metacarpophalangeal
  milkmaid's elbow
  Monteggia
  Nélaton ankle
  nonreducible
  nontraumatic
  old
  open
  Otto pelvis
  partial
  patellar
  pathologic fracture
  perilunate carpal
  peroneal tendon
  posterior hip
  primitive
  radial head
  recent
  recurrent
  simple
  Smith
  subastragalar
  subcoracoid shoulder
  subglenoid shoulder
  subspinous
  swivel
  talar
  tarsal
  tarsometatarsal
  tendon
  teratologic
  transscaphoid perilunate
  traumatic
  triquetrolunate
  volar semilunar wrist
dislocation factor
dislocation fracture
dislocations of time and space
  perception
disorder
  acute labyrinthine
  apperceptive
  apraxic

disorder *(continued)*
  attention deficit (ADD)
  attention deficit hyperactivity
    (ADHD)
  autosomal dominant
  cerebral
  choreic movement
  conversion
  convulsive
  cubist d. of visual perception
  cumulative trauma (CTD)
  cyclothymic
  demyelinative
  end-stage
  extrapyramidal
  factitious
  functional
  gait
  hemodialysis-related spine
  hyperkinetic motor
  idiopathic tic
  labyrinthine
  lilliputian disorder of visual
    perception
  median nerve
  motor
  movement
  multifocal seizure
  neurogenic
  peripheral nerve
  peroxisomal
  perseverative
  personality
  pointilliste disorder of visual
    perception
  post-traumatic stress
  potential cumulative trauma
  seizure
  sleep
  sleep arousal
  somatization
  somatoform
  supranuclear disorder of ocular
    movement
  syntactical
  target

disorder *(continued)*
  thalamic
  vestibular nerve
  zoom disorder of visual perception
disorder of initiating and maintaining
  sleep (DIMS)
disorder of visual perception
disorganization, spatial
disorganized pattern
disorientation
  geographic
  right-left
  spatial
  visuospatial
disoriented patient
disparate
disparity
displaced fat pad sign
displaced intra-articular fracture of
  tarsal navicular
displacement
  brain stem
  Ellis Jones peroneal
  fracture fragment
  interhemispheric fissure
  Laurin lateral patella
  midbrain
  radial epiphyseal
  spinal column
  vertebral body
display, stereoscopic head-mounted
disproportion, fiber-type
disrupted syndesmosis
disruption
  extensor mechanism
  facet capsule
  joint
  leptomeningeal venous
  ligamentous
  syndesmotic
  transverse ligament
  traumatic
dissecans
  osteochondritis (OD)
  osteochondrosis
dissect

dissected out
dissecting hematoma
dissecting intracranial aneurysm
dissecting subcutaneous extrafascial
  infection
dissection
  aneurysmal
  arterial
  blunt
  bone
  cervical artery
  cranial nerve
  extracapsular
  extracranial cervicocephalic arterial
  field of
  finger
  fingertip
  interfascial
  intraneural fascicular
  microsurgical
  sharp
  spontaneous arterial
  spontaneous extracranial
  subperiosteal
  vertebral artery
dissector
  aneurysm neck
  Angell James
  angled
  ball
  bunion
  Cavitron
  Clodius
  Creed
  Crile
  Crile gasserian ganglion knife and
  Crile nerve hook and
  Davis dura
  dura
  Effler-Groves
  endarterectomy
  Fager pituitary
  Feild suction (*not* Field)
  golf stick
  grooved
  Hajek-Ballenger
  hand

dissector *(continued)*
  Hardy pituitary
  Herbert
  hockey stick
  Holinger endarterectomy
  Howarth
  Jannetta aneurysm neck
  Kennerdell-Maroon
  Kleinert-Kutz
  Kocher
  Lewin bunion
  MacDonald
  Malis
  Marino transsphenoidal
  Maroon-Jannetta
  micro
  Milligan
  nerve root
  Oldberg
  Olivecrona dura
  Penfield (No. 1, 2, 3, 4, 5)
  pituitary
  Rayport dural and knife
  Rhoton ball
  Rhoton spatula
  Rochester lamina
  round
  Schmieden-Taylor
  Scoville
  sesamoidectomy
  Smithwick
  spatula
  suction
  teardrop
  Toennis-Adson
  Toennis dura
  transsphenoidal
  West hand
  Woodson
  Yasargil micro
disseminated disease
disseminated sclerosis
disseminated tuberculosis
disseminated-type pigmented
  villonodular synovitis
dissipate
dissociated (ataxic) nystagmus

dissociated sensory loss
dissociation
    albumino-cytologic (in Guillain-
      Barré)
    scapholunate
    segmental sensory
dissociative state
distal Akin phalangeal osteotomy
distal articular set angle (DASA)
distal branches
distal denervation
distal humeral physeal separation
distal interphalangeal (DIP) joint
distal L osteotomy
distally
distal medial crease
distal oblique osteotomy
distal phalanx, duplicated
distal phocomelia
distal radioulnar articulation
distal radioulnar joint
distal tandem disease
distal third of shaft
distal tibial physes
distal ulna ballottement
distalward
distance
    intercaudate
    interelectrode
    interlaminar
    internuclear
    interopercular
    interorbital
    interpedicular
    interpediculate
    interridge
    interspinous
distant metastases
distend
distended
distensibility
distensible
distention, hydraulic
disto-occlusal
distorted synaptic input
distortion
    curvilinear

distortion *(continued)*
    geometric
    image
    spatial
    visual-spatial
distortion trauma
distract, distracting
distractibility
    easy
    heightened
distractible
distraction
    callus
    fracture fragment
    hyperflexion injury
    joint
    mechanical
    physeal
    segment
    small step
    soft tissue
    transpedicle
distraction bar
distraction-flexion stage (DFS)
distraction frame
distraction gap
distraction hyperflexion injury
    congenitally short metatarsal
distraction osteogenesis
distraction phase
distractor
    Acufex ankle
    Anderson
    Bliskunov implantable femoral
    DeBastiani
    femoral
    Ilizarov
    Kessler metacarpal
    Monticelli-Spinelli
    Orthofix M-100
    Pinto
    Santa Casa
    turnbuckle
    Wagner
distribution
    anatomic
    anomalous

distribution *(continued)*
　centrilobular
　diffuse
　field of
　glovelike
　infarct
　lateral
　lateralized
　mottled
　myotomal
　onion skin
　regional
　rimlike calcium
　stocking
　stocking glove
　stocking-like
　uniform
distribution of activity
disturbance
　articulation
　cognitive
　endocrine
　focal neurologic
　functional
　gait
　high level perceptual
　oculomotor
　sphincter
　visual
　visual field
　disturbed ion homeostasis
disturbed orientation
disuse
　demineralization from
　lesser atrophy of
disuse atrophy
disuse osteoporosis
dive bomber discharges on
　electromyogram
dive bomber sound on electro-
　myography
divergence, ocular
divergent dislocation
diverging collimator
diver paralysis
diving reflex
divisional block

divisionary line
divot
Divry-van Bogaert familial cortico-
　meningeal angiomatosis
Dix-Hallpike maneuver
dizziness, orthostatic
dizzy
DJD (degenerative joint disease)
DMA (distal metatarsal angle)
DMARDs (disease-modifying anti-
　rheumatic drugs)
DMD (Duchenne muscular dystrophy)
DMD gene
DMD phenotype
DMI orthopedic bed
dMRI (dynamic magnetic resonance
　imaging)
DNA flow cytometry
DNA index
DNA ploidy pattern
D.O. (doctor of osteopathy)
DOA (diagnostic and operative
　arthroscopy)
Doane knee retractor
docility
Dockery procedure
doctor of chiropractic (D.C.)
doctor of osteopathy (D.O.)
doctor of podiatric medicine (D.P.M.)
doctor of podiatry (D.P.)
Doctor's First Report of Injury
doctrine, Monro-Kellie
dodecafluoropentane (DDFP) imaging
　agent
DOES (disorders of excessive sleep)
doffing prosthesis (taking it off)
dog ear
Dohn-Carton brain retractor
Dohrmann-Rubin cannula
dolichocephaly
dolichoectasia, vertebrobasilar
dolichoectatic dissecting aneurysm
dolichostenomelia
Doll trochanteric reattachment
　technique
doll's eye reaction
doll's eye reflex

doll's eyes
doll's eye sign
doll's head maneuver
dolorimeter
dome
    anterior talar
    shoulder
    talar
    weightbearing acetabular
dome of aneurysm
dome osteotomy
Domen laminoplasty
dome proximal tibial osteotomy
dome screw
dome to neck ratio of aneurysm
domiciliary setting
dominance
    cerebral
    lack of clear-cut cerebral
    left hemisphere
    left/right hemisphere
    mixed cerebral
    right hemisphere
dominant hemisphere lesion
dominant sinus
dominant waking frequency
DOMS (delayed-onset muscle
    soreness)
Donaghy angled suture needle holder
donation, preoperative autologous
    blood
Donati suture
DonJoy Gold Point knee brace
DonJoy knee splint
DonJoy Quadrant shoulder brace
DonJoy Ultrasling shoulder
    immobilizer
DonJoy Universal ankle brace
DonJoy wrist splint
donning (putting on) prosthesis
donor site morbidity
donor team
donut support brace
Dooley nail
doorbell sign
dopa-decarboxylase
dopamine

dopamine agonist
dopamine D1 agonist
dopamine D2 receptor
dopamine energy neurons
dopamine levels in corpus striatum
dopaminergic-cholinergic balance
dopaminergic receptor
dopaminergic system
dopamine transporter
dopa-responsive dystonia (DRD)
Dopascan injection
Doplette monitor
Doppler
    color flow
    continuous wave
    contrast-enhanced
    duplex
    duplex B-mode
    gray scale
    pocket
    pulsed-wave
    range-gated pulsed
    range-gated transcranial
    real-time
    transcranial
Doppler ankle systolic pressure
Doppler blood flow monitor
Doppler blood flow velocity signal
Doppler blood pressure
Doppler calf systolic pressure
Doppler color flow mapping
Doppler color spectral analysis
Doppler flowmetry
Doppler flow probe study
Doppler flow signal
Doppler imaging
Doppler insonation
Doppler Intra-Dop intraoperative
    device
Doppler laser flowmetry
Doppler phenomenon
Doppler pulse
Doppler real-time two-dimensional
Doppler Resistive Index (DRI)
Doppler shift principle
Doppler signal enhancers
Doppler spectral analysis

Doppler spectral waveform analysis
Doppler study
Doppler thigh systolic pressure
Doppler tissue imaging (DTI)
Doppler ultrasonic blood flow detector
Doppler ultrasonic velocity detector
Doppler ultrasonography
Doppler ultrasound, high frequency
  (HFD)
Doppler ultrasound segmental blood
  pressure testing
Doppler venous examination
Doppler waveform analysis
dopey feeling (also dopy)
Doral (quazepam)
Dorello canal
Dorrance hand prosthesis
dorsal aponeurotic expansion hood
dorsal calcaneocuboid ligament
dorsal capsulodesis
dorsal carpal capsulitis
dorsal carpal ligament
dorsal carpometacarpal ligament
dorsal closing wedge metatarsal
  osteotomy
dorsal cochlear nucleus
dorsal column stimulator (DCS)
dorsal cuboideonavicular ligament
dorsal cuneocuboid ligament
dorsal cuneonavicular ligament
dorsal digital nerves
dorsal intercalated segment instability
dorsal interosseous muscles
dorsal interosseous nerve
dorsalis pedis fasciocutaneous flap
dorsalis pedis pulse
dorsal lateral cutaneous nerve
dorsal medial cutaneous nerve
dorsal medial nucleus of the thalamus
dorsal medulla
dorsal metacarpal ligament
dorsal metatarsal ligament
dorsal muscles
dorsal nerve
dorsal nucleus of vagus
dorsal pedal bypass
dorsal pedal pulse

dorsal position
dorsal proximal synovial recess
dorsal radiocarpal ligament
dorsal ramus of spinal nerve
dorsal recumbent position
dorsal root entry zone (DREZ) lesion
dorsal root ganglia (DRG)
dorsal root rhizotomy
dorsal rotation flap
dorsal sacrococcygeal muscle
dorsal sacroiliac ligament
dorsal scapular nerve
dorsal spine (D1-D12)
dorsal spinocerebellar tracts
dorsal subaponeurotic space
dorsal subcutaneous space
dorsal talonavicular ligament
dorsal transposition flap
dorsal wing fracture
dorsal wrist ligament
dorsalis pedis
dorsalis pedis myofascial flap
dorsalis pedis pulse
dorsalis tabes
dorsalward
Dorsey dural separator
Dorsey separator
Dorsey ventricular cannulas
dorsiflexed
dorsiflexion
  active
  neutral
  passive
dorsiflexor
dorsiflexion stop brace
dorsiflexion torque
dorsoanterior
dorsocephalad
dorsolateral and medial capsulotomy
dorsomedial incision
dorsopalmar translation
dorsoplantar talonavicular angle
dorsoplantar view
dorsoposterior
dorsoradial
dorsorostral
dorsum sellae

dose volume relationship
Dostinex (cabergoline)
dothiepin HCl (Prothiaden)
double anterior horn sign
double arthrodesis
double athetosis
double-bladed knife
double bubble flushing reservoir
double bundle PCL reconstruction
  technique
double camelback sign
double clamping
double consecutive coma of epidural
  hematoma
double contrast arthrography
double contrast laryngography
double contour
double crush syndrome
double dose delay (DDD)
double dose gadolinium imaging
double drape
double echo three-point Dixon method
  fat suppression
double fracture
double hemiplegia
double hollow nail
double-jointed
double leg raise test
double leg stance phase of gait
double-looped semitendinosus gracilis
  graft
double lumen sign
double minute chromosomes
double pearl-face hip joint
double photon absorptiometry (DPA)
double simultaneous sensory
  stimulation
double simultaneous stimulation
  tactile
  visual
double spin-echo proton spectroscopy
double stem silicone lesser MP
  implant
double strand, intracellular DNA
double-threaded Herbert screw
Dougados Functional Index
doughnut, foam

doughnut magnet
Douglas ligament
Douglas skin graft
douloureux, tic (trigeminal neuralgia)
Dow Corning Wright prosthesis
dowager's hump
dowel, doweling
  bone
  bone bank
  calf bone
  cylindrical
  graft
  iliac
  iliac crest
dowel arthrodesis
dowel cutters, Cloward
dowel graft technique
doweling spondylolisthesis technique
dowel spinal fusion
Dowling intracranial cyst removal
  technique
downbeat (downbeating) nystagmus
Down epiphyseal knife
Down syndrome
Downey hemilaminectomy retractor
Downey object recognition stereognosis test
Downey texture discrimination test
downgoing toes
Downing cartilage knife
Downing retractor
Down syndrome
doxacurium chloride (Nuromax)
doxepin (Sinequan)
doxorubicin (Adriamycin)
doxycycline (Vibramycin)
Doyen bone mallet
Doyen costal rasp
Doyen cylindrical drill
Doyen rib elevator or rasp
Doyen spherical bur
Doyle Combo nasal airway splint
Doyle Shark nasal splint
DPA (double [or dual] photon absorp-
  tiometry)
DQOL (Diabetic Quality of Life)
  score

DRA (digital rotational angiography)
DRA (distal reference axis)
draggy, feeling (or draggy feeling)
Dragstedt skin graft
drain
    Becker external
    Charnley suction
    Davol
    external ventricular (EVD)
    Hemovac
    Hemovac Hydrocoat
    Heyer-Schulte wound
    Jackson-Pratt
    lumbar
    monofilament nylon
    Nélaton rubber tube
    nylon threads as
    Penrose
    rubber
    Shirley
    Silastic drip
    spinal
    suction
    Surgivac
    ventriculoperitoneal
    ventriculostomy
    wound
    Wound-Evac
drainage
    fish mouth
    leptomeningeal venous
    lumbar
    mucopurulent
    purulent
    ventricular
Drake aneurysm clip
Drake scale
DRAM (de-epithelialized rectus
    abdominis muscle) flap
drape
    adhesive
    double
    fenestrated
    foot
    head
    impervious
    Ioban Vi-Drape

drape *(continued)*
    isolation
    lint-free
    Loban adhesive
    NeuroDrape surgical
    Opmi microscope
    Opraflex incise
    plastic
    povidone-iodine (Betadine)
        impregnated
    3M skin
draped out
Draw a Bicycle test
Draw a Flower test
Draw a House test
Draw a Person test
drawer sign (at ankle or knee)
drawn ankle clonus
DRD (dopa-responsive dystonia)
dream, dreaming
dreamless sleep
dreamy state
Drennan metaphyseal-epiphyseal angle
Dressinet netting bandage
dressing (see also *bandage*; *packing*)
    ABD
    ABD pad
    ACU-derm wound
    Adaptic
    Aeroplast
    Allevyn
    Aquaphor
    Aquasorb hydrogel
    Avitene "flour"
    Betadine
    Bioclusive transparent
    bulky
    Bunnell
    calcium alginate
    Coban
    cold compressive
    collagen-alginate wound
    collodion
    Comfeel Ulcus occlusive
    compression wrap
    compressive
    Conform

dressing *(continued)*
  corrective soft
  cotton
  Covaderm Plus adhesive barrier
  Coverlet adhesive surgical
  Cover-Roll adhesive gauze
  Cryo/Cuff ankle
  dry
  DuoDerm
  elastic salve
  elasticized gauze
  Elastikon
  Elastomull
  Elastoplast
  EndoAvitene
  Esmarch
  Fabco gauze bandage
  Fellonet ointment gauze
  felt
  figure of 8 (or figure 8)
  Flexinet
  fluff
  foam gauze
  4 x 4 gauze
  Fuller shield
  Furacin gauze
  gauze
  Glasscock ear
  hydrogel
  hydrophilic powder
  Inerpan flexible burn
  iodoform gauze
  Jelonet (paraffin-soaked tulle)
  Jones
  Kalginate calcium alginate
  Kaltostat
  Kerlix
  Kling adhesive
  Koch-Mason
  Lyofoam
  Microfoam
  Mills
  Mitraflex SC sacral
  modified Robert Jones
  moleskin
  moleskin strips

dressing *(continued)*
  Mother Jones (modified Robert
    Jones)
  Multidex hydrophilic powder
  nonadherent gauze
  Nu Gauze
  O'Donoghue
  occlusive
  Op-Site
  Owen gauze
  palm-to-axilla
  patch
  pledget
  Polyderm hydrophilic polyurethane
    foam
  polyurethane foam (PFD)
  pressure
  Reston
  rigid
  Robert Jones
  Schanz
  silk mesh gauze
  Snugs
  Sof-Rol
  Sof-Wick
  soft bulky
  stent
  sterile
  Steri-Strips
  Stimson
  Suture-Self
  SyringeAvitene
  Tegaderm
  Telfa gauze
  toe-to-groin modified Jones
  T strap in single-bar ankle brace
  Tubex gauze
  Tubigrip
  Velpeau
  Vigilon
  Webril
  wet-to-dry
  wide-mesh petroleum gauze
  Xeroform gauze
dressing and bathing ability
dressing apraxia

Dreyer formula
Dreyer test
DREZ (dorsal root entry zone) lesion
DREZ modification of Eriksson
  technique
DREZ-otomy, microsurgical
DREZ procedure
DRG (dorsal root ganglia)
Dr. Grip writing devices
Driessen hinged plate
drift, drifting
  arm
  eye
  finger pursuit
  finger-to-nose exam
  leg
  medial metatarsal
  navicular
  pronator
  ulnar
drill, drilling
  Acra-Cut wire pass
  Adson twist
  air
  air-powered cutting
  Anspach power
  archimedean hand
  battery-driven hand
  biflanged
  Black and Decker
  bone
  Bosworth
  brace
  Bunnell hand
  cannulated
  Cebotome
  Cement Eater
  centering
  cervical
  Championnière bone
  Charnley centering
  Charnley femoral condyle
  Cherry-Austin
  Children's Hospital hand
  chuck
  Cloward
  Coballoy twist

drill *(continued)*
  Codman wire pass
  Collison
  cortex
  cortical
  cranial
  Crutchfield hand
  Cushing flat
  Cushing perforator
  D'Errico perforating
  dental
  Elan-E power
  femoral condyle
  fingernail
  flat
  flex
  Gray
  Hall air
  Hall large bore
  Hall Micro E
  Hall Surgairtome
  Hall Versipower
  hand
  hand-operated
  high-speed twist
  hip fracture compaction
  Hudson brace
  Hudson cranial
  Kirschner hand
  Kirschner wire
  Küntscher (Kuentscher)
  Mam
  Mathews hand
  McKenzie perforating twist
  Micro-Aire
  microsurgery
  Mira Mark III cranial
  Moore hand
  Osteone air
  otologic
  patellar
  Pease bone
  penetrating
  Penn fingernail
  perforating twist
  Phoenix cranial
  Pilot

drill *(continued)*
  pneumatic
  Ralk hand
  Raney cranial
  Raney perforator
  right-angle dental
  Shea
  Smedberg hand
  Smedberg twist
  Smith automatic perforator
  Smith cranial
  spiral
  step
  Stille bone
  Stille cranial
  Stille hand
  Stille-Sherman bone
  Stryker microsurgery
  subchondral
  Synthes
  Toti trephine
  Treace
  trephine
  Trinkle
  twist
  wire
  wire pass
  Xomed
  Zimmer hand
drill bit
  cannulated
  hip fracture compaction
  Howmedica Microfixation System
  Leibinger Micro System
  Luhr Microfixation System
  Storz Microsystems
  Synthes Microsystem
drill bushing
drill flat
drill guide
  ACL (anterior cruciate ligament)
  Adson
  neutral and load
drill hole
drill point
  cannulated
  carbon steel

drill point *(continued)*
  Crutchfield
  Raney-Crutchfield
  Stille
drill points, burs, and trephine
drill/reamer, Micro-Aire
drill set, Hudson cranial
drive
  Jacobs chuck
  worm
driven equilibrium imaging
driver
  blade plate
  bullet
  Flatt
  Hall
  Harrington hook
  Jewett
  K-wire
  Küntscher (Kuentscher) nail
  Linvatec
  Lloyd nail
  Massie
  Micro Series wire
  nail
  Orthoairtome wire
  Paramax angled
  plate
  power
  prosthesis
  staple
  supine position
  Sven-Johansson
  Teflon-coated
driver-bender-extractor, Rush
driver-extractor
  Hansen-Street
  Ken
  McReynolds
  Sage
  Schneider
  Zimmer
driving, photic
driving response
Dr. Joseph's Original Footbrush
dromedary gait
dronabinol (Compassia)

drooling
droop, facial
droopy shoulder thoracic outlet
  syndrome
drop
  foot
  navicular
  wrist
drop arm test
drop attack, akinetic
drop finger
dropfoot
dropfoot gait
drop Lasègue sign
droplets, lipid
dropout, neuronal
drowsiness
  excessive daytime
  postictal
  state of
  transition to
drowsy feeling
drug delivery pump system (see *pump*)
drug delivery system, DUPEL
  iontophoretic
drug holiday, therapeutic
drug-induced lupus erythematosus
  (DILE)
drug-induced nystagmus
drug-induced parkinsonism
drugs (see also *medications*)
  absorption of
  addictive potential of
  administration of
  adrenergic
  aerosolized
  alternate-day steroids
  aminoglycoside
  amphetamine
  analgesic
  anaphylactic
  anesthetic
  antianxiety
  antibiotic
  anticholinergic
  anticonvulsant
  antidepressant

drugs *(continued)*
  antidote for overdose
  antiemetic
  antifungal
  anti-infective
  anti-inflammatory
  antimetabolite
  antineoplastic
  antiparkinsonian
  antipruritic
  antipsychotic
  antipyretic
  antiseizure
  antiseptic
  antispasmodic
  antitussive
  antiviral
  antiyeast
  anxiolytic
  bactericidal
  bacteriostatic
  barbiturate
  barbiturate hypnotic
  benzodiazepine
  beta blocking
  blood screen for
  branched chain amino acids
    (BCAA)
  broad-spectrum antibiotic
  calcium channel blocking
  CNS-stimulating (central nervous
    system)
  cephalosporin
  chemotherapy
  cholinergic
  combination
  corticosteroid
  CR (controlled release)
  curare-like
  dextrorotatory
  disease-modifying antirheumatic
    (DMARDs)
  disinfectant
  diuretic
  emergency
  epidural anesthetic
  fibrinolytic agents

drugs *(continued)*
    fractionalized fish oil
    general anesthetic
    gold salts
    half-life of
    heterocyclic antidepressant
    high-dose
    hydantoin
    hypnotic
    ICV (intracerebroventricular)
        administration of
    illicit
    inhalation of
    insomnia
    intolerance of
    intracavitary chemotherapy
    intradiscal
    intramuscular (IM)
    intranasal
    intrathecal
    intratumoral chemotherapy
    intravenous (IV)
    investigational
    isomer
    LA (long-acting)
    levorotatory
    loading dose of
    local anesthetic
    maintenance dose of
    MAO (monoamine oxidase)
        inhibitor
    monoclonal antibody
    monocyclic antidepressant
    muscle relaxant
    musculoskeletal relaxant
    naphthylalkalone
    narcotic
    narcotic agonist
    narcotic analgesic
    narcotic antagonist
    neuroleptic
    neurological
    neuromuscular blocking
    neuroprotector
    nonbarbiturate hypnotic
    non-narcotic analgesic

drugs *(continued)*
    nonsteroidal anti-inflammatory
        (NSAIDs)
    nootropics
    oral
    over-the-counter (OTC)
    peak and trough levels of
    peak level of
    peripheral vasodilating
    phenothiazine
    placebo
    prescription
    prophylactic
    psychiatric
    psychotic
    SA (sustained action)
    salicylate
    sedative
    sedative/hypnotic
    skeletal muscle relaxant
    SL (sublingual)
    slow-release (SR)
    spinal anesthetic
    SR (slow release, sustained release)
    stepwise increase in dosage of
    steroid
    succinimide
    sulfa
    sulfonamide (sulfa)
    sustained release (SR)
    systemic
    tapering doses of
    tetracyclic antidepressant
    tetracycline
    therapeutic effects of
    therapeutic index of
    titrated dose of
    tolerance of
    topical
    topical antiviral
    toxic effects of
    tranquilizer
    tricyclic antidepressant
    trough level of
    vasoconstrictor
    vasodilating
    vasopressor

drug-seeking behavior
drug-withdrawal seizure
DRUJ (distal radioulnar joint)
　prosthesis
Drummond button
Drummond hook holder
Drummond wire technique
drunken sailor gait
Dry Flotation wheelchair cushion
dry gangrene
dryness (Chinese medicine term)
Dryspell cast cover
Drytex RocketSoc ankle brace
DSA (digital subtraction angiography)
　frameless stereotaxic
　intra-arterial
　intravenous
DSC (dynamic susceptibility contrast)
　MR imaging
DSI (dynamic stability index)
DSI camera
DSP Micro Diamond-Point micro-
　surgery instruments
DST&G (doubled semitendinosus and
　gracilis) autograft
DTICH (delayed traumatic intracere-
　bral hemorrhage)
DTRs (deep tendon reflexes)
DTs (delirium tremens)
DTT (dynamic transverse traction)
　screw
dual-channel stimulator
dual energy x-ray absorptiometry
　(DEXA) scan
Dualer inclinometer
Dualer Plus system
dual-head gamma camera system
dual-head SPECT
dual-isotope scanning
dual-isotope single-photon emission
　CT
dual-lock hip prosthesis
dual-lock total hip replacement system
dual-photon absortiometry (DPA)
dual-photon densitometry test for
　osteoporosis
dual x-ray absorptiometry (DXA)

Duane retraction syndrome
Dubecq-Princeteau angulating needle
　holder
Dubini chorea
Dubini disease
Duchenne-Aran spinal muscular
　atrophy
Duchenne-Erb palsy
Duchenne muscular dystrophy (DMD)
　duck waddle gait in
　wasp tail deformity in
Duchenne sign
duck gait
duck waddle gait
duck waddle test
duct, aberrant
ductal architecture
ductal carcinoma in situ (DCIS)
ductal constriction
ductal dilatation
ductal ectasia
ductal epithelial hyperplasia
ductal hyperplasia
ductal pattern
ductal remnant
ductular
ductule
Dudley Morton syndrome
Dugas test
dull trocar
Dumbach cranial titanium mesh
dumbbell neurofibroma tumor
dumbbell schwannoma
dumbbell-shaped shadow on x-ray
dumbbell tumor
dumbbell-type neuroblastoma
Duncan prone rectus test
Dunlop-Shands view
Dunlop traction
Dunn-Brittain foot stabilization
　technique
Dunnet two-sided test
Dunn fracture device
Dunn-Hess trochanteric osteotomy
Dunn hip procedure
Duo-Cline bed wedge
DuoDerm dressing

Duo-Driv screw
Duografin contrast medium
Duo-Lock
Duopress guide
Dupaco knee control
DUPEL iontophoretic drug delivery
    system
Duplay disease
duplex Doppler scan
duplex Doppler sonography (DS)
duplex imaging, color flow
duplex pulsed-Doppler sonography
duplex scan, color flow
duplex screening test
duplex ultrasound
duplicated distal phalanx
duplicated metacarpal
duplicated proximal phalanx
DuPont CRONEX x-ray film
DuPont Rare Earth Imaging System
Dupré muscle
Dupuytren contracture release
Dupuytren fasciitis
Dupuytren fracture
dura
    attenuated
    bulging
    clival
    freeze-dried
    lyophilized
Duracon prosthesis
Duracon total knee system
Duract (bromfenac sodium)
Dura-Flex back brace
DuraGen absorbable dural graft matrix
Dura-Kold wrap
dural arteriovenous fistula
dural arteriovenous malformation
        (DAVM)
    classic
    extrasinusal-type
    sinusal-type
dural attachment
dural collar
dural dissector and knife
dural elevator
dural fold

dural guard
dural hook
dural hook knife
dural impingement
dural leaf or leaflet
Duraloc acetabular liner
dural puncture
dural retractor
dural ring
dural root pouches
dural sac
dural scar
dural scissors
dural separator
dural separator spatula
dural sheath
dural sinus thrombosis (DST)
dural tear
dural trail sign
dural venous sinus thrombosis
dura mater of the brain
dura mater of the spinal cord
Duran-Houser wrist splint
Duran passive mobilization
Duran regimen
Durapatite bone replacement material
duraplasty, decompressive
DuraPrep
Durasul acetabular insert
Duray-Read gouge
Duret hemorrhage
Duret lesion
Durham flatfoot
Durie and Salmon classification of
    multiple myeloma
Durkan CTS (carpal tunnel syndrome)
    gauge
durotomy
Dusard syndrome
DUS (diagnostic ultrasound) machine
DUS (diagnostic ultrasound
    of shoulder)
Dutch Vocational Handicap Question-
    naire
duToit-Roux staple capsulorrhaphy
Duval elevator
Duverney fracture

Duverney muscle
DuVries arthroplasty
DuVries condylectomy
DuVries deltoid ligament
reconstruction technique
DuVries hammer toe repair
DuVries-Mann bunionectomy
DuVries modified McBride hallux
valgus operation
DuVries phalangeal condylectomy
DuVries technique for overlapping toe
dV/dt (contractility)
DVI (deep venous insufficiency)
DVI Simpson atherocath
DVI (device independent)
DVI (digital vascular imaging)
DVP (draining vein pressure)
DVR (Department of Vocational
Rehabilitation)
DVRT (differential variable reluctance
transducer)
DVT (deep venous thrombosis)
dwarfism
achondroplastic
chondroplastic
deprivation
diastrophic
Langer mesomelic
Lorain-Lévi
mesomelic
pituitary
Russell-Silver
short limb
Walt Disney
Dwyer cable and screw
Dwyer cable for correction of scoliosis
Dwyer clawfoot operation
Dwyer osteotomy
Dwyer-Wickham electrical stimulation
DXA (dual x-ray absorptiometry),
Hologic
Dycal base
Dycem devices
Dyck-Lambert classification
Dy-DTPA-BMA imaging agent
dye (see *imaging agent*)
dye fluorescence index (DFI)

dying bug range-of-motion exercise
Dyke-Davidoff-Masson syndrome
DynaGraft bioimplant
Dynagrip blade handle
Dyna knee splint
Dyna-Lok spinal instrumentation
system
dynamic activity
dynamic ambulatory balance
dynamic aphasias
dynamic compression plating
dynamic computerized tomography
dynamic condylar screw
dynamic conformal therapy
dynamic contrast-enhanced subtraction
study
dynamic entrapment of vertebral
artery
dynamic equinus contracture
dynamic external fixation
Dynamic Flotation pressure control
zone therapy
dynamic friction
dynamic gait
dynamic graciloplasty
dynamic hip screw
dynamic load
dynamic locking nail system
dynamic pedobarography
dynamic radiotherapy
dynamic snapshot
Dynamic Spatial Reconstructor (DSR)
scanner
dynamic splint
dynamic stability index (DSI)
dynamic standing balance
dynamic stress view
dynamic susceptibility contrast (DSC)
magnetic resonance imaging
dynamic tagging magnetic resonance
angiography
dynamic tendon gripping (DTG)
technique
dynamic ultrasound of shoulder (DUS)
dynamic visual acuity test
dynamic volume-rendered display
dynamic volumetric SPECT

dynamic wedge
dynamics, foot
dynamization collar
dynamometer
  ballistic
  Biodex
  bulb
  Collins
  Cybex II
  hand
  isokinetic
  Jamar hand
  Jamar hydraulic pinch-gauge
Dynaplex knee prosthesis
Dynasplint knee extension unit
Dynasplint shoulder system
DynaSport athletic tape
Dyno-Cinch lumbosacral support
Dynorphin A
DyoCam 550 arthroscopic video camera
Dyonics arthroplasty bur
Dyonics arthroscopic blade
Dyonics arthroscopic instruments
Dyonics cannula
Dyonics Golden Retriever magnet
Dyonics rod-lens endoscope
Dyonics shaver
Dyonics shaving system
DyoVac suction punch
dysarthria
  apraxic
  ataxic
  cerebellar
  clumsy hand
  hypophonic
  labial
  laryngeal
  lingual
  moderate
  pharyngeal
  severe
dysarthric speech
dysautonomia, familial
dysbaric
dyscalculia, developmental
dyschondroplasia
dyscollagenosis

dysconjugate eye movement (also
  disconjugate)
dyscrasia, dyscratic
dyscrasic fracture
dysdiadochokinesia
dysdiadochokinesis
dysdiadochokinetic
dysequilibrium syndrome
dyserethesia
dyserethism
dysergia
dysesthesia
  burning
  painful
dysesthetic sensation
dysesthetic skin
dysfluency (stammering or stuttering)
dysfunction
  age-related neurologic
  autonomic
  bilateral cerebral
  bilateral hemisphere
  bilateral upper motor neuron
  bowel and bladder
  brain
  brain stem
  cerebral
  cognitive
  cortical neuronal
  corticospinal motor system
  diffuse brain
  eighth nerve
  fiber tract
  frontal lobe
  hemispheral
  higher cerebral (HCD)
  higher cortical
  language
  lingual airway
  lumbopelvic
  midbrain
  minimal brain
  neuroendocrine
  neuroimmune
  neurologic
  neuromotor
  oculomotor

dysfunction *(continued)*
  parietal lobe
  positional
  posterior tibial tendon
  post-traumatic cortical
  premotor areas of cerebral cortex
  progressive rostral-caudal brain
    stem
  severe diffuse brain
  somatic
  spinal
  subcortical neuronal
  supranuclear (bilateral upper motor
    neuron)
  swallowing
  sympathetic
dysgenesis
  alar
  anorectal
  callosal
  corticocallosal
  epiphyseal
  gonadal
dysgeusia
dysgnosia
dysgraphia with dyslexia
dyshormonogenesis
dysinhibition, emotional
dysjunctive eye movement
dysjunctive gaze
dyskinesia
  anteroapical
  choreic
  facial
  faciobuccolingual
  L-dopa-induced
  neuroleptic-induced
  oral-buccal-lingual
  orofacial
  regional
  tardive
  tardive oromandibular
  withdrawal emergent
dyskinetic
dyskoimesis
dyslalia

dyslexia
  developmental
  dyseidetic
  dysphonetic
  mixed dysphonetic-dyseidetic
dyslexia with (or without) dysgraphia
dyslexic
dyslogia
dysmaturity
dysmemory
dysmetria
  cerebellar
  lower limb
  ocular
  truncal
dysmetric overshoot of eye movement
dysmimia
dysmnesia
dysmnesic
dysmorphia, muscle
dysmorphophobia
dysmyelinatus, status
dysmyotonia
dysnomia
  amnestic
  literal paraphasic
  paraphasic
  verbal paraphasic
dysosteogenesis
dysostosis
  cleidocranial
  craniofacial
  metaphyseal
dysostosis multiplex
dysphagia
dysphasia
  concomitant
  global
  motor
  sensory
dysphasic
dysphonia
dysplasia
  acropectorovertebral
  bone
  cleidocranial

dysplasia *(continued)*
  congenital d. of hip (CDH)
  congenital hip
  cranioskeletal
  developmental
  diaphyseal
  epiarticular osteochondromatous
  familial arterial fibromuscular
  fibromuscular (FMD)
  fibrous
  foot
  Kniest
  mesomelic
  metaphyseal
  metatrophic
  microscopic cortical
  Mondini
  monostotic fibrous
  multiple epiphyseal
  Namaqualand hip
  oculoauriculovertebral (OAV)
  odontoid
  osseous
  osteofibrous
  perimedial
  polyostotic fibrous
  progressive diaphyseal
  sphenoid wing
  Sponastrine
  spondyloepiphyseal
  Streeter
dysplasia with associated lesion or
  mass (DALM)
dysplastic osteoarthritis
dysplastic spondylolisthesis
dyspnea on exertion
dyspractic movement
dyspraxia
  ideational
  ideomotor
  innervatory
  limb kinetic
  sympathetic
  vocal
dysprosody

dysraphism
  closed spinal
  occult spinal
  spinal
dysreflexia, autonomic
dysrhythmia
  anterior slow
  cerebral
  slow anterior
dysrhythmic movement
dysrhythmic, scattered, slow activity
dysrhythmic speech
dyssynergia
  Ramsay Hunt cerebellar myoclonic
  segmental
dyssynergia cerebellaris myoclonica
  syndrome
dyssynergy
dystasia, hereditary areflexic
dysthymia
dystocia
  fetal
  shoulder
dystonia
  autosomal dominant myoclonic
  body
  dopa-responsive (DRD)
  facial
  focal
  focal appendicular
  kinesogenic
  nonkinesogenic
  spasmodic
  tardive
  torsion
dystonia-parkinsonism, rapid-onset
dystonic pain
dystonic posture
dystonic posturing
dystopia
dystopic
dystrophic calcification
dystrophic changes
dystrophic gait
dystrophin

dystrophy
  adiposogenital
  Becker-Kiener
  Becker muscular (BMD)
  Becker-type of muscular
  Becker variant of Duchenne
  benign X-linked muscular
  benign X-linked recessive muscular
  cerebromacular
  congenital muscular
  congenital myotonic
  distal muscle
  Duchenne muscular (DMD)
  Emery-Dreifuss
  Erb muscular
  faciohumeral muscular
  facioscapulohumeral (FSH)
    muscular
  Fröhlich (Froehlich) adiposogenital
  Gowers muscular
  humeroperoneal muscular
  infantile neuroaxonal

dystrophy *(continued)*
  juvenile muscular
  juvenile neuroaxonal
  Kiloh-Nevin ocular form of
    progressive muscular
  Landouzy-Dejerine
  limb-girdle muscular
  minor reflex
  muscular
  myopathic
  myotonic muscular
  ocular muscular
  oculopharyngeal muscular
  postinjection reflex sympathetic
  pseudohypertrophic muscular
  reflex sympathetic (RSD)
  scapuloperoneal
  sympathetic reflex
  Thomsen
  Welander muscular
  X-linked recessive muscular

E, e

EADL (extended activities of daily living)
Eagle arthroscope
eagle's beak bone-cutting forceps
Eagle straight-ahead arthroscope
Eales disease
ear
    cauliflower
    scrum (in rugby players)
    swimmer's
    wrestler's
early dementia
early traumatic epilepsy
early ulnar nerve paresis
ear reference montage
EAST (external rotation abduction stress test)
eastern equine viral encephalitis
Eastman Kodak scanner
East-West retractor
Easy-Pull sock aide device
Eater, Anspach Cement
Eaton-Lambert syndrome
Eaton-Littler technique
Eaton-Malerich fracture-dislocation technique
Eaton prosthesis
EBCT (electron beam computed tomography)

Eberle contracture release technique
EBI (Electro-Biology, Inc.) bone healing system
EBIORT (electron beam intraoperative radiotherapy)
EBI SpF-T bone stimulator
EBI SpF-2 implantable bone stimulator
EBI spinal fusion (SpF) stimulator
EBL (estimated blood loss)
EBRT (external beam radiation therapy)
EBT (electron beam tomography)
eburnated area
eburnated bone
eburnation, bony
EBV (Epstein-Barr virus)
EC (endothelial cell) adhesion molecule-1
ECA (external carotid artery)
eccentric axis of rotation
eccentric hamstrings
eccentric ledge
eccentric lesion
eccentric muscle training
eccentric quadriceps contraction
eccentric stenosis
eccentric vessel
ecchondroma
ecchondrotome

ecchymosis
   periorbital (raccoon eye sign)
   postauricular (Battle sign)
eccrine angiomatous hamartoma
eccrine carcinoma
Echlin duckbill rongeur
Echlin laminectomy rongeur
Echlin-Luer rongeur
echo (pl. echoes)
   bright
   dense
   highly mobile
   homogeneous
   inhomogeneous
   internal
   linear
   metallic
   navigator
   shower of
   solid
   sonographic
   spin
   swirling smokelike
   thick
   ultrasonographic
   ultrasound
echo characteristics on ultrasound
echo contrast
echo delay time (TE)
echo dense (or echodense)
echo density
echoencephalogram
echoencephalography
EchoEye 3-D ultrasound imaging
   system
echo FLASH MR
echo-free area
echo-free central zone
echo-free space
EchoGen imaging agent (dodeca-
   fluoropantane)
echogenic
echogenicity
echogram, echography
echoic
echoicity
echolalia

Echols retractor
EchoMark angiographic catheter
echo pattern
   homogeneous
   inhomogeneous
echo planar imaging
   FLAIR
   MR (magnetic resonance)
   multi-shot
   one-shot
   pulse sequence
   sequence
echopraxia
echo reflectivity
echo reverberation
echo sign
echo signature
echospeed platform
echo tagging technique
echo texture (also echotexture)
echo time (TE)
echo train length (ETL)
ECHO (enteric cytopathic human
   orphan)
ECHO therapy
ECHO virus
Echovar Doppler system
Echovist (SHU 454) imaging agent
ECI (electrocerebral inactivity)
ECIC (extracranial-intracranial) arterial
   bypass
Ecker-Lotke-Glazer tendon reconstruction technique
Eckert-Davis classification of peroneal
   tendon subluxation
ECLAM score
Eclipse ankle brace
Eclipse TENS unit
ECM (extracellular matrix)
ECoG (electrocorticogram)
ecological validity of rehabilitation
   testing
economic dependence
economy ROM brace
EconoSoc ankle brace
Econo-Wave cervical pillow
E-cotton bandage

ECR (evoked cortical response)
ECRB (extensor carpi radialis brevis)
  muscle
ECRB (extensor carpi radialis brevis)
  tendon
ECRL (extensor carpi radialis longus)
  muscle
ECRL (extensor carpi radialis longus)
  tendon
ECS (electrocerebral silence)
ECT (electroconvulsive therapy)
ECT (European compression
  technique) bone screw
ECT internal fracture fixation
ectasia
  basilar artery
  diffuse arterial
  segmental
  vascular
ectoderm, embryonic neural
ectopic bone growth in joint
ectopic foci of seizures
ectopic marrow
ECTR (endoscopic carpal tunnel
  release)
Ectra carpal tunnel instruments
Ectra endoscopic release
ectrodactyly
ECU (extensor carpi ulnaris) muscle
ECU (extensor carpi ulnaris) tendon
EDAMS (encephaloduroarterio-
  myosynangiosis)
EDAS (encephaloduroarteriosynangiosis)
EDB (extensor digitorum brevis)
  muscle
EDB (extensor digitorum brevis)
  tendon
EDC (extensor digitorum communis)
  muscle
EDC (extensor digitorum communis)
  tendon
EDCP (eccentric dynamic compression
  plate)
eddy (pl. eddies)
eddy current artifact
eddy formation

edema
  angioneurotic
  antral
  brain
  cerebral
  circumscribed
  collateral
  compressive
  cyclic idiopathic
  cyclical
  dependent
  diffuse
  fingerprint
  focal
  idiopathic
  inflammatory
  internal capsular
  intracompartmental
  leg
  local(ized)
  malignant brain
  mild
  mushy
  nerve root
  nonpitting
  optic disk
  papilledema
  passive
  patchy
  perilesional
  periorbital
  peripheral
  peritumoral brain
  perivascular
  pitting
  plerocephalic
  pretibial
  radiation
  scalp
  stasis
  terminal
  trace
  vasogenic
edema fluid
edematous brain tissue
edematous stump
Eden-Hybbinette arthroplasty

Eden-Lange procedure
Eden test
Eder-Puestow metal olive dilator
EDF scoliosis cast
EDG (electrodynogram)
Edgarton-Grand thumb adduction
edge
  boundary
  leading
  rough
  sawtooth
  sternal
  tentorial
edge detection angiography
edge effect
edge overgrowth
EDH (epidural hematoma)
EPI (echo planar imaging)
Edinburgh-2 Coma Scale (E-2CS)
Edinburgh Rehabilitation Status Scale
  (ERSS)
Edinger-Westphal complex
Edinger-Westphal nucleus
EDiT (electric differential therapy)
EDL (extensor digitorum longus) muscle
EDL (extensor digitorum longus) tendon
Edna towel clamp
EDQ (extensor digiti quinti) muscle
EDQ (extensor digiti quinti) tendon
edrophonium (Tensilon) test
EDSS (Expanded Disability Status
  Scale)
Education, Foundation for Chiro-
  practic (FCE)
educed EEG electrode array
Edwards D-L modular fixator
Edwards D-L modular screw rod
Edwards hook
Edwards-Levine hook
Edwards-Levine rod
Edwards-Levine sleeve
Edwards procedure
Edwards syndrome
EEA (end-to-end anastomosis) stapler
EEG (see *electroencephalogram*)
EEG focus

EEG frequency
  alpha
  beta
  delta
  theta
EEG leads, nasopharyngeal
EEG telemetry
EFA (Epilepsy Foundation of
  Amercia)
EFF (electromagnetic focusing field)
  probe
efface
effacement
  cistern
  dural sac
  nerve root sheath
  sulcus
  ventricle
effect
  adverse
  anisotropic
  attenuation
  boxcar (with arterial emboli to the
    retinal vessels)
  copper wire (in arteriosclerosis of
    the retina)
  cumulative
  deleterious
  demagnetization field
  doorstopper
  edge
  extrapyramidal side
  fetal alcohol (FAE)
  flow-related enhancement
  halo effect on x-ray
  hemispheral mass
  hemodynamic
  lag
  magnetization transfer
  mass
  neuroprotective
  neurotoxic
  on-off effect of L-dopa in
    parkinsonism
  putative
  reservoir

effect *(continued)*
   side
   silver wire
   trapdoor
   washboard effect on myelography
     in cervical spondylosis
   wearing-off effect of drugs
efferent digital nerve
Effexor XR (venlafaxine hydrochloride) extended-release capsules
efficacious
efficacy
   clinical
   drug therapy
   treatment
Effler-Groves dissector
Effler-Groves hook
effleurage (neuromuscular massage
   therapy)
effusion
   bloody
   hemorrhagic
   inflammatory joint
   joint
   noninflammatory joint
   recurrent
   subdural
effusion artifact
Eftekhar broken femoral stem
   technique
Egawa sign
EGFP (enhanced green fluorescent
   protein)
Eggcrate mattress
Eggers plate
Eggers screw
Eggers splint
Eggers tendon transfer technique
egress of arthroscopic fluid
egress of blood
Eggsercizer CTS exerciser
eggshell border of aneurysm
eggshell-like calcification
égoïsme à deux phenomenon
EHL (extensor hallucis longus) muscle
EHL (extensor hallucis longus) tendon
Ehlers-Danlos syndrome

Ehrenfeld disease
Eicher femoral prosthesis
18F-fluorodeoxyglucose
18F-fluorodopa
18F fluoro-m-tyrosine positron
   emission tomographic scan
eighth cranial nerve (auditory and
   vestibular divisions)
eighth nerve dysfunction
EIL (internal elastic lamina)
EIP (extensor indicis proprius) muscle
EIP (extensor indicis proprius) tendon
EIS (Emotional Intimacy Scale)
Eisenmenger complex
Eisenmenger syndrome
ejector, Cloward dowel
Ekbom restless leg syndrome
Elan-E power drill
elastic bandage
Elastic Foam bandage
elasticity, modulus of
elastic knee sleeve brace
elastic stable intramedullary nailing
   (ESIN)
elastic subtraction spiral CT
   angiography
Elastikon elastic tape
elastin
elastofibroma dorsi
Elasto-Gel shoulder therapy wrap
elastohydrodynamic lubrication
elastomer, thermoplastic (TPE)
Elastomull elastic gauze bandage
Elastomull splint
elastomyofibrosis
Elavil (amitriptyline)
elbow
   baseball pitcher's
   boxer's
   floating
   golfer's
   javelin thrower's
   Little Leaguer's
   milkmaid's
   nursemaid's
   pulled
   reverse tennis

elbow *(continued)*
 Sorbie-Questor total
 tennis
 thrower's
 wrestler's
elbow bone (olecranon process of
 ulna)
elbow joint
elbow prosthesis
elbow replacement
elbow-wrist-hand orthosis
Eldepryl (selegiline)
elective mutism
 complete
 relative
elective surgery
electrical impedance
electrically generated pain management techniques
electrical potential
electrical stimulation of bone
electrical stimulation of calf muscles
electrical stimulation therapy
electrical stimulation train
electric differential therapy (EDiT)
electric galvanic stimulation
Electri-Cool cold therapy system
electric joint fluoroscopy
electric wheelchair
electric zone
electro-acupuncture
 Acu-Treat
 Electro-Acuscope
Electro-Acuscope electro-acupuncture
electrocautery
 Aspen
 ArthroCare
 Oratec
electrocerebral activity
electrocerebral inactivity (ECI)
electrocerebral silence (ECS)
electrocoagulation, radiofrequency
 (RFE)
electroconvulsive therapy (ECT)
electrocorticogram (ECoG)
electrocorticographic electrode
electrocorticographic evaluation

electrocorticography
electrode (pl. electrodes)
 A (auricular)
 A_1
 A_2
 active recording
 AF (anterior frontal)
 AF_3
 AF_4
 AF_7
 AF_8
 AF_z
 Ag-AgCl (silver-silver chloride)
 anterior temporal surface
 ArthroCare
 Aspen laparoscopy
 auricular (A)
 average potential reference of
 average reference
 ball
 bar
 basal
 bipolar
 bipolar depth
 C (central)
 C_1-C_6
 C_z
 chains of
 chlorided silver
 clip
 coaxial
 common reference
 concentric
 Copeland fetal scalp
 cortical
 CP (centroparietal)
 CP_1-CP_6
 CP_z
 DBS (deep brain stimulating)
 deep brain stimulating
 delta
 depolarizing
 depth
 dermal
 diamond-shaped
 disc
 disposable

electrode *(continued)*
earlobe
EEG
electrocorticographic
electroencephalogram (EEG)
electromyogram (EMG)
epidural
epidural peg
equipotential
exploring
F (frontal)
F_1-F_{10}
F_z
FC (frontocentral)
FC_1-FC_6
FC_z
FF (frontopolar-frontal)
4-contact strip
Fp (frontopolar)
Fp_1-Fp_2
Fp_z
FpF (frontopolar-frontal)
frontal (F)
frontocentral (FC)
frontopolar (Fp)
frontotemporal (FT)
FT (frontotemporal)
FT_7-FT_{10}
G_1
G_2
gold
gold bulb
gold-coated
Goldmann-Offner reference of
grid of
ground
grounding
impedance of
inactive
indifferent
interhemispheric
intracerebral
I_z
International 10-20
Levin thermocouple cordotomy
loop
M_1 (mastoid)

electrode *(continued)*
M_2 (mastoid)
mandibular angle
mastoid (M)
metal cup
metal surface
Mitek Vapr T
monopolar
multipolar
Nashold TC
nasopharyngeal
neck muscle
needle
neighboring
neutral
Nichrome cylindrical
noncephalic reference
nonpolarizable
N_z
O (occipital)
O_1
O_2
O_z
P (parietal)
P_1-P_{10}
P_z
pad
peak N9
peak N20
peak N22
peak P14
peak P38
peg
pipe cleaner
placement of EEG
platinum
platinum-coated
PO (parieto-occipital)
PO_3
PO_4
PO_7
PO_8
PO_z
prefrontal
Radionics radiofrequency
recording
reference recording

electrode *(continued)*
  resistance of
  ring
  rod
  scalp
  scalpel
  scout
  silver ball
  silver chloride-coated
  silver-silver chloride
  Silverman placement of
  Sluyter-Mehta thermocouple
  sphenoid(al)
  stainless steel
  Stephenson-Gibbs reference
  stereotactic or stereotaxic
  sternospinal reference
  stick-on
  stigmatic
  stimulating
  subdural
  suction
  surface
  T (temporal)
  T_7-T_{10}
  temporal (T)
  10-20 System of
  tin-coated
  TP (temporal-posterior)
  TP_7-TP_{10}
  transverse tripolar
  true anterior temporal
  21 recording
  unchlorided silver
  uninsulated tip of
  VPL (ventroposterolateral) thalamic
  watchband
  zero potential reference
electrode grid
electrode headband
electrode insertion point
electrode monitoring
electrode paste
electrode placement
electrode polarization
electrodecremental seizure
electrodesiccated bleeding points

electrodiagnostic examination
electrodynogram (EDG)
electrodynography
electroencephalogram (EEG) (see also
  montage, potential, wave)
  absolute band frequency on
  absolute band value on
  absolute peak frequency on
  after-discharge on
  age-related changes on
  alerting maneuver during
  aliasing on
  all-night sleep recording with
  alpha activity on
  alpha blocking on
  alpha coma pattern on
  alpha frequency range on
  alpha rhythm on
  alpha spindles on
  alpha variant rhythm on
  alphoid rhythm on
  ambulatory recording of
  amplifier drift on
  anachronism on
  anterior slow dysrhythmia on
  aperiodic waves (or complexes) on
  apiculate waveform on
  arceau rhythm on
  arch-shaped waves on
  arrhythmic delta activity on
  arrhythmical repetitive
  arrhythmical waves on
  artifact-free
  artifact on
  asymmetric waveforms on
  asynchronous bursts of activity on
  asynchronous delta waves on
  asynchronous epileptiform activity on
  asynchronous sleep spindles on
  asynchronous slow waves on
  asynchronous spindles on
  asynchronous waves on
  attack-specific potential on
  attenuation of alpha rhythm on
  attenuation of background rhythm on
  atypical spike and wave complexes
    on

electroencephalogram *(continued)*
    delta brush pattern on
    delta focus on
    delta index on
    delta occipital pattern on
    depth (DEEG)
    desynchronization of
    desynchronized pattern on
    diagnostic
    diffuse delta pattern on
    diffuse distribution of activity on
    diffusely low voltage
    digital
    digital signal analysis of
    diphasic spikes on
    diphasic wave on
    direct current (DC-EEG)
    discontinuous activity on
    disorganized electrical activity on
    disorganized pattern on
    double-banana montage on
    driving response on
    drowsiness during
    dysmaturity on
    dysrhythmia on
    dysrhythmic delta activity on
    dysrhythmic pattern on
    ear reference montage on
    ear reference recording during
    electrocardiogram during
    electrocerebral inactivity (ECI) on
    electrocerebral silence (ECS) on
    electrodecremental seizure on
    electrode-popping artifact on
    electrographic maturation seen on
    electrolyte gel for
    electrolyte jelly for
    electrolyte paste for
    electro-oculogram (EOG) during
    electroretinogram and
    EMG by submental monitor during
    encoches frontales on
    epileptiform activity on
    epileptiform burst discharges on
    epileptiform event on
    epileptiform pattern on
    epileptiform spike on

electroencephalogram *(continued)*
    epileptiform waveform on
    epileptogenic burst on
    epileptogenic focus on
    epochs on
    evoked potential (EP) mapping of
    extracerebral activity on
    eye blinks on
    eye closing on
    eye movement (EM) monitor on
    eye opening and closing maneuver
    eye opening on
    eye position monitoring on
    eyelid flutter on
    fast alpha variant rhythm on
    fast alpha variants on
    fast Fourier transform (FFT) analysis
    fast waves on
    FIRDA (frontal intermittent
        rhythmic delta activity)
    flash stimulation on
    flat
    flatline
    flattening of tracing on
    focal activity on
    focal epileptiform discharges on
    focal interictal epileptiform activity
    focal parietal theta rhythm on
    focal periodic pattern on
    focal sharp waves on
    focal slow waves on
    focal slowing on
    frequency domain mapping of
    frontal beta rhythm on
    frontal rhythmic theta activity on
    frontal sharp transient
    frontal sharp waves on
    frontocentral slow waves on
    fused alpha wave morphology on
    Galileo evoked potential
    galvanic skin response during
    gamma rhythm on
    generalization on
    generalized asynchronous slow
        waves on
    generalized background slowing on
    generalized distribution of activity on

electroencephalogram *(continued)*
  generalized epileptiform activity on
  generalized epileptiform discharges
  generalized fast waves on
  generalized flattening on
  generalized paroxysmal fast activity
  generalized periodic pattern on
  generalized slow
  generalized spike and wave
    discharges on
  generalized spikes
  glissando photic stimulation during
  glossokinetic artifact on
  grape juice for hypoglycemia during
  hand movement monitoring during
  high amplitude
  high amplitude transients on
  high filter frequency (HFF) on
  high voltage complexes on
  high voltage pattern on
  high voltage slow pattern on
  horizontal dipoles on
  hypersynchronous
  hyperventilation during
  hypnagogic hypersynchrony during
  hypoglycemic changes on
  hypsarrhythmia on
  hypsarrhythmia pattern on
  ictal epileptiform activity on
  ictal focal epileptiform discharges on
  ictal focal slow waves on
  ictal pattern on
  impedance pneumogram used during
  in-phase waves on
  independent waves on
  indeterminate sleep during
  infantile pattern of spikes on
  instrumental phase reversal on
  interburst interval measurement on
  interference on
  interhemispheric synchrony on
  interictal continuous spikes on
  interictal epileptiform activity on
  interictal focal epileptiform
    discharges on
  interictal focal slow waves on
  interictal generalized epileptiform

electroencephalogram *(continued)*
    waves on
  interictal spike
  interictal temporal lobe spikes on
  intermittent focal spikes on
  intermittent rhythmical delta activity
  intermittent slowing on
  intermittent temporal slow waves on
  intermixed spike pattern on
  intracerebral
  intracranial
  invariant pattern on
  ipsilateral reference montage on
  IRDA (intermittent rhythmic delta
    activity) on
  isoelectric pattern on
  isopotential line on
  Janz response on
  jaw jerks on
  juvenile pattern of spikes on
  K complex on
  kappa rhythm on
  lambda waves on
  Laplacian montage on
  larval spike and slow waves on
  lateral rectus spike on
  lateralized activity on
  lateralized distribution on
  lateralized epileptiform activity on
  lateralized slowing on
  lateralizing epileptiform discharges
  left-sided lead on
  lid flutter on
  linear
  linked ear reference montage on
  local slow waves on
  localized evoked potentials on
  longitudinal bipolar (LB) montage on
  low amplitude spikes on
  low filter frequency (LFF) on
  low voltage activity on
  low voltage pattern on
  low voltage slow waves on
  M-type (minimal) alpha rhythm on
  mean peak frequency on
  medium voltage slow waves on
  methohexital given during

electroencephalogram *(continued)*
    MFD (monorhythmic frontal delta)
        waves on
    midline focus of
    midline theta rhythm on
    midtemporal discharges on
    miniblinks on
    mirror foci on
    monomorphic waves on
    monophasic sharp waves on
    monorhythmic activity on
    monorhythmic frontal delta (MFD)
        waves on
    monorhythmic frontal slowing
    monorhythmic pattern on
    monorhythmic sinusoidal delta
        activity on
    monorhythmic waves on
    MSTs (multifocal sharp transients)
    multichannel
    multifocal independent spikes on
    multifocal sharp transients (MSTs)
    multifocal spike discharges on
    multifocal spikes on
    multiple sleep latency test (MSLT)
        with
    multiple spike and slow wave
        complexes on
    multiple spike complexes on
    mu (μ) rhythm on
    nasal thermistor used during
    negative vertex spike on
    neonatal
    non-REM sleep periods on
    noncephalic reference montage on
    noncerebral activity on
    nonepileptiform activity on
    nonphysiologic artifact on
    nonspecific diffuse slowing on
    nonspecific reaction to stimuli on
    normalization of
    notched rhythmic theta activity on
    NREM (nonrapid eye movement)
        sleep on
    O waves on
    occasional periodic discharges on
    occipital negative

electroencephalogram *(continued)*
    occipital rhythm on
    occipital spikes of blind person on
    occipital spikes on
    occipital waveforms on
    OIRDA (occipital intermittent
        rhythmic delta activity) on
    Omni Prep electrolyte gel for
    on and off response on
    onset bursts on
    opposite polarity of signals on
    oral thermistor used during
    out-of-phase waves on
    overreading of
    oversampling on
    P-type (persistent) alpha rhythm on
    paper stop artifact on
    paradoxical alpha rhythm on
    paradoxical μ (mu) rhythm on
    paroxysmal activity on
    paroxysmal alpha activity on
    paroxysmal beta activity on
    paroxysmal delta activity on
    paroxysmal discharges on
    paroxysmal hypnagogic hyper-
        synchrony on
    paroxysmal pattern on
    paroxysmal rhythmical waves on
    paroxysmal theta activity on
    paste for
    pattern sensitivity on
    PDA (polymorphic delta activity) on
    peak of wave on
    pentylene tetrazol given during
    period between complexes on
    periodic complexes on
    periodic discharges on
    periodic generalized sharp waves on
    periodic lateralizing epileptiform
        discharges (PLEDs)
    periodic slow waves on
    persistent alpha rhythm slowing on
    perspiration artifact on
    phantom spike and wave pattern on
    phase angle on
    phase lag on
    phase reversal on

electroencephalogram *(continued)*
  photic driving with
  photic stimulation during
  photoconvulsive response on
  photometrazol test during
  photomyoclonic jerking on
  photomyoclonic response on
  photoparoxysmal response on
  photosensitivity during
  physiologic artifact on
  PLEDs (periodic lateralized
    epileptiform discharges) on
  plotting field of potentials on
  polymorphic delta activity on
  polymorphic slow activity on
  polymorphic waves on
  polyphasic sharp wave on
  polyphasic spike on
  polyphasic transients on
  polyphasic waves on
  polyrhythmic waves on
  polyspike and slow wave complexes
  polyspike and wave complexes on
  polyspike and wave discharges on
  polyspike complexes on
  positive bursts on
  positive occipitital spike-like sleep
    waves on
  positive sharp waves on
  positive spikes on
  posterior beta rhythm on
  posterior dominant activity on
  posterior slow waves of youth on
  posterior theta rhythm on
  postictal alpha rhythm slowing on
  postictal bisynchronous slow waves
  POSTS (positive occipital sharp
    transients) on
  potentials on
  projected rhythms on
  prominent flash evoked response
    during
  propagation of activity on
  pseudoepileptiform activity on
  pseudoepileptiform pattern on
  pulse wave artifact on
  quadrant on

electroencephalogram *(continued)*
  quadriphasic waves on
  quantitative analysis of
  quantitative (QEEG)
  quasiperiodic waves on
  quiet sleep during
  quiet wakefulness during
  R-type (reactive) alpha rhythm on
  radiotelemetry
  rapid eye movements (REM)
    during sleep on
  recruiting response on
  reduction of amplitude on
  referential alternating montage on
  referential block montage on
  referential montage on
  referential recording of
  relative band frequency on
  relative band value on
  REM sleep periods on
  repetitive flashes of light used on
  repetitive spikes on
  repetitive waves on
  respiratory monitoring during
  resting wakefulness during
  reversal of polarity on
  rhythmic activity on
  rhythmic artifacts on
  rhythmic temporal theta waves on
  rhythmic theta burst of drowsiness
  rhythmic theta pattern on
  rhythmical midtemporal discharges
  rhythmical repetitive
  rhythmical slow waves on
  rhythmical waves on
  rhythmicity of
  right-sided lead on
  RMTDs (rhythmical midtemporal
    discharges) on
  rolandic dip on
  rolandic sharp transient on
  rolandic sharp waves on
  rolandic spike on
  runs of sharp theta activity on
  saccadic eye movements on
  salt bridges connecting electrodes
    during

electroencephalogram *(continued)*
    sampling rate on
    sawtooth waves on
    scalp (SEEG)
    scalp-scalp montage on
    SDEEG (stereotaxic depth)
    seizure focus on
    seizure pattern on
    SEMs (slow lateral eye movements)
    serial recording of
    sharp and slow wave discharges on
    sharp transients on
    sharp wave complexes on
    sharp wave focus on
    sharp waves on
    sharply contoured waveform on
    shut eye waves on
    sigma rhythm on
    signal analysis of
    simultaneous opposite polarities on
    simultaneous video monitoring
      during
    simultaneous waves on
    sinusoidal appearing sleep spindles
    sinusoidal waves on
    sleep
    sleep-deprived
    sleep onset REM period
      (SOREMP) on
    sleep spindle on
    slow alpha variant on
    slow alpha variant rhythm on
    slow anterior dysrhythmia on
    slow lateral eye movements
      (SLEMs) on
    slow spike and wave complex on
    slow spike and wave discharges on
    slow wave sleep during
    slow waves on
    small sharp spikes (SSS) on
    somatosensory stimulation during
    SOREMP (sleep onset REM period)
    spatial resolution on
    spectral analysis of
    spectral averaging on
    spectral edge frequency on
    spicules on

electroencephalogram *(continued)*
    spike and dome complexes on
    spike and wave complex on
    spike and wave discharges on
    spike averaging on
    spike focus on
    spike-like artifact on
    spike wave discharges on
    spikes on
    spiking activity on
    spiky transients on
    spindle bursts on
    spindle coma pattern on
    spindle-like activity on
    spindle-shaped activity on
    spindles on
    sporadic generalized slow waves on
    sporadic waves on
    squeak phenomenon on
    SREDA (subclinical rhythmic epi-
      leptiform discharges of adults) on
    SSS (small sharp spike) on
    stage I (drowsiness) sleep on
    stage II (light sleep) sleep on
    stage III (deep sleep) sleep on
    stage IV (very deep sleep) sleep on
    stage W (wakefulness) sleep on
    startling noise used during
    startling stimulus used during
    stepwise photic stimulation during
    stereotactic (SEEG) (or stereotaxic)
    stereotactic depth (SDEEG)
    stereotyped spikes on
    stimulus artifact on
    stroboscopic flashes of light used on
    subclinical rhythmical discharge on
    subclinical seizure
    submental EMG activity monitor
      used during
    superimposed on
    suppression-burst pattern on
    surface electromyogram (EMG)
      during
    synchronous bursts of
    synchronous waveforms on
    synchronous waves on
    tactile stimulation during

electromyogram *(continued)*
  short potentials on
  single-fiber (SFEMG)
  small amplitude polyphasic motor
    units on
  SNAP (sensory nerve action
    potential) on
  spikes without baseline crossings on
  SSR (sympathetic skin response) on
  stimulus-evoked
  superficial peroneal nerve sensory
    study on
  surface
  sural nerve sensory study on
  terminal latencies on
  tibial nerve motor/sensory study on
  triphasic wave on
  turns on
  ulnar nerve motor/sensory
electromyographic feedback
electromyographic incomplete
  interference pattern
electromyographic insertion study
electromyographic potentials
electromyographic recording
electromyographic study
electromyography (EMG)
electron and x-ray diffraction patterns
electron arc therapy
electron beam boost
electron beam computed tomography
  (EBCT)
electron beam CT scanner
electron beam intraoperative radiotherapy (EBIORT)
electron beam therapy
electron bolus
electron dosimetry
electroneuromyography
electron equilibrium loss
electronic portal imaging
electron linear accelerator
electron photon field matching
electron production, secondary
electron spin resonance (ESR)
electronystagmogram
electronystagmography (ENG)

electro-oculogram (EOG)
electro-oculographic analysis
electrophoresis
  fluorophore-coupled oligosaccharide
  temperature gradient gel
electrophoretic mobility shift assay
  (EMSA)
electrophysiologic integrity (of nerve
  impulse)
electrophysiological localization of
  nerve lesions
electrophysiological mapping
electrophysiologic arousal response
electrophysiologic test
electrophysiology nerve study
electroplethysmography
electroretinogram (ERG)
  flash
  pattern
electrostatic potential
electrostimulation for nonunion of
  fracture
electrotherapy, Staodyn TENS
electrotherapy unit, Dial Away Pain 400
electrothermal arthroscopy
electrothermally assisted capsular shift
  (ETAC)
electrothermal technology
Elekta stereotactic head frame (*not*
  Elektra)
element
  neoplastic destruction of spinal
  posterior
  subluxation of
elemental calcium
elephantiasis neurofibromatosa
elevate on pillows
elevation, head
Elevations shoe build-up
elevation of extremity
elevator
  Adson periosteal
  angular
  Aufranc periosteal
  Bennett bone
  Bethune periosteal
  Blair

elevator *(continued)*
  blunt
  bone
  Bowen periosteal
  Bristow periosteal
  Brophy periosteal
  Buck
  Buck periosteal
  Cameron-Haight periosteal
  Campbell periosteal
  Carroll-Legg periosteal
  Chandler bone
  Cheyne periosteal
  chisel
  chisel edge
  Cloward osteophyte
  Cloward periosteal
  Cobb periosteal
  Cobb spinal
  Cohen periosteal
  Converse periosteal
  Coryllos-Doyen periosteal
  Cottle-MacKenty
  Crawford dural
  Crego
  curved periosteal
  Cushing-Hopkins periosteal
  Cushing Little Joker
  Cushing periosteal
  Cushing pituitary
  Cushing staphylorrhaphy
  D'Errico periosteal
  Darrach
  Davidson-Sauerbruch-Doyen
    periosteal
  Dawson-Yuhl-Key
  Dawson-Yuhl periosteal
  Doyen rib
  duckbill
  dural
  Duval
  Endotrac
  Farabeuf periosteal
  Fomon periosteal
  fracture reducing
  Frazier dural
  Freer periosteal

elevator *(continued)*
  Freer septal
  Gardner
  Hajek-Ballenger septal
  hand
  Harrington spinal
  Henahan
  Herczel rib
  Hibbs chisel
  Hoen periosteal
  Iowa University periosteal
  Jannetta duckbill
  joker periosteal
  Joseph periosteal
  J-periosteal
  Kahre-Williger periosteal
  Kennerdell-Maroon
  Key periosteal
  Kirmission periosteal
  Kleinert-Kutz periosteal
  Kocher
  Lambotte
  lamina
  Lane periosteal
  Langenbeck periosteal
  Lempert periosteal
  Lewis periosteal
  liberator
  Locke
  Love-Adson periosteal
  lumbosacral fusion
  MacKenty periosteal
  Malis
  Matson-Alexander
  Matson rib
  McGlamry
  Mead periosteal
  Molt periosteal
  Moore bone
  nasal
  OSI Extremity
  osteophyte
  Penfield
  periosteal
  Phemister
  Presbyterian Hospital staphylor-
    rhaphy

elevator *(continued)*
  Ray-Parsons-Sunday staphylorrhaphy
  Rhoton
  rib
  Roberts-Gill periosteal
  Rochester lamina
  Rochester spinal
  Rosen
  round-tapped periosteal
  Sauerbruch rib
  Sayre periosteal
  Scott-McCracken periosteal
  Sebileau periosteal
  Sedillot periosteal
  septal
  Sheffield hand
  Sisson fracture reducing
  spinal
  staphylorrhaphy
  straight periosteal
  Sunday staphylorrhaphy
  Swanson
  T handle
  Tegtmeier
  Tenzel
  Tronzo
  von Langenbeck periosteal
  Ward periosteal
  Wiberg periosteal
  wide periosteal
  Willauer-Gibbon periosteal
  Williger periosteal
  Woodson
  Yankauer periosteal
  Yasargil
elevator dissector
elevator muscle
elevator periosteotome
elevatus
  iatrogenic
  metatarsus
  metatarsus primus
eleventh cranial nerve (spinal accessory nerve)
Eligoy metal alloy
Elihorn Maze Test
elimination kinetics

elipridil
ELISA (enzyme-linked immunosorbent assay) test
Elite Farley retractor for spinal surgery
Elite knee brace
Elizabethtown method osteotomy
Elliott femoral condyle blade plate
Elliott plate
ellipsoid joint
elliptical
ellipticity index
Ellis classification
Ellis Jones peroneal tendon technique
Ellison lateral knee reconstruction
Ellis technique for Barton fracture
Ellman International Surgitron
Elmslie-Cholmeley foot procedure
Elmslie peroneal tendon operation
Elmslie-Trillat patellar procedure
Elmslie triple arthrodesis
elongation derotation flexion
elongation, tissue
eloquent areas of brain
eloquent cortex
ELP broach
ELP femoral prosthesis
ELP stem for hip arthroplasty
Elsberg brain cannula
Elsberg ventricular cannula
Elscint Twin CT scanner
Ely heel-to-buttock test
EM (eye movement) monitor used during EEG
EMA (epithelial membrane antigen) antibody
EMA immunostain
embarrassment
  circulatory
  cord
  midbrain function
  nerve root
  respiratory
embarrassment of midbrain function
embedding of stent coils
embolectomy, percutaneous balloon
embolic cerebral infarction

embolic event
embolic gangrene
embolic material, nidus of
embolic obstruction
embolic occlusion
embolic phenomenon
embolic shower
embolic stroke
embolism
  air
  arterial
  arterial stenosis
  bone marrow
  cancer
  catheter-induced
  cerebral
  cerebral fat
  cholesterol
  direct
  fat
  foam
  gas
  gas nitrogen
  intracranial
  massive
  miliary
  multiple
  obturating
  oil
  pantaloon
  peripheral
  polyurethane foam
  pulmonary (PE)
  pyemic
  recurrent
  retinal
  retrograde
  riding
  septic
  septic pulmonary
  silent cerebral
  straddling
  thrombus
  trichinous
  tumor

embolization
  alcohol
  balloon
  balloon and coil
  balloon therapeutic
  coil
  endovascular coil
  flow-directed
  Gelfoam powder
  Ivalon
  microvascular
  percutaneous transvenous
  Silastic bead
  stent
  super selective
  therapeutic coil
  transarterial
  transvenous
embolus (pl. emboli) (see *embolism*)
embouchure
EMBP (estramustine binding protein)
embryonal tumor
embryonic artery
embryonic communication
embryonic mesencephalic transplant
embryonic mesencephalon
embryonic neural ectoderm
embryonic stem cells
EMC (encephalomyocarditis)
  encephalitis
Emed-F foot force measurement system
EMED scanner
emergency closed manipulative measure
emergency department
emergency muscles
emergency room area, minor (MERA)
emergent, emergently
Emery-Dreifuss disease
Emery-Dreifuss dystrophy
emetic center
EMG (electromyogram, electromyography) (see *electromyography*)
EMG biofeedback
EMI CT scanner

eminence
  arcuate
  articular
  collateral
  cruciate
  cruciform
  deltoid
  facial
  frontal
  hypothenar
  iliopectineal
  iliopubic
  intercondylar
  intercondyloid
  medial
  median
  occipital
  pyramidal
  thenar
  tibial
  wasting of hypothenar
  wasting of thenar
EMLA cream
Emmon osteotomy
emotional deficits
emotional dependence
emotional dysinhibition
Emotional Intimacy Scale (EIS)
emotional indifference
emotional lability
empirical therapy
empty sella syndrome
empyema
  intracranial tuberculous subdural
  spinal
  subdural
empyematic scoliosis
EMS (encephalomyosynangiosis)
EMS (eosinophilia-myalgia syndrome)
EMSA (electrophoretic mobility shift
    assay)
emulsified
EMX2 gene
en bloc laminectomy
en bloc resection
en bloc turning in parkinsonism
en face view

en plaque, meningioma
ENA (extractable nuclear antigen) test
ENA-713 (Exelon)
enarthrodial joint
Enbrel (etanercept)
encapsulated brain abscess
encapsulated radioactive seeds
encasement, vessel
encephalalgia
encephalatrophy
encephalauxe
encephalic nerves
encephalitic
encephalitis (pl. encephalitides) (see
    also *encephalitis, viral*)
  acute disseminated
  acute necrotizing
  benign myalgic
  brain stem
  bulbar
  California
  Central European
  chronic subcortical
  CMV (cytomegalovirus)
  Colorado tick fever
  cortical
  Coxsackie A
  Coxsackie B
  cytomegalovirus (CMV)
  Dawson inclusion body
  dengue
  diffuse necrotizing
  eastern equine
  EMC (encephalomyocarditis)
  epidemic
  Epstein-Barr virus
  focal
  fulminant
  Hayem
  hemorrhagic
  herpes simplex virus (HSV)
  herpes zoster
  herpetic
  HSV (herpes simplex virus) type II
  Ilheus
  infantile
  infectious hepatitis

encephalitis *(continued)*
  infectious mononucleosis
  influenza
  influenzal
  Japanese
  Japanese B
  LaCrosse virus
  lead
  Leichtenstern
  limbic
  louping ill
  lymphogranuloma venereum
  measles
  mumps
  Murray Valley (Australian X)
  Mycoplasma pneumoniae
  necrotizing
  optic
  poliomyelitis
  postinfectious
  postvaccinal
  psittacosis
  purulent
  pyogenic
  rabies
  Rasmussen
  rubella
  rubeola
  Schilder
  St. Louis
  Strümpell-Leichtenstern
  subacute inclusion body
  suppurative
  tick-borne
  toxoplasmic
  vaccinal
  van Bogaert
  varicella zoster
  Venezuelan equine
  viral
  West Nile
  western equine
  yellow fever
encephalitis, viral (see also *encephalitis*)
  Australian X
  California
  Colorado tick fever

encephalitis, viral *(continued)*
  Coxsackie A
  Coxsackie B
  Creutzfeldt-Jakob
  cytomegalovirus (CMV)
  dengue
  eastern equine
  ECHO (enteric cytopathic human
    orphan)
  encephalomyocarditis (EMC)
  herpes simplex (HSV)
  herpes zoster
  Ilheus
  infectious hepatitis
  infectious mononucleosis
  influenza
  Jakob-Creutzfeldt
  Japanese B
  kuru
  louping ill
  lymphocytic choriomeningitis
  measles
  mumps
  Murray Valley
  poliomyelitis
  progressive multifocal leuko-
  J encephalopathy (PML)
  rabies
  slow virus
  St. Louis
  subacute sclerosing panencephalitis
    (SSPE)
  tick-borne
  Venezuelan equine
  West Nile
  western equine
  yellow fever
encephaloarteriography
encephalocele
  anterior fontanelle
  cranial vault
  ethmoidal
  frontoethmoidal
  frontosphenoidal
  interfrontal
  interparietal
  intranasal

encephalocele *(continued)*
  middle fossa
  nasoethmoidal
  nasofrontal
  naso-orbital
  occipital
  posterior fontanel
  sphenoethmoidal
  sphenomaxillary
  spheno-orbital
  suboccipital
  temporal
  transethmoidal
  transsphenoidal
encephalocele with cranium bifidum
encephaloclastic lesion
encephalocystocele
encephalodialysis
encephaloduroarteriosynangiosis
  (EDAS)
encephalodysplasia
encephalogram
encephalography
encephaloid
encephalolith
encephaloma
encephalomalacia
  cystic
  macrocystic
encephalomeningitis
encephalomeningocele
encephalomeningopathy
encephalometer
encephalomyelitis
  acute disseminated (ADEM)
  acute hemorrhagic
  ascending
  benign myalgic
  disseminated
  granulomatous
  Leigh subacute necrotizing
  paraneoplastic (PEM)
  postinfectious
  postmeasles
  postvaccinal
  rabies postvaccinal
  toxoplasmic

encephalomyelitis *(continued)*
  varicella zoster
  viral
encephalomyeloneuropathy
encephalomyelopathy
  postinfection
  postvaccinal
  subacute necrotizing
encephalomyeloradiculitis
encephalomyeloradiculopathy
encephalomyeloradiculoneuritis
encephalomyocarditis (EMC)
  encephalitis
encephalomyocarditis (EMC) viral
  encephalitis
encephalomyopathy, mitochondrial
encephalomyosynangiosis (EMS)
encephalon
encephalonarcosis
encephalopathic parkinsonism
encephalopathic process, diffuse
encephalopathy
  AIDS
  allergic
  amyotrophic type of spongiform
  anoxic
  biliary
  bilirubin
  bovine spongiform ("mad cow
    disease")
  childhood
  demyelinating
  diabetic
  dialysis
  diffuse
  Heidenhain type of spongiform
  hepatic (HE)
  HIV
  hypernatremic
  hypertensive
  hypoglycemic
  hyponatremic
  hypoparathyroid
  hypoxic-ischemic (HIE)
  idiopathic
  ischemic-hypoxic
  lead

encephalopathy *(continued)*
   Leigh necrotizing
   limbic
   metabolic
   myoclonic
   Nevin-Jones subacute spongiform
   painter's
   pancreatic
   portal-systemic (PSE)
   postanoxic
   postinfectious
   postshunt
   post-traumatic
   postvaccinal
   progressive subcortical
   progressive traumatic
   punch-drunk
   renal
   saturnine
   spongiform
   static
   subacute arteriosclerotic
   subacute necrotizing
   subacute spongiform
   thiamine deficiency (TDE)
   toxic
   transmissible spongiform viral
   traumatic
   uremic
   viral
   Wernicke
   Wernicke-Korsakoff
encephalopuncture
encephalopyosis
encephalorachidian
encephaloradiculitis
encephalorrhagia
encephalosclerosis
encephaloscope
encephaloscopy
encephalosepsis
encephalosis
encephalospinal
encephalothlipsis
encephalotome
encephalotomy
encephalotrigeminal angiomatosis

encerclage
enchondral ossification
enchondroma protuberans
enchondromatosis
encircle, encircled
encirclement
encircling
encoches frontales on EEG
encoding task
encopresis
Encore Orthopedics
   instruments/devices
encroachment
   bony
   foraminal
encroachment on the spinal cord
endarterectomized vessel
endarterectomy
   carotid (CEA)
   carotid artery
   carotid bifurcation
   eversion
   vertebral
   vertebral artery
end-biting forceps
Ender femoral fracture technique
Ender nail
Ender rod fixation
endfeel (physiotherapy)
end-inspiratory pressure
Endius spinal endoscopic camera
EndoAvitene
Endobutton button
Endobutton FM
Endobutton tape
endocavitary applicator system
endochondral bone
endochondral ossification
endocranium
endocrine disturbance
endocrine fracture
endocrine-inactive pituitary microadenoma
endocrine myopathy
endocrinological cure
endocrinological remission
endocrinopathy

EndoFix bioabsorbable interference
   screw
endogenous callus formation
endogenous depression
endoluminal scaffold
endolymphatic hydrops
endolymphatic shunt
Endo-Model rotating knee joint
   prosthesis
endomysium
endoneural
endoneurial
endoneuritis
endoneurium
endoneurolysis
endonuclease
Endopearl fixation device
endoperineuritis
endophlebitis
Endo-P-Probe
endoprosthesis (see *prosthesis*)
end organs, proprioceptive
endosaccular coil
endoscope
   Desormaux
   Dyonics rod-lens
   Endius spinal endoscopic camera
   Hopkins rigid glass lens
   MED
   PercScope percutaneous diskectomy
   rigid-lens
   SpineScope percutaneous
   stereotaxic
   Surgenomic
   SurgiScope
endoscope-assisted microneurosurgery
endoscope-controlled microneurosurgery
endoscopically
endoscopic carpal tunnel release
   (ECTR)
endoscopic correction of scoliosis
endoscopic division of incompetent
   perforating veins
endoscopic endonasal transsphenoidal
   surgery
endoscopic fasciotomy

endoscopic neurosurgery
endoscopic plantar fasciotomy
endoscopic quadrature RF coil
endoscopic retrocalcaneal decompression procedure
endoscopic retroperitoneal thoracoabdominal approach
endoscopic sclerosing therapy
endoscopic strip craniectomy
endoscopic ultrasound (EUS)
endoscopic washing pipe
endoscopic water pick
endoscopist
endoscopy (see *endoscope*)
   posterior fossa
   spinal canal
   thoracoscopic spine surgery
   virtual
endoskeleton
endosteal revascularization
endosteal surface
endosteum
Endostatin
endosteal callus
endosteal hypertrophy
endosteal revascularization
endosteal surface
Endo Stitch suturing device
ENDOtec instruments/devices
endotenon
endothelial cell (EC) adhesion
   molecule
endothelial cell chemotactic factor
endothelialization of stent
endothelial nitric oxide synthase
   (eNOS)
endothelin-1 (ET-1)
endotheliomatous meningioma
Endotrac instruments
endovascular coil
endovascular coil embolization
endovascular flow wire study
endovascular glue
endovascular interventionalist
endovascular scar
endovascular stent
endovascular stent-graft

endovascular therapy
endovascular ultrasonography
endplate
    hyaline cartilage
    vertebral body
endpoint, measurable
endpoint of orthopedic tests
endpoint (physiologic) nystagmus
end post
end-pressure artifact
end-range limitation of motion
end-stage coxarthrosis
end-stage disorder
end-to-end anastomosis (EEA) stapler
end-to-end sutures
Endurance bone cement
endurance, rhythmic handgrip
Enduron acetabular liner
energy
    beam
    kinetic
    low photon
    strain
energy-absorbing capability of knee
enervation
ENG (electronystagmography)
engagement levels
Engel classification of postoperative
    seizures
Engelhardt femoral prosthesis
Engelmann disease
Engelmann splint
Engel-May nail
Engel plaster saw
Engel-Recklinghausen disease
Engen palmar finger orthosis
Engen palmar wrist splint
Engh total hip replacement
engineering
    biomedical
    rehabilitation (RE)
    tissue
English brace
enhanced green fluorescent protein
    (EGFP)
enhanced imaging
enhanced scan

enhancement
    contrast medium
    Doppler flow signal
    nonhomogeneous
    signal
    vascular MR contrast
enhancement morphology
enhancement pattern
enhancement rate, instantaneous
enhancing lesion
enhancing mass (on CT or MRI scan)
Enker brain retractor
enlarged frontal horns
enlarged vascular channels
enlargement, ventricular
Enlon-Plus (atropine and edro-
    phonium)
Enneking staging of malignant soft
    tissue tumor
enophthalmic
enophthalmos, unilateral
eNOS (endothelial nitric oxide
    synthase)
enoxaparin (Lovenox)
ENP (extractable nucleoprotein)
ensemble of epochs
entacapone (Comtan)
enteric cytopathic human orphan
    (ECHO) viral encephalitis
enterogenous cyst
enterovirus
enthesitis
enthesopathy
enthesophytes, subacromial
entrapment
    lateral
    nerve
    patellar
    PIN (posterior interosseous nerve)
    popliteal
    posterior tibial nerve
    soft tissue
    suprascapular nerve
    ulnar nerve (at the elbow)
entrapment mononeuropathy
entrapment myopathy
entrapment neuropathy

entrapment syndrome
entrapped plantar sesamoid
entry zone
enucleate, enucleated
enucleation
enucleator
  Hardy
  Hardy micro
  Marino transsphenoidal
  Rhoton
  transsphenoidal
envelope
  soft tissue
  stem
Envelope arm sling
Enview camera system
environmental assessment
enzyme
  cholinergic
  lysosomal
  proteolytic
EOG (electro-oculogram)
eosinophilia-myalgia syndrome (EMS)
eosinophilic adenoma
eosinophilic granuloma
epaulet
EPB (extensor pollicis brevis) muscle
EPB (extensor pollicis brevis) tendon
ependyma
ependymal cells
ependymitis
  granular
  purulent
ependymoblastoma
ependymoma
  malignant
  myxopapillary
  spinal cord
ependymoma tumor
ephaptic conduction
EPI (echo planar imaging)
epicerebral space
epicondylar fracture
epicondyle
epicondylectomy
epicondylitis
epicortical lesion

epicranial aponeurosis
epicranial muscle
epicritic function
epicritic two-point sensation
epidemic Kaposi sarcoma
epidermoid cyst of brain
epidermoid, posterior fossa
epidermoid tumor
epidermolysis bullosa
epidural abscess
epidural block anesthesia
epidural blood
epidural blood patch
epidural catheter
epidural cavity
epidural electrode
epidural hematoma
epidural hemorrhage
epidural implant
epidural injection
epidural invasion
epidural macroabscess
epidural mass
epidural pressure
epidural space
epidural spinal abscess
epidural spinal cord compression
  (ESCC)
epidural steroid block
epidural venography
epidurogram
epidurography
epiduroscopy
epigastric sensation (prior to seizure)
epihyal ligament
epilemmal
epilepsy (see also *seizure*)
  abdominal
  absence
  acquired
  activated
  alcohol-precipitated
  alcoholic
  amygdalar
  anterior polar-amygdalar
  arithmetical
  automatic

epilepsy *(continued)*
  benign childhood
  benign familial myoclonic
  benign focal
  benign rolandic
  Bravais-jacksonian
  centrencephalic
  centrotemporal (rolandic)
  childhood
  chronic
  cingulate
  clouded state
  communicating
  cortical
  cryptogenic myoclonic
  cursive
  dacryocystic
  Dark Warrior
  dementia in
  deterioration
  diencephalic autonomic
  diurnal
  dorsolateral
  early traumatic
  essential
  extrinsic
  familial progressive myoclonic
  focal
  focal cerebral
  focal motor with march
  frontal lobe
  gelastic (laughing seizures)
  generalized
  genetic
  glassy stare of petit mal
  grand mal
  GTC (generalized tonic-clonic)
  haut mal
  hippocampal
  hysterical
  idiopathic generalized
  impulsive petit mal
  insular
  intractable
  intrinsic
  Jackson
  jacksonian

epilepsy *(continued)*
  juvenile
  juvenile myoclonic
  Koshevnikoff
  Lafora inclusion body
  larval
  laryngeal
  late traumatic
  latent
  Lundborg myoclonic
  major
  matutinal
  menstrual
  mesiobasal limbic
  minor
  motor cortex
  musicogenic
  myoclonic
  myoclonic-astatic
  myoclonus
  Nintendo
  nocturnal
  occipital
  occipital paroxysms with
  opercular
  orbitofrontal
  organic
  paroxysmal patterns of
  pattern-induced
  perceptive
  petit mal
  photic
  photogenic
  photosensitive
  physiologic
  postanoxic
  posttraumatic
  precipitation of
  primary reading
  primary rhinencephalic psychomotor
  procursive
  progressive familial myoclonic
  progressive myoclonic
  provocative tests for
  psychic
  psychomotor
  psychomotor variant of

epilepsy *(continued)*
   quiritarian
   reading
   reflex
   rolandic
   running
   secondary reading
   sensorial
   sensory
   serial
   situation-related
   spinal
   supplementary motor
   symptomatic
   tardy
   television-induced
   temporal lobe (TLE)
   temporolimbic
   thalamic
   tonic
   tornado
   traumatic
   uncinate
   Unverricht-Lundborg myoclonus
   Unverricht myoclonic
   versive
   vestibulogenic
   visual
   xanthine derivatives-induced
Epilepsy Foundation of America
   (EFA)
epileptic
epileptic attack
epileptic automatism
epileptic diathesis
epileptic discharge
epileptic equivalent
epileptic focus
epileptic fugue state
epileptic mania
epileptic march
epileptic neuron
epileptic neuronal aggregate
epileptic prodrome
epileptic syndrome

epilepticus
   focal status
   furor
   globus
   status
epileptiform abnormalities
epileptiform activity
epileptiform event
epileptiform pattern
epileptiform response
epileptiform spike
epileptiform wave form
epileptiform waves on
epileptogenesis
epileptogenic burst
epileptogenic focus
epileptogenic lesion
epileptogenic stimulation
epileptogenic temporal lesion
epileptogenic zone
epileptogenicity, hemispheral
epileptogenous
epileptoid
epileptologist
epileptology
epimeric muscle
epimysium
epineural covering
epineural repair
epineurial neurorrhaphy
epineurium
epineurolysis, volar
epineurosis
epineurotomy
epiphora, in migraine
epiphyseal *or* epiphysial
epiphyseal arrest
epiphyseal bracket
epiphyseal chondroblastic growth
epiphyseal coxa vara
epiphyseal disk
epiphyseal extrusion index
epiphyseal fracture
epiphyseal fragility
epiphyseal growth

epiphyseal hyperplasia
epiphysealis
epiphyseal plate
epiphyseal porosis
epiphysial *or* epiphyseal
epiphysiodesis
  Blount
  bone peg
  percutaneous
  spontaneous post-fracture
epiphysiolysis, distraction
epiphysis (pl. epiphyses)
  annular
  atavistic
  capital
  capital femoral
  capitular
  hypertrophy of
  Perthes
  pressure
  slipped
  slipped capital femoral (SCFE)
  slipped upper femoral (SUFE)
  stippled
  tibial
  traction
epiphysitis
Epipoint elbow support
episode
  confusional
  convulsive
  gray-out
  silent ischemic
  sleep onset
episode, syncopal
episodic confusion
episodic memory
episodic vertigo
epispinal space
Epistar subtraction angiography
epistaxis (nosebleed), spontaneous
epitendineum
epitenon
epipteric bone
epithelialization, creeping

epithelial malignancy
epithelial membrane antigen (EMA)
  antibody
epithelial-myoepithelial carcinoma
epithelioid hemangioepithelioma of
  bone
epithelioid neurofibroma
epithelioid sarcoma
epitope spreading
Epitrain knitted elbow support
Epitrain Viscoped support
epitrochlea
epitrochlear
epitrochleoanconeus muscle
EPL (extensor pollicis longus) muscle
EPL (extensor pollicis longus) tendon
E plane
Epley canalith repositioning procedure
Epley maneuver
epoch length
epochs
  averaged
  ensemble of
epochs of wakefulness
eponychium
Eppright dial osteotomy
EPR dosimetry
EPSP (excitatory postsynaptic potential)
Epstein-Barr virus
Epstein bone rasp
Epstein curet
Epstein neurological hammer
EQP (extensor quinti proprius) muscle
EQP (extensor quinti proprius) tendon
Equalizer Pro massager
Equi-Flow hydrocephalus valve
equilibratory ataxia
equilibrium, Hardy-Weinberg
equilibrium reactions
Equilizer short leg walking cast
equine encephalitis
  eastern
  Venezuelan
  western
equine gait

equinocavovarus
equinovalgus
  pes
  spastic
equinovalgus rearfoot deformity
equinovarus hindfoot deformity
equinovarus of spastic paralysis
equinovarus, talipes
Equinox EEG neuromonitoring system
equinus
  calcaneal
  metatarsus
  talipes
equinus contracture (in cerebral palsy)
equinus deformity
equinus, gastrocnemius
equinus hamstring tightening
equipment
  adaptive
  interventional
  real-time
equipment artifact
equipotential line
equivalent
  epileptic
  migraine
equivocal findings
equivocal plantar reflex
equivocal reflex
ER (evoked response)
Erb disease
Erb-Duchenne-Klumpke injury to
  brachial plexus
Erb-Duchenne palsy
Erb-Duchenne paralysis
Erb-Goldflam disease
Erb injury to brachial plexus
Erb-Landouzy disease
Erb muscular dystrophy
Erb palsy
Erb paralysis
Erb point
Erb sign
Erb spastic paraplegia
Erdheim-Chester disease
ERE (external rotation in extension)
erector muscle of spine

erect position
erect view
ERF (external rotation in flexion)
ERG (electroretinogram)
ergometer, handgrip
ergometry, bicycle
ergonomically correct chair
ergonomically designed transducer
ergonomics
Erich splint
Erichsen sign
Erickson-Leider-Brown technique
Eriksson cruciate ligament
  reconstruction
Eriksson knee prosthesis
Eriksson ligament technique
Eriksson muscle biopsy cannula
ERM proteins
erosion
  articular surface
  bony
  linear
  osteoclastic
  pedicle
  tumor
erosion of articular surface
erosion of dorsum sellae on x-ray
erosive osteoarthritis
errors
  aphasic
  paralexic
ERSS (Edinburgh Rehabilitation Status
  Scale)
erysipelas
erythema migrans
erythema of joint
erythematosus, systemic lupus
erythematous
erythrasma (from *Corynebacterium
  minutissimum*)
erythrocyte sedimentation rate (ESR)
erythromycin
erythroprosopalgia
ESCC (epidural spinal cord compression)
eschar
escharotic

escharotomy
escharotomy and fasciotomy
ESCS (epidural spinal cord stimulator)
E-selectin
ESFAS (European Society of Foot and
  Ankle Surgeons)
ESIN (elastic stable intramedullary
  nailing)
Esmarch bandage
Esmarch plaster knife
Esmarch plaster scissors
Esmarch plaster shears
Esmarch tourniquet
esodic nerve (afferent nerve)
esophagus, corkscrew (diffuse
  esophageal spasm)
esophoria
ESR (erythrocyte sedimentation rate)
  test
essential cerebellar tremor
essential myoclonus
essential tremor
essential ultra trace elements (in
  nutrition)
Esser skin graft
Essex-Lopresti axial fixation technique
Essex-Lopresti calcaneal fracture
  classification
Essex-Lopresti fixation of calcaneal
  fracture
estazolam
Esterom
esthesia
esthesiometer
  Semmes-Weinstein
  Weber
esthesiometry, depth-sense
esthesioneuroblastoma
estimated blood loss (EBL)
estramustine-binding protein (EMBP)
Estridge biopsy needle
ETAC (electrothermally assisted
  capsular shift)
etanidazole
ETA receptor
état criblé (atrophy of cerebral tissue)
état lacunaire (multiple small strokes)

état marbré (marble state)
ETB1 receptor
ETB2 receptor
ethanol injection, percutaneous
EthBr (ethidium bromide) stain
Ethibond suture
ethidium bromide (EthBr) stain
Ethiflex suture
Ethilon suture
Ethiodane contrast medium
ethiodized oil
Ethiodol contrast medium
ethmoidal canal
ethmoidal foramen
ethmoidal meningoencephalocele
ethmoidal nerve
ethmoidal notch
ethmoid bone
ethmoid sinus
Ethodian (iophendylate) radiopaque
  contrast medium
ethylene vinyl alcohol (EVAL)
ethyl 2-cyanoacrylate
etidronate (Didronel)
etiology undetermined
etiology unknown
ETL (echo train length)
ETL 3D FSE imaging
etodolac (Lodine, Ultradol)
etodolac extended-release (Lodine XL)
E-TOF (time of flight) detecting
  module
etomidate
E-2CS (Edinburgh-2 Coma Scale)
Eucalyptamint 2000 gel
eukinesis
EULAR (European League Against
  Rheumatoid) Response Criteria for
  Rheumatoid Arthritis
Eulenburg disease
Euler angle of wrist motion
eumycetoma
euphoria
Euroglide MKII slide board
European Society of Foot and Ankle
  Surgeons (ESFAS)
Euroqol questionnaire

eurysternum
eustachian muscle
eutectic mixture
evacuation of blood clot
evacuation of hematoma
evacuator
   hematoma
   Hemo-Drain
   Reichert-Mundinger hematoma
EVa HiRES motion analysis device
EVAL (ethylene vinyl alcohol)
evaluation
   functional
   home
   Hughston knee
   initial staging
   morphometric
   neurosurgical
   NK hand
   noninvasive soft tissue
   orthopedic
   orthoptic
   postneurosurgical
   posttreatment neuropsychologic
   preneurosurgical
   pretreatment neuropsychologic
   rehabilitation
   Smith physical capacities (PCE)
   strain gauge
   vocational (VE)
evanescent
Evans ankle joint instability operation
Evans ankle reconstruction technique
Evans-Burkhalter rehabilitation
Evans calcaneal distraction wedge
   osteotomy
Evans calcaneal lengthening procedure
Evans fracture classification system
Evans tenodesis
Evazote foam
EVD (external ventricular drain)
even distribution of echoes in ultra-
   sonography
eventration
events, recall of
Eve procedure
Evers diet for multiple sclerosis

Evershears surgical instrument
eversion of rearfoot
eversion sprain of the ankle
evert, everted
everyday memory questionnaire
EX-FI-RE external fixation system
evoked potential recording
evoked potentials
evoked response (ER)
evolution, stroke in
Evolution hip prosthesis
evolving hematoma
evolving stroke
Ewald score
Ewald total elbow replacement
Ewald-Walker kinematic knee
   arthroplasty
EWHO (elbow-wrist-hand orthosis)
Ewing sarcoma, estraosseous
Ewing tumor
exacerbate, exacerbated
exacerbation, acute
exacerbation of pain
Exactech instruments/devices
Exact-Fit ATH hip replacement
   system
exam (examination)
exametazime imaging agent
examination (see also *test*)
   biomechanical
   Boston Diagnostic Aphasia
   electrodiagnostic
   Folstein Mini-Mental Status
   intact neurologic
   mental status
   Mini-Mental State Examination
   Neurobehavioral Cognitive Status
   neurological
   nonfocal neurologic
   ophthalmoscopic
   physiologic neurologic
   SCORE (Simple Calculated Osteo-
     porosis Risk Estimation)
   shear
   Simple Calculated Osteoporosis
     Risk Estimation (SCORE)
   visual field

examiner, certified disability
Examining for Aphasia test
exarticulation
excavatum, pectus
Excedrin Migraine (acetaminophen,
    aspirin, caffeine)
excellent prognosis
Excel polyester suture
excessive diffuse low and medium
    wave beta activity (on EEG)
excessive joint play
exchange, liner
excimer (from "excited dimer") laser
excision (see *operation*)
    split-thickness skin (STSE)
    wedge
    wide
excision arthroplasty
excision of intervertebral disk
excision of osteochondroma
excitation
    TCR rebound
    wave of
excitation function measurement
excitation light
excitation profile
excitation-spoiled fat-suppressed
    T1-weighted SE images
excitatory lesion
excitatory postsynaptic potential
    (EPSP)
excitatory synapse
excitomotor cortex
excitoreflex nerve
excitor nerve
excitotoxic cascade
excoriation
excrescence, bony
excretion, SIADH (syndrome of
    inappropriate antidiuretic hormone)
excursion
    calcaneus
    hindfoot
    range of
executive function
Exelon (rivastigmine tartrate,
    ENA-713)

exercise (pl. exercises)
    active assisted range of motion
    active range of motion (AROM)
    aerobic
    ankle pump
    aquatic
    AROM (active range of motion)
    Brandt-Daroff vertigo
    Buerger Allen exercise
    Calleja
    chain reaction
    chin tuck
    closed-chain kinetic
    Codman
    contract/relax
    Cooksey-Cawthorne
    Crane shoulder
    DeLorme
    dying bug
    external rotation
    gastroc-resistive (gastrocnemius)
    graded
    hamstring-setting
    heel cord stretching
    heel raises
    heel rocks
    hip abductor strengthening
    hook-fist positioning
    hook-lying pectoral stretch
    horizontal shoulder abduction
    internal rotation
    inversion-eversion
    isokinetic passive mode
    isometric
    isotonic
    knee extension
    knee pump
    lower abdominal pelvic tilt
    MacKenzie
    muscle-setting
    muscle-strengthening
    myofascial stretching
    parallel squat
    passive assistive
    passive range of motion (PROM)
    passive stretch
    pelvic tilt

exercise *(continued)*
 pendulum
 Pilates method
 plyometric
 PNF (proprioceptive neuromuscular facilitation)
 PREs (progressive resistive)
 progressive resistive
 PROM (passive range of motion)
 prone scapular retraction
 pulley
 quad-set (quadriceps-setting)
 quad-strengthening
 range of motion
 Regen flexion
 resistive strengthening
 seated scapular retraction
 self-monitored
 short-arc progressive resistance
 straight leg raising
 strengthening
 strenuous
 supported extension
 Tai Chi Chuan
 tai chi
 tendon stretching
 therapeutic
 toe gripping
 toe raises
 translation
 vestibular enhancement
 Williams flexion
 wrist stretch
exercise-induced amenorrhea
exercise-induced myokymia
exercise intolerance
exerciser
 continuous anatomical passive (CAPE)
 CPM (continuous passive motion)
 Cybex II isokinetic
 Cybex II+ isokinetic
 Danniflex CPM
 Digi-Flex finger
 Exer-Cor
 ExtendaFLEX
 finger

exerciser *(continued)*
 JACE shoulder
 jaw
 KineTec clubfoot CPM
 Nelson finger
 NordiCare Enabler
 NordiCare Strider
 Omni-Flexor wrist
 Orthotron
 Powerflex CPM
 Preston Traveler CPM
 strengthening
 Stryker CPM
 Stryker leg
 Thera-Band resistive
 Therabite jaw
 Toronto Medical CPM
 Wilco ankle
 Xercise Bands
 Zimmer continuous anatomical passive
Exercise Self-Efficacy Scale
Exer-Cor exerciser
ExerFlex ball
exertional compartment pressure measurement
exertional compartment syndrome
Exeter bone lavage
Exeter hip prosthesis
Exeter intramedullary bone plug
Exeter stem
exit wound
Exner area
Exner plexus
Exner writing center (in brain)
exoccipital bone
exodic nerve
exogenous depression
exogenous obesity
exogenous reaction, acute
Exogen SAFHS (sonic accelerated fracture healing system)
exon, mutated
exophthalmos
 bilateral
 pulsatile
 unilateral

exophytic adenocarcinoma
Exo-static cervical collar
exostectomy
exostosis, exostoses
  blocker's
  bony
  epiphyseal
  hereditary multiple
  hypertrophic
  impingement
  marginal
  retrocalcaneal
  tackler's
  traction
  turret
exotoxin tetanospasmin
Expanded Disability Status Scale
  (EDSS)
expander
  acetabular
  hetastarch plasma volume
  hydroxyethylstarch plasma volume
  Mentor tissue
  tissue
expanding intracranial mass
expansile lytic lesion
expansion, colloid volume
expenditure, resting energy (REE)
Expert-XL densitometer
exploration and debridement
exploration and revision
exploration, posterior fossa
explosivity of behavior
eXpose retractor
exposure
  bone-tendon
  extensile
expression
  Ki-67
  muscles of
expressive aphasia
expressive aphasic disorder
exquisite detail
exsanguinate, exsanguinated
exsanguination
exstrophy

ExtendaFLEX CPM exerciser
extended activities of daily living
  (EADLs)
extended ADLs
extended tibial in situ bypass
extender
  nail
  stem
Extend total hip system
extensile exposure
extension
  basal
  Buck
  capital
  cervical
  Codivilla
  extra-axial
  flexion and
  headrest
  Hittenberger halo
  intracavitary
  medial
  outward
  parietal
  range of
  sitting knee
  suprasellar (of tumor)
  tumor
  toe plate
  volitional resisted
extension bias neutral
extension injury
extension lock splint (ELS)
extensive dissection
extensometer, strain-gauge
extensometry testing
extensor (pl. extensors)
  apparatus (of fingers and toes)
  mechanism (of hand and foot)
  radial
  ulnar
  wrist
extensor brevis arthroplasty
extensor carpi radialis brevis (ECRB)
  muscle
extensor carpi radialis brevis (ECRB)
  tendon

extensor carpi radialis longus (ECRL)
  muscle
extensor carpi radialis longus (ECRL)
  tendon
extensor digitorum brevis manus
extensor digitorum communis (EDC)
  muscle
extensor digitorum communis (EDC)
  tendon
extensor digitorum longus (EDL) muscle
extensor digitorum longus (EDL) tendon
extensor hallucis longus (EHL) muscle
extensor hallucis longus (EHL) tendon
extensor indicis proprius (EIP) muscle
extensor indicis proprius (EIP) tendon
extensor mechanism disruption
extensor muscle
extensor pollicis brevis (EPB) muscle
extensor pollicis brevis (EPB) tendon
extensor pollicis longus (EPL) muscle
extensor pollicis longus (EPL) tendon
extensor quinti proprius (EQP) muscle
extensor quinti proprius (EQP) tendon
extensor reflex
extensor retinaculum
extensor wad of three
external acoustic meatus, nerve of
external beam radiation therapy
  (EBRT)
external carotid artery (ECA)
external carotid nerves
external carotid steal syndrome
external collateral ligament
external fixation
external hyperthermia treatment
external immobilization
external intercostal muscles
external jugular vein
external ligament
external neurolysis
external oblique muscle
external obturator muscle
external pterygoid muscle
external respiratory nerve of Bell
external rotation in extension (ERE)
external rotation in flexion (ERF)
external rotation recurvatum test

external saphenous nerve
external ventricular drain (EVD)
external wire fixation
extinction of stimulus
extinction phenomenon
extirpation
  microsurgical
  radical
  trigeminal neuroma
  tumor
extra-articular arthroscopy
extra-articular fracture
extra-articular resection
extracapsular dissection
extracapsular fracture
extracapsular ligament
extracellular glutamate concentration
extracellular matrix
extracellular protective glycocalyx
extracerebral activity
extracerebral intracranial glioneural
  hamartoma
extracerebral potential
extracorporeal heat exchanger
extracorporeal photochemotherapy
extracranial carotid occlusive disease
extracranial cerebral circulation
extracranial cervicocephalic arterial
  dissection
extracranial-intracranial bypass (ECIC)
extracranial sectioning of cranial
  nerves
extracranial vessel
extraction
  CTAB
  proteinase-K
  Qiaex gel method
  transcranial oxygen
extractor
  Austin Moore
  bone
  bone plug
  break screw
  Cherry
  cloverleaf pin
  corkscrew femoral head
  femoral head

extractor *(continued)*
 FIN
 Jewett
 Küntscher
 Kalish Duredge wire
 Massie
 metatarsal head
 Moore prosthesis
 Nicoll
 Rousek
 staple
 Sven-Johansson
extractor-driver, Schneider
extractor-impactor, Fox
extradural abscess
extradural artery
extradural compartment
extradural defect
extradural space
extradural tumor
extradural vertebral plexus of veins
extraforaminal disk herniation
extramedullary hemangioma
extramedullary hematopoiesis
extraneous material
extraocular muscles
extrapial plane
extrapontine myelinolysis
extrapulmonary tuberculosis
extrapyramidal symptoms
extrapyramidal tract
extraskeletal chondroma
extraskeletal osteosarcoma
extra-striate cortex
extrasynovial tissue

extrathecal nerve roots
extravasated blood
extravasated contrast
extravasation
 contrast
 dye
 joint fluid
 radiopaque fluid
extraventricular obstruction
extremity (pl. extremities)
 lower (LE)
 upper (UE)
extrinsic lesion
extrinsic muscles
extrude
extruding
extrusion, disk
exuberant granulation tissue
exudate
exudation of fibrin-rich fluid
exudative consolidation
exudative effusion
ex vacuo, hydrocephalus
ex vivo magnetic resonance imaging
eye-view 3D-CRT
eyeball muscles (extraocular muscles)
eyelet, rod
EZ Bend sponges
E-Z Flap neurosurgery mini-plate
 system
E-Z reacher device
ezrin, radixin, and moesin (ERM
 proteins)
EZ "T" orthopedic shirt
EZ-Up inversion table

F, f

FA (femoral anteversion)
Fabco gauze bandage dressing
FAB (Fear Avoidance Behavior)
  Questionnaire
fabella
fabellofibular complex
fabere (flexion, abduction, external
  rotation, extension)
fabere sign
fabere test
Fabry disease
FAC (Functional Ambulation
  Categories)
face, en
face-hand test
facet (also facette)
  articular
  atlas
  capitate
  clavicular
  costal
  flat
  hamate
  inferior
  Lenoir
  locked
  lunate
  medial
  patellar

facet *(continued)*
  scaphoid
  squatting
  superior
  transverse
facetal imbrication
facet capsule disruption
facet dislocation
facetectomy, O'Donoghue
facet fusion
facet injection
facetious
facet joint vacuum
facet surface of vertebra
facet syndrome
facet tropism
face validity of rehabilitation testing
facial and masticatory muscles
facial bipartition
facial bones
facial dystonia
facial fracture
facial expression, muscles of
Facial Grading System (FGS)
    for Bell palsy
facial grimaces, repetitive
facial hemiplegia
facial movement weakness
facial muscles

249

facial myoclonia
facial myokymia
facial nerve (seventh cranial nerve)
facial nerve canal
facial nerve reanimation
facial nerve reconstruction
facial nerve schwannoma
facial nucleus
facial palsy, persistent
facial paralysis
  contralateral
  ipsilateral
facial paresthesia
facial recognition test
facial reflexes
facial spasm of Meige
facies (pl. facies)
  birdlike
  hatchet
  mask (of parkinsonism)
  masklike
  moon
  myasthenic
  myopathic
  myotonic
  parkinsonian
  swan-neck
facilitation, proprioceptive neuromuscular (PNF)
Facilities, Health-Related (HRF)
facility, skilled nursing (SNF)
facing of metacarpal heads
facioauriculovertebral (FAV) syndrome
faciobrachial hemiplegia
faciobuccolingual dyskinesia
faciohumeral dystrophy
faciolingual hemiplegia
facioplegic migraine
facioscapulohumeral muscular
  dystrophy (FSHD)
faciostenosis
faciotomy, medial
factitious attack
factitious disorder
factitial

factor (pl. factors)
  basal endothelium-derived relaxing
  Boltzmann
  brain-derived neurotrophic (BDNF)
  dislocation
  endothelial cell chemotactic
  endothelium-derived relaxant
    (EDRT)
  epidermal growth
  equilibrium
  fibroblast growth
  glial-derived neurotrophic (GDNF)
  growth hormone releasing (GRF)
  IgA-RF class-specific rheumatoid
  IgG-RF class-specific rheumatoid
  IgM-RF class-specific rheumatoid
  insulin-like growth factor binding
    protein-3 (IGFBP-3)
  insulin-like growth factor-1 (IGF-1)
  nerve growth (NGF)
  putative
  RA (rheumatoid arthritis)
  recurrent human granulocyte
    colony stimulating (r-met
    HuG-CSF)
  rheumatoid (RF)
  skeletal growth
  technical
  tumor necrosis (TNF)
  tumor necrosis factor alpha
    (TNF-a)
  wedge
factor I, insulin-like growth
factor V Leiden
factor VIII deficiency
factor IX deficiency
facultative pacemaker theory
fad therapy
fadir (flexion, adduction, internal
  rotation)
fadir sign
fadir test
FAE (fetal alcohol effects)
Fager pituitary dissector
Fahey-Compere pin

Fahey-O'Brien procedure
Fahey retractor
Fahr disease
FAI (Frenchay Activities Index)
failed back surgery syndrome (FBSS)
failure of conservative management
failure, pure autonomic
Fairbanks changes on x-ray
Fairbanks-Sever procedure
Fajersztajn crossed sciatic sign
fakie (snowboard move)
falciform ligament
falcine region
falcotentorial meningioma
falcula, falcular
falling attack
falling out
fallopian ligament
fallout, signal
false aneurysm
false channel
false joint
false localizing sign
false negative result
false neuroma
false positive result
false sac
falx
    calcification of
    cerebral
falx cerebri
falx meningioma
familial amyotrophic lateral sclerosis
familial articular hypermobility
    syndrome
familial avascular necrosis of
    phalangeal epiphysis
familial cavernous malformation
familial dysautonomia
familial frontotemporal dementia
familial gliomatosis cerebri
familial hypophosphatemic rickets
familial parkinsonism
familial visceral neuropathy
familial paroxysmal choreoathetosis
familial sensory radicular neuropathy
familial spastic ataxia

familial spastic paraplegia
familial tremor
fan-beam x-ray absorptiometry
Fanconi syndrome
Fanelli guide
fan, macular
fanning of toes
fan-shaped view
fan sign
FAP (femoral artery pressure)
Farabeuf bone-holding forceps
Farabeuf bone rasp
Farabeuf-Collin rasp
Farabeuf-Lambotte bone-holding
    forceps
Farabeuf-Lambotte raspatory
Farabeuf periosteal elevator
Farabeuf rasp
Faraday catheter
Faraday shield
faradic current stimulation
Farber syndrome
far field
Farmer operation
farnesyl protein transferase inhibitor
farnesylation
farnesyltransferase inhibition
Farrior wire-crimping forceps
Farr test for systemic lupus erythema-
    tosus
FAS (fetal alcohol syndrome)
fascia
    antebrachial
    bicipital
    brachial
    cervical
    clavipectoral
    Colles
    crural
    deep
    deltoid
    iliac
    infraspinous
    interthenar
    investing
    lumbar
    lumbodorsal

fascia *(continued)*
  medial geniculate
  palmar
  plantar
  psoas
  quadratus femoris
  rim of
  Sibson
  superficial temporalis
  superficial temporoparietal
  thoracolumbar
fascia cruris
fascia lata *(but* tensor fasciae latae)
fascial arthroplasty
fascial band
fascial plane
fascial release
fascial rent
fascial sling
fascial thickening
fascial tract
fasciaplasty (also fascioplasty)
fasciatome
  Masson
  Moseley
fascicle, nerve
fascicular repair, grouped
fasciculations, muscle-wasting
fasciculi of the cord
fasciculus (pl. fasciculi)
  arcuate (AF)
  fibrous palmar
  palmar fibrous
  lenticular
  longitudinal
  longitudinalis medialis
  medial longitudinal (MLF)
fasciectomy, partial
fasciitis
  Dupuytren
  necrotizing
  nodular
  plantar
fasciocutaneous island flap
fasciodesis
fasciogram

fascioplasty (also fasciaplasty)
fasciorrhaphy
fascioscapulohumeral muscular
  dystrophy
fasciotomy
  compartment
  decompression
  endoscopic
  minimal incision plantar
  open plantar
  plantar
  subcutaneous palmar
  superficial
FAST (Frenchay Aphasia Screening
  Test)
FASTak suture anchor system
fast component of nystagmus
fast dynamic volumetric x-ray CT
Fastex proprioceptive and agility test
fast flow lesions
fast flow malformation
fast flow vascular anomaly
fast Fourier spectral analysis
fast Fourier transform (FFT) analysis
  of EEG
fastigial pressor response (FPR)
FASTIN threaded anchor
fast muscle (white muscle)
F.A.S.T. 1 intraosseous infusion
  system
fast PC cine MR sequence with
  echo-planar gradient
FasTracker microcatheter
Fas-Trac strips
fast routine production
fast SE (FSE) imaging
fast SE and fast IR (FMPIR) imaging
fast SE train
fast short tau inversion recovery
  (STIR)
fast spin echo MR imaging
fast spin echo T2-weighted image
fast spoiled-gradient-recalled MR
  imaging
fast STIR (short tau inversion
  recovery)

fast twitch fibers
fat
    retrolaminar
    Siri formula for percentage of body
    subcutaneous
FAT (Frenchay Arm Test)
fatal familial insomnia
fatal PE (pulmonary embolus)
fat embolism, cerebral
fat embolism syndrome (FES)
fat-fluid level (on x-ray)
fat-free (body) mass (FFM)
fathometer
fatigability, muscular
fatigue
    arousal-attentional
    intentional
fatigue characteristics of bone grafts
fatigue curve
fatigue fracture
fatigue strength
fatigue stress
fat pad
    foveal
    heel
    Hoffa
    infrapatellar
    scalene
fat pad sign
fat-suppressed 3D spoiled gradient-
    echo imaging
fat-suppressed proton density fast
    spin-echo imaging
fat-suppressed T2-weighted fast
    spin-echo imaging
fat suppression technique
fatty degeneration
fatty filum terminale
fatty streak
fatty tumor
fauces (pl. of faux)
    anterior pillar of
    arch of
    muscles of
faucial sensation
Faulkner curet
fault, sagittal plane

faux (pl. fauces)
faveolate
favor the injured part
Fazio-Londe disease
Fazio-Londe syndrome
FB cast cushion
FBN1 (protein monomers of fibrillin)
FBS (failed back syndrome)
FBSS (failed back surgery syndrome)
FC (frontocentral) electrode
    (FC_1-FC_6, FC_z)
FCE (Foundation for Chiropractic
    Education)
FCE (Functional Capacity Evaluation)
FCL (fibular collateral ligament)
FCR (flexor carpi radialis) muscle
FCR (flexor carpi radialis) tendon
FCR 9501HQ high resolution storage
    phosphor imaging agent
FCS (full cervical spine) x-ray series
FCU (flexor carpi ulnaris) muscle
FCU (flexor carpi ulnaris) tendon
FDA ([U.S.] Food and Drug
    Administration)
FDC (flexor digitorum communis)
    muscle
FDC (flexor digitorum communis)
    tendon
FD-43 microdissector
FDI (first digital interosseous) muscle
FDI (first digital interosseous) tendon
FDIM (fluorescence digital imaging
    microscopy)
FDL (flexor digitorum longus) muscle
FDL (flexor digitorum longus) tendon
FD PET (fluorodopa PET scan)
FDP (fibrin degradation products)
FDP (flexor digitorum profundus)
    muscle
FDP (flexor digitorum profundus)
    tendon
FDQ (flexor digiti quinti) muscle
FDQ (flexor digiti quinti) tendon
FDQB (flexor digiti quinti brevis)
    muscle
FDQB (flexor digiti quinti brevis)
    tendon

FDS (flexor digitorum sublimis) muscle

FDS (flexor digitorum sublimis) tendon

FDS (flexor digitorum superficialis) muscle

FDS (flexor digitorum superficialis) tendon

Fear Avoidance Behavior Questionnaire (FAB)

Feather-Lite reacher device

fecal incontinence

febrile convulsion

febrile seizure

Fédération International de Chiropractic Sportif (FICS)

feebleminded, feeblemindedness

feedback

    electromyographic (EMG)

    power

feeder arteries

feeder veins

feeding artery to aneurysm

feeding branch of artery

feeding mean arterial pressure (FMAP)

feeding vessel

Feild blade (not Field)

Feild-Lee brain biopsy needle

Feild suction dissector

Feingold diet

Feiss line

F (frontal) electrode

F_1-F_{10} electrode

felbamate (Felbatol)

Feldene (piroxicam)

felon, fingerstick

felon infection

Fellonet ointment gauze

felt

    orthopedic

    rolled

    Teflon

felt collar splint

felt dressing

felt patch

Felty syndrome

femoral above-knee popliteal bypass

femoral aligner

femoral anteversion (FA)

femoral artery

femoral bone

femoral cam

femoral canal restrictor

femoral capital epiphysis

femoral condylar defect

femoral condyle

femoral cutaneous nerve

femoral cutter

femoral-femoral bypass graft

femoral-femoral crossover

femoral head amputation

femoral head and neck

femoral head deformity

femoral head, Matroc

femoral head vascularity

femoral ligament

femoral jig

femoral muscle

femoral myelocavity file

femoral neck

femoral nerve stretch test

femoral nerve traction test

femoral-peroneal in situ vein bypass graft

femoral-popliteal bypass surgery

femoral-popliteal Gore-Tex graft

femoral prosthesis

femoral pulse

femoral pusher

femoral shaver

femoral tuberosity

femoral venoarterial bypass

femoral view

femoroaxillary bypass

femorocrural graft

femorodistal bypass procedure

femorodistal popliteal bypass graft

femorodistal PTFE graft (polytetrafluoroethylene)

femorofemoral approach

femorofemoral bypass

femorofemoropopliteal

femoroiliac thrombophlebitis

femoropatellar joint
femoroperoneal bypass graft
femorotibial angle (FTA)
femorotibial bypass graft
femorotibial joint (FTJ)
FemoStop femoral artery compression
   arch
fem-pop (slang for femoral-popliteal)
   bypass
femur (pl. femora)
   apex of head of
   body of
   greater trochanter of
   head and neck of
   head of
   lesser trochanter of
   neck of
   nutrient artery of
femur button graft complex
femur-fibula-ulna syndrome
femur length (FL)
fender fracture
fenestra (pl. fenestrae)
fenestrated Drake clip
fenestrated drape
fenestration of cyst
fenestration of dissecting aneurysm
fenestration, pars interarticularis
fenestration saw
Fenlin total shoulder system
fenoprofen (Nalfon)
Fenton bolt
Ferciot-Thomson excision
Ferguson bone-holding forceps
Ferguson brain suction tip
Ferguson-Frazier suction tube
Ferguson hip reduction
Ferguson-Thompson-King two-stage
   osteotomy
Fergusson method for measuring
   scoliosis
Ferkel torticollis technique
Fernandez osteotomy
Ferrein ligament
Ferris Smith bone-biting forceps

Ferris Smith intervertebral disk
   rongeur
Ferris Smith-Kerrison disk rongeur
Ferris Smith-Kerrison laminectomy
   rongeur
Ferris Smith pituitary jaw rongeur
Ferris Smith rongeur forceps
Ferris Smith-Spurling disk rongeur
Ferris Smith tissue forceps
ferritin, glycosylated
ferrocalcinosis, familial cerebral
ferromagnetic relaxation
ferrugination
FES (fat embolism syndrome)
FES (functional electrical stimulation)
festinant quality in parkinsonian
   speech
festinating gait
festination
fetal alcohol effects (FAE)
fetal alcohol syndrome (FAS)
fetal cortical tissue graft
fetal hydrops
fetal lobulation
fetal malformation
fetal pig cell transplantation
fetal sonography
fetal substantia nigra implants
fetal tissue transplantation
fetal ultrasonography
fetal ultrasound
fetal ventral mesencephalic tissue
   transplantation
Fett carpal prosthesis
FF (frontopolar-frontal) electrode
FFC (fixed flexion contracture)
FFI (Foot Function Index)
F-4500 fluorescence spectrophotometer
FFM (fat-free [body] mass)
FFT (fast Fourier transform) analysis
   of EEG
FFT (fast Fourier transform) image
FGS (Facial Grading System)
FHB (flexor hallucis brevis) muscle
FHB (flexor hallucis brevis) tendon

FHL (flexor hallucis longus) muscle
FHL (flexor hallucis longus) tendon
fiber (pl. fibers)
  anchoring
  annular
  annulospiral
  cerebellar
  collagen
  commissural
  contractile
  corticobulbar
  corticospinal
  degeneration of muscle
  demyelinated nerve
  denervated muscle
  extrafusal
  fast twitch
  frontopontine
  general somatic efferent (motor)
  ghost muscle
  intrafusal (spindle system)
  mossy
  motor (general somatic efferent)
  muscle
  myelinated nerve
  nerve
  nerve root
  parasympathetic pupillary constrictor
  pontocerebellar
  postganglionic gray
  pupillomotor
  ragged-red
  regenerating peripheral
  regeneration of muscle
  retinacular
  secretomotor (parasympathetic)
  Sharpey
  skeletal muscle
  slow C
  somatesthetic
  somatic alpha
  somatic nerve
  spinal sympathetic
  tendinous
  thalamofrontal
  trihelical collagen

fiber *(continued)*
  type I muscle
  type II muscle
  unmyelinated nerve
  white
fiber formation, Rosenthal (in
  leukodystrophy)
fiberglass cast
Fiberlase flexible system for CO_2
  surgical laser
fiberoptic headlamp
fiberoptic intracranial pressure monitor
fiberoptic light source
fiber tract dysfunction
Fiblast (trafermin)
Fibrijet surgical sealant
fibrillary matrix
fibrillation
fibrillogenesis
fibrils of connective tissue
fibrin clot formation
fibrin degradation products (FDP)
fibrin glue, percutaneous
fibrin mass
fibrin membrane
fibrinogen
  radiolabeled
  technetium 99mTc-labeled
fibrinogen degradation
fibrinoid exudate
fibrinoid necrosis
fibrinolysis, intraventricular
fibrinolytic agents
fibrinolytic treatment
fibrin sealant
fibrin split products
fibroadenoma
fibroadipose tissue
fibroarthrosis
fibroblast growth factor
fibroblast metabolism
fibroblast radiosensitivity
fibroblastic meningioma
fibroblastoma, perineural
fibrocalcific cusps
fibrocalcification

fibrocartilage
  circumferential
  intra-articular plates of
  triangular
fibrocartilaginous disk
fibrocartilaginous plate
fibrocartilaginous tissue
fibrocollagenous connective tissue
fibrodysplasia ossificans progressiva
  (FOP)
fibroma
  aponeurotic
  cementifying
  cemento-ossifying
  chondromyxoid (CMF)
  desmoplastic
  juvenile ossifying
  meningeal
  nonossifying
  nonosteogenic
  ossifying
  osteogenic
  periosteal
  subcutaneous
fibroma molle
fibroma molluscum
fibromatosis
  fascial
  infantile dermal
  irradiation
  palmar
fibromatosis colli
fibromuscular disease
fibromuscular dysplasia (FMD)
fibromuscular lesion
fibromuscular ridge
Fibromyalgia Impact Questionnaire
fibromyalgia joint pain
Fibromyalgia Self-Efficacy Scale
fibromyalgia syndrome (FMS)
fibromyoma
fibromyositis
fibromyxoid sarcoma
fibronectin, cellular
fibronectin-positive mesenchymal cells
fibro-osseous tunnel
fibrosarcoma

fibrosclerotic
fibrosed muscles
fibrosis
  arachnoid
  basilar
  leptomeningeal
  mediastinal
  meningeal
  periarticular
  peridural
  perimuscular
  postradiation
  posttraumatic
  radiation-induced
  replacement
fibrositis, periarticular
fibrotic cavitating pattern
fibrotic tissue
fibrous dysplasia ossificans progressiva
fibrous histiocytoma
fibrous joint
fibrous nonunion
fibrous palmar fasciculi
fibrous union
fibroxanthoma
fibroxanthosarcoma
fibula
  apex of head of
  nutrient artery of
fibular bone
fibular collateral ligament (FCL)
fibular head resection
fibular hemimelia
fibular joint disruption
fibular muscle
fibular nerve
fibular notch
fibular ostectomy
fibular physes
fibulocalcaneal
fibulotalar ligament
fibulotalocalcaneal (FTC) ligament
Ficat classification of femoral head
  osteonecrosis
Ficat-Marcus grading system
Ficat operation
Ficat stage of avascular necrosis

FICS (Fédération International de
Chiropractic Sportif)
FID (free induction decay)
fiducial box
fiducial localization system attached to
stereotactic frame
fiducial marker
fiducial movement
fiducial plate
field (pl. fields)
altitudinal loss of visual
blind spot in visual
bloodless
Brodmann cytoarchitectonic
central visual
chiasmal visual
concentric visual
confrontation visual
curtain pulled across visual
disk to magnetic
EEG potentials plotting
high power
irregular loss of visual
low power
nasal retinal visual
oscillating magnetic
peripheral
pulsating electromagnetic (PEMF)
pulsed electromagnetic
rf *or* RF (radiofrequency)
temporal visual
tesla (T)
vertical meridian of visual
visual
window shade pulled down
on visual
field defect
field gradient
field H of Forel
Fielding-Magliato classification of
subtrochanteric fracture
field lock
field of dissection
field of distribution
field of view (FOV) imaging
field stretcher
fifth compartment

fifth cranial nerve (trigeminal nerve)
mandibular division
maxillary division
ophthalmic division
fifth rib
fighter's fracture
figure 4 position (figure of 4)
figure 8 cast (figure of 8)
figure 8 dressing
figure 8 interscapular bandage
figure 8 ring harness
figure 8 suture
fila of nerve roots
file
bone
femoral myelocavity
McCain TMJ
filed
filgrastim (Neupogen)
filiform
Fillauer bar
Fillauer night splint
filler, shoe
filling defect
filling factor
filling
venous
vessel
film (see also *position, projection,
view*)
Accu-Flo dura
AP (anteroposterior)
chiropractic
comparison
cross-table lateral
decubitus
digital subtraction
DuPont Cronex x-ray
Knuttsen bending
lateral decubitus
low contrast
oblique
overhead
PA (posteroanterior)
plain
portable
preliminary

film *(continued)*
  prone
  scout
  skull
  spot
  stress
  suboptimal
  subtraction
  supine
  upright
film-based viewing
filmless imaging
filter
  bird's nest percutaneous IVC
  caval
  compensation (x-ray)
  Gianturco-Roehm bird's nest vena
    caval
  Greenfield vena caval
  inferior vena cava (IVC)
  Kalman
  Kimray-Greenfield caval
  Mobin-Uddin umbrella
  percutaneous inferior vena cava
    (IVC)
  prophylactic IVC
  Simon nitinol percutaneous IVC
  umbrella
  Venatech percutaneous IVC
filtered-back projection
Filtzer interbody rasp
filum, fatty
filum terminale
FIM (Functional Independence
  Measure)
fin of prosthetic stem, lateral
FIN pin extractor
FIN pin guide
final handicap
finder
  angle
  Dasco Pro angle
  gravity-driven angle
  pedicle
finding (pl. findings)
  angiographic
  characteristic

finding *(continued)*
  equivocal
  focal
  lateralizing
  no discernible
  ominous
  pathognomonic
  salient physical
  specious
  spurious
fine-angled curet
fine calcifications
fine needle
fine-needle biopsy, ultrasound-guided
fine tactile discrimination
fine tactile sensations
finger (pl. fingers)
  angle
  baseball
  base of
  bolster
  clubbed
  Dasco Pro angle
  football
  gravity-driven angle
  index
  jammed
  jersey
  little
  long
  mallet
  middle
  pedicle
  pulp of
  pulley of
  replantation of
  replanted
  ring
  sausage
  spade
  speck
  spider
  stoved
  trigger
  webbed
finger agnosia
finger agnosis

Finger Blocking Tree
finger count test
fingerbreadth
finger dexterity
fingerdrop
finger extrinsics
finger fillet flap
finger fracture dissection
finger intrinsics
fingernail
 base of
 circumferential
finger of tumor
finger opposition
finger pad
finger pursuit drift
finger splint
 malleable metal
 Joint-Jack
fingerstick felon
fingertip
fingertip amputation
fingertip dissection
fingertip pad
finger-to-finger test
finger-to-nose test (F to N)
fingertrap
 Chinese
 Japanese
fingertrap phenomenon
fingertrap suspension
finisher
 Küntscher
 Sven-Johansson
Finkelstein sign for synovitis
Finkelstein test
Finn hinged knee replacement
 prosthesis
Finochietto laminectomy retractor
Finochietto rib spreader
FIRDA (frontal intermittent rhythmic
 delta activity)
fire (Chinese medicine term)
firing of neuron
Firm D-Ring wrist splint
FirmFlex custom orthotic
first compartment

first cranial nerve (olfactory nerve)
first dorsal interosseous
FIRST knee prosthesis
first metatarsal angle
first ray instability
first ray insufficiency
first ray stabilizers (muscles)
first rib resection
first temporal gyrus
first-toe Jones repair
FIRST total knee instrumentation
first-trimester nuchal translucency
Fisch bone rongeur
Fisch dural hook
Fischer frame
Fischer ring
Fischer tendon stripper
Fischer ventricular cannula
Fisch micro hook
Fisch rongeur
Fish cuneiform osteotomy technique
Fisher exact test
Fisher guide
Fisher rasp
Fisher syndrome
fish-mouth drainage
fish-mouth incision
Fiskars Softouch scissors
FISP (gradient echo sequence)
fissuration
fissure
 anterior median (of cord)
 antitragohelicine
 auricular
 brain
 calcarine
 callosomarginal
 central
 cerebellar
 cerebellopontine or cerebellopontile
 cerebral
 choroidal
 displacement of interhemispheric
 glaserian
 hippocampal
 inflammatory process of the superior
  orbital

fissure *(continued)*
  interhemispheric
  lateral
  longitudinal
  neoplastic process of the superior
    orbital
  occipital
  rolandic
  superior orbital
  supraorbital
  sylvian
fissure fracture
fissure of Rolando
fissure of Sylvius
fisticuffs
Fist-Palm-Side Test
Fist-Ring Test
fistula
  arteriovenous (AVF)
  basilar cavernous
  carotid-cavernous sinus
  cerebral arteriovenous
  cerebrospinal fluid
  congenital
  CSF (cerebrospinal fluid)
  dural arteriovenous (AVF)
  durocutaneous
  iatrogenic
  intradural arteriovenous
  intradural retromedullary
    arteriovenous
  parietal
  premedullary arteriovenous
  spinal dural arteriovenous
  tangle of
  transdural
  trigeminal cavernous
fistulogram
fistulography
fistulous formation
fistulous tract
fit (epileptic seizure)
Fitnet joint testing system
Fitron
Fits-All supports

fitting
  immediate postsurgical (IPSF)
  prosthetic
  Velcro
5-aminolevulinic-acid-induced
  porphyrin fluorescence
5 Degree of Freedom robotic manipulator arm
five-in-one knee repair
fix and focus attention
fixateur (see *fixator*)
Fixateur Interne fixation system
Fixateur Interne rod
Fixateur Interne screw
fixation (see also *fixator*; *operation*)
  Ace-Fischer
  Ace Unifix
  atlantoaxial
  atlantoaxial rotatory
  Barbour cervical
  Biofix absorbable
  BioStinger low profile
  bolt
  bone ingrowth
  Calandruccio triangular compression
  cementless
  circumferential wire loop
  Cole tendon
  contoured loop
  dynamic
  dynamic external
  ECT (European compression
    technique) internal fracture
  Ender nail
  Ender rod
  Endopearl
  EX-FI-RE external
  external wire
  four-bar external
  four-point
  fracture
  Galveston sacral
  Georgiade visor halo
  greenstick
  Hammer external

fixation *(continued)*
  Herbert bone screw
  Hoffmann external
  hook-pin
  hook-plate
  horizontal interosseous wire loop
  hybrid
  hydroxyapatite
  internal fracture
  intrapedicular
  K wire (Kirschner)
  LPPS hydroxyapatite
  Luque loop
  Luque rod
  Luque segmental
  Magerl hook-plate
  Magerl transarticular screw
  Meniscus Arrow
  Minerva
  minifragment plate
  monofilament wire
  Monticelli-Spinelli leg
  nail
  NeuroPro rigid
  Olerud transpedicular
  open reduction and internal (ORIF)
  Orthofix
  OrthoSorb pin
  PDS (poly-p-dioxanone) pin
  pedicle screw
  Pennig dynamic wrist
  pin
  Polarus Plus humeral
  poly-p-dioxanone (PDS) pin
  postural
  Precision Osteolock
  primary metallic
  primary rigid
  Rezinian external
  rigid internal
  Rogozinski spinal
  screw
  screw and keel
  screw and plate
  screw and wire
  screw plate
  segmental spinal

fixation *(continued)*
  Seidel intramedullary
  SmartTack
  spinal pedicle
  spring
  Stableloc II external
  staple
  static
  suprasyndesmotic
  Suretac shoulder
  suture bridge
  tension band
  TiMesh implantable hardware
  Torus external
  transarticular screw
  TransFix ACL system
  transpedicular
  transsyndesmotic screw
  triangular external ankle
  True/Lok external
  Tylok high tension cerclage cabling
  variable screw plate (VSP)
  Varigrip spine
  Versa-Fx femoral
  Versalok low back
  Vidal-Adrey modified Hoffmann
  wedge
  wire
  Wolvek sternal approximation
  Wrightlock posterior
  Xact ACL graft
  Zickel nail
  ZMS intramedullary
  ZPLATE-ATL anterior spinal
fixation device
fixation muscles
fixation nystagmus
fixation of a scoliosis
fixation peg
fixation reflexes
fixation system
fixation wire
fixator
  Ace-Colles external
  Ace-Fischer external
  Agee external
  AO internal

fixator *(continued)*
  articulated
  cantilever external
  circular external
  Claiborne external
  Clyburn Colles fracture
  D-L internal
  DeBastiani external
  dynamic axial (DAF)
  Edwards D-L modular
  external
  external spinal skeletal (ESSF)
  hinged articulated
  Hoffmann external
  Ilizarov
  Ilizarov external
  Kessler external
  mini-Hoffmann external
  mini-Kessler external
  mini-Orthofix
  Monofixateur external
  Monticelli-Spinelli
  Olerud internal
  one-bar external
  Orthofix external
  Orthofix miniature
  Oxford
  Pennig dynamic wrist
  ReFix stereotactic head
  ring external
  thin wire Ilizarov
  Thomas
  Vermont spinal (VSF)
  Wagner external
  Wiltse
fixator-augmented nailing
fixed-bearing knee implant
fixed bony planus
fixed intracavitary filling defect
fixed mass
fixed neurologic deficit
fixed perfusion defect
fixed pupils
fixed sagittal imbalance
fixer, Wagner
FL (femur length)

flabby heart
FL/AC ratio (femur length to
  abdominal circumference)
flaccid hemiplegia
flaccidity
flaccid paralysis
flaccid paraplegia
flaccid weakness
Flagg Fiberglass knee brace
flail digit
flail foot
flail joint
flail shoulder
FLAIR (fluid-attenuated inversion
  recovery) sequences
FLAIR-FLASH imaging
flake avulsion fracture
flaking of cartilage
Flanagan-Burem apposing hemicylin-
  dric graft
Flanagan spinal fusion gouge
flange
flank bone (ilium)
flap (pl. flaps)
  abdominal
  advancement
  anconeus muscle
  artery island
  Atasoy-Kleinert
  Atasoy palmar
  Atasoy triangular advancement
  axial flag
  axial pattern
  bilobed
  bipedicle
  bone
  bursal
  butterfly
  Chinese
  cross finger
  cross leg
  Dandy myocutaneous scalp
  digital
  dorsalis pedis fasciocutaneous
  dorsalis pedis myofascial
  dorsal rotation

flap *(continued)*
   dorsal transposition
   DRAM (de-epithelialized rectus
     abdominis) muscle
   entry
   extended
   extensor carpi radialis longus
   fascial
   fasciocutaneous island
   finger fillet
   free
   free fasciocutaneous
   free fibular harvest
   free latissimus dorsi
   free temporal
   galeal
   gastrocnemius sliding
   gracilis muscle
   groin
   hemipulp
   horseshoe-shaped
   iliac osteocutaneous free
   iliofemoral pedicle
   interdigitating skin
   island pedicle
   Kutler digital
   latissimus dorsi musculocutaneous
     free
   lumbrical muscle
   microsurgical free
   Moberg
   modified dorsalis pedis myofascial
   muscle
   musculocutaneous free flap
   musculotendinous
   myocutaneous
   myofascial
   necrotic
   neurocutaneous island
   neurovascular island pedicle
   nutrient
   osteocutaneous free
   osteoplastic
   palmar advancement
   parascapular
   pectoralis major
   pedicle

flap *(continued)*
   pedicled muscle-tendon
   pericranial
   peroneal island
   pulp
   radial-based
   radial forearm
   rectus abdominis
   rectus abdominis musculocutaneous
     free
   rectus muscle
   remote pedicle
   rotational
   rotator
   scalp
   scapular
   segmented
   skin
   subscapularis muscle
   Tait
   tensor fasciae latae
   thenar
   three-square
   transposition
   triangular
   triceps
   tumbler
   turned-down tendon
   V-Y advancement
   vascularized
   wraparound
flap congestion
flap graft, Kutler V-Y
flapping tremor
flap tear
flap viability
flare
   axon
   condylar
   metaphyseal
   tibial
   trochanteric
flare phenomenon
flareup of disease
flareup of pain
FLASH (fast low-angle shot)
FLASH 3D sequence

FLASH images
flashback
flashes per second of photic stimulation
flashlamp pulsed dye laser
flash stimulation on EEG
flash visual evoked response
flat acromion
flat affect
Flatau-Schilder disease
flatback deformity
flat bone
flat EEG recording
flat (isoelectric) EEG record
flatfoot
   acquired
   adult
   calcaneovalgus
   congenital
   Durham procedure for
   hypermobile
   Kidner
   neonatal
   pathologic
   peroneal spastic
   physiologic
   pronated straight
   rigid
   rockerbottom
   spastic
flatfoot deformity
flatfootedness
flatfoot pathomechanics, juvenile
flat-hand test
flatline EEG
flat nasolabial fold
Flatt finger/thumb prosthesis
flattened longitudinal arch of foot
flattening, generalized
flattening of EEG tracing
flattening of normal lumbar curve
flaval ligament
flavum, pleating of ligamentum
flawed image
Flechsig bundle
Flechsig tract
Fleck sign
Fleischmann bursa

Fleischner disease
Fleischner sign
flesh
   live
   proud
flesinoxan
flex against gravity
flexer (see *flexor*)
Flexeril
Flex-Foam bandage
Flexfoot foot prosthesis
FLEX H/A total ossicular prosthesis
flexibility, waxy
flexible spastic equinovarus deformity
flexible stent
flexible surface coil-type resonator
   (FSCR)
Flexicair bed
Flexi-Grip exercise putty
Flexilite conforming elastic bandage
flexion
   dorsiflexion
   elongation-derotation
   forced plantar
   neutral
   plantar
   range of
   resisted active
   Riordan finger
   spasmodic
   toe
   uninhibited
   volitional resisted
flexion against resistance
flexion and extension
flexion bias
flexion contracture
flexion crease
flexion deformity
flexion distraction chiropractic table
flexion distraction injury
flexion distraction therapy
flexion maneuver
flexion reflex
flexion-rotation-compression
   maneuvers
flexion rotation injury of spine

flexion teardrop injury
flexion test
Flexisplint flexed arm board
Flex-Master bandage
Flex-Node AcuVibe massager
flexometer, Moeltgen
flexor (pl. flexors)
  capital
  hallux
  snapping thumb
  toe
  X-TEND-O knee
flexor carpi ulnaris (FCU) muscle
flexor carpi ulnaris (FCU) tendon
flexor digitorum profundus (FDP)
  muscle
flexor digitorum profundus (FDP)
  tendon
flexor digitorum superficialis (FDS)
  muscle
flexor digitorum superficialis (FDS)
  tendon
flexor hallucis longus (FHL) muscle
flexor hallucis longus (FHL) tendon
flexor muscle
flexor palmar plates
flexor pollicis longus (FPL) muscle
flexor pollicis longus (FPL) tendon
flexor pronator slide therapy
flexor reflex
flexor retinaculum
flexor tendon graft
flexor tenosynovium
flexor wad of five
flexorplasty
  Bunnell modification of Steindler
  Eyler
  Steindler
flexors and extensors
FlexStrand cable
FlexTech knee brace
FlexTip intervertebral rongeur
flexural modulus properties
flexure
  cephalic
  cerebral

flexure *(continued)*
  cervical
  cranial
F. L. Fischer microsurgical
  neurectomy bayonet scissors
flip angle
flipped meniscus sign
flipper hand
floating elbow forearm fracture
floating traction
floating time (in gait)
floccillation
flocculent foci of calcification
flocculonodular lobe of cerebellum
flocculonodular tumors
flocculus of cerebellum
Flood ligament
floor effect in rehabilitation testing
floor of acetabulum
floor of ventricle
floor, sellar
floppy infant
floppy infant syndrome
florid reactive periostitis
florid synovitis
Florida cervical brace
Florida J-24 brace
Florida J-35 brace
Florida J-45 brace
Florida J-55 brace
Flotan thumb
flottant, pouce (floating thumb)
flow
  axoplasmic
  cerebral blood (CBF)
  cerebral brain
  cerebrospinal fluid (CSF)
  collateral blood
  compromised
  decreased cerebral blood
  regional cerebral blood (rCBF)
  reversed vertebral blood (RVBF)
  total cerebral blood (TCBF)
flowable polymer
flow-compensated gradient-echo
  sequence

flow-compromising lesion
flow cytometry
flow-dependent obstruction
flow effect artifact
Flower bone
flow images
flowmetry
  blood
  Doppler laser
  laser Doppler (LDF)
  Parks 800 bidirectional Doppler
  pulsed Doppler
flow of cerebrospinal fluid
flow scan, radionuclide
flow void
Floyd classification of peripheral
  nerves
FLP (Functional Limitation Profile)
fluasterone (synthetic dehydroepiandrosterone, DHEA)
fluconazole
fluctuant mass
fludeoxyglucose F-18 PET
fluent aphasic speech
fluent paraphasic speech
fluffy rarefaction of Paget disease (on
  x-ray)
fluid
  bursal
  cerebrospinal (CSF)
  egress of arthroscopic
  high signal (on MRI) intratendinous
    collection of
  joint
  leakage of cerebrospinal
  loculated
  serosanguineous
  serous
  spinal
  subgaleal cerebrospinal
  synovial
fluid accumulation in tissues
FluidAir bed
fluid-attenuated inversion recovery
  (FLAIR) imaging
fluid barrier boot
fluid collection, loculated

fluid prosthesis
fluid shear stress
fluorapatite
fluorescein angiography
fluorescein perfusion monitoring
fluorescein uptake
fluorescence
  5-aminolevulinic-acid induced
    porphyrin
  laser-induced
  tissue
fluorescence digital imaging
  microscopy (FDIM)
fluorescence spectroscopy
fluorescent porphyrins
fluorescent treponemal antibody (FTA)
  test
fluorine (F)
  18F (fluorine-18, F-18)
  18F 2-deoxyglucose (18FDG)
    uptake on PET scan
  18F estradiol (FES)
  18F fluoro-DOPA
  18F fluorodeoxyglucose PET scan
  18F fluorotamoxifen
  18F labeled derivatives of
    m-tyrosine
  18F labeled HFA-134a
  18F labeled polyfluorinated ethyl
  18F N-methylspiperone
  18F spiperone
  18F uptake
  18FDG (fluorine-18 2-deoxy-D-
    glucose) PET scan
fluorodeoxyglucose (FDG) radioactive
  tracer
fluorodopamine accumulation
fluorodopa PET scan (FD PET)
fluorophore-coupled oligosaccharide
  electrophoresis
fluorometry
  fiberoptic
  image intensification
  portable C-arm image intensifier
  two-plane
  video
FluoroPlus angiography

FluoroPlus Roadmapper digital
    fluoroscopy system
FluoroScan mini C-arm imaging
fluoroscope (see *fluoroscopy*)
fluoroscopic assistance
fluoroscopic control, advanced under
fluoroscopic diskectomy
fluoroscopic guidance
fluoroscopic localization
fluoroscopic road-mapping technique
    in angioplastic vascular procedures
fluoroscopic stress view (x-ray)
fluoroscopic view
fluoroscopy
    C-arm digital
    digital
    electric joint
    FluoroPlus Roadmapper digital
    real-time CT
fluoroscopy-guided condylar lift-off
fluoroscopy-guided subarachnoid
    phenol block (SAPB)
Fluoro Tip cannula
fluoxetine hydrochloride (Prozac)
flupertine maleate
flurry of myoclonic jerks
flush
    heparinized saline
    peroxide
flutes of cannulated screw
flutter
    eyelid
    lid
    ocular
fluxmetry, laser Doppler
fly-catching movements of the tongue
Flynn technique
FMA cephalometric measurement
FMD (fibromuscular dysplasia)
FMH (first metatarsal head)
FMPIR (fast SE and fast IR) imaging
FMPSPGR (fast multiplanar spoiled
    gradient-recalled) sequence
FMR (functional MR) imaging
fMRI or FMRI (functional magnetic
    resonance imaging)
FMS (fibromyalgia syndrome)

FO (foot orthosis)
foam
    Evazote
    Plastazote
    Supazote
    velvet
foam cell
foam embolus
foaming at the mouth during seizure
focal abnormality
focal activity
focal area of hemorrhage
focal calcification
focal cerebral epilepsy
focal changes
focal damage
focal deficit
focal degenerative change
focal delta slow wave activity
focal demyelinating disease
focal distortion
focal eccentric stenosis
focal edema
focal finding
focal lesion
focal mass
focal motor seizure
focal neurologic sign
focal plaque-like defect
focal sclerosing osteomyelitis
FocalSeal-S neurosurgical sealant
focal sensory seizure
focal sign
focal status epilepticus
focal stenosis
focal weakness
focal white matter signal abnormalities
foci of abnormal epileptic neurons
foci of calcification
foci of tumor
focus (pl. foci)
    anaplastic
    asynchronous
    bilateral
    centrotemporal paroxysmal
    ectopic seizure
    EEG

focus *(continued)*
  epileptic
  epileptogenic
  hemorrhagic
  junctional
  mesial frontal
  midline parasagittal
  mirror
  multiple
  occipital
  resection of epileptogenic
  rolandic paroxysmal
  seizure
  sharp wave
  shifting
  spike
  stationary
  unilateral
focus of activity
  midline
  unilateral
Foerster forceps
Fogarty arterial embolectomy catheter
Foix-Alajouanine disease
Foix-Alajouanine syndrome
Foix syndrome
fold
  asymmetric thigh
  flat nasolabial
Folius muscle
following ability of eyes
following movements
Folstein Mini-Mental Status
  Examination
Foltz catheter
Foltz flushing reservoir
fomentation therapy
Fomon chisel
Fomon periosteal elevator
Fomon periosteotome
Fomon rasp
Fonar Stand-Up MRI scanner
fontanel (fontanelle)
  anterior
  anterolateral
  bregmatic
  bulging

fontanel *(continued)*
  closed
  cranial
  frontal
  fused
  Gerdy
  mastoid
  occipital
  open
  overriding sutures of
  posterior
  posterolateral
  sagittal
  sphenoid
  tense
  triangular
Food and Drug Administration (FDA)
foot (pl. feet)
  anesthetic
  arch of
  architecture of the
  arcuate artery of
  articulations of
  athlete's
  axial compression of the
  ball of
  bones of
  burning
  calcaneocavus
  calcaneovalgus
  cavovarus
  cavus
  Charcot
  clawfoot
  contralateral
  cosmetically acceptable
  deconditioned
  diabetic Charcot
  digital artery of
  drop
  flail
  flatfoot
  flat calcaneovalgus
  flat flexible
  flat neonatal
  flat pronated straight
  flat rigid

foot *(continued)*
  Friedreich
  functional disability of the
  hollow (pes cavus, pes arcuatus,
    clawfoot)
  hypoflexibility of
  insensate
  ischemic
  Kidner flatfoot
  lateral wedges for sole or heel of
  lift-off of
  lobster claw
  longitudinal arch of
  Madura
  march
  monodactylous cleft
  Morton
  neuroarthropathic
  perforating artery of
  peroneal spastic flatfoot
  phalanges of
  planovalgus
  plantigrade
  polydactylous cleft
  pronated
  propulsive
  push-off of
  Quantum
  revascularization of
  rigid
  rocker (rockerbottom flatfoot)
  rockerbottom
  SACH (solid-ankle, cushioned heel)
  SAFE (stationary attachment
    flexible endoskeletal)
  serpentine
  single-axis
  skew
  sole of
  splay
  split
  supporting
  Syme prosthetic
  tabetic
  valgus
  venous pump of the
  Z

foot-ankle assembly
foot-ankle complex
footballer's ankle
football finger
footdrop
  paralytic peroneal
  postpartum
  steppage gait due to
footdrop of central origin
footdrop of peripheral origin
footdrop splint
foot dynamics
foot dysplasia
foot fall measurement
Foot Function Index (FFI)
Foot Health Status Questionnaire
foot intrinsic muscle strength
foot ischemia
foot joint
Foot Levelers orthotics
foot orthosis (FO)
foot piece
  Bunker
  traction
footplate, metal
foot pound
footprint
  dynamic
  static
footprint analysis
footprint index
foot progression angle (FPA)
foot prosthesis
foot roller reflexology device
foot slap
foot stagnation (Chinese medicine
  term)
foot strain
foot strike phase of gait
foot-to-hand transfer
footwear
FOP (fibrodysplasia ossificans
  progressiva)
forage procedure
foramen (pl. foramina)
  arachnoidal
  Bichat

foramen *(continued)*
  blind
  carotid
  cecal
  cranial
  emissary sphenoidal
  ethmoidal
  frontal
  great sacrosciatic
  greater palatine
  greater sciatic
  intertransverse
  interventricular
  intervertebral
  Luschka
  Magendie
  Monro
  Morgagni
  neural
  sacrosciatic
  spinous
  stylomastoid
  vertebral
foramen magnum herniation
foramen magnum of skull
foramen magnum pressure coning
foramen of Froesch
foramen of Luschka
foramen of Magendie
foramen of Monro
foramen ovale
foramina (pl. of foramen)
foraminal encroachment
foraminal space
foraminiferous
foraminotomy, keyhole
foraminulum
Forbes-Cori disease
Forbes disease
Forbes modification of Phemister graft
  technique
force (pl. forces)
  axial compression (loads on spine)
  daltons of (SI units)
  ground reaction
  impact
  intradural hydraulic

force *(continued)*
  lateral tensile
  lateral translation
  linear translation
  medial compressive
  Newton
  pascals of (SI units)
  propulsive
  rotational
  shearing
  tension
  torque
  torsional impaction
  transverse plane
forced plantar flexion
forcefully wedged
force/motion synchronization
force platform
forceps
  Acland clamp-applying
  Acufex curved basket
  Acufex rotary biting basket
  Adson bayonet dressing
  Adson bipolar
  Adson-Brown tissue
  Adson clip-introducing
  Adson dressing
  Adson dura protecting
  Adson hemostatic
  Adson hypophyseal
  Adson micro tissue
  Adson-Mixter neurosurgical
  Adson rongeur
  Adson tissue
  adventitial
  Aesculap bipolar cautery
  alligator
  alligator grasping
  Allis tissue
  Angell James hypophysectomy
  Angell James reverse-action
    hypophysectomy
  angled-down
  angled-up
  anterior
  AO reduction
  arthroscopy basket

forceps *(continued)*
  arthroscopy grasping
  Asch
  Backhaus towel
  Bacon rongeur
  Baer bone cutting
  Bane rongeur
  Bangerter muscle
  Bardeleben bone-holding
  basket
  bayonet
  bayonet-shaped
  Berens muscle
  Beyer rongeur
  biarticular bone-cutting
  biopsy
  bipolar cautery
  Bircher-Ganske cartilage
  Bishop-Harmon
  blunt
  Boies
  bone-biting
  bone-breaking
  bone-cutting
  bone-grasping
  bone-holding
  bone punch
  bone-splitting
  brain
  brain clip
  brain spatula
  brain tumor
  Brand tendon-holding
  Brand tendon-passing
  Brand tendon-tunneling
  Brigham brain tumor
  Brown-Adson tissue
  Brown-Cushing
  Brown tissue
  Cairns hemostatic
  capsular release
  Carroll bone-holding
  Carroll dressing
  Carroll tendon-pulling
  Carroll tissue
  cartilage
  Caspar alligator

forceps *(continued)*
  cervical punch
  Chandler spinal perforating
  Charnley wire-holding
  Cherry-Kerrison laminectomy
  Citelli punch
  clamp-applying
  Cleveland bone-cutting
  clip-applying
  clip-bending
  clip-cutting
  clip-introducing
  Cloward punch
  Cloward rongeur
  coagulating
  Cone skull punch
  Cone wire-twisting
  cranial rongeur
  Crile artery
  cup
  cupped-jaw
  curved
  Cushing bipolar
  Cushing dressing
  Cushing monopolar
  Cushing rongeur
  Cushing tissue
  cutting
  Dandy scalp hemostatic
  Davis coagulating
  Davis monopolar
  Dawson-Yuhl-Kerrison rongeur
  Dawson-Yuhl-Leksell rongeur
  DeBakey
  Decker alligator
  Decker microsurgical
  DeMartel scalp flap
  Demel wire-tightening
  Demel wire-twisting
  D'Errico bayonet pituitary
  D'Errico hypophyseal
  D'Errico pituitary
  D'Errico tissue
  DeTakats-McKenzie brain clip
  DeVilbiss rongeur
  Dingman bone-holding
  disk

forceps *(continued)*
    dissecting
    dressing
    dura protecting
    eagle's beak bone-cutting
    ear
    Echlin rongeur
    ethmoid
    extracting
    Farabeuf bone-holding
    Farabeuf-Lambotte bone-holding
    Farrior wire-crimping
    Ferguson bone-holding
    Fergusson
    Ferris Smith-Kerrison
    Ferris Smith rongeur
    Ferris Smith tissue
    fine-tip
    Foerster
    Fox bipolar
    Friedman rongeur
    gall duct
    Gardner bone
    Gerald bipolar
    Gerald dressing
    Gerald tissue
    Gildenberg biopsy
    glenoid-reaming
    grasping
    Greene
    Greenwood bipolar and suction
    Gruenwald ear
    Gruppe wire-crimping
    Gunderson bone
    Gunderson muscle
    Hajek-Koffler bone punch
    Halsted artery
    Halsted mosquito
    Hardy bipolar
    Hardy dressing
    Hardy microbipolar
    Hardy sella punch
    Harrison bone-holding
    Hartmann mosquito
    Heermann alligator
    hemostatic
    Hibbs bone-cutting

forceps *(continued)*
    Hinderer cartilage
    Hirsch hypophysis punch
    Hoen angular
    Hoen scalp hemostatic
    Horsley bone-cutting
    Horsley-Stille bone-cutting
    Housepan clip-applying
    Howmedica Microfixation System
    Hudson
    Hunt tumor
    Hunt-Yasargil pituitary
    Hurd bone-cutting
    hypophyseal
    hypophysectomy
    hypophysis punch
    Ingraham skull punch
    intervertebral disk
    Jackson tendon-seizing
    Jacobson dressing
    Jacobson micro mosquito
    Jacobson mosquito
    Jannetta alligator
    Jannetta bayonet
    Jansen-Middleton septal
    Jansen monopolar
    Jarell
    Jarit brain
    Jarit tendon-pulling
    jeweler's
    Johnson brain tumor
    Johnson tumor
    Juers-Lempert rongeur
    Kelly artery
    Kern bone-holding
    Kern-Lane bone
    Kleinert-Kutz bone-cutting
    Kleinert-Kutz rongeur
    Kleinert-Kutz tendon
    Knight bone-cutting
    knotting
    Kocher
    Lalonde hook
    Lambotte bone-holding
    laminectomy punch
    Landolt spreading
    Lane bone-holding

forceps *(continued)*
   Lane screw-holding
   Lane self-retaining bone-holding
   Langenbeck bone-holding
   Larsen tendon-holding
   Leibinger Micro System plate-holding
   Leksell rongeur
   Lempert rongeur
   LeRoy clip-applying
   LeRoy scalp clip-applying
   Lester muscle
   Lewin bone-holding
   Lewin spinal-perforating
   ligamentum flavum
   lion
   lion-jaw
   Liston bone-cutting
   Liston-Key bone-cutting
   Liston-Littauer bone-cutting
   Liston-Stille bone-cutting
   Littauer-Liston bone-cutting
   Llorente dissecting
   Lore suction tube and tip-holding
   Love-Gruenwald alligator
   Love-Gruenwald intervertebral disk
   Love-Gruenwald pituitary
   Love-Kerrison rongeur
   Lowman bone-holding
   Luer rongeur
   Luer-Whiting rongeur
   Luhr Microfixation System plate-holding
   Malis angled-up bipolar
   Malis bipolar cautery
   Malis bipolar coagulation
   Malis irrigation
   Malis-Jensen microbipolar
   Malis jeweler bipolar
   Markwalder rib
   Martin cartilage
   Mayfield
   McCain TMJ
   McGee-Priest wire
   McGee wire-crimping
   McIndoe rongeur
   McKenzie brain clip

forceps *(continued)*
   McKenzie clip-applying
   McKenzie clip-bending
   McKenzie clip-introducing
   meniscus
   microartery
   microbipolar
   Micro-One dissecting
   microsurgery
   Micro-Two
   microvascular
   Miltex tendon-pulling
   Mixter
   mosquito
   Moynihan
   nail-pulling
   Nicola
   Niro bone-cutting
   Niro wire-twisting
   Oldberg pituitary
   Olivecrona clip-applying and removing
   Olivecrona-Toennis clip-applying
   Overholt clip-applying
   Pean
   peapod intervertebral disk
   perforating
   Perman cartilage
   pick-up
   Pierce
   pinch-band
   pituitary
   plain tissue
   plate-holding
   Poppen
   Potts-Smith dressing
   Preston ligamentum flavum
   pulpiform nucleus
   punch
   Raimondi hemostatic
   Raimondi infant scalp hemostatic
   Raimondi scalp
   Raney coagulating
   Raney rongeur
   Raney scalp clip-applying
   Rhoton bipolar
   Rhoton cup

forceps *(continued)*
  Rhoton-Cushing
  Rhoton dissecting
  Rhoton-Tew bipolar
  rib
  Riches artery
  Richter laminectomy punch
  ring
  Rochester-Carmalt
  Rochester-Ochsner
  Rochester-Pean
  rongeur
  Rowe disimpaction
  Rowe glenoid-reaming
  Rowe-Harrison bone-holding
  Rowe modified-Harrison
  Ruskin bone-splitting
  Ruskin-Liston bone-cutting
  Ruskin rongeur
  Ruskin-Rowland bone-cutting
  Russian
  Samuels
  Sauerbruch rib
  scalp clip
  scalp flap
  Scharff microbipolar and suction
  Scheicker laminectomy punch
  Schlesinger cervical punch
  Schlesinger rongeur
  Schnidt
  Schwartz clip-applying
  Schwartz temporary clamp-applying
  Scoville brain clip-applying
  Scoville brain spatula
  screw-holding
  seizing
  self-centering bone-holding
  sella punch
  Selverstone rongeur
  Semb bone
  Semb rib
  Semkin tissue
  septal
  sequestrum
  Sewall brain clip
  Sewall clip-applying
  Shutt Mantis retrograde

forceps *(continued)*
  skull punch
  Smithwick clip-applying
  smooth-tipped jeweler's
  spatula
  Spence rongeur
  spinal perforating
  sponge-holding
  spreading
  Spurling-Kerrison rongeur
  Steinmann tendon
  Stevenson alligator
  Stevenson grasping
  Stille-Horsley bone
  Stille-Liston bone-cutting
  Stille-Luer rongeur
  Stiwer bone-holding
  Storz Microsystems plate-holding
  straight
  Synthes Microsystems plate-holding
  Takahashi
  Take-apart
  taper-jaw
  tenaculum-reducing
  tendon
  tendon-holding
  tendon-passing
  tendon-pulling
  tendon-retrieving
  tendon-seizing
  tendon-tunneling
  termite
  three-edge cutting
  thumb
  tissue
  titanium microsurgical bipolar
  Toennis tumor
  tonsil
  toothed tissue
  transsphenoidal bipolar
  Tudor-Edwards bone-cutting
  tumor-grasping
  tying
  Ulrich bone-holding
  Ulrich-St. Gallen
  Van Buren sequestrum
  vascular

forceps *(continued)*
   Verbrugge bone-holding
   Walter-Liston
   Walton-Ruskin
   Walton wire-pulling
   Weller cartilage
   Wiet cup
   Wilde
   Wilde ethmoid
   Wilde rongeur
   wire
   wire-crimping
   wire-cutting
   wire-extracting
   wire-holding
   wire-pulling
   wire-tightening
   wire-twisting
   Yasargil artery
   Yasargil bayonet
   Yasargil clip-applying
   Yasargil hypophyseal
   Yasargil knotting
   Yasargil micro
   Yasargil tumor
forceps major
forceps minor
forceps occipitalis
forceps posterior
forceps speculum
force regimen for osteosynthesis
force-strain relationship
Ford Hospital ventricular cannula
forearm, one-bone
forearm compartment syndrome
forearm fascial hernia
forearm lengthening procedure
forearm lift-assist on prosthesis
forebrain
forefinger
forefoot
   angulation of the
   mid- and
   narrowing of
   splaying of
forefoot adductovarus
forefoot adduction correction test

forefoot adductus
forefoot angulation
forefoot cavus
forefoot digital amputation
forefoot peak pressure
forefoot splaying
forefoot striker
forefoot-to-rearfoot loading
forehead
   free-floating
   prominence of
foreign body (FB)
   metallic
   retained
foreign body reaction
foreign material artifact
Forel, field H of
Forestier bowstring sign
Forestier disease
forgetful
forgetfulness, benign senescent
fork
   carotid
   double-prong
   Gardiner-Brown tuning
   Hardy three-prong
   implant application
   Jannetta
   Rhoton
   three-prong
   tuning
forking of sylvian aqueduct
forks of the circle of Willis
fork strap prosthetic support
formalin, 10% neutral buffered
format
   three-dimensional
   two-dimensional
formation
   brain stem reticular
   bunion
   callosal
   callus
   Chiari
   gray reticular
   hippocampal
   lateral reticular

formation *(continued)*
  marginal osteophyte
  mesencephalic reticular
  midbrain reticular (MRF)
  new bone
  osteophyte
  palisade
  paramedian pontine reticular
  periosteal bone
  pontine parareticular (PPRF)
  reticular
  rouleaux
  saccular
  spur
  thrombus
  villus
  white reticular
forme fruste (pl. formes frustes)
forme tardive
formication
formula
  Abercrombie neuronal cell count
  Dreyer
  Siri
forniceal rupture
fornix (pl. fornices)
Forrester-Brown head halter
Forrester splint
Forte distal radius plate system
Forte harness
Fortical (salmon calcitonin)
fortification scotomata
fortification spectrum during migraine
49er knee brace
forward-biting basket
forward-head posture
forward subluxation
Fosamax (alendronate)
fosphenytoin
fossa (pl. fossae)
  acetabular
  amygdaloid
  anconeal (also anconal)
  antecubital
  articular
  bony
  condylar

fossa *(continued)*
  coronoid
  cranial
  cubital
  digital
  femoral
  glenoid
  iliac
  infraspinous
  infrasternal
  infratemporal
  intercondylar
  intercondyloid
  interpeduncular
  Jobert
  lateral cerebral
  middle cerebral
  middle cranial
  navicular
  olecranon
  patellar
  pituitary
  popliteal
  posterior
  pterygopalatine
  radial
  rhomboid
  sphenoidal
  Sylvius
  temporal
fossa of Rosenmüller
fossa of Sylvius
Foster bed
Foster frame
Foster-Kennedy maneuver
Foster-Kennedy syndrome
Foster splint
Foundation, Epilepsy F. of America
  (EFA)
Foundation for Chiropractic Education
  (FCE)
Foundation total knee and hip systems
4-aminopyridine
4-azido-2-([14C]-methylamino) tri-
  fluorobenzonitrile imaging agent
four-bar fixation device
four-flanged nail

four-flap Z-plasty
four-in-one arthroplasty
four-corner fusion
four-dimensional (4D) image
Fourier pulsatility index
Fourier transform imaging
Fourier two-dimensional (2D) imaging
Fournier test for ataxic gait
four-part fracture
4-point IROM brace
4-point SuperSport functional knee
  brace
four-point walker
four-poster cervical orthosis
four-strand Savage suture technique
fourth branchial cleft pouch
fourth compartment
fourth cranial nerve (trochlear nerve)
fourth lumbar nerve
fourth ventricle tumor
four-vessel cerebral angiography
fovea, basistyloid
foveal fat pad
foveal vision
FOV (field of view) imaging
Foville fasciculus
Foville syndrome
Fowler maneuver
Fowles dislocation technique
Fox bipolar forceps
Fox-Blazina knee procedure
Fox extractor-impactor
foxphenytoin (Cerebyx)
Fox splint
FP (frontopolar) artery
FP electrode (FP$_1$, FP$_2$, F$_z$)
FPA (foot progression angle)
    forefoot
    hindfoot
FPB (flexor pollicis brevis) muscle
FPB (flexor pollicis brevis) tendon
FpF (frontopolar-frontal) electrode
FPL (flexor pollicis longus) muscle
FPL (flexor pollicis longus) tendon
FPR (fastigial pressor response)
Frac-Sur splint

fraction
    ejection
    linear
    S-phase
    transchondral
fractionated radiation therapy
fractionated stereotaxic radiation
    therapy
fractionation
fraction dose
Fractura Flex
Fractura Flex bandage
Fractura Flex cast
fracture
    abduction
    acute avulsion
    adduction
    agenetic
    Aitken epiphyseal
    alveolar bone
    anatomic
    angulated
    ankle mortise
    annular
    AO ankle
    apophyseal
    articular
    atrophic
    avulsion
    avulsion chip
    axial compression
    backfire
    Barton radial
    basal neck
    basal skull
    baseball finger
    basilar femoral neck
    basilar skull
    basocervical
    bending
    Bennett basic hand
    Berndt-Harty transchondral
    bicondylar
    bimalleolar ankle
    bipartite
    birth

fracture *(continued)*
- blow-in
- blow-out
- boot-top
- Bosworth
- both-bone
- boxer's
- Boyd type II
- bucket-handle
- buckle
- bumper
- bunk bed
- burst
- bursting
- butterfly
- buttonhole
- Canale-Kelly talar neck
- capitate
- carpal bone
- carpal navicular
- carpal scaphoid bone
- cartwheel
- Cedell talus
- cemental
- cementum
- cervical
- cervicotrochanteric
- Chance
- Chance spinal
- chauffeur's
- chevron
- chip
- chisel
- circumferential
- clay shoveler's
- cleavage
- closed
- closed break
- Colles
- Colles radial
- collicular
- comminuted
- comminuted bursting
- comminuted intra-articular
- comminuted teardrop
- complete
- complex

fracture *(continued)*
- complicated
- composite
- compound
- compression
- condylar
- condylar compression
- condylar split
- congenital
- contrecoup
- corner
- cortical
- Cotton ankle
- cough rib
- crack
- craniofacial dysjunction
- crush
- cuboid
- cuneiform
- dancer's
- Danis-Weber ankle
- Darrach-Hughston-Milch
- dashboard
- decompression of
- Denis (A, B, C, D, or E) spinal
- dens
- dentate
- depressed
- depressed and compound
- depressed skull
- de Quervain navicular
- derby hat
- diacondylar
- diaphyseal
- diastatic
- die punch
- direct
- dishpan
- dislocation
- displaced
- displaced intra-articular
- dogleg
- dome
- dorsal wing
- double
- Dupuytren
- Duverney iliac

fracture *(continued)*
dyscrasic
endocrine
epicondylar
epiphyseal slip
Essex-Lopresti calcaneal
extra-articular
extracapsular
facial
fatigue
femoral neck
fender
fighter's
finger
fissure
flake hamate
flexion burst
flexion compression
flexion distraction
floating arch
floating elbow forearm
four-part
fragility
Freiberg
Frykman radial
fulcrum
Galeazzi radial
Garden femoral neck
Gosselin tibial
graft
greenstick
grenade thrower's
gross
growing cranial
growth plate
Guérin facial bone
Gustilo tibial
gutter
Hahn-Steinthal capitellum
Hansen
hairline
hamate tail
hangman's
Hansen
Hawkins (I-IV)
Hawkins talar neck
healed

fracture *(continued)*
heat
hemicondylar
Herbert scaphoid bone
Hermodsson
hickory stick
hockey stick
horizontal
horizontal maxillary
humeral head-splitting
hyperextension teardrop
hyperflexion
hyperflexion teardrop
hyperparathyroidism-induced stress
idiopathic
impacted subcapital
impacted valgus
impression
incomplete
indented skull
indirect
inflammatory
infraction
insufficiency
intercondylar
internally fixed
interperiosteal
intertrochanteric
intra-articular
intracapsular
intraperiosteal
intrauterine fetal
irreducible
ischioacetabular
Jefferson burst
joint
joint depression
Jones
Jones fifth metatarsal
juvenile Tillaux
juxta-articular
Kapandji radial
Kocher
Kocher-Lorenz capitellum
lateral column calcaneal
laterally displaced
lateral vertebral body wedge

fracture *(continued)*
- Lauge-Hansen ankle
- Lauge-Hansen stage II supination-eversion
- lead pipe
- LeFort maxillary (I-III)
- linear and depressed skull
- Lisfranc metatarsal
- local compression
- local decompression
- long bone
- longitudinal
- loose
- lorry driver's
- low T humerus
- lunate
- Maisonneuve fibular
- malar
- Malgaigne pelvic
- mallet
- malunited
- mandibular
- march
- maxillary
- Mayo elbow
- medial column calcaneal
- medial epicondyle
- medial malleolar
- Melone
- midfacial
- midshaft
- minimally displaced
- monomalleolar ankle
- Monteggia ulnar
- Montercaux
- Moore radial
- Müller humerus
- multangular ridge
- multipartite
- multiple
- nasal
- navicular body
- naviculocapitate
- neck
- Neer shoulder
- neoplastic
- neurogenic

fracture *(continued)*
- neuropathic
- neurotrophic
- nightstick
- nonarticular radial head
- nondisplaced
- oblique
- occipital
- occult
- odontoid
- Ogden epiphyseal
- old
- olecranon tip
- one-part
- open
- open-break
- osteochondral
- Pais
- panfacial
- paratrooper
- parry
- patellar
- pathologic
- Pauwel femoral neck
- pedicle
- pelvic rim
- pelvic ring
- perforating
- periarticular
- peripheral
- periprosthetic
- pertrochanteric
- phalangeal
- physeal plate
- Piedmont radial
- pillion
- pillow
- pilon
- ping-pong
- plafond
- plastic bowing
- plateau tibial
- pond
- posterior element
- postmortem
- Pott ankle
- pressure

fracture *(continued)*
  proximal end tibia fracture
  puncture
  pyramidal
  Quervain (de Quervain)
  radial head
  radial styloid process
  resecting
  retrodisplaced
  reverse Barton
  reverse Colles
  rib
  ring
  Rolando metacarpal
  rotation-burst
  Ruedi-Allgower tibial plafond
  sacral insufficiency
  Salter
  Salter-Harris-Rang epiphyseal (I-V)
  sandbagging long bone
  Sanders computed tomography
  scaphoid
  seat-belt
  secondary
  segmental
  Segond tibial avulsion
  senile subcapital
  SER (supination, external rotation-
    type fracture) I-IV
  shaft
  shear
  Shepherd astragalus
  sideswipe elbow
  silver fork
  simple
  simple skull
  skier's
  Skillern radial
  sleeve
  slice
  small
  Smith radial
  Sneppen talar
  snowboarder's
  spiral
  splintered
  split compression

fracture *(continued)*
  spontaneous
  sprain
  Springer
  sprinter's
  stable
  stairstep
  Steida femoral
  Steinert epiphyseal
  stellate
  stellate undepressed
  step-off of
  straddle
  strain
  stress
  stress-type
  subcapital
  subcutaneous
  subperiosteal
  subtrochanteric
  supination-adduction
  supination-eversion
  supination, external rotation-type
    (I-IV)
  supracondylar femoral
  surgical neck
  T
  T condylar
  T-shaped
  talar osteochondral
  teardrop
  teardrop-shaped flexion compression
  temporal bone
  thalamic calcaneal
  thoracolumbar "burst"
  three-part
  through-and-through
  tibial pilon
  tibial plafond
  tibial plateau
  tibiofibular
  Tillaux
  Tillaux-Kleiger
  Tillaux tibial
  tongue
  tongue-type
  Torg

fracture *(continued)*
  torsion
  torus
  torus-type buckle
  total condylar depression
  transcapitate
  transcervical femoral
  transchondral talar
  transcondylar
  transepiphyseal
  transhamate
  transscaphoid
  transtriquetral
  transverse
  traversing the
  trimalleolar ankle
  triplane
  triquetral
  trophic
  tuberosity avulsion
  tuft
  two-part
  ulnar styloid
  undisplaced
  unilateral
  unstable
  ununited
  vertebra plana
  vertebral wedge compression
  vertical
  vertical shear
  V-shaped
  wagon wheel
  Wagstaffe malleolar
  Watson-Jones navicular
  Watson-Jones spinal
  Weber A–C
  wedge, wedged
  wedge compression
  wedge flexion compression
  willow
  wrist guard top
  Y
  Y–T
  Zickel
  zygomatic-malar complex (ZMC)
fracture blister

fracture by contrecoup
fracture circumferential
fracture classification
fracture deformity
fracture dislocation, perilunate (PLFD)
fracture en coin
fracture en rave
fracture fragment
fracture frame
fracture in close apposition
Fracture Intervention Trial (FIT)
fracture line
fracture nonunion
  elephant-foot
  horse-hoof
  oligotrophic
  torsion wedge
fracture splint
fracture trauma
fracture zone
fragility
  epiphyseal
  hereditary bone
fragility fracture
Fragmatome tip
fragment (pl. fragments)
  alignment of fracture
  articular
  avulsed fracture
  avulsion
  bone
  bony
  butterfly fracture
  capital
  chondral
  cortical
  disk
  displaced
  displacement of fracture
  fracture
  free
  free-floating cartilaginous
  loose
  major fracture
  osteochondral
  overriding of fracture
  retrolisthesed

fragment *(continued)*
    retropulsed bony
    Thurston-Holland
fragmentation of apophysis
fragment-in-notch sign
frail elderly patient
frame
    Ace-Colles fracture
    Ace-Fischer fracture
    Ace-Fischer ring
    Alexian Brothers overhead
    Boehler-Braun leg
    Boehler fracture
    Boehler reducing
    Balkan fracture
    Bradford fracture
    Braun
    Brooker
    Brown-Roberts-Wells stereotactic
        head
    Budde-Greenberg-Sugita stereotactic
        head
    Charest head
    Chick CLT operating
    CircOlectric
    claw-type basic
    Codman spinal
    Cole fracture
    Cole hyperextension
    Cosman-Roberts-Wells (CRW)
        stereotactic head
    Crawford head
    DeBastiani
    DePuy rainbow
    DePuy reducing
    double-ring
    Elekta stereotactic head
    Fischer
    fixation
    Foster turning
    four-poster
    fusion
    Garches
    Gardner-Wells fixation
    gNomos head
    Goldthwait
    Granberry

frame *(continued)*
    Hastings
    head
    Heffington lumbar seat spinal
        surgery
    Herzmark
    Hibbs
    Hitchcock stereotactic head
    Hoffmann-Vidal double
    Ilizarov
    ISAH stereotactic immobilization
    Jones abduction
    Jordan
    Kessler traction
    Komai stereotactic head
    Laitinen stereotactic head
    laminectomy
    Leksell D-shaped stereotactic
    Leksell-Elekta stereotactic
    Leksell gamma stereotactic
    Leksell Model G stereotactic
    Leksell stereotactic coordinate
    Lex-Ton spinal
    Malcolm-Lynn C-RXF cervical
        retractor
    Mayfield fixation
    Monticelli-Spinelli
    Mundinger-Reichert stereotactic
    OBT stereotactic
    Olivier-Bertrand-Talairach
        stereotactic head
    Patil stereotactic head frame
    Pearson attachment to Thomas
    Pelourus stereotactic
    phantom
    Pittsburgh pelvic
    Radionics CRW stereotactic head
    Radionics stereotactic
    Reichert-Mundinger-Fischer
        stereotactic head
    Relton-Hall
    robotics-controlled stereotactic
    scoliosis operating
    Slatis pelvic fracture
    spine
    stereotactic coordinate
    stereotactic (or stereotaxic) head

frame *(continued)*
  Stryker fracture
  Stryker turning
  Sugita head
  Talairach stereotactic
  Taylor spinal
  Thomas
  Thompson
  Todd-Wells stereotactic
  triangular ankle fusion
  Wagner
  Whitman
  Wilson
  Wilson convex
  Wingfield
  Wolfson
  Zimmer laminectomy
frameless navigation
frameless stereotaxic DSA
frameless stereotaxic guidance tools
frameless stereotaxic system
frameless stereotaxy
frame placement for stereotactic
  surgery
Framer finger extension bow
Framer splint
Framer tendon passer
Framer tendon-passing needle
frameshift
frank dislocation
frank hemorrhage
Fränkel (Fraenkel) classification of
  spinal cord injury
Fränkel sign
Fränkel white line
Frankfort horizontal plane
Frankfort mandibular incisor angle
Frank Noyes function questionnaire
frank pus
Frank sign
Frank vectorcardiogram (VCG)
fraught with error
fray, frayed, fraying
fraying of edges
fraying of meniscus
fraying of tendon
Frazer wrist brace

Frazier brain-exploring cannula
Frazier brain trocar
Frazier cordotomy knife
Frazier dural elevator
Frazier dural hook
Frazier dural scissors
Frazier dural separator
Frazier-Ferguson suction tube
Frazier laminectomy retractor
Frazier lighted brain retractor
Frazier nerve hook
Frazier pituitary knife
Frazier retractor
Frazier scissors
Frazier separator
Frazier suction tip
Frazier suction tube
Frazier ventricular cannula
Frazier ventricular needle
free beta test
Freedom arthritis support for hand
free-floating cartilaginous fragment
free fibular harvest flap
free flap of cartilage
free flap transfer
free-floating osteotomy
free fluid
free fragments
freehand interventional sonography
freehand ultrasound
Freehand prosthesis system
Freehand surgically implanted neuroprosthetic device
free induction decay (FID)
free induction signal
free inferior limb
free latissimus dorsi flap
free lower limb
Freeman femoral component with
  Rotalok cup
Freeman modular total hip prosthesis
Freeman-Swanson knee prosthesis
free muscle graft
free phalangeal base autograft for
  hallux limitus
free radicals
Freer chisel

Freer elevator dissector
free revascularized autograft
Freer periosteal elevator
Freer septal elevator
Freer-Swanson ganglion knife
free tissue transfer (FTT)
free toe transfer
free-walking velocity
freeze-drying
freezing of movement
freezing phenomena
Freiberg cartilage knife
Freiberg craniotome
Freiberg disease
Freiberg infraction
Freiberg-Kohler disease
Freiberg meniscectomy knife
Frejka cast
Frejka jacket
Frejka pillow
fremitus
French Alzheimer Collaborative
  Group
Frenchay Activities Index (FAI)
Frenchay Aphasia Screening Test
  (FAST)
Frenchay Arm Test (FAT)
French brain retractor
French fracture technique
French MBIH catheter
French pigtail catheter
French scale for caliber of catheter
French scale for sizing catheters
French shaft balloon
frenectomy
frenulum
Frenzel lens
frequency
  absolute peak
  alpha
  dominant waking
  EEG spectral edge
  high filter (HFF)
  low filter (LFF)
  mean peak
  treatment

frequency analysis of Doppler signal
frequency-dependent conduction block
frequency domain imaging (FDI)
frequency encoding
frequency-related peak
frequency measured in cycles per
  second
frequency measured in hertz (Hz)
frequency range
freshen the surface
freshened surfaces
freshening of bone
Fresnel prism
F response
FRIA (Friends and Relatives of the
  Institutionalized Aged)
friability
friable feeder arteries
friable lesion
friable mass
friable mucosa
friable tumor
friable vegetation
friable wall
friction
  deep transverse
  dynamic
friction-reducing polymer
friction rub in knee
friction syndrome, iliotibial band
Friedel Pick syndrome
Fried-Green foot procedure
Fried-Hendel tendon technique
Friedman bone rongeur
Friedman brace
Friedman elbow support
Friedman splint
Friedreich ataxia
Friedreich disease
Friedreich foot
Friedreich sign
Friends and Relatives of the
  Institutionalized Aged (FRIA)
Fries score for rheumatoid arthritis
Frigitronics probe
Frimodt-Moller syndrome
fringe, synovial

Frisium (clobazam)
frogleg view
frog splint
Fröhlich adiposogenital dystrophy
Frohse, arcade of
Frohse ligamentous arcade
Froimson-Oh arm procedure
Froin syndrome
FROM (full range of motion)
Froment paper sign
Froment sign or test
frond-like appearance
frond, synovial
frontal ataxia
frontal bone
frontal defect
frontal foramina
frontal gyrus
frontal horn of lateral ventricle
frontal horns, enlarged
frontal irregular rhythmic delta activity
   (FIRDA)
frontal lobe contusion
frontal lobe damage
frontal lobe disease
frontal lobe dysfunction
frontal lobe hypometabolism
frontal lobe lesion
frontal lobe personality
frontal lobe reflex
frontal lobe sign
frontal lobe syndrome
frontal lobe tumor
frontal neoplasm
frontal nerve
frontal notch
frontal plane growth abnormalities
frontal plane loop
frontal pole
frontal release sign
frontal sinus obliteration
frontal suture
frontal view
frontocentral (FC) electrode
frontocentral convexity
frontocentral head region
frontoethmoidal encephalocele

fronto-orbital advancement
frontoparietal suture
frontopolar region
frontosphenoid suture
frontosphenoidal encephalocele
frontopontine fiber
frontopontine tract
frontopontocerebellar pathway
frontosphenoid suture
frontosphenoidal encephalocele
frontotemporal (FT)
frontotemporal atrophy
frontotemporal craniotomy
frontotemporal dementia
frontotemporal muscle
frontotemporal electrode
frontotemporal region
frontotemporoparietal craniotomy
frontozygomatic region
frontside snowboard stance
frost, synovial
Frost posterior tibialis tendon
   lengthening
Frost foot procedure
Frost stitch
frostbite injury
frovatriptan (Miguard)
frozen radiated wedge allograft
frozen section diagnosis
frozen shoulder
F.R. Thompson femoral prosthesis
Fruehevald splint
Frykholm bone rongeur
Frykman classification of hand and
   wrist fractures
FS-BURST MR imaging
F-Scan foot pressure analysis
FSCR, flexible surface coil-type
FSE (fast SE) imaging
FSE-T2 with fat suppression to detect
   ligamentous abnormalities
FSH (facioscapulohumeral) dystrophy
FSI (Functional Status Index)
FSQ (Functional Status Questionnaire)
FTA (femorotibial angle)
FTA (fluorescent treponemal antibody)
   test

FTC (fibulotalocalcaneal) ligament
FT electrode (frontotemporal)
  (FT_9-FT_{10})
FTJ (femorotibial joints)
F to N (finger-to-nose) test
FTSG (full-thickness skin graft)
FTT (free tissue transfer)
Fuchs-Rosenthal counting chamber for
  CSF cells
FUdR (5-fluorouracil deoxyribo-
  nucleoside)
fugax, amaurosis
fugue state
  epileptic
  hysterical
Fuji FCR9000 computed radiology
  (CR) system
Fujita snake retractor
Fujita suction retractor
Fukushima retraction system
Fukushima C-clamp
Fukuyama congenital muscular dystrophy
Fukuyama disease
fulcrum fracture
fulcrum, joint
fulgurate, fulgurated
Fulkerson oblique tibial tubercle
  osteotomy
Fulkerson osteotomy
full circle goniometer
full recruitment pattern
full scan (FS) method/projection
full scan with interpolation (FI)
  method/projection
full spectrum reflexology
full thickness injury to articular
  cartilage
full thickness skin graft (FTSG)
full width at half maximum (FWHM)
fully jacketed (handgun) missiles
fulminant cerebral lymphoma
fulminant course of disease
fulminant encephalitis
fulminant hydrocephalus
fulminate
Fulton laminectomy rongeur

Fulton rongeur
function (pl. functions)
  brain stem
  bundle
  caloric test for vestibular
  cognitive
  cortical
  discrepant intellectual
  embarrassment of midbrain
  epicritic
  executive
  higher cerebral
  higher cortical
  higher integrative
  higher level cognitive
  independent
  neuro-ophthalmologic
  position of
  prefrontal
  verbally mediated
functional abnormality
Functional Ambulation Categories
  (FAC)
Functional Assessment Staging
  (FAST)
functional aphonia
functional axial rotation
functional brain imaging
Functional Capacity Evaluation (FCE)
functional disability of the foot
functional disorder
functional disturbance
functional electrical stimulation (FES)
functional evaluation
functional grip
functional gym stabilization evaluation
functional impairment
functional hyperlordosis
functional inattention
Functional Independence Measure
  (FIM)
Functional Limitation Profile (FLP)
functional loss
functional magnetic resonance imaging
  (fMRI)
functional movements
functional outcome

functional overlay
functional paralysis
functional posterior rhizotomy
Functional Rating Score
functional recovery
functional splint
Functional Status Index (FSI)
Functional Status Questionnaire (FSQ)
functional training
functional units of spine
fundamental aspects of mobility
fundiform ligament
fund of information
fund of knowledge
fundus (pl. fundi)
   aneurysmal
   ocular
   optic
funduscopically
fungal cultures on Sabouraud medium
fungal meningitis
fungating
fungoides, mycosis
fungus (see *pathogen*)
fungus ball
funicular suture
funiculus (pl. funiculi)
funnel chest
funnel deformity
Funsten splint
Funston congenital cervical rib
   syndrome
Funston syndrome
FUO (fever of undetermined origin)
furcal nerve (fourth lumbar nerve)
Furlong tendon stripper
Furnas bayonet osteotome
Furnas-Haq-Somers technique
furor epilepticus
Fuscger analysis
fused ankle
fused commissures
fused papillary muscle
fused physis
fusiform aneurysm
fusiform dilatation
fusiformis

fusiform spindle-shaped muscle
fusiform narrowing of arteries
fusiform shadow
fusiform swelling
fusiform widening of duct
fusimotor nerves
fusion (see also *operation*)
   Albee lumbar spinal
   ankle
   anterior cervical (ACF)
   anterior cervical body
   anterior spinal
   atlanto-occipital
   Blair ankle
   Blair talar body
   Bohlman triple-wire
   bone (bony)
   Bosworth lumbar spinal
   Brooks-Gallie cervical
   Brooks-Jenkins cervical
   calcaneotibial
   carpal-metacarpal (CMC)
   carpometacarpal
   cervical interbody
   chevron
   Cloward back
   diaphyseal-epiphyseal
   diskectomy with Cloward
   dowel spinal
   extra-articular hip
   facet
   four-corner
   Gallie atlantoaxial
   Gallie cervical
   Gallie wire
   Hatcher-Smith cervical
   Horwitz ankle
   hyperostotic bony
   interbody
   interphalangeal
   interspinous process
   intertransverse
   intra-articular knee
   joint
   McKeever metatarsophalangeal
   metatarsocuneiform joint
   metatarsophalangeal joint

fusion *(continued)*
   multilevel
   occipitocervical
   pantalar
   posterior cervical
   posterior lumbar interbody (PLIF)
   posterior spinal
   posterolateral
   Robinson-Riley spinal
   Rowe
   screw
   Smith-Robinson interbody
   spinal
   subaxial posterior cervical spinal
   subtalar distraction bone block
   symmetric vertebral
   talar body
   talocrural
   tibiocalcaneal
   tibiotalar

fusion *(continued)*
   tibiotalocalcaneal
   transfibular
   transforaminal lumbar interbody
     (TLIF)
   transpedal multiplanar wedge
     osteotomy/fusion
   triple-wire
   two-stage
fusion defect
fusion of vertebral segments
fusion frame
fusion, two-stage
Futuro braces and supports
fuzziness, mental
F wave measurements
F wave on electromyogram
F wave response
fx (fracture)

G, g

Ga (gallium)
GABA (gamma-aminobutyric acid)
GABA-BN complex
gabapentin (Neurontin)
GABA-T (GABA-transaminase)
Gabitril (tiagabine)
gadobenate dimeglumine imaging
   agent
gadobutrol
gadodiamide imaging agent
gadolinium (Gd)
   Gd-BOPTA/Dimeg imaging agent
   Gd-DOTA contrast medium
   Gd-DOTA-enhanced subtraction
      dynamic study
   Gd-DTPA/Dimeg imaging agent
   Gd-DTPA-enhanced turbo FLASH
      MRI
   Gd-DTPA imaging agent
   Gd-DTPA-labeled albumin
   Gd-DTPA-labeled dextran
   Gd-DPTA PGTM imaging agent
   Gd-DTPA with mannitol contrast
   Gd-enhanced imaging agent
   Gd-EOB-DTPA imaging agent
   Gd-FMPSPGR imaging
   Gd-HIDA chelate
   Gd-Hp-DO3A imaging agent

gadolinium *(continued)*
   Gd-153 imaging agent
   Gd oxide contrast medium
gadolinium complex
gadolinium-enhanced MRI arthrogram
gadopentetate dimeglumine imaging
   agent
gadoteridol contrast
Gaeltec catheter-tip pressure transducer
Gaenslen sign
Gaenslen split heel incision
Gaenslen test
Gaffney ankle prosthesis
Gaffney joint orthosis
Gage sign
Gage-Winter radiographic criteria for
   avascular necrosis
Gagnon splint
gag reflex
gain (as a result of illness)
   primary
   secondary
gait
   abductor lurch
   antalgic
   apraxic
   astasia-abasia
   ataxic

gait *(continued)*
- avoidance
- batrachian (frog)
- broad-based
- cadence of
- calcaneal
- calcaneous
- cerebellar
- Charcot
- Charlie Chaplin type of
- choreatic
- clumsy
- cogwheel
- crab
- cross-leg, cross-legged
- dancing
- dancing bear
- double-leg stance phase of
- double-step
- double-tap
- drag-to
- dromedary
- dropfoot
- drunken sailor
- duck's waddle
- dynamic
- dystrophic
- equine
- festinating
- floating
- foot-strike phase of
- four-point
- free-swinging knee
- glue-footed
- gluteal
- gluteus maximus
- gluteus medius
- heel
- heel-and-toe
- heel-contact phase of
- heel-off phase of
- heel-strike phase of
- heel-to-toe
- heel-toe
- helicopod
- hemiplegic
- high steppage

gait *(continued)*
- hobbling
- hysterical
- instability
- intermittent double-step
- intoeing
- jerky
- listing
- lurching
- marche à petits pas
- narrow-base
- Oppenheim
- opposite foot strike phase of
- opposite toe-off phase of
- parkinsonian
- petit pas
- Petren
- pigeon-toeing
- propulsion
- propulsion of
- propulsive phase of
- push-off phase of
- quality of
- reeling
- retropulsion of
- reversal of fore-aft shear phase of
- rigid
- scissor-leg
- scissors
- scraping-toe
- shuffling
- slap-foot
- slapping
- spastic
- speed of
- stable
- staggering
- stance phase of
- steppage
- stiff
- stiff-legged
- stride length of
- strike phase of
- stuttering (in parkinsonism)
- swaying
- swing phase of
- swing-through

gait *(continued)*
  swing-to
  tabetic
  tandem
  Thorazine shuffle
  three-point
  tiptoe
  toe-in
  toe-off phase of
  toe-out
  toe-walking
  tottering
  Trendelenburg
  two-point
  uncoordinated
  unsteadiness of
  unsteady
  waddling
  wide-based
Gait Abnormality Rating Scale
  (GARS)
gait analysis
gait and mobility
gait and station, unsteadiness of
gait apraxia
gait ataxia
gait biomechanics
gait cycle
  stance phase of
  swing phase of
gait determinants
  combined ankle and knee motion
  knee flexion during stance phase
  pelvic rotation
  pelvic shift
  pelvic tilt
gait adaptation
Gait Arms Legs and Spine (GALS)
  screening
gait deviations
gait disturbance
Gaiter cast
gait initiation
gait instability
gait lock splint (GLS) brace
Gaitmat II device
gait pathomechanics

gait plate
GAIT (great toe arthroplasty implant
  technique) spacer
gait training
galactography
galactosylceramide
Galant sign
Galante hip prosthesis
galea aponeurotica
galeal extension of tumor
Galeazzi fracture
Galeazzi patellar operation
Galeazzi sign
Galen, great cerebral vein of
Galen nerve
Galileo evoked potential electro-
  encephalograph
Gallagher rasp
Gallannaugh bone plate
Gallie ankle arthrodesis
Gallie atlantoaxial arthrodesis
Gallie atlantoaxial fusion technique
Gallie cervical fusion
Gallie fusion-using cable
Gallie H-graft
Gallie wire fixation technique
gallium (Ga)
  ^{67}Ga bone scan (also gallium-67)
  ^{67}Ga citrate radioactive imaging
  ^{67}Ga imaging agent
  ^{68}Ga GABA uptake carrier
gallium-arsenid (GaA) laser
gallium scanning, with ^{67}Ga
gallium scintigraphy
Gallo traction
GALOP (gait disorder, autoantibody,
  late-age, onset, polyneuropathy)
  syndrome
GALS (Gait Arms Legs and Spine)
  screening
Galt hand trephine
Galt skull trephine
galvanic body sway test (GBST)
galvanic stimulation
galvanic skin response (GSR) on EEG
galvanometer, EEG pen
Galveston metacarpal brace

Galveston Orientation and Awareness
  Test (GOAT)
Galveston sacral fixation
game knee
game leg
gamekeeper's thumb
gamma-aminobutyric acid (GABA)
gamma camera
gamma counter
gamma efferent system
gamma globulin elevated in CSF
gamma hydroxybutyrate (GHB)
gamma irradiation
Gamma radiosurgery knife
gamma locking nail
gamma loop nervous system
gamma motor neurons
gamma probe
gamma ray attenuation
gamma rhythm on EEG
gamma spectrometric analysis
gamma unit
gammopathy, monoclonal
ganaxolone (CCD 1042)
ganglia (pl. of ganglion)
gangliated nerve
ganglioglioma
gangliolysis, radiofrequency
ganglion (pl. ganglia)
  aberrent
  acousticofacial
  Acrel
  auditory
  auricular
  basal
  calcification of basal
  cervical
  cervicothoracic
  ciliary
  coccygeal
  diffuse
  dorsal root (DRG)
  gasserian
  geniculate
  intraosseous
  marbled appearance of basal
  otic

ganglion (continued)
  palmar
  paravertebral
  petrosal
  posterior root
  prevertebral
  radiocapitellar joint
  scapholunate
  Scarpa
  sensory
  sphenopalatine
  spinal
  submandibular
  sympathetic
  trigeminal
  vestibular
  Wrisberg
ganglion cells
  degeneration of
  shrinkage of
  vacuolation of
ganglioneuroma
ganglioneuromatosis
ganglion hook, Cushing gasserian
ganglionic cyst in synovial tendon
  sheath
ganglion scissors, Adson
ganglioradiculitis
ganglioside GM_1 and GM_2
gangliosidosis
  acute infective
  dry
  gas
  ischemic
  Meleney synergistic
  peripheral
  wet
gangrene
Ganley modification of Keller
  arthroplasty
GANS (granulomatous angiitis of the
  nervous system)
Ganser syndrome
Gant hip arthrodesis
Gant osteotomy
gantry angulation
gantry of CT scanner

gantry room
gantry tilt
Gantzer muscle
gap, air-bone
gap formation
Garceau-Brahms arthrodesis
Garceau cheilectomy
Garceau tendon technique
Garches frame
Garcia criteria for wrist laxity
Garcin syndrome
Garden angle
Garden femoral neck fracture
Gardiner-Brown tuning fork
Gardner bone forceps
Gardner chair
Gardner elevator
Gardner neurosurgical skull clamp
Gardner skull clamp pin
Gardner-Wells fixation frame
Gardner-Wells headrest
Gardner-Wells skull traction tongs
Garré disease
Garré, sclerosing osteomyelitis of
Garrett technique and instrumentation
GARS (Gait Abnormality Rating
    Scale)
Gartland supracondylar fracture
gas CT cisternography
gasless retroperitoneal video-assisted
    spine surgery
gas nitrogen embolism
gasserian ganglion tumor
gas, subcutaneous tissue
Gastaut HHE (hemiconvulsion, hemi-
    plegia, and epilepsy) syndrome
gastric nerves
gastroc (gastrocnemius muscle)
gastrocnemius muscle
gastrocnemius recession procedure
gastrocnemius reflex
gastrocnemius-soleus complex
gastrocolic ligament
gastroc-resistive exercises
gastroc/soleus contractures
gastrodiaphragmatic ligament
gastrohepatic ligament

gastrolienal ligament
gastropancreatic ligament
gastrophrenic ligament
gastrosplenic ligament
Gatch bed
gatched bed
gate clamp
gate clip
gate control pain treatment
Gatellier-Chastang ankle approach
Gaucher disease
gauge
    acetabular
    B&L pinch
    bone screw ruler
    Charnley femoral condyle radius
    Charnley socket
    Cloward depth
    Cobb
    depth
    elasticized
    foam
    isometric strain
    measuring
    Philips toe force
    pinch
    Preston pinch
    rosette strain
    screw depth
    socket
    strain
gauge of wire
gauntlet
    Jobst
    leather lacer
gauntlet splint
gauss
gauze (see also *dressing*)
    Aquaphor
    elasticized
    foam
    Nu Gauze
    Owen
    Sofrature
    tantalum
Gavard muscle
Gaynor-Hart position

gaze
  cardinal directions of
  conjugate
  conjugate fixed
  conjugate horizontal
  consensual
  disconjugate (or dysconjugate)
  down
  dysjunctive
  field of
  fixed
  following
  horizontal
  ipsilateral tonic conjugate
  lateral
  paresis of
  pontine center for
  preference of
  refixational shift of
  up
  vertical
gaze center in brain (pontine)
gaze coordinating aggregate
gaze deficit
gaze impairment
gaze mechanism in brain stem
gaze palsy
gaze paralysis
gaze paresis
gaze-paretic nystagmus
gaze preference
GBM (glioblastoma multiforme)
GBS (Guillain-Barré syndrome)
GBST (galvanic body sway test)
GCS (Glasgow Coma Scale)
GCSF (granulocyte colony stimulating
  factor)
GCT (germ cell tumor) of the central
  nervous system
GCTSPS (germ-cell tumor with
  synchronous lesions in pineal and
  suprasellar regions)
Gd (gadolinium)
GDC (Guglielmi detachable coil)
Gd-DOTA (gadolinium tetra-azacyclo-
  dodecanetetraacetic acid) contrast
  medium for MRI

Gd-DTPA contrast medium used in
  MRI scan
GDF-1 (growth differentiation factor-1)
GDNF (glial cell-derived neurotrophic
  factor)
GDS (Geriatric Depression Scale)
GE (General Electric) scanners (see
  scanner)
Geckler screw
gegenhalten
Geiger counter
Geiger rongeur
gel
  Adcon L Adhesion Control barrier
  alginate-collagen
  atelocollagen
  electrolyte EEG
  Lectron II electrode
  Omni Prep electrolyte EEG
gelastic epilepsy
gelatin foam, thrombin-soaked
gelatinous debris
gelatinous hematoma
gel cast
Gelfoam
  thrombin-soaked
  wafer of
Gelfoam cookie
Gelfoam pack
Gelfoam powder embolization
gelling phenomenon
Gelman foot procedure
Gelocast Unna boot compression
  dressing/wrap
gel pads
Gelpi pediatric retractor
gemellus (pl. gemelli) muscle
Gemini chiropractic table
Gemini hip system
Gemini MKII mobile-bearing knee
  implant
Gem total knee system
gender-related tumor
gene
  amyloid precursor protein
  cystatin B
  EMX2

gene *(continued)*
  GTP cyclohydrolase I (GCH-I)
  neurofibromatosis 1 (NF1)
  neurofibromatosis 2 (NF2)
  osteoblast-related
  P450 2D6
  p53
  TNF (tumor necrosis factor)
  tumor necrosis factor (TNF)
gene delivery imaging
general pattern matching
General Electric scanner (see *scanner*)
general endotracheal anesthesia
General Health Questionnaire (GHQ)
generalization on EEG
generalized convulsive seizure with (or
  without) focal onset
generalized delta activity
generalized nonconvulsive seizure
generalized osteoarthritis
generalized slowing
generalized theta activity
generalized tonic-clonic seizure
general paresis
general somatic efferent (motor) fibers
General Well-Being Schedule
Generation II Unloader ADJ knee
  brace
Generation II Unloader Select knee
  brace
generator, RFG-3CF radiofrequency
gene sequencing
Genesis arthroplasty hardware
genesis, crystal
Genesis knee prosthesis
Genesis II mobile-bearing knee
  implant
gene therapy
genetic epilepsy
genetic locus (pl. loci)
genetics, molecular
genial tubercle of mandible
genicular artery
genicular position
geniculate body
geniculate ganglion
geniculate herpes zoster

geniculate neuralgia
geniculate nucleus
geniculocalcarine region
geniculocalvarium
geniculocortical pathway
geniculum
genioglossal muscle
geniohyoid muscle
genitofemoral nerve
genitoinguinal ligament
Gennari
  band of
  line of
  stripe of
genome screen
genomic deletion
genomic instability
genomic sequence
genotype, genotyping
  apolipoprotein E (apo E)
  proband
gentamicin-impregnated polymethyl-
  methacralate (PMMA) beads
Gentle Threads interference screw
genuarthritis, medial
Genucom ACL laxity analysis system
Genucom arthrometer
Genucom knee flexion analysis system
genu recurvatum
Genutrain PE patellar realignment
Genutrain P3 knee brace
genu valgum deformity
genu varum deformity
Genzyme tissue repair (GTR)
  (NeuroCell)
Geoffrey criteria for Friedreich ataxia
geographic disorientation
Geomedic total knee prosthesis
geometric total knee prosthesis
geometry, aneurysm
George line on x-ray
Georgiade visor cervical collar/support
Georgiade visor halo fixation apparatus
geotropic nystagmus
gepirone Hcl
Gerald bipolar forceps
Gerald dressing forceps

Gerald tissue forceps
geranylgeranylation
geranylgeranyltransferase inhibition
Gerard prosthesis
Gerard resurfacing procedure
Gerbode-Burford rib spreader
Gerdy ligament
Gerdy tubercle in knee
geriatric
Geriatric Depression Scale (GDS)
germ cell tumor (GCT)
germinal matrix
germinoma
 basal ganglia
 medulla oblongata
 neurohypophyseal
 pineal
 suprasellar
germline mutation
Gerontological Society
gerontologist
Gerota capsule
Gerster traction bar
Gerstmann-Straussler-Scheinker
 disease
Gerstmann-Straussler syndrome
Gertzbein classification of seat-belt
 injury
Gerzog bone mallet
gestalt
gestural automatism
Getty decompression technique
GFAP (glial fibrillary acidic protein)
 antibody
GFAP immunostain
G5 Fleximatic massager/percussor
G5 ProPower massager
Ghajar guide
GHL (glenohumeral ligament)
Ghon-Sachs complex
Ghormley arthrodesis
Ghormley shelf procedure
ghosting artifact
ghost muscle fibers
GHQ (General Health Questionnaire)
Giannestras modification of Lapidus
 technique

Giannestras step-down modified
 osteotomy
giant aneurysm
giant cell arteritis, Horton
giant cell carcinoma
giant cell granulomatous hypophysitis
giant cell malignant tumor of soft tissue
giant cell reparative granuloma
giant cell tumor
giant neurons
giant pyramidal Betz cells
Gianturco prosthesis
Gianturco-Roehm bird's nest vena
 caval filter
Gianturco-Roubin flexible coil stent
Gianturco-Wallace venous stent
Gianturco wool-tufted wire coil stent
GIA stapler
gibberish
gibbous deformity
Gibbs artifact
Gibbs random field
gibbus (hump)
Gibney bandage
Gibson approach
Gibson bandage
Gibson-Piggott osteotomy
Gibson splint
giddy feeling
giddy headache
Giebel blade plate
Giertz rib shears
Giertz-Shoemaker rib shears
Giertz-Stille scissors
GIF (graphics interchange format)
Gifford mastoid retractor
gigantism, cerebral
Gigli saw blade
Gigli saw guide
Gigli wire saw
Gilbert-Tamai-Weiland technique
Gilchrest test
Gildenberg biopsy forceps
Giliberty bipolar femoral head
Giliberty device
Giliberty femoral prosthesis
Gilles de la Tourette syndrome

Gillespie syndrome
Gillette joint orthosis
Gillette modification of ankle-foot
    orthosis
Gillette suspensory ligament
Gilliat-Summer nerve-damaged hand
Gillies bone hook
Gillies-Dingman hook
Gillies graft
Gillies-Millard cocked-hat technique
Gillies pollicization
Gillies suture
Gillis test
Gill-Manning-White spondylolisthesis
    technique
Gill modification of Campbell ankle
    operation
Gillquist joint instruments
Gill shelf procedure
Gill sliding graft technique
Gill-Stein arthrodesis
Gilmer splint
Gillquist-Lysholm score
Gilvernet retractor
Gimbernat ligament
gimpy leg
gin-clear cerebrospinal fluid
gingival hyperplasia
gingivodental ligament
Gingrass and Messer pins
Ginkgo biloba extract
girdle
    limb
    pectoral
    pelvic
    shoulder
    superior limb
Girdlestone arthroplasty
Girdlestone pseudarthrosis
Girdlestone resection arthroplasty
Girdlestone-Taylor procedure
Girdlestone tendon transfer
Gissane angle
Gissane spike
gitter cells
give-way phenomena
giving way of ankle

giving way of knee
glabella
glabella reflex
glabellar tap
glabellar tapping
gladiatorum, herpes
gland
    calcification of pineal
    haversian
    interscapular
    lacrimal
    pineal
    pituitary
    von Ebner
glandular toxoplasmosis
Glaser automatic laminectomy retractor
Glaser laminectomy retractor
Glasflex material
Glasgow Assessment Schedule
Glasgow Coma Scale (GCS)
Glasgow Outcome Scale (GOS)
Glasgow screw
Glasgow sign
Glass-Bessen transfixion screw
glassy-eyed stare
glassy stare of petit mal epilepsy
glatiramer acetate
G-lengthening of semitendinosus tendon
glenohumeral articulation
glenohumeral glide
glenohumeral joint subluxation
glenohumeral ligaments (GHL)
glenoid cavity
glenoid component, keel of
glenoid fossa
glenoid labrum
glenoid ligament
glenoid process
glenoplasty
Gliadel implant
Gliadel wafer
glial-derived neurotrophic factor
    (GDNF)
glial disease
glial fibrillary acidic protein (GFAP)
    antibody

glial fibrillary acidic protein immunoreactivity
glial nodule
glial reaction
glial scarring
glial tumor
GliaSite radiation therapy system
glide, glenohumeral
glide hole
gliding contusion
glioblast
glioblastoma multiforme (GBM)
glioma
    anaplastic cerebral
    brain stem
    butterfly-type
    cerebral
    high grade
    intracranial
    low grade
    malignant
    non-anaplastic
    optic
    optic nerve
    optic pathway
    pontine
    precentral
    rolandoparietal
    supratentorial
glioma tumor
gliomatosis, meningeal
glioneural hamartoma
gliosarcoma
gliosis
    astrocytic
    progressive subcortical
    reactive
gliosis of sylvian aqueduct
Glisson capsule
Glisson sling
global amnesia
global aphasia
global cerebral hypometabolism
global cerebral hypoperfusion
global cerebral ischemia
global cortical defect
Global Deterioration Scale (GDS)

global distress
global hypokinesis
global hypometabolism
Global total shoulder arthroplasty
system
globe, optic
globe-orbit relationship
globoid cell leukodystrophy
globose cell
globulin, gamma (elevated in CSF)
globus epilepticus
globus hystericus
globus pallidus internus
glomerular basement membrane
glomeruloid formation
glomi of choroid plexus
glomus arteriovenous malformation
glomus jugulare tumor
glomus of choroid plexus
glomus (subungual) tumor
glomus-type arteriovenous malformation (AVM)
glossoepiglottic ligament
glossokinetic artifact
glossokinetic potential
glossopalatine muscle
glossopharyngeal muscle
glossopharyngeal nerve
glossopharyngeal neuralgia
glove (pl. gloves)
    antivibratory
    Biobrane
    Bio-Form
    carpal tunnel
    Handeze fingerless
    Isotoner
    Jobst
    SoftFlex computer
    Tubigrip
    Valeo lifting
glove-and-stocking anesthesia
distribution
glovelike distribution
GLS (gait lock splint) brace
GLS suture anchor
Gluck rib shears
glucocorticoid therapy

glucosamine, chondroitin, manganese
(Cosamine DS)
glucosamine sulfate
glucose metabolic tracer
glue
biomedical
cyanoacrylate
endovascular
fibrin
Hemaseel HMN tissue
percutaneous fibrin
skin
Tissucol fibrin
glue-footed gait
"glued-to-the-floor" phenomenon
glutamate excitotoxicity
glutamate inhibitor
glutamine/glutamate/creatine ratio
glutamine synthetase
gluteal bonnet
gluteal lines
gluteal lurch
gluteal muscle
gluteal nerve
gluteal punch test
gluten-free diet for multiple sclerosis
Gluterex
glutethimide intoxication
gluteus maximus tensing muscle
gluteus maximus tensing test
gluteus medius gait
gluteus medius muscle
gluteus minimus muscle
glycocalyx, extracellular protective
glycogen supersaturation, muscle
glycosaminoglycan
glycosylated ferritin
glycosylated hemoglogin
Glynn-Neibauer technique
GM-1 ganglioside (Sygen)
GM_1 gangliosidosis
GM_2 gangliosidosis
gNomos head frame
GOAT (Galveston Orientation and
Awareness Test)
Godfrey test
Goethe bone

Golaski graft
Golay coil
GoldenEye arthroscope
Goldenhar syndrome
Golden Period for primary closure in
infected wounds
Goldflam disease
Goldmann-Offner reference of
electrode
Goldmar opponensplasty
Goldner-Clippinger technique
GoldPoint ACL functional knee brace
GoldPoint hinged knee brace
GoldPoint knee brace
gold salts therapy
gold standard of diagnosis
Goldstein spinal fusion technique
Goldthwait brace
Goldthwait-Hauser procedure
Goldthwait sign
golfer's elbow
Golgi apparatus
Golgi organs
Golgi reflex
Golgi system
Gombault degeneration
Gomori stain
gonalgia
gonarthrosis
medial
unicompartmental
Golda reflex
G1 (grid 1) on EEG
gonial angle
goniometer
electronic
finger
full-circle
Polk finger
Scerratti
Sedan
gonion-gnathion plane
gonococcal arthritis
Gooch splint
Goode wraps
Good Grips utensils
GoodKnight 318 sleep monitoring
system

Goodman orthopedic bed
Good rasp
goofy-footed snowboard stance
Gordon-Broström technique
Gordon knee phenomenon
Gordon reflex
Gordon sign
Gordon splint
Gordon-Taylor technique
Gore bit
Gore Smoother Crucial Tool
Gore-Tex cast liner
Gore-Tex catheter
Gore-Tex interpositional arthroplasty
Gore-Tex graft
Gore-Tex knee prosthesis
Gore-Tex nonabsorbable surgical
    suture
Gore-Tex surgical membrane
Gorham disease
GOS (Glasgow Outcome Scale)
Gosselin fracture
Gosset, spiral band of
Gouffon hip pin fixation
gouge (see also *chisel*)
    Abbott
    Acufex
    Alexander
    Andrews
    Army bone
    arthroplasty
    Aufranc
    Bishop
    bone
    Buch-Gramcko
    Campbell
    Capner
    Cobb spinal
    curved
    Dawson-Yuhl
    Duray-Read
    Flanagan spinal fusion
    gooseneck
    Guy
    Hibbs spinal fusion
    Hoen
    Hoen lamina

gouge *(continued)*
    Jewett
    Killian
    Lexer
    Lucas
    Metzenbaum
    Meyerding curved
    mini-Lexer
    Moe
    motorized
    Murphy
    oscillating
    Partsch
    Read
    Ruben
    Sheehan
    Smith-Petersen curved
    Smith-Petersen straight
    Smith-Peterson gooseneck
    spinal fusion
    Stille bone
    straight
    swan-neck
    tendon
    U.S. Army
    Watson-Jones bone
    West
    West bone
    Zielke
    Zimmer
Gould Statham pressure transducer
Goulet retractor
gourmand syndrome
gout
    abarticular
    acute
    articular
    calcium
    chalky
    idiopathic
    intercritical
    interval
    latent
    lead
    masked
    monarticular
    overhanging edges or margins in

gout *(continued)*
  oxalic
  polyarticular
  primary
  pseudogout
  rheumatic
  secondary
  tophaceous
gouty arthritis
gouty diet
gouty tophus
Gowers bundle in cerebellum
Gowers column
Gowers fasciculus
Gowers maneuver
Gowers muscular dystrophy
Gowers phenomenon
Gowers sign
Gowers syndrome
Gowers tract
grab bars
grabber, disk
Graber-Devernay hip procedure
Grace method of ratio of metatarsal
  length
gracilis muscle flap
graciloplasty, dynamic
grade (see *grading system*)
grade 1–3 tear
Gradenigo syndrome
grades of movement
gradient
  amplitude
  anterior-posterior amplitude
  frequency-amplitude
  posterior dominant amplitude
gradient coil
gradient echo imaging sequence
gradient echo MR with magnetization
  transfer
gradient echo phase image
gradient echo pulse sequence
gradient echo sequence imaging
gradient magnetic field
gradient-recalled acquisition in a
  steady state (GRASS)
gradient-recalled echo (GRE)

gradient sheet coils
gradient waveforms
grading scale or system
  Boston Children's Hospital
  Campanacci giant cell tumor
  Dallas
  Facial Grading System (FGS)
  Köhler hip protrusion
  Modic
  osteoarthritis
graduated compression stockings
Graf classification of infant hips
Graflex material
graft
  ACL
  adipose
  adrenal medulla
  advancement flap
  Albee bone
  allogeneic bone
  allogenous bone
  anterior iliac crest
  anterior sliding tibial
  articular cartilage autograft
  autochthonous
  autogenous bone
  autogenous inlay
  autologous crest bone
  autologous reverse
  Banks bone
  bicortical iliac bone
  bicortical ilial strip
  BioPolyMeric
  bone chip
  bone peg
  bone-retinaculum-bone autograft
  bone-tendon-bone
  Bonfiglio bone
  bovine collagen
  Boyd dual onlay bone
  BPB (bone-patellar ligament-bone)
    autologous
  BPB (bone-patellar tendon-bone)
    autologous
  Braun skin
  bridge
  cable

graft *(continued)*
  Calcitite
  calvarial free bone
  Campbell onlay
  cancellous and cortical bone
  cancellous chip bone
  carbon fiber
  cartilage
  chip
  Chuinard autogenous bone
  clothespin spinal fusion
  Codivilla bone
  Collagraft bone graft matrix
  composite
  consolidated
  cortical strut
  corticocancellous bone
  corticocancellous chip
  cranial bone
  cutaneous
  Dacron
  Daniel iliac bone
  Davis muscle-pedicle
  demineralized bone
  devitalized bone
  diamond inlay
  Douglas skin
  dowel
  Dragstedt skin
  DST&G (doubled semitendinosus
    and gracilis) autograft
  DTAFA (descending thoracic
    aorta-to-femoral artery) bypass
  dual onlay bone
  dural
  Esser skin
  extra-articular
  fascia lata
  femorocrural
  femorodistal PTFE
  fetal cortical tissue
  fetal substantia nigra
  fillet local flap
  Flanagan-Burem apposing
    hemicylindric
  flexor tendon
  free

graft *(continued)*
  free fat
  free muscle
  free skin
  freeze-dried
  freeze-dried bone
  fresh frozen
  full-thickness skin
  fusion
  Gillies bone
  Golaski
  Gore-Tex vascular
  gracilis muscle
  Haldeman bone
  Harris superior acetabular
  harvesting of
  Hemashield enhanced
  hemicylindrical bone
  Henderson onlay bone
  Henry bone
  heterogeneous (heterogenous)
  Hey-Groves-Kirk bone
  Hoaglund bone
  homogeneous (homogenous)
  homologous
  H-shaped
  human meniscal allograft
  Huntington bone
  iliac crest bone
  iliotibial band
  impaction
  Inclan bone
  inlay bone
  in situ vein
  intercalary
  interfascicular nerve
  interposition bone
  interposition saphenous vein
  intramedullary
  Isotec patellar tendon
  Judet
  jump
  keystone
  Krause-Wolfe skin
  Kutler V-Y flap
  Langenskiöld bone
  Lee bone

graft *(continued)*
  Leibinger Micro Dynamic mesh
  lyophilized bone
  Massie sliding
  matchstick
  McFarland bone
  McMaster bone
  medullary bone
  morselized (morcellized) bone
  morcelized bone
  myocutaneous
  nerve
  neuroplasty fat
  neurovascular island
  Nicoll cancellous bone
  nontubed closed distant flap
  nontubed open distant flap
  Ollier thick split free
  Ollier-Thiersch skin
  onlay
  onlay cancellous iliac
  Opteform 100HT bone
  OP-1 implant
  osteoarticular
  osteocartilaginous
  osteochondral
  osteoperiosteal
  Osteoset bone graft substitute
  Overton dowel
  Papineau
  particulate
  patellar tendon
  pedicle
  pedicle bone
  peg
  percutaneous autogenous dowel
    bone
  PerioGlas bone graft material
  peroneus brevis
  Phemister onlay bone
  polyester tripled hamstring
  polyglactin mesh dural
  porous polyethylene
  postage stamp
  powdered bone
  Pro Osteon 500 bone graft
    substitute

graft *(continued)*
  prosthetic femorodistal
  proud
  PTFE (polytetrafluoroethylene)
  Reverdin epidermal free
  Russe bone
  Ryerson bone
  sandwiched iliac bone
  saphenous vein extracranial-
    intracranial bypass
  segmental
  semitendinosus
  short vessel
  single onlay cortical bone
  skin
  skull bone
  sliding inlay
  Soto-Hall bone
  split calvarial bone
  split-thickness skin
  strut bone
  subclavian-external carotid artery
  Tait
  temporal fascia
  Thiersch medium split free
  Thiersch thin split free
  Thomas extrapolated bar
  three-strand semintendinosus tendon
  tricortical bone
  tricortical ilial strip
  tube flap
  tumbler
  vein
  Wilson bone
  Wolfe full-thickness free
  Wolfe hand surgery
  Wolfe-Kawamoto bone
  wraparound flap bone
  Z-plasty local flap
graft copolymer
graft delamination
graft elongation
graft enhanced with collagen
graft fracture
grafting
graft loading pattern
graft loosening

graft morselizer
Grafton demineralized bone matrix
   putty
graft patency
graft pre-tensioning
graft sizer
graft slippage
graft tensioner
graft tensioning
graft-versus-host disease (GVHD)
Graham nerve hook
gram-positive sulfur-containing fila-
   mentous bacteria
Granberry frame
Granberry splint
Granberry traction
grand mal seizure (tonic-clonic)
Grantham classification of femur
   fracture
granular cell tumor
granular chromophobe cell
granulation tissue
granulations, pacchionian
granules, pigment
granulocyte colony stimulating factor
   (GCSF)
granuloma (pl. granulomata)
   calcified
   cholesterol
   eosinophilic
   fishtank
   foreign body
   frontoethmoidal giant cell
      reparative
   giant cell reparative
   intrathecal
   lethal midline
   malarial
   Mignon
   silicotic
   stellate
   swimming pool
granulomatous giant cell angiitis
granulosa-theca cell tumor
granulous fibrous tissue in rheumatoid
   arthritis
granulovacuolar change in hippocampus

granulovacuolar degeneration
graphanesthesia
graphesthesia
graphic impairment
graph, Moseley straight line
Grashey aphasia
grasper
   pituitary
   Questrus Leading Edge
grasping loop suture
grasping power
grasp reflex
GRASS (gradient-recalled acquisition
   in a steady state)
GRASS MR imaging
GRASS pulse sequence
grate, grating
Gratiolet convolutions
Gratiolet, optic radiation of
Graton bone matrix/marrow combination
gravidarum, chorea
gravis, myasthenia
gravity
   center of (CG)
   flex against
gray (Gy)
gray commissure of spinal cord
gray horns in spinal canal
graying of vision in multiple sclerosis
gray matter
gray radiation absorbed dose (Gy rad)
Gray reamer
gravity equinus
Gray drill
gray horns in the spinal canal,
   posterior
gray matter of central nervous system
gray-out episode
Gray Panthers
gray-scale Doppler
gray-scale images
gray-scale range
gray-scale ultrasound
Grayson ligament in hand
gray-to-white-matter activity ratio
gray-to-white-matter utilization ratio

gray-white differentiation on CT
gray-white matter junction
GRE (gradient-recalled echo)
great adductor muscle
great auricular nerve
greater multangular bone
greater occipital nerve
greater palatine nerve
greater pectoral muscle
greater petrosal nerve
greater posterior rectus muscle
greater psoas muscle
greater rhomboid muscle
greater saphenous vein
greater sciatic notch
greater splanchnic nerve
greater superficial petrosal nerve
greater trochanter
greater tuberosity osteotomy
greater zygomatic muscle
great toe push-off
great vein of cerebrum
Green-Anderson growth table
Green-Banks technique
Greenfield IVC (inferior vena cava)
    filter
Green-Joynt sign
Green-Laird modification of the
    Reverdin osteotomy
Green muscle hook
Green procedure
Green transfer
Greenberg clamp
Greenberg hand rest
Greenberg Universal retractor
Greene forceps
Greenfield classification of spino-
    cerebellar ataxia
Greenfield disease
Greenfield filter
Greenfield osteotomy
greenstick fracture
Greenwood bipolar and suction forceps
Greig cephalopolysyndactyly syndrome
grenade thrower's fracture
Grenoble-Paris-Rennes (GPR) robot
    neurosurgical microscope

Grenoble stereotactic robot
grenz ray
Greulich and Pyle, bone age
    according to
grey (see *gray*)
Grice-Green correction of hindfoot
    valgus deformity
Grice-Green extra-articular subtalar
    arthrodesis
grid
    AdTech electrode
    epidural electrode
    megavoltage
    subdural electrode
grid lead
grid 1 (G1) and grid 2 (G2) on EEG
grid therapy
Grierson tendon stripper
Griesinger sign
grimace, facial
grimace test
grimacing
Grimelius stain
grind, grinding
grinder, DePuy calcar
grinding and locking of knee joint
grip
    functional
    handle lift
    key
    pistol
    Posey
    power
    precision
Gripper acetabular cup prosthesis
grip pinch testing
grip strength
grip test, Jamar
GripTrack Commander strength tester
Grisel syndrome
griseofulvin
Gristina-Webb total shoulder
    arthroplasty
grit-blasted prosthesis
Gritti-Stokes distal thigh amputation
Gritti-Stokes knee prosthesis
grommet, titanium

groove
  annular
  anterolateral
  anteromedian
  basilar
  biceps
  bicipital
  carotid
  carpal
  cavernous
  deltopectoral
  digastric
  femoral
  fibular
  flexor
  Harrison
  infraorbital
  intercollicular
  intercondylar
  intertubercular
  meningioma of the olfactory
  neural
  olfactory
  parasagittal
  paravertebral
  patellar
  patellofemoral
  peroneal
  radial
  radial neck
  Ranvier
  sagittal
  spiral
  spiral humeral
  trochlear
  trochleocapitellar
  ulnar
  vertebral
grooved titanium rod
grooving of articular surface
groping reaction
Grosse-Kempf interlocking medullary
  nailing
Grosse-Kempf nail
Gross Motor Function Measure scale
ground-reaction forces
ground substance

group b arboviruses
group, muscle
Grover meniscotome
Grover meniscus knife
Groves-Goldner technique
Groves opponensplasty
growing cranial fracture
growth
  abnormal epiphyseal
  anchorage-dependent
growth arrest line
growth center of bones
growth curves, standardized
growth factor I, insulin-like
growth hormone antibody
growth hormone releasing factor
  (GRF)
growth plate arrest
growth plate, cartilaginous
growth plate fracture
growth spurt
Gruber fossa
Gruber suture
Gruca lower leg procedure
Gruenwald bayonet dressing forceps
Gruenwald neurosurgical rongeur
grumous debris
grumous tissue
Gruppe wire-crimping forceps
gryphotic
GSB (Gschwind-Scheier-Bahler) elbow
  prosthesis
GSPECT (gated SPECT)
GSR (galvanic skin response) on EEG
G suit
GSW (gunshot wound)
GSWH (gunshot wound to head)
GTC (generalized tonic-clonic)
GTC convulsions
GTC epilepsy
GTC seizures
G to A substitution
GTP cyclohydrolase I (GCH-I) gene
GTR (Genzyme tissue repair)
  (NeuroCell)
GTS great toe two-piece implant
  system

G2 anchor
G2 (grid 2) on EEG
G-II (Generation II)
G-II EasyAnchor
G-II Snap-Pak anchor
G-II Unloader knee brace
guanfacine (Tenex)
guard
  ankle
  dural
  eye
  knee
  McDavid ankle
  McDavid hinged knee
Guardian Red Dot walker
guarding, muscle
Guardsman femoral screw
Gubler hemiplegia/paralysis
Gudden atrophy
Gudden, nucleus of
Gudden tract
Gude tunneler
Guérin fracture
Guepar hinge-knee prosthesis
Guglielmi detachable coil (GDC)
guidance
  active biplanar MR imaging
  fluoroscopic
  microelectrode recording
  radiologic
  under fluoroscopic
guide
  Accu-Line
  acetabular
  ACL drill
  Acufex tibial
  adjustable angle
  Adson drill
  Adson dural protector
  Adson saw
  alignment
  Arthrex femoral
  Arthrex tibial
  Bailey-Gigli saw
  ball-tipped Küntscher (Kuentscher)
  barrel
  Blair saw

guide *(continued)*
  bone wire
  Bullseye
  calibrated pin
  Cloward drill
  Cushing-Gigli saw
  Cushing saw
  Davis saw
  DePuy femoral acetabular overlay
  drill
  Duopress
  eccentric drill
  Fanelli
  femoral intermedullary
  FIN pin
  Fisher
  Ghajar
  Gigli saw
  Hall-Dundar drill
  Hewson cruciate
  Hewson drill
  Hoffmann pin
  Howell tibial
  intercondylar drill
  intermedullary
  Lebsche saw
  ligature
  long axial alignment
  nail rotational
  neutral and load drill
  neutral drill
  patellar drill
  PCA cutting
  PCA medullary
  picket fence
  Pinn.ACL
  Poppen Gigli saw
  Raney saw
  Reese osteotomy
  Richards angle
  saw
  stationary angle
  Synthes wire
  T-bar
  telescopic wire
  tibial cutter
  tibial cutting

guide *(continued)*
    tibial drill
    Todd-Wells
    tube
    tunnel drill
    wire
    XMB tibial reaming
    Yasargil ligature
guide bushing
guide pin
    ball-point
    ball-tip
    calibrated
guide sleeve
guideline
    Hartel
    Böhler (Boehler)
    Letournel
guidewire introducer
guidewire, steerable
Guild Memory Test
Guilford cervical brace
Guillain and Mollaret, triangle of
Guillain-Barré-Strohl syndrome
Guillain-Barré syndrome (GBS)
Guillain-Garcin syndrome
Guillain-Mollaret triangle
Guilland sign
guillotine, Charnley femoral inlay
Guleke bone rongeur
Guleke-Stookey approach
Gulf War syndrome
Guller resection
Gumley classification of seat-belt
    injury
gumma (pl. gummas *or* gummata)
gumma of rib
gun
    cement
    CMW cement
    Harris cement
    Lidge cement
    power-driven staple
    staple
Gunderson bone forceps
Gunderson muscle forceps
Gunn jaw winking

Gunning splint
gunshot wound (GSW)
gunshot wound to head (GSWH)
GunSlinger shoulder orthosis
gun-stock deformity
Gunston-Hult knee prosthesis
Günz (Guenz) ligament
Günzberg (Guenzberg) ligament
Guppe forceps
gurney
gustatory aura
gustatory nerves
gustatory seizure
gustatory symptom
Gustilo-Anderson classification of
    tibial plafond fracture
Gustilo classification of puncture
    wounds
Gustilo classification of tibial fractures
Gustilo knee prosthesis
Gustilo-Kyle cementless total hip
    arthroplasty
Guthrie bacterial inhibition test
Guthrie muscle
gutter
    lateral
    sacral
gutter fracture
guttering
Guttmann subtalar arthrodesis
Guy gouge
Guyon canal
Guyon tunnel release
guy suture
G/W Heel Lift
Gy (gray) radiation absorbed dose
Gymnic ball
gymnast's wrist
Gypsona cast material
gyral crest
gyration
gyri cerebri
gyriform calcification
Gyro-Flex upper extremity exerciser
gyromagnetic ratio
Gyroscan, Philips
Gyroscan S15 scanner

gyrus (pl. gyri)
  angular (AG)
  annectant
  ascending parietal
  Broca
  callosal
  central
  cingulate
  contiguous supramarginal
  dentate
  fasciolar
  first temporal
  flattening of
  frontal
  fusiform
  Heschl transverse
  hippocampal
  inferior frontal
  inferior temporal
  infracalcarine
  insular
  lamination of
  lateral occipitotemporal
  lingual
  marginal
  medial occipitotemporal
  middle frontal
  middle temporal
  occipital
  occipitotemporal
  olfactory

gyrus *(continued)*
  orbital
  paracentral
  parahippocampal
  paraterminal
  parietal
  postcentral
  posterior central
  precentral
  preinsular
  quadrate
  short insular
  subcallosal
  subcollateral
  superior frontal
  superior parietal lobule
  superior temporal
  supracallosal
  supramarginal
  temporal
  transverse temporal
  Turner marginal
  uncal
  uncinate
gyrus callosus
gyrus cerebelli
gyrus cingulatus
gyrus cinguli
gyrus isthmus fornicatus
gyrus rectus

H, h

Haacker sling
Haas osteotomy
Haas paralysis
habenula
habenular nucleus
habitus, spondylolisthetic
HAC (hydroxyapatite)
Hachinski Ischemic Score for
    Dementia
hacksaw
HA (hydroxyapatite) coating
Haddad-Riordan arthrodesis
Hadfield hand board
Haemonetics Cell Saver
Haemophilus influenzae meningitis
Hagie pin
Hagie sliding nail plate
HAGL (humeral avulsion of gleno-
    humeral ligaments) lesion
Haglund disease
Haglund foot deformity
Haglund-Stille plaster spreader
Haglund syndrome
Hagner disease
Hahn bone nail
Hahn screw
Hahn-Steinthal classification of
    capitellum fracture
Haid cervical plate

Haid UBP (universal bone plate) system
Haight-Finochietto rib spreader
Haight rib spreader
Haines-McDougall medial sesamoid
    ligament
hairline crack in bone cortex
hairline fracture
Hajek antrum rongeur
Hajek-Ballenger dissector
Hajek-Ballenger septal elevator
Hajek chisel
Hajek-Koffler bone punch forceps
Hajek-Koffler laminectomy rongeur
Hajek mallet
Hakansson bone rongeur
Hakim-Cortis ventriculoperitoneal
    shunt
Haldeman bone graft
half-and-half nails
half-base syndrome
half-Fourier acquisition single-shot
    turbo spin-echo (HASTE)
half-Fourier imaging (HFI)
half-Fourier three-dimensional tech-
    nique
half-hitch arthroscopic knot
half-pipe snow ramp
half ring
half-scan (HS) method/projection

half-scan with extrapolation (HE)
method/projection
half-scan with interpolation (HI)
method/projection
half-shoe
Halifax interlaminar clamp
halistatin-1 (H1) imaging agent
Hall air-driven oscillating saw
Hall driver
Hall-Dundar drill guide
Halle bone curet
Halle dura knife
Halle nasal speculum
Halle speculum
Hallermann-Streiff-François syndrome
Hallervorden-Spatz disease
Hallister heel cup
Hall large bore drill
Hall Micro E drill
Hall Micro E oscillating saw
Hall Micro E reciprocating saw
Hall Micro E sagittal saw
Hall Micro E wiredriver
Hall neurosurgical craniotome
Hall rod
Hall Surgairtome drill
hallucal pronation
hallucal sesamoids
hallucination
  auditory
  gustatory
  hypnagogic
  hypnopompic
  nocturnal
  olfactory
  simple
  structured
  tactile
  visual
hallucinatory component
hallucinosis
  alcoholic
  organic
  peduncular
hallux abductovalgus
hallux elevatus
hallux extensus

hallux flexus deformity
hallux interphalangeal (IP) joint
  arthrodesis
hallux interphalangeal joint
hallux interphalangeus angle
hallux limitus (HL)
hallux limitus/rigidus
hallux malleus deformity
Hallux Metatarsophalangeal-
  Interphalangeal Scale
hallux migration
hallux nail
hallux rigidus deformity
hallux valgus (HV), unilateral
hallux valgus angle (HVA)
hallux valgus interphalangeus angle
hallux valgus-metatarsus primus varus
  complex
hallux varus correction, Johnson-
  Spiegl
hallux varus deformity
Hall Versipower drill
Hall Versipower oscillating saw
Hall Versipower reamer
Hall Versipower reciprocating saw
halo
  Bremer
  Brown-Roberts-Wells head ring
  Houston
  Ilizarov
  Lerman
  Philadelphia
  pulsating visual
  Twin Cities Lo-Profile
halo body jacket
halo cast
halo crown system, Bremer
halo effect
halo immobilization
halo ring
halo sign
halo traction
halo vest
Halsey nail scissors
Halsey needle holder
Halstead-Reitan Battery
Halstead-Wepman Aphasia Screening
  Test

Halsted artery forceps
Halsted mosquito forceps
halter
   Cerva Crane
   DePuy
   Diskard head
   flannel head
   foam head
   Forrester-Brown head
   head
   Redi head
   Repro head
   Upper 7 head
   Zimfoam head
   Zimmer head
halter traction, cervical
hamartoma
   cartilaginous
   chondromatous
   eccrine angiomatous
   glioneural
   subependymal
   vascular
   ventromedial hypothalamic
hamartomatous lesion
hamartomatous polyp
Hamas prosthesis
hamate bone, hook of
hamate, capitate
hamate tail fracture
Hamilton bandage
Hamilton Rating Scale for Depression
Hamilton ruler test
Hamilton screw
Hamilton test
Hamilton traction
Hamman sign
hammer
   Babinski percussion
   Berliner percussion
   Buck neurological
   Buck percussion
   Cloward
   Davis percussion
   Dejerine-Davis percussion
   Dejerine percussion
   Epstein neurological

hammer *(continued)*
   Küntscher
   neurological
   percussion
   Rabiner neurological
   slotted
   Taylor percussion
   Traube neurological percussion
   Trömner percussion (Troemner)
Hammer external fixation
hammer-marked skull
hammer toe (or hammertoe)
   dynamic
   fixed
hammer toe repair
hammocking of conventional mattresses
hammock ligament
Hammond foot procedure
Hammond splint
hamstring fixation technique
hamstring lengthening operation
hamstring muscle
hamstring/quadriceps torque ratio
hamstring release operation
hamstring spasm
hamstring stain
hamstring strain
hamstring tendon
hamstring, tight
Hamus wrist arthroplasty
hand
   all-ulnar
   ape
   apelike
   articulations of
   bear's paw
   bones of
   claw
   cleft
   digital artery of
   dorsum of
   flipper
   Gilliat-Summer nerve-damaged
   hemiplegic
   intrinsic plus
   lobster claw
   mirror

hand *(continued)*
   Myobock artificial
   oath
   obstetrician's
   opera glass
   phalanges of
   preferential use of right/left
   prosthetic
   psychoextended
   psychoflexed
   radial club
   spastic
   split
   web area of
   web border of
handbreadth
hand-carpal unit
hand drill, Children's Hospital
handedness, right/left
H&E (hematoxylin and eosin) stain
Handeze fingerless gloves
hand, foot, and mouth disease
hand-foot syndrome
hand-foot-uterus syndrome
Hand Functional Index (HFI)
hand-glove prosthesis
handgrip ergometer
handgrip exercise
handheld assist
handheld template
handheld weights (HHW)
Hand Helper
handicap
   final
   mobility
handle
   Bard-Parker
   Beaver blade
   bladeless scalpel
   cup holder
   Dynagrip blade
   multisided blade
   Ortho-Grip silicone rubber
   surgical knife
handlebar palsy
handle lift grip
hand preference

hand prosthesis
Hand-Schüller-Christian disease
Hands Free knee retractor system
hand sign, alien
hand-wringing, repetitive
Handy-Buck traction
hanging arm cast
hangman's fracture
hang-up
Hang Ups gravity boots
Hank buffered saline solution
Hanna night splint
Hannover Polytrauma score
Hansen classification of fractures
Hansen-Street driver-extractor
Hansen-Street nail
Hansen-Street pin
Hansen-Street plate
Hapad (shoe insert)
Hapad heel pad
Hapad medial arch pad
Hapad metatarsal arch
Hapad metatarsal insole
Hapad scaphoid arch
haplotype, paternal
Hapset hydroxyapatite bone graft
   plaster
haptic ability
HAQ (Health Assessment Question-
   naire) Index
Harada, syndrome of
hard disk herniation
Harding criteria for Friedreich ataxia
Hardinge femoral approach
Hardinge vastus lateralis operation
Hardt-Delima osteotome
hardware, orthopedic
Hardy bipolar forceps
Hardy-Clapham sesamoid classification
Hardy classification of pituitary
   tumors
Hardy spinal retractor
Hardy curet
Hardy dissector
Hardy dressing forceps
Hardy enucleator
Hardy hypophysectomy instruments

Hardy-Joyce triangle
Hardy micro bipolar forceps
Hardy micro dissector
Hardy micro enucleator
Hardy pituitary dissector
Hardy pituitary spoon
Hardy sellar punch forceps
Hardy speculum
Hardy suction tube
Hardy three-prong fork
Hardy-Weinberg equilibrium
Hare device
"hare's eye" (lagophthalmos)
Hare pin
Hare traction splint
Harken rib spreader
Hark foot procedure
Harlow plate
harmonic imaging
harmonics of waveform
Harmon transfer technique
Harm posterior cervical plate
harness
    acromioclavicular
    EEG head
    figure 8 ring
    immobilizer
    Pavlik
    weight-relieving Forte
Harpenden calipers
Harpoon suture anchor
Harrington compression rod
Harrington distraction outrigger
Harrington distraction rod
Harrington fixation device
Harrington hook
Harrington-Kostuik distraction device
Harrington-Luque
Harrington retractor
Harrington rod clamp
Harrington rod to correct scoliosis
Harrington spinal elevator
Harrington spreader
Harris-Beath arthrodesis
Harris-Beath axial hindfoot x-ray
Harris-Beath footprint mat
Harris broach

Harris-CDH hip prosthesis
Harris Design 1 (or 2) femoral
    prosthesis
Harris footprint mat
Harris-Galante acetabular component
Harris-Galante hip prosthesis
Harris HD (or HD-2) hip prosthesis
Harris hip line
Harris hip nail
Harris hip scale
Harris hip score
Harris-Smith cervical fusion
Harrison bone-holding forceps
Harrison-Nicolle polypropylene peg
Hartel guideline
Hartmann bone rongeur
Hartmann mosquito forceps
Hartnup disease
Hartshill rectangle rod
Hart sign
Hart splint
Harvard Criteria for Brain Death
harvester, tubular
harvesting
    bone
    graft
Harvey wire-cutting scissors
HA 65101 implant metal
Hass procedure
Hassmann-Brunn-Neer elbow
    technique
HAST (In-Home Alzheimer Screening
    Test)
Hastings bipolar hemiarthroplasty
Hastings frame
Hastings prosthesis
Hatcher pin
Hatcher-Smith cervical fusion
hatchet-head deformity
Hatfield bone curet
Hauser ambulation index
Hauser bunionectomy
Hauser heel cord procedure
Hauser patellar tendon procedure
Hausted orthopedic bed
Haverfield-Scoville hemilaminectomy
    retractor

haversian canal
haversian gland
Hawiva test
Hawkeye suture needle
Hawkins classification of talar neck
  fractures
Hawkins impingement sign
Hawkins line
Hawkins II-IV talar neck fracture
Hawkins-Warren shoulder score
Hayem encephalitis
Hayes retractor
Haygarth node
Hay-Groves shelf procedure
Haynes brain cannula
Haynes-Stellite 21 (HS-21) implant
  metal
Hays hand retractor
HBCT (helical biphasic contrast CT)
H-benzapine imaging agent
H buttress support patellofemoral
  brace
HCD (higher cerebral dysfunction)
HCFA (Health Care Financing
  Administration)
HCTH (helical CT holography)
HDI (HDTV-interlaced)
HDI (high definition imaging) 3000
  ultrasound system
HD II (or HD-2) total hip prosthesis
HE (hepatic encephalopathy)
head (pl. heads)
  Biolox ceramic ball for hip replace-
    ment
  cartilaginous cap of phalangeal
  clavicular
  Continuum bipolar acetabular head
  doll's
  femoral
  first metatarsal (FMH)
  forward positioning of
  humeral
  long
  metatarsal
  nerve
  radial
  Series-II humeral

head (continued)
  short
  terminal
  tower
  ulnar
  Zirconia orthopedic prosthetic
headache (pl. headaches)
  alarm-clock
  band-like
  benign exertional
  bifrontal
  bilateral
  bioccipital
  blind
  blood patch for post lumbar
    puncture
  cataclysmic
  chronic
  cheese reaction
  cluster
  combination
  conditions that precipitate a
  cough
  disabling
  dull
  duration of
  essential
  evening
  exertional
  frequency of
  frontal
  generalized
  giddy
  histamine
  Horton
  hot dog
  ice cream
  ice pick
  ipsilateral
  leakage
  matutinal (morning)
  migraine
  migraine-like
  mixed
  morning
  muscle contraction
  nitrite

headache *(continued)*
  nonpulsating
  persistent
  post-LP (lumbar puncture)
  postconcussion
  postictal migrainous
  posttraumatic
  psychogenic
  pulsating
  recurrent
  recurring
  seasonal
  sentinel
  severe
  severity of
  sex
  sinus
  suboccipital
  sudden onset
  Symonds
  temporal
  tension
  tension-type
  tension-vascular
  throbbing
  thunderclap
  traumatic
  unilateral
  unusual
  vacuum
  vascular
  vasodilator
  vasomotor
  weekend
  whole cranial
  Willis
  Wolff
headache-free interval
headache syndrome
head and neck, femoral
headband, electrode
head bobbing
head circumference size
head cradle
head dislocation, radial
head elevation

head fracture, radial
headframe
  Kannon
  Sugita
  thousand-hands Kannon universal
head halter
head holder
head-injured patient
head injury (HI)
head injury instructions
head lag
headlamp, fiberoptic
headlight
head-mounted LCD screen
head nodding
headrest
  Gardner-Wells
  horseshoe
  Light-Veley
  Mayfield horseshoe
  Mayfield-Kees
  Mayfield neurosurgical
  Multipoise
  pediatric
  pin
  pin fixation
  Reston foam-padded
  three-point
  Veley
headrest extension
head rotation test
head-shaking nystagmus test
head thrust test
head sheet
head subluxation, radial
head trauma
healing by primary intention
healing by secondary intention
healing
  therapeutic ultrasound for tendon
  tuberosity
Healos bone-grafting material
Health and Labor Questionnaire
Health Assessment Questionnaire
  (HAQ)
Health Assessment Questionnaire for
  Spondyloarthropathies (HAQ-S)

Health Care Financing Administration
(HCFA)
health-handicapped child
health maintenance organization
(HMO)
Health-Related Facilities (HRF)
heart blood deficiency (Chinese medicine term)
heart qi deficiency (Chinese medicine
term)
heart yin deficiency (Chinese medicine
term)
heat
  application of
  moist
heat expandable stent
heat fracture
heat-generating source
Heath mallet
heating unit, Hydrocollator
heat labile hydrogen bond
heat shock protein
heat in the blood (Chinese medicine
term)
heat toxin (Chinese medicine term)
heave, parasternal
heavy feeling
heavy metal neuritis
heavy particle irradiation
Heberden disease
Heberden node
hebosteotomy
hebotomy
Hebra blade
Hector, tendon of
Hedblom rib retractor
Hedley-Hungerford hip prosthesis
Hedrocel cup
Hedrocel porous tantalum
Hedrocel titanium screw
Hedrocel trabecular metal
Hedspa
heel
  anterior
  black-dot
  cucumber
  high prow

heel *(continued)*
  painful
  prominent
  reverse Thomas
  rubber walking
  SACH (solid ankle, cushioned
    heel) orthopedic
  Sorbol
  Thomas
  valgus
  varus
  walking
Heelbo decubitus heel/elbow protector
heel bone
heel contact phase of gait
heel cord advancement
heel cord stretching exercise
heel cradle
heel cup
heel height
heel lift in shoe
heel lock
heel-off phase of gait
heel pad thickness
heel pads ("cookies")
heel spur syndrome
heel-strike phase of gait
heel tendon
heel-to-knee test
heel-to-shin test
heel-toe gait
heel-toe runners
heel-walking
Heerfort syndrome
Heerfordt syndrome
Heermann alligator forceps
Heffington lumbar seat spinal surgery
frame
Heidenhain-type of spongiform
encephalopathy
Heifetz cranial perforator
Heifetz procedure
Heifitz clip
height, heel
heightened attention, state of
heightened awareness, state of
Hein rongeur

Heiss soft tissue retractor
Helal osteotomy
Helbing sign
Helenca bandage
Helfet test
helical biphasic contrast-enhanced CT
(HBCT)
helical coil stent
helical computed tomography (CT)
helical CT holography (HCTH)
helical CT scanner
helical pattern
helical platinum leads
helical thin-section CT scan
helical-tip Halo catheter
helicopod gait
Heliodorus bandage
Helios diagnostic imaging system
heliotrope rash
Helistat collagen sponge
helium-filled balloon catheter
helium ion Bragg peak
helium ion particle beam radiosurgery
Helix camera
helmet-molding therapy
helmet, Sheffield collimator
Helmholtz axis ligament
Helmholtz coil
helminthic infection
helminth larva
heloma (pl. helomata)
heloma durum
heloma molle
HELP (heparin-induced extracorporeal
low density lipoprotein/fibrinogen
precipitation)
hemal arch
hemangioblastoma, cerebellar
hemangioblastoma tumor
hemangioendothelioma, Masson
vegetant intravascular
hemangioma
capillary
cavernous
extramedullary
leptomeningeal

hemangioma (continued)
trigeminal
verrucous
hemangiomatosis
hemangiopericytoma
Hemaquet PTCA sheath with
obturator
hemarthrosis
Hemaseel HMN tissue glue
Hemashield enhanced graft
hematogenous dissemination
hematogenous osteomyelitis
hematogenous spread of metastases to
brain
hematoma
acute intramural
aneurysmal
balancing subdural
carotid plaque
chronic subdural (CSDH)
dural
encapsulated subdural
epidural (EDH)
evacuation of
evolving
extracerebral
extradural
gelatinous
hemispheral
hypertensive
intracerebral
intracranial
intramural
intraparenchymal
intraventricular
nasal septum
organized
posterior fossa
primary intracerebral
retromembranous
scalp
spinal epidural
spinal subdural
spontaneous
subcapsular
subdural

hematoma *(continued)*
  subgaleal
  subungual
  traumatic
hematoma evacuator
hematomyelia
hematopoiesis, extramedullary
hematopoietic reticulum of marrow
hematoxylin and eosin (H&E) stain
hemeralopia (blurred vision in bright light)
hemiagenesis
hemianesthesia, contralateral
hemianopia
  absolute
  altitudinal
  bilateral homonymous
  binasal
  binocular
  bitemporal
  complete
  congruous
  contralateral
  crossed
  dense
  heteronymous
  homonymous
  horizontal
  incomplete
  incongruous
  ipsilateral
  lateral
  macular
  nasal
  paracentral
  partial
  quadrant
  quandrantic
  relative
  temporal
  unilateral
hemianopsia (see *hemianopia*)
hemiarthroplasty
  Bateman
  Austin Moore
  I-beam
  Neer

hemiataxia
hemiatrophy
hemiaxial view
hemiballism, hemiballismus
hemibasal syndrome
hemic calculus
hemicallotasis
hemichondrodiasthesis
hemichorea-hemiballism syndrome
hemichorea, vascular
hemichoreic
hemiconvulsions, hemiplegia, and epilepsy (HHE syndrome)
hemicorpora
hemicorporectomy
hemicrania, chronic paroxysmal
hemicraniectomy
hemicraniotomy
hemicranium
hemidecortication, cerebral
hemidepot form of triamcinolone for joint injections
hemidiaphyseal debridement
hemidystonia
hemiepiphyseodesis
hemifacial microsomia
hemifacial spasm
hemifacial weakness
hemifield of vision
hemifield loss
hemihypertrophy
hemihypesthesia
hemi-inattention
  auditory
  tactile
  visual
hemijoint arthroplasty
hemiknee, Savastano
hemilaminectomy
  partial
  segment
  unilateral
hemilaminectomy retractor, Scoville-Haverfield
hemimelia
  fibular
  paraxial (complete and incomplete)

hemiparalysis, contralateral
hemiparesis
  ataxic (AH)
  contralateral
  dense
  hemiparetic
  paradoxical ipsilateral
  pure motor (PMH)
  residual
  spastic
hemiparesthesia
hemiparetic hemiparesis
hemiparkinsonism
hemipelvectomy
hemipelvis
hemiphalangectomy, Johnson
hemiplegia
  acutely acquired
  alternating oculomotor
  ascending
  capsular
  cerebral
  contralateral
  crossed
  dense
  double
  facial
  faciobrachial
  faciolingual
  flaccid
  Gubler
  hysterical
  infantile
  left
  motor
  puerperal
  pure motor
  right
  spastic
  spinal
  Wernicke-Mann spastic
hemiplegia alternans
hemiplegic gait
hemiplegic hand
hemiplegic migraine headache
hemisacrectomy with hemipelvectomy

hemisection of spinal cord
hemisensory loss
hemisensory syndrome
Hemi Sling for shoulder subluxation
hemisoma
hemisomatognosia
hemispheral dysfunction
hemispheral gaze deficiency
hemispheral mass
hemispheral mass effect
hemisphere
  cerebellar
  cerebral
  dominant
  left
  mesial
  nondominant
  right
hemisphere atrophy
hemisphere damage
hemispherectomy
hemisphere damage
hemisphere dominance, left/right
hemisphere lesion, dominant
hemisphere stroke
hemispherical contact probe
hemitremor
hemivertebra
  balanced
  unbalanced
hemizygosity
hemoclamp
hemoclip
hemodialysis-related spine disorder
Hemo-Drain evacuator
Hemo-Drain needle
hemodynamics
  limb
  microvascular
hemogenesis
hemoglobin, glycosylated
hemophilia A
hemophilia B
hemophilia, classic
hemophiliac
hemophilic joint

hemorrhage
 aneurysmal
 anticoagulant-induced
 arterial
 brain stem
 capillary
 central nervous system
 cerebellar
 chronic parenchymal
 concealed
 delayed traumatic intracerebral
  (DTICH)
 diffuse subarachnoid
 Duret
 eight-ball
 epidural
 extradural
 flame-shaped
 focus of
 frank
 hypertensive
 hypothalamic
 intertrabecular
 intracerebral (ICH)
 intracranial
 intramural arterial
 intraparenchymal
 intraplaque (IPH)
 intraventricular (IVH)
 life-threatening
 lobar intracerebral
 meningeal
 neonatal intracranial
 nondominant putaminal
 nontraumatic epidural
 old
 parenchymal
 parenchymatous
 periaqueductal
 petechial
 pontine
 putaminal
 retrobulbar
 slit
 spinal epidural (SEH)
 spinal subarachnoid
 spinal subdural (SSH)

hemorrhage *(continued)*
 splinter
 striate
 subacute
 subarachnoid (SAH)
 subdural (SDH)
 subependymal
 subhyaloid preretinal
 subhyaloid retinal
 thalamic
 thrombolysis-associated intracerebral
 traumatic meningeal
 venous malformation
hemorrhagic consolidation
hemorrhagic conversion
hemorrhagic infarct
hemorrhagic necrosis
hemorrhagic stroke
hemorrhagic zone, pyramidal
hemorrheology
hemostasis
hemostat (see also *forceps*)
 Allis
 Avitene microfibrillar collagen
 curved
 Hoen scalp
 Kelly
 Mixter
 mosquito
 tonsil
 Vapr
hemotympanum
Hemovac Hydrocoat drain
Hemovac suction tube
Henahan elevator
Hendel correction of scaphocephaly
Hendel guided osteotome
Henderson-Jones chondromatosis
Henderson lag screw
Henderson onlay graft
Henle, ligament of
Henley carotid retractor
Hennessy knee brace
Henning cast spreader
Henning mallet
Henning meniscal retractor

Henning plaster spreader
Henoch chorea
Henoch-Schönlein purpura
(Schoenlein)
Henry
master knot of
vertebral artery by
Henry acromioclavicular technique
Henry and Wrisberg, ligaments of
Henry-Geist spinal fusion technique
Henschke-Mauch SNS knee prosthesis
Hensing ligament
heparin
low molecular weight
unfractionated
heparin-induced extracorporeal
low density lipoprotein/fibrinogen
precipitation (HELP)
heparinization
heparinized blood
heparinized Ringer's injection, lactated
heparinized Ringer's irrigation
heparinoid
hepatic coma
hepatic encephalopathy
hepatic encephalopathy tremor
hepatocerebral disease
hepatolenticular degeneration
Heplock catheter
herald bleed
Herbert dissector
Herbert-Fisher fracture classification
system
Herbert jig or saw
Herbert knee prosthesis
Herbert screw fixation
Herbert-Whipple bone screw
Hercules plaster shears
Herczel rib elevator
Herczel rib rasp
hereditary areflexic dystasia
hereditary motor sensory neuropathy
hereditary multiple exostoses
hereditary progressive arthro-ophthalmology
hereditary sensory radicular neuropathy
hereditary spastic ataxia

hereditary spastic paraplegia
heredoataxia
heredofamilial tremor
heredopathia atactica polyneuritiformis
Hering sinus nerve
Hermodsson fracture
Hermodsson internal rotation
technique
Hernandez-Ros bone staple
Herndon-Heyman foot procedure
hernia, forearm fascial
herniated cerebellar tonsil
herniated cervical disk
herniated disk
herniated intervertebral disk (HID)
herniated nucleus pulposus (HNP)
herniation
brain
brain stem
central
cerebellar tonsil
cerebral
cingulate
concentric
disk
extraforaminal disk
fatal
foramen magnum
frank disk
hard disk
hindbrain
hippocampal
impending
internal disk
intraspongy nuclear disk
lumbosacral intervertebral disk
phalangeal
soft disk
subfalcine (subfalcial)
subligamentous disk
supraligamentous disk
temporal lobe
tentorial notch
thoracic intervertebral disk
tonsillar
transtentorial
uncal

herniation of brain tissue
herniation of lumbosacral intervertebral
disk
herniation of nucleus pulposus
herniation of temporal lobe into orbit
herniation of thoracic intervertebral disk
herniorrhaphy
herpes encephalitis
herpes gladiatorum
herpes simplex encephalitis
herpes simplex myelitis
herpes zoster encephalitis
herpes zoster viral encephalitis
herpes zoster virus
herpetic whitlow
Herring lateral pillar classification
(pillars A-C)
hersage (Fr. "combing")
hertz (Hz) (cycles per second)
Hertzler rib retractor
Herzmark frame
Heschl convolution
Heschl transverse gyrus
hesitation test
Hesselbach ligament
Hessel-Nystrom pin
hetastarch plasma volume expander
heterogeneous (or heterogenous)
heterogeneous appearance
heterogeneous hyperattenuation
heterogeneous isodense enhancement
heterogeneous microdistribution
heterogeneous perfusion pattern
heterogeneous system degeneration
heterogeneous system disease
heterogeneous uptake
heterogenesis
heterografts, porcine
heterologous graft
heterotopia, gray matter
heterotopic bone formation
heterotopic gray matter
heterotopic ossification
heterozygote point mutation
heterozygous
Heubner, recurrent artery of
Heubner syphilitic endarteritis

Heuter-Volkmann law
Hewlett-Packard phased-array imaging
system
Hewson cruciate guide
Hewson ligament button
Hewson suture passer
Hexabrix contrast medium
hexadactyly
hexamethylpropyleneamine oxime
Hexcelite cast
Hexcel total condylar k nee system
Hex-Fix fracture fixation system
hex nut
hex screw
Hey amputation
Heyer-Schulte antisiphon device
(ASD)
Heyer-Schulte bur hole valve
Heyer-Schulte neurosurgical shunt
Heyer-Schulte wound drain
Hey-Groves-Kirk bone graft
Hey-Groves ligament reconstruction
Hey ligament
Heyman-Herndon clubfoot operation
Heyman-Herndon procedure
Heyman-Herndon-Strong technique
HFD (high frequency Doppler) ultra-
sound
HFF (high filter frequency)
HFI (Hand Functional Index)
HG Multilock hip prosthesis
HGO (hip guidance orthosis)
HHA (homonymous hemianopia)
HHE syndrome (hemiconvulsions,
hemiplegia, and epilepsy)
HHS (Harris Hip Score)
HHW (hand-held weights)
HI (head injury)
HIAD (high impact aerobic dance)
hiatus, popliteal
Hibbs blade
Hibbs bone-cutting forceps
Hibbs chisel elevator
Hibbs curet
Hibbs gouge
Hibbs-Jones spinal fusion procedure
Hibbs mallet

Hibbs metatarsocalcaneal angle
Hibbs osteotome
Hibbs retractor
Hibbs spinal curet
Hibbs spinal fusion gouge
Hibbs-Spratt spinal fusion curet
Hibbs test
Hibiclens scrub
Hibiclens solution
hickory stick fracture
Hicks lugged plate
HID (herniated intervertebral disk)
hidradenoma, poroid
HIE (hypoxic-ischemic encephalopathy)
hierarchical information
hierarchical scales of ADLs
hierarchical scanning pattern
HIF (higher integrative functions)
HIFU (high intensity focused ultrasound)
high air-loss bed
high attenuation
high caliber, low velocity handgun
  injury
high contrast film
high definition imaging (HDI) 3000
  ultrasound system
high density linear array
high density polyethylene
high dose hook effect
high energy gunshot wound
high energy imaging
high energy protons
high energy trauma
higher cerebral dysfunction (HCD)
higher cognitive functions
higher cortical dysfunction
higher cortical functioning
higher integrative functions (HIF)
higher integrative language processing
higher level cognitive functions
higher order association cortex
high field open MRI scanner
high field strength magnet
high field strength MR imaging
high field system
high flow cannula

high frequency Doppler ultrasound
high frequency miniature probe
high frequency therapeutic ultrasound
high frequency ultrasound imaging
high grade astrocytoma tumor
high grade stenosis
high impact activities
high impact aerobic dance (HIAD)
high level motor problem
high level perceptual disturbance
high manganese diet
high muscular resistance bed
high osmolar contrast media
high-pitched bruit
high pontine lesion
high power athlete
high resolution B-mode imaging
high resolution coronal cuts
high resolution CT (HRCT) scan
high resolution diffraction
high resolution EEG
high resolution infrared (HRI) imaging
high resolution, low speed radiography
high resolution magnification
high resolution storage phosphor
  imaging
high resolution ultrasound scanning for
  foreign bodies
high-riding patella
high-risk sports
high-signal intratendinous collection of
  fluid
high signal mass
high steppage gait
high temporal resolution cine CT
  (HTRCCT)
high temporal resolution mode (multi-
  time point imaging)
high tibial osteotomy (HTO)
high-tide walking brace
high torque (see *Hi-Torque*)
high torque bur
high velocity gunshot wound
high velocity jet
high voltage pulsed galvanic stimulator
high voltage slow and sharp activity
high voltage stimulation (HVS)

high volt biphasic stimulator
high volt inferential stimulator
Hilgenreiner angle
Hilgenreiner horizontal Y line
Hilgenreiner line
Hilgenreiner-Pauwel line
Hilgenreiner-Perkins line
Hilger facial nerve stimulator
Hilight Advantage System CT scanner
Hill-Nahai-Vasconez-Mathes technique
Hill-Rom orthopedic bed
Hill-Sachs (posterior-superior humeral
   head) defect
Hill-Sachs shoulder lesion
hillock, axon
Hillock arch
Hilton law
Hilton muscle
hilum, hilar
hindbrain deformity
hindbrain herniation
Hinderer cartilage forceps
hindfoot arthrodesis
hindfoot excursion
hindfoot instability
hindfoot joint complex
hindfoot kinematics
hindfoot motion
hindfoot valgus
hinge
   Arizona Health Sciences Center-
      Volz
   Bahler
   Compass
   Dee elbow
   flail-elbow
   implant
   Kinematic rotating
   Kudo
   Lacey
   Noiles
   Quengel
   Rancho swivel
   stabilizing
hinged Ilizarov device
hinged implant
hinge joint, stable

hip
   CDH (congenital dislocation of hip)
   CDH (congenital dysplasia of hip)
   DDH (developmental dysplasia of
      hip)
   dislocated
   hanging
   pillow orthosis for
   Precision total
   snapping
   Senegas approach to
hip abduction stress test
hip arthroplasty, Mark II Sorrells
hip axis length
hip bone (os coxae)
hip bump
hip dislocation
hip dysplasia measurements in children
      with cerebral palsy:
   AA (acetabular anteversion)
   AAI (axial acetabular index)
   AD/FHD (ratio of acetabular depth
      to femoral head diameter)
   AI (acetabular index)
   CEA (center-edge angle) of Wiberg
   FA (femoral anteversion)
   MI (migration index
   NSA (neck-shaft angle) of femur
   SMAI (superior-medial acetabular
      index)
HIPciser abduction splint
hip fracture compaction drill and drill
   bits
hip hinging
hip joint
hip-knee-ankle-foot orthosis (HKAFO)
HipNav (navigation) computer-assisted
   process in hip replacement surgery
Hippel-Lindau syndrome (von Hippel-
   Lindau syndrome)
hip pinning
hippocampal-amygdala complex
hippocampal atrophy
hippocampal blood flow
hippocampal commissure
hippocampal cooling, intraoperative
hippocampal formation

hippocampal gyrus
hippocampal herniation
hippocampal infarction
hippocampal MR volumetry
hippocampal region
hippocampal sclerosis
hippocampal seizure
hippocampal volume
hippocampus
    CA1, CA2, CA3 subfields of
    dentate granule subfield of
    granulovacuolar change in
    hilar subfield of
    hippocampal
    Sommer sector of
Hippocrates bandage
Hippocrates manipulation
hip pointer
hip prosthesis
hip replacement
hip skid
hip spica cast
hippotherapy
Hippuran contrast medium
Hirano bodies
HiRider motorized/lift wheelchair
Hirsch hypophyseal punch
Hirsch hypophysis punch forceps
Hirschberg sign
Hirschhorn compression approach
Hirschtick splint
hirudin, recombinant
His-Haas muscle transfer
HiSpeed CT scanner
Hi Speed Pulse Lavage
hissing respiration in uremic coma
histamine cephalalgia
histamine headache
Hi-Star midfield MRI system
histinemia
histiocytic origin
histiocytoma
    angiomatoid
    benign fibrous
    fibrous
    low-grade malignant
    malignant fibrous

histiocytosis, sinus
histiocytosis X group of diseases
Histoacryl glue
histological tendon changes
histolytica, Torula (earlier name for
    Cryptococcus neoformans)
Histoplasma capsulatum meningitis
history of seizures
history of trauma or unusual activities
His-Werner disease
Hitachi imaging systems
hitch
    ankle
    bunting
Hitchcock arm procedure
Hitchcock stereotactic head frame
Hitchcock tendon technique
Hi-Top foot/ankle brace
Hi-Top foot/ankle walker
Hittenberger halo extension
Hittenberger prosthesis
HIV dementia complex
HIV encephalopathy
HIV viral antigen
HJB (high jugular bulb)
HKAFO (hip-knee-ankle-foot orthosis)
HL (hallux limitus)
HLA-B27 molecule
HLA-DQ
HLA (horizontal-long axial) images
HLA subtype
HMPAO (hexamethyl propylene
    amine oxime) SPECT scan
HMSN (hereditary motor and sensory
    neuropathy)
HMT (Hodkinson Mental Test)
HNA (hypothalamoneurohypophyseal
    axis)
HNB angiographic catheter
HNP (herniated nucleus pulposus)
Hoaglund bone graft
Hobb view
hobble, hobbling
hockey stick incision
Hodes, surface method of
Hodgen splint
Hodgkin lymphoma, intracranial

Hodgkin tumor
Hodkinson Mental Test (HMT)
Hoehn-Yahr staging of Parkinson
    disease
Hoek-Bowen cement removal system
Hoen angular forceps
Hoen clamp
Hoen dural separator
Hoen hemilaminectomy retractor
Hoen intervertebral disk rongeur
Hoen lamina gouge
Hoen laminectomy rongeur
Hoen nerve hook
Hoen periosteal elevator
Hoen scalp hemostat
Hoen scalp retractor
Hoen skull plate
Hoen ventricular needle
Hoffa disease
Hoffa fat pad
Hoffa tendon shortening
Hoffa test
Hoffer-Daimler cast spreader
Hoffer ankle procedure
Hoffman-Mohr unicoronal cranial
    sysnostosis repair
Hoffmann atrophy
Hoffmann-Clayton operation
Hoffmann external fixation device
Hoffmann metatarsal operation
Hoffmann mini-lengthening fixation
    device
Hoffmann monosynaptic reflex
    (H reflex)
Hoffmann reflex
Hoffmann sign or syndrome
Hoffmann-Vidal double frame
Hogg chair
Hohl tibia condylar fracture
    classification
Hohmann bone retractor
Hohmann osteotomy
Hohmann-Thomasen metatarsal
    osteotomy
Hoke Achilles tendon lengthening
    operation
Hoke lumbar brace/corset

Hoke-Martin traction
Hoke osteotome
Hoke procedure for tibial palsy
Hold-and-Hold positioner
Holdaway ratio
holder
    acetabular cup
    Adson dural needle
    Adson needle
    Aesculap head
    Alvarado knee
    Alvarado leg
    arm
    arthroscopic leg
    Ayers needle
    Barraquer needle
    Böhler-Steinmann pin (Boehler)
    bone
    Castroviejo needle
    CBI stereotactic head
    Charnley trochanter
    Crile-Wood needle
    cup
    Donaghy angled suture needle
    Drummond
    Drummond hook
    Ferguson bone
    Halsey needle
    head
    Jacobson needle
    knee
    leg
    LH1000 arthroscopic leg
    lithotomy leg
    Low Profile leg
    Malis needle
    Mayfield skull-pin head
    Mayo-Hegar needle
    microneedle
    microsurgery needle
    Micro-Two needle
    needle
    neurosurgical needle
    operative leg
    OSI Arthroscopic Leg
    Patil stereotactic head
    pin

holder *(continued)*
    Prep-Assist leg
    ReFix stereotactic head
    Rhoton needle
    Ryder needle
    Schmidt rod
    shell
    skull-pin head
    staple
    Surbaugh leg
    Surg-Assist leg
    tibial track
    trochanter
    Wangensteen
    Webster needle
    well-leg
    Yasargil needle
    Zollinger leg
Holdsworth classification of spinal
    injury
hole
    acetabular seating
    anchor
    anchoring
    bur (or burr)
    centering
    drill
    glide
    guide
    offset drill
    pullout
hole cutter
holiday, drug (therapeutic)
Holinger endarterectomy dissector
holistic approach
Hollingshead Index
Holl ligament
hollow bone
hollow foot
hollow mill Asnis cannulated screw
hollow-point bullet
Hollywood bed extension hook set
Holmes-Adie pupil
Holmes-Adie syndrome
Holmes cortical cerebellar degeneration
Holmes degeneration

holocord intradural lipoma
holocrania
Hologic DXA device
Hologic scanner
hologram
holography
    3-D
    MEVH (multiple-exposure
        volumetric)
    volumetric multiplexed transmission
    Voxgram multiple exposure
holoprosencephaly
Holscher nerve root retractor
Holt bolt
Holt nail
Holt-Oram syndrome
Holt plate
Holzheimer retractor
Homans sign
home assessment
home evaluation
homeostatic balance
Homer-Wright pseudorosette
homocystinuria
homogeneity
homogeneous appearance
homogeneous echo pattern
homogeneous graft
homogeneous perfusion
homogeneous soft tissue density
homograft
homolateral fracture-dislocation
homologous graft
homologue, meniscus
homonymous defect
homonymous hemianopsia (HHA)
homonymous scintillating scotomata
homozygous
homozygosity
Honda sign on tomography
H1 spectroscopy
honeymoon palsy
hood
    dorsal aponeurotic expansion
    extensor
    retinacular

hook
  Acufex nerve
  Adson dissecting
  Adson dural
  Adson nerve
  André
  APRL (Army Prosthetics Research
    Laboratory)
  Austin Moore
  Barr
  bifid
  Blair palate
  blunt
  blunt nerve
  Bobechko
  bone
  Boyes-Goodfellow
  button
  buttressed
  C-D
  Carroll skin
  caudal
  cautery
  clawed pedicle
  Cloward cautery
  Cloward dural
  compression
  cordotomy
  corkscrew dural
  Cotrel-Dubousset
  Crile nerve
  Culler
  Cushing dural
  Cushing gasserian ganglion
  Cushing nerve
  Dandy nerve
  DePuy nerve
  dissecting
  distraction
  double
  Drummond
  DTT (dynamic transverse traction)
  dura
  dural
  Edwards
  Edwards-Levine
  Effler-Groves

hook *(continued)*
  Fisch dural
  Fisch micro
  Frazier dural
  Frazier nerve
  ganglion
  garment
  Gillies
  Gillies bone
  Gillies-Dingman
  Graham muscle
  Graham nerve
  Green muscle
  Harrington
  Hoen nerve
  Isola
  Jameson muscle
  Jannetta
  jig
  Joseph
  Küntscher nail extracting
  Keene compression
  Kennerdell-Maroon
  Kilner
  Kirby muscle
  Knodt
  Krayenbuehl (Krayenbühl)
  Lahey Clinic dural
  Lahey Clinic nerve
  Lambotte bone
  laminar
  Leatherman
  Love nerve root
  Lucae nerve
  Malis nerve
  Marino transsphenoidal
  meniscus
  micro
  micro dural
  micronerve
  Micro-One
  Miltex tissue twist
  Moe spinal
  Moe square-ended
  Moss
  muscle
  nail-extracting

hook *(continued)*
  nerve
  O'Brien rib
  pedicle
  prosthetic
  Rhoton
  rib
  right-angle
  Rogozinski
  Rosser crypt
  Sachs dural
  Scoville nerve
  Scoville nerve root
  Selby II
  Selverstone cordotomy
  sharp
  shoe of the
  side opening
  skin
  sliding barrel
  Smithwick button
  Smithwick nerve
  Smithwick sympathectomy
  Speare dural
  spring
  straight dura
  Strully dural
  suture
  sympathectomy
  T-handled
  tendon
  Toennis dura
  traction
  transsphenoidal
  transverse
  transverse process
  Trautman Locktite prosthetic
  TSRH (Texas Scottish Rite
    Hospital)
  twist
  Tyrell
  vessel
  Volkmann
  Volkmann bone
  Weary nerve
  Yasargil spring
  Zielke

hook *(continued)*
  Zimmer caudal
  Zuelzer
hooked acromion
hooked bone
hook-fist positioning exercise following tendon repair
Hook hemi-harness shoulder
  immobilizer
hooklike osteophyte formation
hook-lying position
hook-plate fixation
hook-rod
  Cotrel-Dubousset
  Isola
  TSRH (Texas Scottish Rite
    Hospital)
hook tip coagulator
Hooper Visual Organization Test
Hoover sign
Hoover test
Hopkins plaster knife
Hopkins telescope/rigid glass lens
  endoscope
Hopkins Verbal Learning Test
Hoppenfeld-Deboer technique
hop, single-leg horizontal
horizontal fracture
horizontal gaze
horizontal interosseous wire loop
  fixation
horizontal long axial images (HLA)
horizontal long-axis SPECT image
horizontal loop suture technique for
  meniscal repair
horizontal plane
horizontal shoulder abduction exercises
hormone
  growth
  luteinizing
  prolactin
  thyrotropin
horn
  Ammon
  anterior
  central
  dorsal spinal cord

horn *(continued)*
  enlarged frontal
  frontal
  lateral
  meniscal
  occipital
  posterior
  posterior gray
  projectile
  spinal cord
  spinal dorsal
  splaying of frontal
  temporal
Horner muscle
Horner syndrome
  congenital
  neonatal
horn of ventricle
horse, charley
horseshoe abscess of hand
horseshoe appearance
horseshoe patellofemoral brace
horse-tail appearance of ruptured
  Achilles tendon
Horsley bone-cutting forceps
Horsley bone rongeur
Horsley dural separator
Horsley saw
Horsley separator
Horsley-Stille bone-cutting forceps
Horsley-Stille rib shears
Horton cephalalgia
Horton disease
Horton giant cell arteritis
Horton headache
Horton histamine cephalalgia
Horton syndrome
Horwitz-Adams arthrodesis
Horwitz ankle fusion
hose, TED (thromboembolic disease)
  (see also *stockings*)
Hospital Anxiety and Depression Scale
Hospital for Sick Children (HSC)
  scales for pain measurement
Hospital for Special Surgery (HSS)
  score

host immune system
hot and cold contrast baths
hot cross bun skull
hot fomentation therapy
Hot/Ice cold therapy cooler therapy
  device
Hot/Ice System III
hot packs
hot shot cervical or brachial plexus
  injury
hot spot on isotope bone scan
hot sulfur baths
Hough hoe
Houghton-Akroyd fracture technique
Hough transform (HT)
Hounsfield calcium density measure-
  ment unit (on CT scan)
hourglass deformity on myelogram
hourglass tumors of the cord
hourglass-type of neurilemmoma
House-Brackmann classification of
  facial nerve function
House-Dieter malleus nipper
House-Fisch dural retractor
House-Fisch dural spatula
housemaid's knee
Housepan aneurysm clips
Housepan clip-applying forceps
House suction irrigation tube
Houston Clinical Score
Houston halo traction cervical collar
  or support
Houston muscle
Hovanian procedure
Howard bone block
Howard spinal curet
Howarth dissector
Howell tibial guide
Howmedica cerclage cable
Howmedica ICS screw
Howmedica Kinematic II knee
  prosthesis
Howmedica Microfixation cranial plate
Howmedica Microfixation System drill
  bit
Howmedica Microfixation System
  plate cutters

Howmedica Microfixation System
 plate-holding forceps
Howmedica Microfixation System pliers
Howmedica-Osteonics instruments/
 devices
Howmedica Universal compression
 screw
Howmedica Vitallium staple
Howmedica VSF fixation system
Howorth-Keillor procedure
Howse total hip replacement
Howtek Scanmaster DX scanner
Ho:YAG (holmium: yttrium-
 aluminum-garnet) laser
Hoyer lift
HP-100 prosthetic finger joint
HPLC test
HPS II hip prosthesis
HRCT (high resolution computed
 tomography) image
H reflex study on electromyography
HRF (Health-Related Facilities)
HRI (high resolution infrared) imaging
H sign (on tomography)
HS (Haynes-Stellite) implant metal
HSC (Hospital for Sick Children)
 scales for pain measurement
HSE (herpes simplex encephalitis)
HSMN (hereditary sensorimotor
 neuropathy)
HSMN III (hereditary sensorimotor
 neuropathy, type III)
HSN (hereditary sensory neuropathy)
HSS (Hospital for Special Surgery)
HSS knee prosthesis
HSS knee score
HSS ligament rating scale
HSV particles on brain biopsy
HTO (high tibial osteotomy)
H2 15O (water O-15) radioactive
 diagnostic agent
H2 15O PET (positron emission
 tomography)
HU (Hounsfield unit)
Hubbard physical therapy tank
Hubbard plate

Huber opponensplasty
Huber needle
Huber transfer of abductor digiti quinti
Huck towel
Huckstep nail
Hudson adapter
Hudson bone bur
Hudson brace drill
Hudson bur
Hudson cerebellar attachment
Hudson cerebellar extension
Hudson chuck adapter
Hudson cranial drill set
Hudson cranial rongeur
Hudson forceps
Hueck ligament
Hueter bandage
Hueter fracture sign
Hueter line
Hughston Clinic classification of injury
Hughston-Degenhardt reconstruction
 technique
Hughston external rotation recurvatum
 test
Hughston-Hauser procedure
Hughston-Jacobson technique
Hughston knee evaluation
Hughston knee score
Hughston-Losee jerk test
Hughston view
human amphiregulin
human autologous chondrocyte
human chondrocyte culture technique
Human Genome Project
human lymphocyte antigen-DQ
human meniscal allograft
human midkine
humeral articulation
humeral bone
humeral head-splitting fracture
humeroperoneal muscular dystrophy
humeroradial articulation
humeroradial joint
humeroulnar articulation
humeroulnar joint
humerus

hump
  buffalo
  dowager's
  hip
humpback
Humphry ligament
hung-up (sustained) knee jerk
Hungerford-Krackow-Kenna knee
  arthroplasty
Hunt disease
Hunter canal
Hunter dural separator
Hunter ligament
Hunter open cord tendon implant
Hunter Silastic rod
Hunter syndrome
Hunter tendon prosthesis
Hunter tendon rod
hunterian ligation of aneurysm
Hunt-Hess aneurysm grading system
Hunt-Hess neurological classification
Hunt-Hess subarachnoid hemorrhage
  scale
Huntington bone graft
Huntington chorea
Huntington disease
Huntington sign
Hunt-Kosnik classification of
  aneurysm
Hunt-Kosnik classification of nuchal
  stiffness
Hunt neuralgia
Hunt paralysis
Hunt tumor forceps
Hunt-Yasargil pituitary forceps
Hurd bone-cutting forceps
Hurler disease
Hurler syndrome
Hurst disease
Hurteau skull plate anvil
Huschke ligament
Husk bone rongeur
Hutchinson pupil
Hutchinson-type neuroblastoma
Hutinel-Pick syndrome
HU-211 (dexanabinol)
HV (hallux valgus)

HVA (hallux valgus angle)
HVO (hallux valgus orthosis) splint
HVS (high voltage stimulation)
Hyalgan (hyaluronic acid)
Hyalgan (sodium hyaluronate)
hyaline articular cartilage
hyaline cartilage endplate of the intervertebral disk
hyalocapsular ligament
hyaluronic acid-derivative injection
hyaluronidase, synovial
Hyams grading system (or criteria) for
  esthesioneuroblastoma
hybrid fixation
hybrid Ilizarov halo apparatus
hybrid MRI imaging agent
hybrid-RARE imaging
hybrid seizure
Hydra-Cadence gait control unit
hydranencephaly (hydrocephalus)
hydrated proteoglycan gel of annulus
  fibrosus
hydraulic distention
hydraulic force
hydrencephalomeningocele
hydrencephaly
hydrocephalic patient
hydrocephalocele
hydrocephalus
  acquired
  acute
  asymptomatic
  bilateral
  chronic
  communicating
  congenital
  delayed
  fulminant
  idiopathic
  infantile
  noncommunicating
  normal pressure (NPH)
  normotensive
  obstructive
  occult
  otitis
  posthemorrhagic

hydrocephalus *(continued)*
    postinfectious
    posttraumatic
    primary
    progressive
    secondary
    symptomatic
    unilateral
    unshunted
hydrocephalus ex vacuo
hydrocephaly
hydrocodone and ibuprofen
    (Vicoprofen)
hydrocollation
Hydrocollator heating unit
Hydrocollator pad
Hydrocollator steam pack
hydrodipsomania
hydrodynamic potential of disk
hydroencephalocele
hydroencephaly
HydroFlex arthroscopy irrigating
    system
hydrogen peroxide
hydroma (see *hygroma*)
hydromyelia
Hydron Burn Bandage
hydrophobia (rabies)
hydrophobic cluster analysis
hydropneumogony
hydrops
    endolymphatic
    labyrinthine
    semicircular canal
Hydro-Splint II
hydrosyringomyelia
hydrotherapy pool
Hydroxial hip prosthesis
hydroxyapatite
    APS (air plasma spray)
    calcium
    coralline
    LPPS (low pressure plasma spray)
hydroxyapatite adhesive
hydroxyapatite bone replacement
    material
hydroxyapatite cement

hydroxyapatite crystals
hydroxyapatite-coated pin
hydroxyapatite-coated porous alumni
    (ceramic)
hydroxychloroquine (Plaquenil)
hydroxyisovaleric aminoaciduria
hygroma
    cystic
    motor oil
    subdural
Hylamer acetabular liner
Hylin rasp
hyoepiglottic ligament
hyoglossal muscle
hyoid bone
hyoscine butylbromide imaging agent
hypalgesia (hypoalgesia)
Hypaque contrast medium
Hypaque myelography
hyperabduction maneuver
hyper-ß-alaninemia
hyperactive behavior
hyperactive deep tendon reflexes
hyperactive dysfunction syndrome of
    cranial nerves
hyperactive reflexes
hyperactive syndrome
hyperactivity
    autonomic
    sudomotor (not pseudomotor)
        autonomic
hyperacusis
hyperacute stroke
hyperalgesia
hyperalgesic
hyperbaric oxygen
hyperbradykininism
hypercalcemia
hypercholesterolemia
hyperdense middle cerebral artery sign
hyperdopaminergic state
hyperdynamic abductor hallucis
hyperechoic region
hyperechoicity
hyperemia test
hyperemic
hyperesthesia, stocking-glove

hyperesthetic
hyperexcitability, central neuronal
hyperextendability, joint
hyperextensibility of joints
hyperextension injury
hyperextension stress
hyperextension teardrop fracture
hyperextension test
hyperfixation
hyperflexion/hyperextension cervical
   injury
hyperflexion injury
hyperflexion teardrop fracture
hyperfractionated radiation therapy
hyperglycemia
   ketotic
   nonketotic
hyperhidrosis
Hypericum perforatum medicinal herb
hyperintense marrow space
hyperintense mass
hyperintense signal
hyperintensity
   cortical
   white matter signal
hyperkeratosis
hyperkeratotic plantar lesion
hyperkinesia
hyperkinesis
hyperkinetic motor disorder
hyperkinetic movement
hyperlaxity
hyperlisenemia
hyperlordosis, functional
hyperlucency
hyperlysinemia
hypermetria
hypermetric saccade
hypermobile first ray
hypermobile joint syndrome
hypermobility
hypermyelination
hypernephroma, cerebral
hyperonychia
hyperostosis
   ankylosing spinal

hyperostosis *(continued)*
   Caffey
   diffuse idiopathic sclerosis (DISH)
   diffuse idiopathic skeletal (DISH)
   idiopathic cortical (ICH)
   infantile cortical
   senile ankylosing
   skull
hyperostosis frontalis interna
hyperostotic lesion
hyperparathyroidism, brown tumor of
hyperparathyroidism-induced stress
   fracture
hyperpathia, thalamic
hyperphalangism, intercalary
hyperpigmented lesion
hyperpituitary state
hyperplasia
   epiphyseal
   gingival
   pituitary
hyperplastic
hyperpneumatization of the cranium
hyperpolarization
hyperpolarize
hyperpolarized helium
hyperpolarized He-3 imaging agent
hyperprolactinemia
hyperprolinemia
hyperpronation
hyperreflexia
   asymmetric
   autonomic
   bilateral
   pathologic
   spastic
   unilateral
hyperreflexic
hypersarcosinemia
hypersensitivity, delayed-type
hypersensitivity reaction to
   anticonvulsants
hypersomnia
hypersomnolence
hypersynchrony, paroxysmal
   hypnagogic

hypertelorism
hypertension
  benign intracranial (BIH)
  idiopathic intracranial (IIH)
  intracranial
  neurogenic
  striate hemorrhage in intracranial
hypertension injury
hypertensive crisis
hypertensive encephalopathy
hypertensive hemorrhage
hypertensive stroke
hypertensive vascular degeneration
hypertensive vascular disease
hyperthermia
  malignant
  volumetric interstitial
  whole body
hyperthermia probe
hyperthermia treatment, ultrasound
hypertonia
hypertonicity
hypertrichosis
hypertrophic infiltrating tenosynovitis
hypertrophic marginal spurring
hypertrophic nonunion
hypertrophic spondylitis
hypertrophic spurring
hypertrophy
  bone
  endosteal
  epiphyseal
  ligamentous-muscular
  muscular
  olivary
  scalenus anticus muscle
  smooth-muscle
hypertylosis of the palms
hyperuricemia
hypervalinemia
hyperventilation
  autonomic
  central neurogenic
  forced
  neurogenic
  psychogenic
  stertorous

hyperventilation as activating
  technique during EEG
hypervigilance
hypesthesia (hypoesthesia)
hypnagogic hallucinations
hypnagogic hypersynchrony on EEG
hypnagogic state
hypnalgia
hypnic jerks
hypnolepsy
hypnopedia
hypnopompic hallucinations
hypoactive deep tendon reflexes
hypoalgesia (hypalgesia)
hypoattenuation
hypocalcemia
hypochondriac region
hypochondriasis
hypocycloidal ankle tomography
hypoechogenic
hypoechoic area on ultrasound
hypoesthesia (hypesthesia)
hypoesthesic
hypoflexibility of foot
hypofunction, vestibular
hypogastric nerve
hypogastric region
hypogeusia
hypoglossal canal
hypoglossal nerve
hypoglossal neuralgia
hypoglycemia
hypoglycemic challenge
hypoglycorrhachia
hypointense signal
hypokinesia
  global
  parkinsonian
  regional
hypokinesis
hypolordosis
hypomelanosis, Ito
hypometria
hypometric saccade
hypomyelination neuropathy
hyponychium
hypo-osmolar glucose solution

hypoparathyroidism
hypoperfused state
hypoperfusion
   global cerebral
   peripheral
   post-ischemic cerebral
hypophonic voice quality
hypophyseal (or hypophysial)
hypophysectomy
   transcranial
   transsphenoidal
hypophysectomy kit, Zervas
hypophysial (or hypophyseal)
hypophysis cerebri
hypophysis, infundibulum
hypophysitis, giant cell granulomatous
hypopituitarism
hypopituitary coma
hypoplasia
   cartilage-hair
   skeletal
hypoplastic horizontal ribs
hypoplastic thumb
hyporeflexia
hyporeflexic
hyposensitization
hypotension
   cerebral
   intracranial
hypothalamic lesion
hypothalamic-pituitary-adrenal axis
hypothalamic-pituitary axis
hypothalamus
   anterior
   rostral
hypothalamus tumor
hypothenar eminence
hypothenar muscle groups of hand
hypothermia
hypothermic circulatory arrest

hypotonia
   benign congenital
   cerebral
   congenital
hypotonic
hypotonic patient
hypoxia
   anemic
   anoxic
   cerebral
   hypoxic
   ischemic
   toxic
hypoxic brain damage
hypoxic encephalopathy
hypoxic injury
hypoxic ischemic encephalopathy
hypoxic ischemic insults
hypsarrhythmia pattern on EEG
   asymmetrical
   unilateral
hypsiloid ligament
hypsokinesis
hysterical aphonia
hysterical blindness
hysterical conversion reaction
hysterical fugue state
hysterical gait
hysterical hemiplegia
hysterical joint
hysterical mutism
hysterical paralysis
hysterical pseudodementia
hysterical seizure
hysterical trance
hysterical tremor
hysterical visual loss
hysterical overbreathing, voluntary
hysteric coma-like state
hystericus, globus
hysteroepilepsy
Hz (hertz or cycles per second)

I, i

IABC (intra-aortic balloon counter-
pulsation)
IADL (instrumental activities of daily
living)
IADSA (intra-arterial digital
subtraction angiography)
IAM (internal auditory meatus)
I&D (incision and drainage)
IAP (intracranial amobarbital
procedure)
IAS (intra-articular shaver)
IAT (intraoperative autologous
transfusion)
iatrogenic carotid-cavernous fistula
iatrogenic dural tear
iatrogenic elevatus
iatrogenic injury
IBCA (n-isobutyl-cyanoacrylate) glue
I-beam, Jergesen
IBF (Insall-Burstein-Freeman) knee
instruments
IBG (iliac bone graft)
IBM (inclusion body myositis)
IBZP (chlorohydroxyiodophenyl-
methyltetrahydro-H-benzapine)
imaging agent for intermittent
catheterization
ICA (internal carotid artery)

ICAM-1 or ICAM-3 (circulating inter-
celluluar adhesion molecule-1 or
molecule-3)
ICBG (iliac crest bone graft)
ICD-9 (International Classification of
Diseases, 9th Revision)
ICD-9-CM (International Classification
of Diseases, 9th Revision, Clinical
Modification)
ICD-10 (International Classification of
Diseases, 10th Revision)
ice, application of
ice cream headache
ICEDP (intracranial epidural pressure)
ice massage
ice water caloric response
ice water irrigation
ICEDP (intracranial epidural pressure)
Iceland (or Icelandic) disease
ICF (Intermediate Care Facilities)
ICH (idiopathic cortical hyperostosis)
ICH (intracerebral hemorrhage)
ichthyosis in Refsum disease
ICIDH (International Classification of
Impairments, Disabilities, Handi-
caps)
ICIDH model of the World Health
Organization

icing, cutaneous
ICLH (Imperial College, London
　　Hospital)
ICLH ankle prosthesis
ICLH double-cup arthroplasty
ICNB (intercostal nerve block)
ICP (intracranial pressure)
ICP catheter
ICP monitor
ICP wave form
ICRS (International Cartilage Repair
　　Society) arthroscopic staging
　　system
ICS (intercostal space)
ICST (isolated cold stress test)
ictal amnesia
ictal automatism
ictal confusional seizure
ictal epileptiform activity
ictal epileptiform pattern
ictal fear preceding temporal lobe
　　seizure
ictal focal epileptiform discharge
ictal hyperperfusion
ictal onset zone
ictal pattern on EEG
ictal period
ictal phase study
ictal SPECT
ictal technetium Tc-99m HMPAO
　　brain SPECT
ictus site
ICV (internal cerebral vein)
IDA index
IDEA (Individuals with Disabilities
　　Education Act)
IDEA (Inventory for Déjà Vu
　　Experiences Assessment)
ideation
　　homicidal
　　suicidal
ideational set-shifting
ideational apraxia
ideational dyspraxia
idée fixe ("ee-day'-feeks")
ideomotor apraxia

ideomotor dyspraxia
IDE protocol
IDET (intradiscal electrothermal)
　　annuloplasty
IDET therapy
IDGH (ischemic disease of the
　　growing hip)
idiocy, mongolian
idioglossia
idiopathic cortical hyperostosis (ICH)
idiopathic encephalopathy
idiopathic epilepsy
idiopathic facial nerve palsy
idiopathic fracture
idiopathic generalized epilepsy
idiopathic gout
idiopathic intracranial hypertension
　　(IIH)
idiopathic polymyositis myopathy
idiopathic polyneuropathy
idiopathic scoliosis
idiopathic seizure
idiopathic tic disorder
idiopathic toe walking
idiopathic tremor
idiot-savant
IDIS (intraoperative digital subtrac-
　　tion) angiography system
IDK (internal derangement of knee)
id reaction
IDSA (intraoperative digital subtrac-
　　tion angiography)
IDSI (Imaging Diagnostic Systems,
　　Inc.) scanner
IDSS (internal decompression for
　　spinal stenosis)
I_z electrode
IES PowerPump 1000
IFA (immunoflourescent antibody)
IFN-g (interferon-gamma)
IgA-RF class-specific rheumatoid fac-
　　tor
IGF-1 (insulin-like growth factor-1)
IGF-BP3 complex (SomatoKine)
IgG-RF class-specific rheumatoid
　　factor

IgM affinity purification test
IgM-RF class-specific rheumatoid
factor
IIH (idiopathic intracranial hypertension)
iiRAD DR1000 digital x-ray device
IJV (internal jugular vein)
IKDC (International Knee Documentation Committee) questionnaire
IKDC rating scale/score
Ikuta fixation device
IL (interleukin)
ILAR classification of arthritis
ileus as response to spinal injury
Ilfeld-Gustafson splint
Ilfeld-Holder deformity
Ilheus viral encephalitis
iliac apophysitis
iliac bone graft (IBG)
iliac compression test
iliac crest bone graft (ICBG)
iliac crest strut graft
iliac dowel
iliac fossa
iliac muscle
iliac osteocutaneous free flap
iliac spine
iliac wing
iliococcygeal muscle
iliocostal muscle
iliocostal space
iliofemoral ligament
iliohypogastric nerve
ilioinguinal nerve
ilioinguinal syndrome
iliolumbar ligament
iliopectineal ligament
iliopsoas muscle
iliosacral implant
iliotibial band augmentation
iliotibial band friction syndrome
iliotibial ligament of Maissiat
iliotrochanteric ligament
ilium
Ilizarov ankle arthrodesis
Ilizarov corticotomy
Ilizarov distractor

Ilizarov external fixator
Ilizarov forearm lengthening procedure
Ilizarov frame
Ilizarov leg lengthening technique
Ilizarov limb lengthening procedure
Ilizarov ring
Ilizarov screw
Ilizarov system
Ilizarov telescoping rod
Ilizarov wire
illicit drug, blood levels of
illness behaviors
illness, progressive dementing
illusion
illusory strabismus
iloperidone (Zomaril)
IM (intermetatarsal) joint
IM (intramedullary) rod
IMA (intermetatarsal angle)
image (see *imaging*)
image acquisition time
image analysis system
image control
imaged
ImageFusion software
image-guided functional neurosurgery
image-guided radiosurgery
image-guided surgery with robotic
assistance
image intensification
image intensifier
image matrix
image noise
image quality degradation
imager (see *scanner*)
image reconstruction
image registration
images, flow
imaging
Accuson 128XP ultrasound
Accuson Sequoia ultrasound
Achilles+ ultrasonometer device
AddOn-Bucky digital
Aloka color Doppler real-time 2D
blood flow imaging with Cine
Memory
Aloka ultrasound

imaging *(continued)*
  AMT-25-enhanced MR
    angiography
  aperiodic functional MR
  Aquilion CT scanner
  arterial flow phase
  arthrography
  Artoscan M
  Aspire continuous (CI)
  ATL real-time Neurosector scan
  attenuation
  axial
  Biopspec Bruker spectroscopy
  blood flow
  blood pool
  body coil
  bone age
  bone density
  bone length
  bone mineral content
  bone phase
  bone scintiscan
  bone ultrasound attenuation (BUA)
  brain scan
  B-scan
  carotid duplex
  CAT (computerized axial
    tomography)
  CDI (color Doppler imaging)
  CECT (contrast enhancement of
    computed tomographic)
  cephalogram
  cerebral perfusion SPECT
  chemical shift
  chemical-selective fat saturation
  chondroitin sulfate iron colloid
    (CSIS)-enhanced MR
  cine
  cine CT (computed tomography)
  cine gradient-echo
  cine PC (phase contrast)
  cineradiography
  cisternography
  collimation
  color amplitude
  color-coded flow

imaging *(continued)*
  color Dopper (CDI)
  color-flow duplex
  column mode sinogram
  combined leukocyte-marrow
  combined multisection diffuse-
    weighted and hemodynamically
    weighted echo planar MR
  combined thallium-Tc-HMPAO
  computed axial tomography (CAT)
  computed tomography (CT)
  computed transmission tomography
  cone-beam
  contiguous
  contrast-enhanced magnetization
    transfer saturation
  contrast material enhanced
  contrast phlebography
  conventional planar (CPI)
  convergent color Doppler
  cross-sectional
  CSF-suppressed T2-weighted 3D
    MP-RAGE MR
  CT (computed tomography)
  CT guidance for cyst aspiration
  CT guidance for needle biopsy
  CT guidance for placement of
    radiation therapy fields
  CTAT (computerized transverse
    axial tomography)
  delayed bone
  DEXA (dual energy x-ray absorp-
    tiometry) bone density scan
  diagnostic ultrasound (DUS)
  diffusion and perfusion magnetic
    resonance
  diffusion magnetic resonance
  diffusion-weighted MR
  digital radiography
  digital vascular (DVI)
  displacement field-fitting MR
  dMRI (dynamic magnetic
    resonance imaging)
  Doppler ultrasonography
  double-dose gadolinium
  double-phase technetium Tc 99m
    sestamibi

imaging *(continued)*
DSC (dynamic susceptibility
contrast) MR
dual energy x-ray absorptiometry
(DEXA)
dual-echo DIET fast SE (spin-echo)
duplex carotid
duplex Doppler
dynamic contrast-enhanced subtraction MR
dynamic scintigraphy
dynamic susceptibility contrast
(DSC) MR
echo-planar (EPI)
echo-planar FLAIR (fluid-attenuated inversion-recovery)
echo-planar MRA
electric joint fluoroscopy
electrodiagnostic
electromagnetic blood flow
electron beam computed
tomography (EBCT)
EPI (echo-planar imaging)
excitation-spoiled fat-suppressed
T1-weighted ST
ex vivo MR
fast Fourier transform (FFT)
fast low-angle shot (FLASH)
fast multiplanar spoiled gradient-
recalled (FMPSPGR)
fast SE and fast IR (FMPIR)
fast spin-echo MR
fast spoiled gradient-recalled MR
fat-suppressed three-dimensional
spoiled gradient-(FDG)
FDG PET
59NP (iodomethylnorcholesterol)
scintigraphy
FLAIR (fluid-attenuated inversion-
recovery)
FLAIR-FLASH
FLASH (fast low-angle shot)
fluid-attenuated inversion-recovery
(FLAIR)
[18F]fluoro-m-tyrosine positron
emission tomographic scan

imaging *(continued)*
FluoroPlus angiography
FluoroPlus Roadmapper digital
fluoroscopy
fluoroscopy-guided condylar lift-off
FMPIR
FMPSPGR
Fonar Stand-Up MRI
four-dimensional (4D)
frequency domain (FDI) in
ultrasound
FS-BURST MR
fSE (functional SE)
functional MR (FMR)
gadolinium (Gd)
gadolinium-enhanced MRI
arthrogram
gallium (Ga)
GE Signa MRI scanner
glucose metabolic tracer
fludeoxyglucose F-18
gradient-echo
gradient-echo phase
gradient-echo sequence
gradient-recalled-echo (GRE) MR
GRASS MR (gradient-recalled
acquisition in steady state)
gray scale
GRE (gradient-recalled echo)
half-Fourier, three-dimensional
technique
Hewlett-Packard phased-array
high definition (HDI)
high energy
high field strength MR
high frequency Doppler ultrasound
high resolution B-mode
HLA (horizontal long axial)
SPECT scan
Hologic QDR 1000W dual-energy
x-ray absorptiometry
holography
H-1 MR spectroscopic
indirect magnetic resonance
arthrography
intracranial

imaging *(continued)*
  intraoperative
  intravenous fluorescein angiography
    (IVFA)
  in vivo
  iodomethylnorcholesterol (59NP)
    scintigraphy
  kinematic MR
  limited
  linear scan
  low field strength MR
  lower extremity
  lower limb venography
  low resolution
  Lunar Expert DXA scanner
  Lunar Expert XL DXA scanner
  magnetic resonance (MRI)
  Magnes 2500 WH (whole head)
  magnetic resonance (MR)
  magnetic resonance angiography
    (MRA)
  magnetic resonance spectroscopy
    (MRS)
  magnetic source imaging (MSI)
  magnetoacoustic
  middle field strength MR
  midsagittal MR
  miniature
  minimum intensity projection
  monoclonal antibody
  MRI (magnetic resonance imaging)
  multi-echo
  multi-echo coronal
  multimodality
  multiorgan
  multiplanar MR
  multiplanar reformatted radio-
    graphic and digitally recon-
    structed radiographic
  multipulse
  multisection diffuse-weighted
  multisection MR
  MUSTPAC ultrasound
  myelography
  native tissue harmonic imaging
    (NTHI)

imaging *(continued)*
  navigated spin-echo diffusion-
    weighted MR
  neurodiagnostic
  neuroradiologic
  noninvasive
  nuclear bone
  nuclear perfusion
  oblique axial MR
  opposed GRE
  opposed-phase GRE
  optical
  orthopantogram
  orthoroentgenogram
  outlet radiographs
  out-of-phase GRE
  oxygenation-sensitive functional
    MR
  P-31 magnetic resonance
    spectroscopy
  panoramic
  Paris ultrasound system
  PC (phase contrast)
  Pediatric Ultrasound Bone
    Analyzer
  Perception 5000 ultrasound
  percutaneous drainage of abscess
  periorbital Doppler
  peripheral quantitative computed
    tomography (pQCT)
  peripheral vascular
  PET (positron emission
    tomography)
  PETT (positron emission transaxial
    tomography)
  phased-array surface coil MR
  phase encode time-reduced acquisi-
    tion sequence
  plain films
  planar (2D)
  positron
  postcontrast MR
  postoperative
  power Doppler (PDI)
  pQCT (peripheral quantitative
    computed tomography)

imaging *(continued)*
  pre-contrast
  preoperative
  pronated grip x-ray
  proton density-weighted
  PSH-25GT transcranial imaging
    transducer
  pulsed electron paramagnetic
  pulsed low intensity ultrasound
  pulsed magnetization transfer MR
  QCT (quantitative computed
    tomography) (for bone loss)
  quantitative fluorescence
  QUS-2 calcaneal ultrasonometer
  radiographically normal
  radioisotope cisternography
  radioisotope gallium
  radioisotope technetium
  radionuclide
  rapid axial MR
  rapid-sequence
  real-time 2D blood flow
  reconstructed radiographic
  rectilinear bone scan
  registration and alignment of 3D
  sagittal gradient-echo
  sagittal oblique
  sagittal T1-weighted image (MRI)
  Sahara clinical bone sonometer
  saline-enhanced MR
  scanogram
  scintigraphic scan
  SE (spin-echo)
  segmenting dual-echo MR
  selective
  sequential
  serial contrast MR
  serial duplex
  shuntogram
  SieScape ultrasound
  Signa Special Procedures (SP)
  simultaneous volume
  single-dose gadolinium
  single-voxel proton brain
    spectroscopy
  sinus tract

imaging *(continued)*
  sliding thin-slab maximum-intensity
    projection CT
  small field-of-view (FOV)
  SmartSPOT high resolution digital
  SoundScan Compact bone
    sonometer
  SoundScan 2000 bone sonometer
  SPECT (single photon emission
    CT) thallium
  spin-echo (SE)
  spin-lock
  spine CT with contrast
  spine CT without contrast
  split-brain
  stacked scans
  STIR (short T1 inversion recovery)
  strain-rate MR
  Stratis II MRI system
  subtraction
  stereotactic CT scan
  31-P magnetic resonance
    spectroscopy
  3DFT (3D Fourier transform)
  3DFT GRASS MR
  3DFT SPGR MR
  3D H-1 MR spectroscopic
  3D reformations of MR
  3D turbo SE (spin-echo)
  2D Fourier transform
  2D gradient-recalled echo
  T1-weighted coronal
  T1-weighted sagittal
  T2-weighted coronal
  T2-QMRI (T2-quantitative
    magnetic resonance imaging)
  TechneScan MAG3
  technetium (see *imaging agent*)
  thallium (Tl)
  thallium, ^{201}Tl SPECT brain
  thallium scintigraphy
  thallium SPECT (thallium 201
    single-photon emission com-
    puted tomographic) imaging
  thick-slice
  thin-collimation

imaging *(continued)*
  thin-slice
  tilted lateral radiograph
  time of flight (TOF)
  tissue Doppler
  tomographic
  Toshiba Aspire continuous
  transaxial
  transcranial imaging transducer
  triple-dose gadolinium
  triple-phase bone scan
  TSPP (technetium stannous
    pyrophosphate) rectilinear bone
  turboFLAIR (fluid-attenuated
    inversion recovery)
  turboFLASH (fast low-angle shot)
  two-dimensional (2D)
  two-phase CT
  ultrafast CT
  ultrasonic tomographic
  ultrasonography
  unenhanced MR
  vascular flow
  venous
  vertical long axial (VLA)
  videofluoroscopy
  video radiography
  Viewing Wand imaging system
  VLA (vertical long axial)
  volume-rendered
  volumetric
  Walker-Sonix UBA 575+ ultra-
    sound
  water selective SE (spin-echo)
  whole body scan
  whole body thallium
  wide beam scan
  xenon-133 (133Xe) SPECT
  xeroradiography
imaging agent (including contrast
    media, radioactive drugs,
    radioisotopes, and technetium)
  air
  Amipaque
  Angio-Conray
  Angiocontrast
  Angiografin

imaging agent *(continued)*
  Angiovist 282, 292, 370
  Ceretec (technetium 99m)
  gadolinium (Gd)
  gallium (Ga)
  Gd (gadolinium)
  Gd-DOTA (gadolinium tetra-
    azacyclododecanetetra-acetic
    acid)
  Isovue nonionic
  Isovue-128; 200; 300; 370
  Isovue-M 200; 300
  Lipiodol myelographic
  Magnevist
  monoclonal (MOAB, MoAb)
    antibody
  myelographic
  Omnipaque
  Omniscan
  Optimark MRI contrast
  technetium-99m bicisate (Neurolite)
  technetium-99m (Ceretec)
  technetium-99 exametazime
  Visipaque
imaging anatomic correlation
imaging-based stereotaxis in tumor
  neurosurgery
imaging criteria
imaging-directed 3D volumetric information on intracranial lesion
imaging pathologic correlation
imaging plane
Imatron C-100 ultrafast CT scanner
Imatron C-150L EBCT scanner
Imatron Fastrac C-100 cine x-ray CT
  scanner
Imatron Ultrafast CT scanner
imbalance
  biomechanical
  fixed sagittal
  muscle
imbecility
imbibition
imbricate
imbrication
  capsular
  facetal

imbrication of facets
IMiG-MRI device
imipramine (Tofranil)
Imitrex (sumatriptan)
immediate memory; recall (short-term
    memory)
immediate postictal period
immediate postsurgical fitting (IPSF)
immersion B-scan ultrasound
immobilization after spinal injury
immobilizer (see also *brace, strap,*
    splint, support)
    cast
    DonJoy Ultrasling shoulder
    external
    halo
    Hook hemi-harness shoulder
    joint
    knee
    Kuz-Medics disposable knee
    long leg
    OEC knee
    postoperative
    Raymond shoulder
    Rowe-Zarin shoulder
    sateen knee
    shoulder
    shoulder abduction
    single-panel knee
    sling and swathe shoulder
    sling
    Slingshot shoulder
    sterno-occipitomanubrial
    Tab-Strap knee
    Trimline knee
    tri-panel knee
    Velcro
    Velpeau shoulder
    Watco 2001 knee
    Westfield acromioclavicular
    Y-strap knee
    Zimmer knee
    Zinco thumb-wrist
immobilization jacket
ImmTher
immune-mediated paraneoplastic
    disorder

immune-mediated systemic reaction
immune modulator
immune system compromise
immune therapy, IR501
immunization, tetanus
immunocompetent
immunocompromised
immunocytochemistry
immuno-electron microscopy
immunoflourescent antibody (IFA)
immunogenic
immunogenicity
immunoglobulin M paraproteinemic
    neuropathy
immunoglobulin, tetanus
immunohistochemical assessment
Immuno 1 Dpd assay
immunoprecipitation assay
immunoreactive chromogranin
immunoreactivity, glial fibrillary
    acidic protein
immunostain
    chromogranin
    cytokeratin
    epithelial membrane antigen (EMA)
    GFAP (glial fibrillary acidic protein)
    pancytokeratin
    proliferating cell nuclear antigen
    S-100 protein
    vimentin
immunostaining
Imount total knee replacement instru-
    ments
IMPA cephalometric measurement
impacted fracture
impacted subcapital fracture
impacted valgus fracture
impact force
impaction graft
Impact total hip prosthesis
impactor
    Austin Moore
    Cloward bone graft
    Dawson-Yuhl
    Küntscher
    Moe
    shell

impactor *(continued)*
   Smith-Petersen
   vertebral body
impactor-extractor, Fox
impactor rod
impaired blood flow
impaired consciousness
impaired venous return
impaired ventilation-perfusion
impaired visuospatial memory
impairment
   anterior horn cell motor
   circulatory
   cognitive
   consciousness
   constructional
   coordination
   disease-specific measure of
   functional
   gaze
   graphic
   intellectual
   memory
   motor
   neurological
   objective symptoms of
   perceptual motor
   peripheral nerve level motor
   reading comprehension
   root level motor
   sensory
   spinal nerve level motor
   subjective symptoms of
   upper motor neuron
   visual
impairment-based measures
IMP-Capello arm support
impedance
   electrical
   electrode
   interelectrode
   ohms
impedance meter
impedance phlebography
impedance plethysmography (IPG)
imperfect regeneration
imperforate aneurysm

impersistence
impinge
impinged upon
impingement
   dural
   lateral
   ligamentous
   nerve root
   talar
   talofibular
impingement exostosis
impingement syndrome
impingement tendinitis
impinging
implant (see also *prosthesis*)
   advanced mobile-bearing knee
   AO-ASIF
   Arenberg-Denver inner-ear valve
   auditory brainstem (ABI)
   BAK/Proximity interbody fusion
   Biocoral
   Biodel
   Biofix biodegradable
   Biomatrix ocular
   cochlear
   COR/T
   CT-based CAD/CAM revision
      femoral
   Custodis
   DePuy orthopedic
   double-stem silicone lesser MP
   Durapatite
   DynaGraft bioimplants
   epidural
   fixed-bearing knee
   Gemini MKII mobile-bearing knee
   Genesis II mobile-bearing knee
   gentamicin
   Gliadel
   Global total shoulder
   Hedrocel proximal tibia
      augmentation
   hinged
   Hunter open cord tendon
   hyaline cartilage
   hydroxyapatite
   iliosacral

implant *(continued)*
    IMEX scleral
    Innovasive COR/T implant system
    Insall-Burstein total knee
    Interax Integrated Secure Assym-
        metric (ISA) mobile-bearing
        knee
    Interpore
    islet cell
    Kinetik great toe
    LaPorta great toe
    LCS Total Knee Systems
    lumbar anterior root stimulator
        (LARSI)
    MBK mobile-bearing knee
    McCutchen press-fit titanium
        femoral
    Medtronic Activa tremor control
        therapy
    methylmethacrylate beads
    Miragel
    mobile-bearing knee
    Moss Miami load-sharing spinal
    NeuFlex metacarpophalangeal joint
    Neuromed Octrode implantable
        device for chronic pain manage-
        ment
    Nexus
    open cord tendon
    Osteonics-HA coated
    PMMA (poly-methylmethacrylate)
    polyglycolide
    polylactide
    Polypin biodegradable pin
    porous-coated
    Profix mobile-bearing knee
    ProOsteon synthetic bone
    Rotaglide knee
    Schuhli implant system
    self-aligning (SAL) mobile-bearing
        knee
    Septacin implant to treat
        osteomyelitis
    Ship hammertoe
    silicone
    silicone elastomer rubber ball
    Sinterlock

implant *(continued)*
    Sutter double-stem silicone
    Swanson metacarpophalangeal
    Synthes Schuhli implant system
    synthetic bone
    System•S soft skeletal
    Techmedica
    Teflon
    TheraSeed
    tobramycin-impregnated PMMA
    total knee
    Total Rotating Knee (TRK) mobile-
        bearing
    Trac II knee
    Translating and Congruent
        (Mobile-Bearing) Knee (TACK)
    vagal nerve
    vagus stimulator
    VDS (ventral derotating spinal)
    Weil-type Swanson-design
        hammertoe
    Zielke VDS (ventral derotating
        spinal)
implantable bone anchor
implantable bone growth stimulator,
    Osteo Stim
implantation
    autologous chondrocyte
    deep brain stimulator
    depth electrodes
    subthalamic nucleus
implant collar
implant hinge
implant metal
Implast bone cement
Implex instruments/devices
Implex ProxiLock femoral stem
impression defect
impression fracture
IMP SPECT scan
IMP Surgical Leg Pedestal
IMP-Turnstile Casting Stand
impulse, simultaneous nerve
impulsive petit mal
impulsiveness
impulsivity
ImuLyme

inability to attend
in-a-chair test
inactivity, electrocerebral (ECI)
inactivation, X-
inappropriate ADH (antidiuretic
  hormone) secretion
inappropriate affect
inappropriate words (paraphrasia)
inattention
  functional
  organic
inattentiveness, momentary
InCare ankle brace
incarial bone
incise
incision
  anteromedial
  battledore (racquet-shaped)
  bifrontal
  bikini skin
  Brunner modified
  Brunner palmar
  Bruser skin (knee)
  capsular
  Charnley
  chevron
  Cincinnati
  circumscribing
  coronal
  coronal scalp
  C-shaped
  Cubbins
  Curtin
  curved
  curvilinear
  deltoid-splitting
  dorsal linear
  dorsomedial
  double
  DuVries
  elliptical
  exploratory
  fascial-splitting
  fiber-splitting
  fish-mouth
  Gaenslen split heel
  H-shaped capsular

incision *(continued)*
  Henderson skin
  Henry
  hockey stick
  J-shaped skin
  Kocher
  Kocher collar
  L-curved
  L-shaped
  lateral
  lateral utility
  lazy-S
  longitudinal
  Ludloff
  Mayfield
  medial
  medial parapatellar
  median parapatellar
  midaxillary line
  muscle-splitting
  oblique
  Ollier
  palmar
  paramedial
  parapatellar
  posterior
  racquet-shaped
  relaxing
  relieving
  S
  S-flap
  S-shaped
  saber-cut
  serpentine
  skin
  split
  stab
  standard
  straight
  T-shaped
  tangential
  transverse
  U-shaped
  V-shaped
  volar
  Wagner skin
  Watson-Jones

infarction *(continued)*
    posterior cerebral territory
    retinal
    root entry zone
    severe
    small, deep, recent (SDRI)
    spinal cord
    subcortical
    subcortical cerebral
    temporal lobe
    thalamic
    thrombotic
    ventral pontine
    vermian
    watershed
    white matter
In-Fast bone screw system
infection
    bone
    brucellosis
    central nervous system
    chronic spinal epidural
    chronic spinal intradural
    closed disk space
    coccidioidomycosis
    cryptococcosis
    disk space
    dissecting subcutaneous extrafascial
    dorsal subaponeurotic
    felon
    helminthic
    Meleney gangrene
    mycotic
    paraspinal
    pin tract
    rickettsial
    slow virus
    soft tissue
    syphilis
    tendon sheath space
    tuberculous cold abscess
infectious hepatitis encephalitis
infectious mononucleosis encephalitis
infectious polyneuritis syndrome
inferior alveolar nerve
inferior basal segment
inferior calcaneonavicular ligament

inferior cerebellar peduncle
inferior cervical cardiac nerve
inferior cluneal nerves
inferior constrictor muscle of pharynx
inferior dorsal radioulnar ligament
inferior facet
inferior frontal gyrus
inferior gemellus muscle
inferior gluteal nerve
inferior hemorrhoidal nerves
inferior laryngeal nerve
inferior lateral brachial cutaneous
    nerve
inferior ligaments
inferior limb
inferior longitudinal muscle
inferior maxillary nerve
inferior oblique muscle of head
inferior parietal lobule
inferior posterior serratus muscle
inferior pubic ligament
inferior pubic ramus (pl. rami)
inferior quadriceps retinaculum
inferior radioulnar joint
inferior rectus muscle
inferior tarsal muscle
inferior temporal gyrus
inferior temporal lobule
inferior tibiofibular joint
inferior tip of scapula
inferior transverse scapular ligament
inferior vesical nerves
INFH (ischemic necrosis of femoral
    head)
infiltrate (infiltration), meningeal
infiltrating tenosynovitis, hypertrophic
infiltration of meninges, leukemic
Infinity hip replacement system
inflame, inflamed
inflammation
    bursal
    calcaneal bursa
    meningeal
    necrotic
    obliterative
    polyarticular symmetric tophaceous
        joint

inflammatory arthropathy
inflammatory fracture
inflammatory granulation tissue
inflammatory process
inflammatory reaction
inflammatory scoliosis
inflate, inflated
inflation
infliximab (Remicade)
inflow connector
inflow portal
influenza encephalitis
influenza viral encephalitis
information
    fund of
    recall of
    tactile
infracalcaneal bursitis
infracalcarine gyrus
infraclavicular pocket
infraction, Freiberg
infragenicular popliteal artery
infragenicular position
infraglenoid tuberosity
infragluteal crease
infrahyoid muscles
infraisthmal
infranuclear lesion
infranuclear paralysis
infranuclear weakness
infraoccipital nerve
infraorbital nerve
infrapatellar contracture syndrome
    (IPCS)
infrapatellar fat pad
infrapatellar tendinitis
infrapopliteal artery occlusion
infrapopliteal vessel
infrared (IR) electronic thermography
infrascapular
infraspinous fossa
infraspinous muscle
infraspinatus tendon
infrasternal angle
infratemporal fossa
infratentorial approach

infratentorial brain tumor
infratentorial compartment
infratentorial Lindau tumor
Infratonic electroacoustical massager
infratrochlear nerve
infundibular stalk
infundibulo-ovarian ligament
infundibulopelvic ligament
infundibulum
    cerebral
    hypophysis
    tumor of the
Infusaid continuous flow drug pump
Infuse-a-port drug delivery system
infusion, Katzman (of radionuclide
    cisternography)
Inge cervical lamina spreader
Inge laminectomy retractor
Inge laminectomy spreader
Inglis-Cooper technique
Inglis-Pellicci elbow arthroplasty
    rating system
Inglis-Ranawat-Straub technique
Ingraham-Fowler tantalum clip
Ingraham skull punch forceps
Ingram-Bachynski classification of hip
    fracture
Ingram osteotomy
Ingram procedure
Ingram-Withers-Speltz motor test
ingress
ingrowth, bone
ingrowing toenail
ingrown toenail
ingrowth, bone
inguinal ligament syndrome
inhaled oxygen brain MR contrast
    agent
inheritance, autosomal dominant
inherited splice mutation
inhibition
    farnesyltransferase
    geranylgeranyltransferase
    periodic interneuron
    reflex
    synchronous interneuron

inhibitor
   COX-2
   cytokine
inhibitory nerve
inhibitory postsynaptic potential (IPSP)
In-Home Alzheimer Screening Test
   (I-HAST)
inhomogeneity
iniencephaly
inion
inion bump
initial double support (of gait)
initiation, gait
initiation of movement
injectable collagenase (Cordase)
injectable hyaluronic acid (Orthovisc)
injection
   Black peroneal tendon sheath
   chymopapain
   corticosteroid
   cortisone
   epidural
   extradural
   facet
   intragluteal
   intraneural phenol
   nerve root
   procaine-phenol motor point
   steroid
   tenosynovial
   thecal
   trigger point
injection of viral vector
injection technique
injector, Medrad power angiographic
injured excitable cells (epileptic foci)
injury (pl. injuries)
   acute stretch
   axial spine compression
   ballistic
   barked
   blunt
   blunt carotid
   brachial plexus
   burst
   cervical spine
   closed head (CHI)

injury *(continued)*
   cocking
   cold-induced brain
   compression flexion
   compression-plus-torque theory of
      cervical
   compressive hyperextension
   contrecoûp
   crush
   decelerative
   degloving
   digit span test of recall after head
   discoligamentous
   distraction hyperflexion
   Erb-Duchenne-Klumpke
   extension
   extensive head
   flexion distraction
   flexion rotation
   flexion teardrop
   forced flexion
   frostbite
   growth plate
   head (HI)
   hyperextension
   hyperflexion
   hyperflexion/hyperextension cervical
   hypertension
   hypoxic
   hypoxic/ischemic
   intercostal nerve
   inversion
   ipsilateral foot
   ischemic
   Klumpke
   lateral bending
   Lisfranc
   low back
   marching band
   matrix
   meniscal
   mild head
   motor vehicle (MVI)
   nerve
   nerve root
   Ontario Cohort Study of Running-
      Related Injuries

injury *(continued)*
  penetrating
  perinatal
  peripheral nerve
  physeal
  plexus
  postnatal
  prenatal
  pronation-external rotation (P-ER)
  radial vascular thermal
  rapid deceleration
  reperfusion
  repetitive strain *or* stress (RSI)
  running-related
  salient antecedents to
  seat-belt
  severe head
  skier's
  snowboarding
  softball sliding
  soft tissue
  soft tissue ankle
  spinal cord (SCI)
  straddle
  strain-sprain
  subliminal
  supination-outward rotation
  three-column
  throwing-arm
  transcutaneous crush
  traumatic
  traumatic brain (TBI)
  traumatic head
  two-column
  ultrasonic assessment of
  weightbearing rotational
  whiplash
  windup
  wringer-type
Injury Scale, Abbreviated
Injury Severity Scale/Score (ISS)
Inland Super Multi-Hite orthopedic
  bed
inlay graft
innermost intercostal muscle
inner stripe of Baillinger

inner table
innervate, innervated
innervation
  crossover
  motor
  parasympathetic
  striatal dopaminergic
  sympathetic
innervatory dyspraxia
Innervision MR scanner
Innomed devices/instruments
innominate aneurysm
innominate angiography
innominate bone
innominate osteotomy
Innovasive COR/T implant system
Innovasive Dart
Innovation Sports bracing products
INO (internuclear ophthalmoplegia)
  syndrome
inoperable brain tumor
in-phase GRE imaging
input
  distorted synaptic (in epilepsy)
  limbic
  sensory
  tonic desynchronizing
INR (international normalized ratio)
INR neurological stent
INRO surgical nails for nail bed
  injuries
Inronail finger prosthesis
Insall-Burstein-Freeman knee
  arthroplasty
Insall-Burstein semiconstrained tricompartmental knee prosthesis
Insall/Burstein II modular total knee
  system
Insall-Crosby rating scale
Insall-Hood reconstruction technique
Insall ligament reconstruction
Insall patella alta method (or ratio)
Insall-Salvati ligament/patella ratio
insensate foot
insensitivity to painful stimuli,
  congenital

insert
  Alimed
  cushioned shoe
  NYU (New York University)
    orthosis
  Poly-Dial
  polypropylene
  silicone gel socket
  sole
  Spenco shoe
  valgus
  viscoelastic
inserter
  Buck cement restrictor
  C-wire
  CDH cup
  cement restrictor
  cement spacer
  cerclage wire
  Kirschner wire
  Massie
  spacer
  staple
  T-shaped
inserter-extractor, compression
inserter-extractor screw-in instrument
insertion
  Alu 1
  anomalous
  Bosworth bone peg
  ligamentous
  percutaneous pin
  tendinous
insertion tendinopathy
inset
insetting
inside-out Bankart shoulder operation
inside-out meniscal repair
insidious onset of symptoms
insight and judgment
insight, preservation of
insipidus, diabetes
in situ pinning
in situ vein graft to ankle
insole
  Aliplast
  Comforthotic

insole *(continued)*
  Darco moldable
  Hapad metatarsal
  Poron
  PPT/Rx firm molded
  viscoelastic
  Viscoped
insomnia, fatal familial
insonation, Doppler
Inspiron
instability
  anterior
  anterolateral rotary knee
  articular
  atlantoaxial
  carpal
  chronic functional
  dorsal intercalary segment (DISI)
  first ray
  hindfoot
  inversion
  joint
  lateral rotatory ankle
  ligamentous
  microsatellite
  multidirectional shoulder
  osseous
  perilunate
  postlaminectomy
  postural
  rotary
  rotary ankle
  rotational
  rotatory
  shoulder joint
  spinal
  subtalar
  sympathetic vascular
  traumatic
  unidirectional
  truncal
  varus-valgus
  vasomotor
  volarflexed intercalated segment
    (VISI)
instability gait
instability while walking

instillation, subarachnoid
InstaScan scanner
InstaTrak 3000 system
institute
   National Institute of Neurological and
      Communicative Disorders and
      Stroke (NINCDS)
   National Institute on Aging (NIA)
   National Institute on Mental Health
      (NIMH)
   Podiatry
Instron 1000 device
instructions, head injury
instrument, instrumentation (see also
   device)
   Accu-Line knee
   Acufex arthroscopic
   Beckman, 20 channel
   CD (Cotrel-Dubousset)
   Collis TDR
   Craig vertebral body biopsy
   craniofacial remodeling
   Dwyer spinal
   Dyonics arthroscopic
   Evershears surgical
   Gamma knife (radiosurgical)
   graft-measuring
   Harrington
   hollow mill
   Howmedica knee
   interspinous segmental spinal (ISSI)
   Kinetix
   Kloehn craniofacial
   Luque
   McElroy
   Midas Rex pneumatic
   Millet neurological test
   Nucleotome Endoflex
   Nucleotome Flex II cannula
   Putti-Platt
   Rancho external fixation
   remodeling
   Richmond subarachnoid screw
   segmental spinal (SSI)
   signature
   Surgi-Tron

instrument *(continued)*
   Wiet graft-measuring
   Zielke
instrumental ADLs (activities of daily
   living) (IADLs) (cooking, house-
   work, shopping, and work)
instrumentation, Garrett
Instrument Makar staples
insufficiency
   autonomic
   basilar
   basilar artery
   brachial-basilar
   cerebrovascular
   muscular
   ray
   transient ischemic carotid
   vertebrobasilar arterial
insufficiency fracture
insufflate, insufflated
insufflation transperitoneal video-
   assisted spine surgery
insula, roof of
insular epilepsy
insular gyrus
insular lobe
insular-opercular syndrome
insular region of brain
insulative development
insulin-like growth factor I (IGF-1)
insulin-like growth factor binding
   protein-3 (IGFBP-3)
insult
   bihemispheral
   cerebrovascular
   mechanical
   occlusive cerebrovascular
   toxic
   vascular
In-Tac bone-anchoring system
intact
   neurologically
   neurovascularly
intact neurologic exam
intact tidemark
integral, center of pressure pattern

integration, matrix
integrative language processing, higher
integrity
    biomechanical
    nervous system
    neurologic
    spinal
Integrity acetabular cup prosthesis
integrity and alignment
integrity of nerve impulse,
    electrophysiologic
integrity of spinal reflex arcs
Intelect Legend ultrasound
intellectual deterioration
intellectual functioning, discrepant
intensifier, image (x-ray)
intensity
    beam
    decreased
    fat signal
    low signal
    maximal
    signal (SI)
    threshold
    variable
intensity-modulated photon beams
intensity windowing
intentional fatigue
intention myoclonus
intention tremor
interaction
    patellofemoral
    surface shoe
    tibiofemoral
interactive electronic scalpel
interactive MR-guided biopsy
interactive visual approach
interarticular disk
interarticularis, pars
interarticular joint
Interax Integrated Secure Assymmetric
    (ISA) mobile-bearing knee implant
Interax total knee system
interbody fusion
interburst interval measurement
intercalary defect
intercalary hyperphalangism

intercapital ligament
intercarotid nerve
intercarpal articulation
intercarpal coalition
intercarpal joint
intercarpal ligament capsulodesis
intercaudate distance
interchondral articulation
interchondral joint
interclavicular ligament
interclavicular notch
interclinoid ligament
intercollicular groove
intercommissural axial plane
intercommissural line
intercompartment difference
intercondylar eminence
intercondylar fossa
intercondylar fracture
intercondylar groove
intercondylar notch
intercondyloid eminence
intercondyloid fossa
intercondyloid notch
intercornual ligament
intercostal ligament
intercostal muscle
intercostal nerve block (ICNB)
intercostal neuralgia
intercostal space (ICS)
intercostal spasm
intercostobrachial nerve
intercostohumeral nerve
intercritical gout
intercuneiform joint
intercuneiform ligament
interdigital clavus
interdigital ligament
interdigital neoplasm
interdigital neuritis
interdigital neuroma
interdigitating coil stent
interdigitating skin flaps
interdigitation of vastus lateralis with
    fascia
interelectrode distance
interelectrode impedance

interface
  acetabular-prosthetic
  acoustic
  bone-cement
  bone-implant
  bony
  cement
  cement-bone
  cement-prosthesis
  electrode-skin
  implant-cement
  joint
  pin-skin
  rotational
  scalp-electrode
  shoe-floor
  skin-electrode
  socket residuum
  socket-stump
  varus-valgus loading
interfascial dissection
interfascicular repair
interference on EEG
interference pattern, EMG incomplete
interference screw
interferential stimulator
interferential, Super Stimm
interferential therapy
interferon-gamma (IFN-g)
interferon-1a (Avonex)
interferon-1b (Betaseron)
interferon tau
interferon therapy
Inter Fix threaded spinal fusion cage
  device
interforniceal approach
interfoveolar ligament
interfoveolar muscle
interfragmental compression
interfragmentary plate
interfragmentary screw
intergluteal cleft
interhemispheric cyst
interhemispheric fissure, displacement of
interhemispheric synchrony
interictal behavior
interictal epileptic personality

interictal epileptiform activity
interictal epileptiform pattern
interictal focal epileptiform discharge
interictal paroxysmal sharp waves
interictal paroxysmal spike waves
interictal PET FDG study
interictal phase
interictal phenomenon
interictal SPECT study
interictal spike discharge
interictal spiking
interlaminal angle
interlaminar clamp system, Halifax
interlaminar distance
interleukin (IL)
interleukin-l receptor antagonist
  (IL-1Ra)
interlimb coordination
interlocking detachable coils
intermaxillary bone
intermediary nerve
intermediate bursa
Intermediate Care Facilities (ICF)
intermediate cuneiform fracture-
  dislocation
intermediate dorsal cutaneous nerve
intermediate great muscle
intermediate nerve of Wrisberg
Intermedics Natural Knee prosthesis
intermediolateral gray column
intermediolateral horn cells
intermedius nerve
intermedullary cavernous malformation
intermedullary guide
intermetacarpal articulation
intermetacarpal joint
intermetacarpal ligament
intermetatarsal angle (IMA)
intermetatarsal angle-reducing
  procedure
intermetatarsal articulation
intermetatarsal joint (IM)
intermetatarsal ligament
intermetatarsal neuroma
intermetatarsal space
intermetatarsophalangeal bursa
intermetatarsophalangeal bursitis

intermittency
intermittent autonomic dysfunction
intermittent catheterization (IC)
intermittent compression pump
(mechanical)
intermittent passive muscle stretch
intermittent pneumatic compression
(IPC)
intermittent shunt failure
intermittent tamponade
intermittent traction
intermixing of wave upon wave
intermuscular septum
internal capsular edema
internal capsule intracerebral hemorrhage
internal carotid artery (ICA)
internal clot
internal collateral ligament
internal decompression for spinal
stenosis (IDSS)
internal derangement of knee (IDK)
internal disk herniation
internal elastic lamina (EIL)
internal femoral rotation
internal intercostal muscle
internal intermuscular septum
internal neurolysis
internal oblique muscle
internal pterygoid muscle
internal rotary component of force
(in gait)
internal rotation in extension (IRE)
internal rotation in flexion (IRF)
internal rotation lag sign
internal snapping hip syndrome
internal speech
internal tibial torsion (ITT)
internal tibiofibular torsion
International Cartilage Repair Society
(ICRS)
International Classification of
Diseases, 10th Revision (ICD-10)
International Classification of
Diseases, 9th Revision, Clinical
Modification (ICD-9-CM)

International Classification of
Epilepsies and Epileptic Syndromes
International Headache Society classi-
fication
International Knee Documentation
Committee (IKDC)
International Knee Ligament Standard
Evaluation questionnaire
international normalized ratio (INR)
International Research Society for
Spinal Deformities (IRSSD)
International Society for Prosthetics
and Orthotics (ISPO)
International Society of Arthroscopy,
Knee Surgery, and Orthopaedic
Sports Medicine (ISAKOS)
International Spinal Development &
Research Foundation (ISDRF)
International 10-20 System for EEG
electrode placement
interneuron, thalamic inhibitory
internuclear distance
internuclear ophthalmoplegia
Inter-Op acetabular prosthesis
interopercular distances
interorbital distance
interosseous cuneocuboid ligament
interosseous cuneometatarsal ligament
interosseous, dorsal
interosseous ligament
interosseous lunotriquetral ligament
interosseous membrane
interosseous metacarpal ligament
interosseous metatarsal ligament
interosseous muscle
interosseous nerve syndrome
interosseous sacroiliac ligament
interosseous space
interosseous talocalcaneal ligament
interosseous tibiofibular ligament
interparietal bone
interpedicular distance
interpediculate
interpeduncular cistern
interpeduncular notch
interpeduncular space

interperiosteal fracture
interphalangeal (IP)
interphalangeal articulation
interphalangeal dislocation
interphalangeal fusion
interphalangeal joint
interphalangectomy
interpleural analgesia
Interpore bone replacement material
Interpore instruments/devices
interposition anchovy of soft tissue
interposition saphenous vein graft
interposition, soft-tissue
interpretation of proverbs test
interpulse time
Inter-Royal frame orthopedic bed
interrupted suture
interscalene block anesthesia (ISB)
interscapular aching
Interseal acetabular cup
intersegmental aberration
intersegmental angle
intersegmental traction chiropractic
    table
interseptal region
intersesamoid ligament
intersigmoid recess
interslice distance
interslice gap
interspace
    ballooning of vertebral
    disk
    vertebral disk
    wedging of vertebral
interspinal ligament
interspinal muscle
interspinous distance
interspinous ligament
interspinous process
interspinous pseudarthrosis
interspinous widening
interspinous wiring
interstices, bone
interstitial fluid hydrostatic pressure
interstitial meniscal tear
interstitial myofasciitis
interstitial nucleus of Cajal

intertarsal articulation
intertarsal joint
interthalamic bridge
interthenar fascia
intertrabecular hemorrhage
intertrabecular soft tissue
intertransverse process arthrodesis
intertransverse fusion
intertransverse ligament
intertransverse muscle
intertrochanteric plate
intertriginous dermatophytosis
intertrigo
intertrochanteric plate
interval
    acromiohumeral (AHI)
    atlantoaxial
    atlantodens (ADI)
    headache-free
    interburst
    lucid (in head trauma)
    supracricoid
interval gout
interval scale in rehabilitation testing
intervention
    nonsurgical
    rehabilitation
interventional limb salvage
interventionalist, endovascular
interventional neuroradiology
interventional radiology
interventricular (IV)
interventricular foramen
intervertebral disk narrowing
intervertebral disk rongeur
    Cushing
    Wilde
intervertebral disk collapse after severe
    lordosis
intervertebral disk narrowing
intervertebral disk space
intervertebral foramen
intervertebral joint
intervertebral ligament
interzone
"in the magnet" (in magnetic reso-
    nance imaging)

intima
in-toeing gait
intolerance, orthostatic
intorting of eye
intorsion
in toto
intoxication
  alcoholic
  anticonvulsant
  carbon dioxide
  carbon monoxide
  glutethimide
  manganese
  water
intra-acetabular
intra-aneurysmal thrombosis
intra-aneurysmal thrombus
intra-aortic balloon counterpulsation
  (IABC)
intra-arterial digital subtraction
  angiography (IADSA)
intra-arterial filling defects
intra-arterial infusion of papaverine
intra-arterial injection of water-soluble
  iodinated contrast agent
intra-arterial intracerebral thrombolysis
intra-arterial thrombus
intra-articular adhesion
intra-articular fracture
intra-articular ligament
intra-articular loose body
intra-articular pigmented villonodular
  synovitis (IPVS)
intra-articular shaver (IAS)
intra-articular sternocostal ligament
intra-articular subscapularis (IASS)
  tendon
intra-auricular muscles
intra-axial brain tumor
intra-axial cyst
intra-axial varix
intracanalicular
intracapsular fracture
intracapsular osteotomy
intracarotid amobarbital speech test
Intracath catheter
Intracath needle

Intracell trigger point massager
Intracell Trigger Wheel
intracerebral electrode
intracerebral hematoma
  basilar
  bulbar
  cerebellar
  cerebral
  cerebromeningeal
  cortical
  internal capsule
  intrapontine
  pontine
  subcortical
  ventricular
intracerebral lesion
intracerebral lymphoma
intrachondrial bone
intracompartmental ischemia
intracondyloid
Intracone intramedullary reamer
intracortical melanoma
intracortical osteogenic sarcoma
intracranial air
intracranial aneurysm
  arteriosclerotic
  congenital
  dissecting
  mycotic
  traumatic
intracranial arterial occlusion
intracranial berry aneurysm
intracranial calcification
intracranial carotid tree
intracranial circulation
intracranial cyst
intracranial electroencephalography
intracranial fat proplase
intracranial glioma
intracranial glossopharyngeal
  rhizotomy
intracranial hemorrhage
intracranial hypertension
intracranial hypotension
intracranial imaging
intracranial lesion
intracranial malformation

intracranial mass
intracranial monitor
intracranial mucocele
intracranial neoplasm
intracranial pressure
intracranial sinus thrombosis
intracranial tumor
intractable pain
intractable plantar keratoses (IPK)
intractable seizures
intracuticular stitch
intradermal angioma
intradermal pedal nevi
intradermal suture
intradiskal pressure
intradural abscess
intradural anastomosis
intradural arteriovenous fistula
intradural extramedullary tumor
intradural nerve root
intradural retromedullary arteriovenous
   fistula
Intraflex intramedullary pin
intraforaminal approach
intrafusal fibers
intragluteal injection
intralaminar thalamus
intramedullary (IM) rodding
intramedullary epidermoid cyst
intramedullary fixation device
intramedullary rasp
intramedullary rod
intramedullary rodding
intramedullary spinal cord tumor
intramedullary spinal lesion
intramedullary tumor
intramuscular injection
intraneural ganglion cyst
intraneural phenol injection
intraneuronal neurofibrillary tangles
intranuclear diskogram
intraoperative autologous transfusion
   (IAT)
intraoperative complications
intraoperative radiation therapy
   (IORT)

intra-orbital air
intraosseous pneumatocyst
intraosseous venography
intrapedicular fixation
intraperiosteal fracture
intraprosthetic
intrasellar Rathke cleft cyst (RCC)
intrasellar tumor
intraspinal adenoma
intraspinal lesion
intraspinal tumor
intraspongy nuclear herniation
intratendinous fluid collection
intrathecal administration of drug
intrathecal roots
intrathecal route of drug administration
intrathecal space
intrauterine cytomegalic inclusion
   disease
intrauterine fracture
intravenous line
intraventricular cannula
intraventricular hemorrhage
intraventricular perineuroma
Intrel II spinal cord stimulator
intrinsic foot muscles
intrinsic muscle spasm in hand
intrinsic-negative runners
intrinsic plus deformity
intrinsic-positive runners
intrinsics, finger
introducer
   Charnley
   ventricular catheter
inturning
intussusception of vein
invagination, basilar
invasion
   arterial
   Aspergillus
   epidural
   neoplastic
   Nocardia
   perineural
   tumoral
   vascular

invasive malignant sheath tumor
inventory
    Battelle Developmental Inventory
      (BDI)
    Beck Depression Inventory
    Vanderbilt Pain Management
      Inventory
    West Haven-Yale Multidimensional
      Pain Inventory
    Wakefield Self-Assessment
      Depression Inventory
Inventory for Déjà Vu Experiences
    Assessment (IDEA)
inverse Argyll-Robertson pupil
inverse Marcus Gunn syndrome
inversion-eversion
inversion injury of the ankle
inversion recovery (IR)
inversion recovery sequence
inversion sprain
inversion time (TI)
InvertaChair traction device
invertors
in vivo degradation
in vivo He-3 MR images
in vivo proton MR spectroscopy
involucrum
involuntary flexor spasm
involuntary movement
involuntary muscles
involvement, cranial nerve
INVOS cerebral oximeter
Inyo nail
Ioban 2 skin prep
Ioban Vi-Drape
iodine-125 therapy
iodixanol (Visipaque)
iodoform gauze
iodophor solution
Iohexol contrast media
IOM (interosseous membrane)
ionic paramagnetic contrast media
iontophoresis, acetic acid
iontophoretic drug delivery system
IORT (intraoperative radiation therapy)
Iowa internal prosthesis
Iowa University periosteal elevator

IP (interphalangeal) joint
IPC (intermittent pneumatic compression)
IPCS (infrapatellar contracture syndrome)
IPG (impedance plethysmography)
IPH (intraplaque hemorrhage)
IPK (indurated plantar keratoma)
IPK (intractable plantar keratoses)
IPL (interpeak latency)
I-Plus humeral brace
IPSF (immediate postsurgical fitting)
ipsilateral autograft
ipsilateral basal ganglia
ipsilateral cerebellar signs
ipsilateral cortical diaschisis
ipsilateral corticospinal tract signs
ipsilateral facial paralysis
ipsilateral facial paresis
ipsilateral foot injury
ipsilateral hemisphere activation
ipsilateral hemispheric carotid TIA
    (transient ischemic attack)
ipsilateral hemianopsia
ipsilateral increase in waveform
    amplitude
ipsilateral loss
ipsilateral monocular blindness
ipsilateral tonic deviation
IPSP (inhibitory postsynaptic potential)
IPVS (intra-articular pigmented
    villonodular synovitis)
IR (infrared electronic thermography)
IRDA (intermittent rhythmic delta
    activity)
IRE (internal rotation in extension)
IRF (internal rotation in flexion)
IR501 immune therapy
iridic muscles
iridocorneal melanoma
iridium-192 seed therapy
iridocyclitis
iridoplegia, reflex
IRIS (intensified radiographic imaging
    system)
IRM spiral arthrosis
IROM bilateral splint

IROM Regal splint
IROM splint with shells
iron, Jewett bending
Ironman Triathlon Pro-Power
   massager
irradiated chondral graft implantation
   arthroplasty
irradiation
   convergent beam
   curative
   external beam
   gamma
   heavy particle
   neutron
   palliative
   partial brain
   proton
   whole brain
   stereotactic proton
   whole brain
irreducible dislocation
irreducible fracture dislocation
irregular bone
irregular nystagmus
irreversible ischemia
irreversible neurologic deficit
irrigation
   antibiotic
   ice water
irrigation of wound
   pulse lavage
   syringe (with deionized sterile
     water)
irrigation with antibiotic solution
irrigator
   Arthro-Flo
   jet
   ophthalmic
   pulse lavage
   Simpulse suction
irritability
   membrane
   muscle
   nerve root
irritation
   meningeal
   nerve root

irritation *(continued)*
   nociceptor
   root
IRSSD (International Research Society
   for Spinal Deformities)
Irvine ankle arthroplasty
Irwin osteotomy
Isaacs syndrome
ISAH stereotactic immobilization
   frame
ISAH stereotactic immobilizing mask
ISAKOS (International Society of
   Arthroscopy, Knee Surgery, and
   Orthopaedic Sports Medicine)
Isch-Dish Plus cushion
ischemia
   anoxic
   anterior circulation
   brachiocephalic
   brain
   brain stem
   carotid artery
   cerebral
   chronic cerebral
   cross-clamp
   cortical
   cortical transient
   foot
   global cerebral
   hypoxic
   intracompartmental
   irreversible
   limb-threatening
   muscle
   myoneural
   neonatal intracranial
   optic nerve head
   rostral brain stem
   spinal cord
   thalamic
   transient brain stem
   transient cerebral
   vertebral-basilar
   vertebrobasilar territory
   Volkmann
   zone of
ischemic area

ischemic attack, transient (TIA)
ischemic brain damage
ischemic change
ischemic contracture
ischemic decompensation
ischemic disease of the growing hip
  (IDGH)
ischemic episode
ischemic event
ischemic foot
ischemic foot ulcer
ischemic forearm exercise test
ischemic gangrene
ischemic hypoxia
ischemic-hypoxic encephalopathy
ischemic infarction
ischemic injury
ischemic instability
ischemic lactic acidosis
ischemic neuritis
ischemic optic neuropathy
ischemic time
ischemic zone
ischial bone
ischial notch
ischial spine
ischial tuberosity
ischiatic scoliosis
ischioacetabular fracture
ischiocapsular ligament
ischiocavernous muscle
ischiofemoral ligament
ischiogluteal bursa
ischium
ISDRF (International Spinal Development and Research Foundation)
ISEDP (intraspinal epidural pressure)
Iselin disease
Ishihara color plate test for multiple
  sclerosis
Ishizuki unconstrained elbow prosthesis
ISIS spectroscopy
island
  bone (or bony)
  Reil
island of impaired vision

island pedicle flap
ISOA questionnaire
Isocam SPECT imaging system
isocenter
isodense appearance
isodense mass
isodensity
isodose shell
IsoDyn knee brace
isodynamic resistance
isoechoic
isoelectric (flat) EEG record
isoform
isointense soft tissue on MRI
isokinetic strength test
isokinetic passive mode exercise
Isola fixation system
Isola hook
Isola rod
Isola spinal instrumentation system
Isola vertebral screw
Isola wire
isolated dislocation of semilunar bone
isolation syndrome
Isoloss AC material
Isometer device
isometric exercise
isometric muscle strength
isometric position
isometry
isopotential line on EEG
isoprene plastic splint
Isotac
Isotec patellar tendon graft
Isotoner gloves
isotonic exercise
isotope bone scan
isotope cisternography
isotopic skeletal survey
isotropic 3D study
isovalericacidemia
Isovue (injectable iopamidol) nonionic
  contrast agent
Isovue contrast series (128, 200, 300,
  370)
Isovue-M contrast series (200, 300)

isoxicam (Maxicam)
ISPO (International Society for
    Prosthetics and Orthotics)
Israel rake retractor
Israel rasp
ISS (inferior sagittal sinus)
ISS (Injury Severity Scale/Score)
Isseis-Aussies scoliosis operation
ISSI (interspinous segmental spinal
    instrumentation)
isthmic spondylolisthesis
isthmus
    femoral
    temporal
IT (iliotibial) band
ITC radiopaque balloon catheter
itraconazole

ITT (internal tibial torsion)
Ivalon embolization
Ivalon particles
Ivalon sponge
IVC (intracerebral-ventricular)
    administration
IVDSA (intravenous digital subtraction
    angiography)
IVFA (intravenous fluorescein
    angiography)
IVH (intraventricular hemorrhage)
ivory osteoma
IVRA (intravenous regional anesthesia)
IWB (Index of Well-Being)
Ixodes pacificus tick
Ixodes scapularis tick
izanidine hydrochloride (Zanaflex)

J, j

J (joule)
Jaboulay amputation
Jaccoud arthritis syndrome
 (cf. *Jacod*)
Jaccoud arthropathy
JACE shoulder exerciser
JACE-STIM electrotherapy stimulation
 unit
JACE W550 CPM device for wrist
jacket
 Boston soft body
 cervicothoracic
 flexion body
 Frejka
 halo body
 immobilization
 Kydex body
 Lexan
 Minerva cervical
 Ortho-Mold lumbar body
 orthoplast
 Prenyl
 Royalite body
 von Lackum transection shift
 Wilmington
jackknife attack
jackknife position
jackknife seizure

Jackson bone clamp
Jackson bone-extension clamp
Jackson compression test
Jackson disk rongeur
Jackson epilepsy
jacksonian attack
 motor
 sensory
jacksonian epilepsy
jacksonian march
jacksonian seizure
Jackson intervertebral disk rongeur
Jackson-Pratt drain
Jackson rod insertion technique
Jackson rongeur
Jackson spinal surgery and imaging
 table
Jackson-Weiss syndrome
Jackson syndrome
Jackson tendon-seizing forceps
Jacob shift test
Jacobs adapter for neurosurgical
 perforators
Jacobs chuck adapter
Jacobs chuck drive
Jacobs distraction rod
Jacobson bulldog clamp
Jacobson dressing forceps

Jacobson endarterectomy spatula
Jacobson hemostatic forceps
Jacobson micro mosquito forceps
Jacobson microneurosurgical scissors
Jacobson microprobe
Jacobson microvascular knife
Jacobson mosquito forceps
Jacobson needle holder
Jacobson nerve
Jacobson-Potts vascular clamp
Jacobson probe
Jacobson scissors
Jacobson suture pusher
Jacobson vessel knife
Jacoby bunion splint
Jacod (neuralgia) syndrome
    (cf. *Jaccoud*)
jacktatio capitis nocturna
jactitation
Jacuzzi
Jadad scale
JAFAR (Juvenile Arthritis Functional
    Assessment Report)
Jäger-Wirth score
Jaffe-Capello-Averill hip prosthesis
Jaffe-Lichtenstein disease
jagged osteophytes
Jahss classification of ankle dislocation
Jahss classification of metatarso-
    phalangeal joint dislocation
jake paralysis (Jamaica ginger)
Jako stimulator
Jakob-Creutzfeldt disease
Jakob-Creutzfeldt viral encephalitis
Jamaica ginger paralysis
jamais entendu (never heard)
jamais vu (never seen)
Jamar grip test
Jamar hand dynamometer
Jamar hydraulic pinch-gauge
    dynamometer
Jameson muscle hook
jammed
jamming forces/trauma
Jamshidi needle
Janecki-Nelson shoulder procedure
Janes fracture frame

Jannetta alligator forceps
Jannetta aneurysm neck dissector
Jannetta bayonet forceps
Jannetta dissector
Jannetta duckbill elevator
Jannetta forceps
Jannetta fork
Jannetta hook
Jannetta knife
Jannetta-Kurze dissecting scissors
Jannetta posterior fossa retractor
Jannetta probe
Jansen bone curet
Jansen disease
Jansen mastoid retractor
Jansen-Middleton septal forceps
Jansen monopolar forceps
Jansen rasp
Jansen rongeur
Jansen scalp retractor
Jansen test
Jansen-Wagner retractor
Jansky-Bielschowsky disease
Jansky-Bielschowsky syndrome
Janz juvenile myoclonic seizure
Janz response
Japanese B viral encephalitis
Japanese fingertrap
Japanese Orthopaedic Association
    (JOA) knee score
Jarcho-Levin syndrome
Jarell forceps
jargon, aphasia
Jarisch-Herxheimer reaction
Jarit brain forceps
Jarit-Kerrison laminectomy rongeur
Jarit-Liston bone rongeur
Jarit rotator
Jarit-Ruskin bone rongeur
Jarit tendon-pulling forceps
Jarjavay ligament
Jarjavay muscle
Javid carotid clamp
Javid shunt
jaw bone
jaw clenching, repetitive
jawed tendon passers

jaw jerk
jaw jerk reflex
jaw joint
Jeanne sign
Jebsen hand function test
Jebsen-Taylor hand function test
Jebsen Taylor score
Jefferson cervical burst fracture
Jeffery classification of radial fracture
Jelanko splint
jelly
    conductive EEG
    EEG electrolyte
jelly nystagmus
Jelonet paraffin-soaked tulle dressing
Jendrassik maneuver
Jenet sign
Jergesen I-beam
Jergesen plate
Jergesen tube
jerk, jerking
    Achilles
    ankle
    biceps
    crossed
    elbow
    flurry of myoclonic
    hypnic
    jaw
    knee (KJ)
    macro square wave
    myoclonic
    nystagmoid
    paretic
    patellar
    photomyoclonic
    quadriceps
    rhythmical
    sleep
    square wave
    supinator
    tendon
    triceps (TJ)
    triceps surae
jerk test
jerky incoordinate movement
jersey finger

Jeter lag/position screws
jet, Ortholav
jet-pilot position
Jette Functional Status Index
jet wire tightener
Jewett bending iron
Jewett bending tool
Jewett-Benjamin cervical orthosis
Jewett brace
Jewett contraflexion brace
Jewett contraflexion orthosis
Jewett driver
Jewett extractor
Jewett gouge
Jewett hyperextension brace
Jewett hyperextension orthosis
Jewett nail
Jewett plate
Jewett postfusion brace
Jewett postfusion orthosis
J-FX bipolar head
jig
    chamfer cut
    Charnley tibial onlay
    cutting
    drilling
    extramedullary tibial alignment
    femoral alignment
    Herbert
    intramedullary
    Miller-Galante
    spacer-tensor
    tibial alignment
jig hook
jing (Chinese medicine term)
jitteriness
jittery response
JOA (Japanese Orthopaedic Association) knee score
JOAS (juvenile onset ankylosing spondylitis)
Jobe relocation test
Jobert de Lamballe fossa
Jobst gloves
Jobst antithrombotic pump
Jobst brassiere
Jobst stocking

Joerns orthopedic bed
Johannesberg staple
Johannson hip nail
Johannson lag screw
John Barnes myofascial release
John C. Wilson arthrodesis
Johns Hopkins bulldog clamp
Johns Hopkins National Low Back
  Pain Study questionnaire
Johnson & Johnson instruments/
  devices
Johnson-Boseker scale
Johnson brain tumor forceps
Johnson hemiphalangectomy
Johnson-Jahss classification of posterior
  tibial tendon tear
Johnson pelvic fracture technique
Johnson resection arthroplasty
Johnson retractor
Johnson-Spiegl hallux varus correction
Johnson tumor forceps
Johnson-Zuck-Wingate motor test
joint
  AC (acromioclavicular)
  acromioclavicular
  atlantoaxial
  bail-lock knee
  ball-and-socket synovial
  basal
  biaxial synovial
  calcaneocuboid
  capitate hamate
  capitolunate
  carpometacarpal
  carpophalangeal
  center of
  Charcot
  Chopart
  chronic recurrent dislocation of the
    ankle
  CMC (carpometacarpal)
  coccygeal
  compound
  compound condylar synovial
  condyloid
  costochondral
  costotransverse

joint *(continued)*
  costovertebral
  cricoarytenoid
  cricothyroid
  Cruveilhier
  cubital
  cuboideonavicular
  cubonavicular
  cuneiform
  cuneocuboid
  cuneometatarsal
  diarthrodial
  DIP (distal interphalangeal)
  distal interphalangeal (DIP)
  distraction of
  double pearl-face hip
  double-stem silicone lesser MP
  elbow
  ellipsoid
  enarthrodial
  facet
  false
  femoropatellar
  femorotibial (FTJ)
  fibrous
  finger
  foot
  flail
  free knee
  Gaffney
  Gillette
  glenohumeral
  gliding
  hallux interphalangeal (IP)
  hemophilic
  hinge
  hip capsule
  HP-100 prosthetic finger
  humeroradial
  humeroulnar
  hyperextensibility of
  hysterical
  immovable
  incudomalleolar
  inferior radioulnar
  interarticular
  intercarpal

joint *(continued)*
    intermetatarsal (IM)
    interphalangeal (IP)
    interchondral
    intercuneiform
    intervertebral
    jaw
    knee
    lateral atlantoaxial
    lesser metatarsophalangeal
    Lisfranc
    lumbosacral
    lunocapitate
    lunotriquetral (LT)
    Luschka
    manubriosternal
    median atlantoaxial
    metacarpal-phalangeal (MCP, MP)
    metacarpophalangeal (MCP, MP)
    metatarsocuneiform (MC)
    metatarsal-phalangeal (MTP)
    metatarsocuboid
    metatarsophalangeal (MPJ, MTP)
    midcarpal
    middle atlantoepistrophic
    middle carpal
    midtarsal
    movable
    multiaxial
    naviculocuneiform
    neurocentral
    neuropathic tarsal-metatarsal
    occipital-axis
    Oklahoma ankle
    petro-occipital
    PIP (proximal interphalangeal)
    pisotriquetral
    pivot
    pivot synovial
    plane synovial
    polyaxial
    posterior intraoccipital
    proximal interphalangeal (PIP)
    proximal radioulnar
    proximal tibiofibular
    radiocapitellar
    radiocarpal

joint *(continued)*
    radiolunate
    radioscaphoid
    radioulnar
    Regnauld degeneration of MTP
    rotary
    rotatory
    sacrococcygeal
    sacroiliac (SI)
    saddle
    scaphocapitate
    scapholunate (SL)
    scaphotrapezoid-trapezial (STT)
    scapulothoracic
    schindyletic
    secondary cartilaginous
    Select
    sesamoidometatarsal
    shoulder
    Silastic finger
    simple
    single pearl-face hip
    single smooth-face hip
    socket
    spheno-occipital
    spheroid
    sternal
    sternoclavicular
    sternocostal
    subtalar
    superior radioulnar
    superior tibiofibular
    surgeon's tarsal
    suture
    Swanson finger
    symphysis sacrococcygeal
    synarthrodial
    synchondrodial
    synchondrosis
    syndesmodial
    synovial
    talocalcaneal
    talocalcaneonavicular
    talocrural
    talofibular
    talonavicular
    tarsal

joint *(continued)*
  tarsal-metatarsal
  tarsometatarsal
  temporomandibular
  thigh
  thoracic
  tibiofibular
  tibiotalar
  transverse tarsal
  trapeziometacarpal
  trapezioscaphoid
  trapeziotrapezoid
  triquetrohamate
  trochoid
  uncovertebral
  uniaxial
  unilocular
  unstable
  wedge-and-groove
  weightbearing
  wrist
  xiphisternal
  zygapophyseal (ZA)
joint arthrography
joint capsule
joint congruency
joint congruity
joint debris
joint depression fracture
joint dislocation
joint effusion
joint fluid aspiration
joint fracture
joint fulcrum
joint hyperextendability
joint hypermobility syndrome
joint immobilization
joint incongruity
joint interface
Joint-Jack finger splint
joint kinematics
joint laxity
joint leveling procedure
joint line pain
joint line tenderness
joint manipulation, chiropractic
joint mice (or mouse)

joint mobilization
joint morphology
joint morphometry
joint mortise
joint play
joint position sense (JPS)
joint proprioception
joint segment
joint space
  cartilage
  metatarsal-phalangeal
  narrowed
  subtalar
  tarsal-metatarsal
  widened
joint stiffness
joint surface realignment
joint survey
joint swelling
joint tenderness
joint warmth
joker periosteal elevator
Jonell splint
Jones abduction frame
Jones-Brackett technique
Jones classification of congenital tibial deficiency
Jones classification of diaphyseal fractures
Jones cock-up toe operation
Jones compression plate
Jones dressing
Jones-Ellison ACL reconstruction
Jones fracture
Jones traction splint
Joplin bunionectomy
Joplin toe prosthesis
Jordan frame
Joseph disease
Joseph elevator
Joseph hook
Joseph periosteal elevator
Joseph periosteotome
Joseph splint
joule (J)
joule shocks
JoyBags therapeutic heat packs

J patellofemoral brace
JPS (joint position sense)
JRA (juvenile rheumatoid arthritis)
J sign (of knee)
J-Tech thrust adjustment device
Judet fracture grading classification
Judet graft
Judet hip prosthesis
Judet hip status system
Judet pelvic x-ray view
judgment and insight
Judgment of Line Orientation
Juers-Lempert rongeur forceps
jugal bone
jugal ligament
jugal suture
jugular bulb
jugular bulb oxygen saturation (SjO_2)
jugular foramen syndrome
jugular nerve
jugular notch
jugular triangle
jugular venous oxygen saturation
jumped facet
jumper's knee position
jumbo acetabular cup
jump sign
jump vein graft
junction
   cervicomedullary
   cervicothoracic
   corticomedullary
   costochondral
   craniocervical
   craniovertebral
   gastrocnemius-soleus
   gray-white matter
   ligament-membrane
   meniscosynovial
   metaphyseal-diaphyseal
   musculotendinous

junction *(continued)*
   myoneural
   myotendinous
   neuromuscular
   occipitocervical
   phrenovertebral
   pontomedullary
   pontomesencephalic
   sternoclavicular
   sylvian/rolandic
   temporal-occipital
   TFA
junction separation
juncture, myofascial periosteal
Jung pyramidal auricular muscle
Jurgan pin ball
jury-rig
Juvara foot procedure
Juvenile Arthritis Functional Assessment Report (JAFAR)
juvenile bunion
juvenile flatfoot pathomechanics
juvenile kyphosis
juvenile myoclonic epilepsy
juvenile nasal angiofibroma
juvenile onset ankylosing spondylitis (JOAS)
juvenile ossifying fibroma
juvenile Paget disease
juvenile paralysis
juvenile rheumatoid arthritis (JRA)
juvenile Tillaux fracture
juxta-articular osteoid osteoma
juxta-articulation
juxtacortical chondroma
juxtacortical sarcoma
juxtafacet cyst
juxtapapillary uveitis
juxtaposition
juxtarestiform body
Juzo braces and supports

K, k

Kadish staging of esthesioneuro-
blastoma
Kaessmann nail
Kaessmann screw
KAFO (knee-ankle-foot orthosis)
Kager triangle
Kahre-Williger periosteal elevator
Kalamchi-Dawe classification of
congenital tibial deficiency
Kalassy ankle brace
kaleidoscope photopsias
Kalginate calcium alginate wound
dressing
Kalish Duredge wire cutter
Kalish Duredge wire extractor
Kalish osteotomy
kallikrein-kinin (KK) system
Kaltostat dressing
Kambin and Gellman lumbar
diskectomy instrumentation
Kampe corset
KAM Super Sucker for arthroscopic
surgery
Kam Vac suction tube
Kanavel brain-exploring cannula
Kanavel cock-up splint
Kanavel four cardinal symptoms
Kanavel sign

Kaneda anterior scoliosis system
(KASS)
Kaneda distraction device
Kaneda rod
Kannon headframe
Kapandji fracture of radius
Kapandji pinning technique
Kapandji-Sauve radioulnar joint repair
Kapel elbow dislocation technique
Kaplan cardinal line
Kaplan-Meier survival curve
Kaplan sign
Kaposi sarcoma
classic
epidemic
kappa rhythm on EEG
Karakousis-Vezeridis resection
Karev technique of pulley reconstruc-
tion
Karfoil splint
Karnofsky performance score (KPS)
Karsch-Neugelbauer syndrome (split-
hand deformity)
Kartchner carotid artery clamp
Kasdan retractor
Kashin-Bek disease
Kashiwagi technique
KASS (Kaneda anterior scoliosis
system)

Kast syndrome
KAT (Kinesthetic Ability Trainer)
Kates forefoot arthroplasty
Kates-Kessel-Kay technique
Katz ADL (activities of daily living)
  Index (KAI)
Katzman infusion of radionuclide
  cisternography
Kaufer tendon technique
Kaufman Adolescent and Adult
  Intelligence Test
Kayser-Fleischer (K-F) ring
Kazanjian splint
K blade
K-Cap to cover end of Kirschner wire
K complex on EEG
Keane Mobility bed
Kearns-Sayre disease
Kearns-Sayre syndrome (KSS)
Kech and Kelly osteotomy
keeled chest
keel-like ridge
keel, McNaught
keel of glenoid component
Keen sign
Keene compression hook
Keene obturator
Kehr sign
Keitel index
Keith needle
Kelikian classification of nail deformity
Kelikian-Clayton-Loseff technique
Kelikian-McFarland procedure
Kelikian modified Z bunionectomy
Kelikian-Riashi-Gleason patellar tendon
  repair
Keller arthroplasty
Keller-Blake half-ring splint
Keller-Brandes procedure
Keller bunionectomy
Keller foot procedure
Keller hallux valgus operation
Keller-Mann resection arthroplasty
Keller resection arthroplasty
Kellgren criteria for grading degenera-
  tive disk disease
Kellgren knee scale

Kellgren-Lawrence (KL) grading
  system
Kellogg-Speed lumbar spinal fusion
Kelly artery forceps
Kelly clamp
Kelly fistula scissors
Kelly forceps
Kelly-Goerss Compass stereotactic
  system
Kelly hemostat
Kelly plication suture
keloid
Kempf internal screw fixation
Kemp test
Ken driver-extractor
Kendall A-V Impulse System
Kendall pneumatic compression sleeve
Kendrick-Sharma-Hassler-Herndon
  technique
Ken nail
Kennedy ligament technique
Kennerdell-Maroon dissector
Kennerdell-Maroon elevator
Kennerdell-Maroon hook
Kennerdell-Maroon orbital retractor
Kenny Howard shoulder sling
Kenny Self-Care Questionnaire
Kerasal
keratan sulfate
keratoderma plantare
keratolytic agents
keratome Beaver blade
keratosis, intractable plantar (IPK)
keratotic lesions
kerf (of saw blade)
kerfs in bone graft
Kerlix bandage
Kerlix cast padding
Kerlix dressing
Kerlix wrap
Kern bone-holding clamp
kernicterus
Kernig sign
Kern-Lane bone forceps
Kernohan classification of astro-
  cytomas and glioblastomas
Kernohan classification of brain tumor

Kernohan grading
Kernohan notch phenomenon
Kernohan notch syndrome
Kerpel bone curet
Kerr-Lagen abdominal support
Kerr sign
Kerr splint
Kerrison curet
Kerrison laminectomy rongeur
Kerrison punch
Kessel-Bonney extension osteotomy
Kessler fixation device
Kessler metacarpal distractor
Kessler posterior tibial tendon transfer
    operation
Kessler prosthesis
Kessler suture
Kessler traction frame
Ketac cement
ketoconazole
ketorolac tromethamine
ketotic hygerglycemia
key
    chuck
    removal
Key-Conwell classification of pelvic
    fracture
keyhole approach
keyhole craniotomy
keyhole neurosurgery
keyhole tenodesis technique
Key intra-articular knee arthrodesis
Key-loc wrench
Key periosteal elevator
Key rasp
Keys-Kirschner traction
Keystone last
keystone of the calcar arch
key the cement
keyway
K-F (Kayser-Fleischer) ring
Khodadad clip
Kickaldy-Willis arthrodesis
Kicker Pavlik harness hip abduction
    brace
Kidde tourniquet
Kidner flatfoot

Kidner procedure for accessory
    navicular
kidney rest
kidney yang deficiency (Chinese
    medicine term)
kidney yin deficiency (Chinese
    medicine term)
Kienböck dislocation
Kienböck lunatomalacia disease
Kiene bone tamp
Kilfoyle classification of condylar
    fracture
Killian gouge
Killian septum speculum
Kilner hook
kilohertz (kHz)
Kiloh-Nevin dystrophy
Kiloh-Nevin ocular form of
    progressive muscular dystrophy
Kiloh-Nevin ocular myopathy
Kiloh-Nevin syndrome
Kim-Ray Greenfield inferior vena
    caval filter
Kimura blink reflex measurement for
    diagnosis of multiple sclerosis
Kimura disease
KinAir bed
Kinamed instruments/devices
kinase assay
kinase C antiglioma monoclonal
    antibody
kinase C protein
Kin-Con device
Kin-Con isokinetic exercise system
kindling phenomenon
Kindt carotid clamp
kinematic indices of McMurtry
kinematic MRI studies
Kinematic rotating hinge knee prosthesis
kinematics, hindfoot
kinematics, joint
kinematics of knee
Kinemax Plus knee prosthesis
kinesigenic attack
kinesiologic testing devices
kinesiology
kinesthesia

Kinesthetic Ability Trainer (KAT)
KineTec clubfoot CPM exerciser
KineTec hip CPM machine
kinetic cervical spine
kinetic chain activities
    closed
    open
kinetic foot pain
kinetic gait analysis
Kinetik great toe implant
Kinetikos instruments/devices
kinetic splint
kinetic strabismus
kinetic tremor
Kinetix instrument for carpal tunnel
    release
Kinetron muscle-strengthening apparatus
King brace
King classification of thoracic scoliosis
King intra-articular hip fusion
King-Moe scoliosis
King operation
King-Richards dislocation technique
Kingsley splint
King-Steelquist technique
King traction
King II scoliosis curves
kinins
Kinnier-Wilson disease
Kinsbourne syndrome
Kirby muscle hook
Kirk distal thigh amputation
Kirk mallet
Kirmission periosteal elevator
Kirmission periosteal rasp
Kirner deformity
Kirschenbaum foot positioner
Kirschner hand drill
Kirschner Medical Dimension hip
    replacement
Kirschner stem
Kirschner tightener
Kirschner traction bow nut
Kirschner wire (K wire)
    fully threaded
    smooth
Kirschner wire cutter

Kirschner wire drill
Kirschner wire traction bow
Ki-67 expression
kissing lesions
kissing spines
Kistler classification of subarachnoid
    hemorrhage
kit
    Qiaex gel extraction
    Shoulder Therapy Kit
    Zervas hypophysectomy
kitchen utensils, one-handed
Kite clubfoot casting
Kite slipper
KJ (knee jerk)
Kjellberg 1% risk line
Kjolbe technique
Klagsbrun harvesting technique
Klebsiella pneumoniae meningitis
kleeblattschädel cloverleaf skull
Kleiger test
Klein cutaneomucous muscle
Klein line
Kleine-Levin syndrome
Kleinert-Kutz bone cutter
Kleinert-Kutz bone-cutting forceps
Kleinert-Kutz dissector
Kleinert-Kutz bone rongeur
Kleinert-Kutz periosteal elevator
Kleinert-Kutz rasp
Kleinert-Kutz rongeur forceps
Kleinert-Kutz synovectomy rongeur
Kleinert-Kutz tendon forceps
Kleinert-Kutz tendon retriever
Kleinert-Ragdell retractor
Kleinert rubber band technique
Kleinert splint
Kleinert technique of pulley recon-
    struction
Klein-Waardenburg syndrome
Klemme laminectomy retractor
Klengall brace
Klenzak spring brace
Klinefelter syndrome
Kling elastic bandage
Klippel-Feil syndrome
Klippel-Trenaunay-Weber syndrome

Klisic-Jankovic technique
Kloehn craniofacial remodeling
    instrument
KLS Centre-Drive screws
Klumpke-Dejerine paralysis
Klumpke injury to brachial plexus
Klumpke palsy
Klumpke paralysis
Klüver-Bucy ablation syndrome
KMC femoral stem
KMP femoral stem
KMW/PC femoral stem
knee
    ACG knee replacement system
    Advance PS total knee system
    Advance total knee system
    Advantim total knee system
    anterior cruciate deficit
    Apollo knee prosthesis system
    Axiom total
    biocompartmental replacement of
    breaststroker's
    Brodie
    corner of
    dislocated
    Duracon total knee system
    floating
    Foundation total knee system
    friction rub in (Renee creak sign)
    game
    Gem total knee system
    gimpy
    hamstrung
    housemaid's
    Insall/Burstein II modular total
        knee system
    internal derangement of the (IDK)
    jumper's
    locked
    MG II total knee system
    Miller-Galante
    motorcyclist's
    Osteonics Scorpio total knee system
    Press-Fit Condylar Total
    Profix total knee system
    runner's
    Scorpio total knee system

knee *(continued)*
    S.O.S. total knee system
    trick
    wrenched
knee-ankle-foot orthosis (KAFO)
knee brace (see *brace*)
kneecap
Kneed-It kneeguard
knee drop test
knee extension
knee extensor forces
knee flexion stress test
knee holder
knee immobilizer
knee jerk, hung-up (sustained)
knee jerk (KJ)
knee joint
knee knob of Osgood-Schlatter disease
kneeling bench test
knee orthosis (see *orthosis*)
knee prosthesis (see *prosthesis*)
KneeRanger hinged knee brace
Knee Signature System (KSS)
Knee Society Score
knee support
Kniest dysplasia
knife (blade)
    acetabular
    Adson dural
    Adson right-angle
    amputation
    angular
    arachnoid
    arthroscopic
    backward-cutting
    Ballenger swivel
    banana
    Bard-Parker
    bayonet
    Beaver-DeBakey
    Bircher meniscus
    Blount
    Bovie
    Bucy chordotomy (or cordotomy)
    cartilage
    Catlin amputating
    chondroplasty

knife *(continued)*
   chordotomy (cordotomy)
   cobalt-60 gamma
   Collin amputating
   cordotomy (chordotomy)
   Crile gasserian ganglion
   Cushing dural hook
   deep blade
   DeMarneffe meniscotomy
   double-bladed
   Down epiphyseal
   Downing cartilage
   dural
   epiphyseal
   Esmarch plaster
   flap
   forward-cutting
   Frazier cordotomy
   Frazier pituitary
   Freer-Swanson ganglion
   Freiberg cartilage
   Freiberg meniscectomy
   full-radius resector
   Gamma (radiosurgical instrument)
   ganglion
   Grover meniscus
   Halle dura
   hemilaminectomy
   hook
   Hopkins plaster
   hot
   interosseous
   Jacobson microvascular
   Jacobson vessel
   Jannetta
   Knifelight surgical knife and light
   Koos microvascular
   Krull acetabular
   Langenbeck flap
   Langenbeck resection
   left-cutting
   Leksell cobalt-60 gamma
   Leksell Gamma
   Lindvall-Stille
   Liston amputating
   Liston phalangeal
   Lowe-Breck cartilage

knife *(continued)*
   Lowe-Breck meniscectomy
   Maltz cartilage
   McKeever cartilage
   meniscotomy
   meniscus
   microvascular
   Midas Rex
   myelotomy
   Neff meniscus
   Olivecrona trigeminal
   Oretorp arthroscopy
   Parasmillie double-bladed
   pituitary
   plaster
   Questrus Leading Edge sheathed
   Rayport dural dissector and
   Reiner plaster
   resection
   retrograde
   Ridlon plaster
   right-angle
   right-cutting
   roentgen
   Salenius meniscus
   semilunar cartilage
   sharp
   skin blade
   Smillie-Beaver
   Smillie cartilage
   Smillie meniscus
   Smith cartilage
   Stecher arachnoid
   Stryker cartilage
   swivel
   tenotomy
   Tiemann Meals tenolysis
   Toennis dura
   201-source cobalt-60 gamma
   vessel
   Weary cordotomy
   Weck
   Yamanda myelotomy
   Yasargil arachnoid
   Yasargil microvascular
Knifelight surgical knife and light
knife/sleeve device

Knight back brace
Knight bone-cutting forceps
Knighton hemilaminectomy retractor
Knighton laminectomy retractor
Knight-Taylor thoracic brace
K9 Scooter
Knobby-Clark procedure
knock, bladder (in distance runners)
knock-knee deformity
knock-out, knocked out (KO)
Knodt compression rod
Knodt hook
knot
    arthroscopic
    half-hitch arthroscopic
    lockable arthroscopic
    Nicky
    ratchet
    sailorman's
    slip
    surfer's
    Tennessee slider
knotless suture anchor
knot of Henry
knot pusher
knot tier and ligature carrier, Retter
knot tightener, Nordt
knowledge, fund of
Knowles nail
Knowles pin
knuckle bender splint
knuckle bone
knuckle-shaped
Knuttsen bending roentgenograms
KO (knock-out, knocked out)
Kocher clamp
Kocher collar incision
Kocher-Cushing sign
Kocher-Debré-Sémélaigne syndrome
Kocher dissector
Kocher elevator
Kocher forceps
Kocher fracture
Kocher-Langenbeck ilioinguinal repair
    of acetabular fracture
Kocher lateral J approach

Kocher-Lorenz classification of
    capitellum fracture
Kocher maneuver
Kocher-McFarland hip arthroplasty
Kocher reduction of shoulder disloca-
    tion
Kocher retractor
Koch-Mason dressing
Kodel knee sling
Koebner phenomenon
Koenig (also König)
Koenig metatarsophalangeal joint
    arthroplasty
Koenig MPJ implant and arthroplasty
Koenig nail-splitting scissors
Koenig rasp
Koenig-Schaefer approach
Koerber-Salus-Elschnig syndrome
Köhler (Koehler) lines to grade hip
    protrusion
Köhler-Pellegrini-Stieda disease
Kohlrausch muscle
Kohs block test
Kolb classification of drug addiction
Komai stereotactic head frame
Konica scanner
König disease (Koenig)
König osteochondritis dissecans
    of the knee
Konstram angle
Kool Kit cold therapy pack
Koos microvascular knife
Korean hand acupuncture
Korn Cage knee brace
Korotkoff method in Doppler
    cerebrovascular examination
Korr neurologic model
Korsakoff amnesia
Korsakoff psychosis
Korsakoff syndrome
Kortzeborn hand procedure
Koshevnikoff epilepsy
Kostuik-Errico classification of spinal
    stability
Kostuik-Harrington spinal instru-
    mentation

Kostuik rod
Kostuik screw
Koutsogiannis-Fowler-Anderson
　osteotomy
Koyter muscle
K pack
K pad
KPS (Karnofsky performance score)
Krabbe diffuse sclerosis
Krabbe disease
Krabbe leukodystrophy
Krackow point
Krackow suture
Krackow whipstitch
Kramer-Craig-Noel osteotomy
　technique
Kramer modification of Hohmann
　osteotomy
Krankendonk pin
Kraske position in surgery
Krause bone
Krause cutaneomucous muscle
Krause ligament
Krause sensory receptor
Krause, suture of
Krause-Wolfe skin graft
Krayenbuehl nerve hook (Krayenbühl)
Kr-81m (krypton) imaging agent
Krempen-Craig-Sotelo tibia nonunion
　technique
Kretschmer syndrome
Kreuscher bunionectomy
Kreuscher scissors
Kristiansen eyelet lag screw
Kronecker aneurysm needle
Kronner external fixation
Krukenberg hand procedure
Krukenberg tumor
Krull acetabular knife
Kruskal-Wallis one-way analysis
krypton (81mKr) imaging agent
KS 5 ACL brace
KSS (Knee Signature System)
KSS (Kearns-Sayre syndrome)
KT1000 knee ligament arthrometer
KTP (potassium titanyl phosphate)
　laser

KTP/532 laser
Kudo unconstrained elbow prosthesis
Kufs disease
Kugelberg-Welander disease
Kugelberg-Welander juvenile spinal
　muscle atrophy
Kugelberg-Welander syndrome
Kuhlman cervical traction
Kumar-Cowell-Ramsey technique
Kumar spica cast technique
Kummel classification for ulnar ray
　deficiency (I-III)
Kümmell disease
Kümmell spondylitis
Küntscher (Kuentscher)
Küntscher awl
Küntscher drill
Küntscher finisher
Küntscher hammer
Küntscher impactor
Küntscher nail
Küntscher nail driver
Küntscher reamer
Küntscher rod
Küntscher nail-extracting hook
Küntscher traction apparatus
Kurosaka fixation screw
Kurtzke disability score
kuru viral encephalitis
Kurze dissection scissors
Kurze suction-irrigator
Kusch'kin Ace wheelchair
Kussmaul aphasia
Kussmaul coma
Kutler digital flap
Kutler V-Y flap graft
Kuz-Medics disposable knee immobi-
　lizer
Kuz-Medics total knee retractor
Kveim test
kVp (kilovolts peak) meter
K wire (Kirschner wire)
K wire driver
K wire fixation
K wire skeletal traction
Kwoh-Young stereotactic robot
Kydex body jacket

Kydex brace
Kyle fracture classification system
kyllosis (clubfoot)
kyphectomy, Sharrard-type
kyphoscoliosis
kyphosis
    Cobb method of measuring
    juvenile
    loss of
    lumbar

kyphosis *(continued)*
    lumbosacral
    postlaminectomy
    Scheuermann juvenile
    spondyloptotic
    thoracic
kyphosis brace
kyphotic angulation
kyphotic pelvis

L, l

L (lumbar vertebra)
Labbé triangle
Labbé, vein of
la belle indifférence in stroke patients
labial dysarthria
lability, emotional
labioglossolaryngeal paralysis
labioglossopharyngeal paralysis
labium
labored breathing
labral injury
labral variant
labrectomy, arthroscopic
labrum
    acetabular
    articular
    glenoid
labrum-ligament complex (LLC)
labyrinth
labyrinthectomy
labyrinthine artery
labyrinthine disorder
labyrinthine hydrops
labyrinthine structures
labyrinthine vertigo
LAC (long arm cast)
laced blucher of shoe
lace-on brace

laceration
    brain
    bursting-type
    chevron
    dural
    stellate
laceration of the spinal cord
lace-up ankle brace
lace-up RocketSoc ankle brace
Lacey knee prosthesis
Lachman maneuver
Lachman sign
Lachman test
Lac-Hydrin
laciniate ligament of ankle
lack of clear-cut cerebral dominance
lacrimal bone
lacrimal nerve
LaCrosse virus encephalitis
lactated Ringer's (LR) injection
lactic dehydrogenase
LactoSorb orthopedic wound material
lacuna (pl. lacunae)
    bone
    cartilage
    osseous
lacunar infarct (infarction)
lacunar ligament

lacunar state
lacunar stroke
lacunar syndrome
Lafora body disease
Lafora inclusion body epilepsy
lag
  adductive
  extension
  head
  lid
  phase
lag screw
lag sign
Lahey clamp
Lahey Clinic dural hook
Lahey Clinic nerve hook
Laing concentric hip cup
Laitinen CT guidance system
Laitinen stereotactic head frame
Laks method
lalling (babbling)
Lalonde hook forceps
Lalonde tendon approximator
lambda wave on EEG
lambdoid suture
Lambert-Eaton myasthenic syndrome
  (LEMS)
Lambert-Lowman bone clamp
Lambert-Lowman chisel
Lambeth Disability Screening
  Questionnaire
Lamb muscle transfer
Lambotte bone-holding forceps
Lambotte bone hook
Lambotte elevator
Lambotte osteotome
Lambotte rasp
Lambrinudi dropfoot operation
Lambrinudi splint
Lambrinudi triple arthrodesis
lamb's wool pad
lamella (pl. lamellae)
lamellar body density (LBD) count
lamellar bone
lamellar reaction

lamina
  medullary
  osseous spiral
lamina chisel, D'Errico
lamina spreader
laminaplasty, Tsuji
laminar air flow system
laminar shear stress
lamination of gyrus
laminectomy
  cervical
  decompressive
  emergency
  multilevel
  osteoplastic
  single-level decompressive
laminectomy frame
laminectomy retractor
  Cloward-Hoen
  Cone
  Meyerding
  Poppen-Gelpi
  Seletz-Gelpi
  Cone
laminectomy rongeur
  Bucy
  Cloward-English
  Codman-Harper
  Codman-Kerrison
  Codman-Leksell
  Codman-Schlesinger cervical
  Echlin
  Ferris Smith-Kerrison
  Fulton
  Hajek-Koffler
  Raney
  Smith-Petersen
  Whitcomb-Kerrison
laminoforaminotomy
laminoplasty, open door
laminotomy, suspension
Lamis patellar clamp
lamp
  stroboscopic
  Wood

Lance-Adams syndrome
lancinating pain
Lancisi, nerve of
land, no man's (in hand)
Landau-Kleffner syndrome
Landau reflex
landmark
   anatomic
   bony
   bony skull
Landolt pituitary speculum
Landolt spreading forceps
Landouzy-Dejerine disease
Landouzy-Dejerine dystrophy
Landry ascending paralysis
Landry-Guillain-Barré-Strohl syndrome
Landsmeer ligament
Landström muscle
Lane bending tool
Lane bone-holding clamp
Lane bone-holding forceps
Lane bone lever
Lane bone screw
Lane periosteal elevator
Lane plate
Lane screw-holding forceps
Lanex screen
Lange Achilles tendon reconstruction
Lange bone retractor
Lange hip reduction
Lange-Hohmann bone retractor
Lange tendon lengthening and repair
Langenbeck bone-holding forceps
Langenbeck flap knife
Langenbeck forceps
Langenbeck metacarpal saw
Langenbeck periosteal elevator
Langenbeck rasp
Langenbeck resection knife
Langenbeck retractor
Langenbeck saw
Langenbeck triangle
Langenskiöld bony bridge resection
Langer axillary arch muscle
Langer-Giedion syndrome
Langer line
Langer mesomelic dwarfism

Langley pilomotor nerve
Langoria sign
language
   emotive
   executive
   expressive
   global loss of
   receptive
language deficit
language dysfunction
language mapping
Lannelongue ligament
Lansing strain (type II poliomyelitis
   virus)
LAO (left anterior oblique) view
lap (laparotomy) sponge
laparoscopic surgeon's thumb
laparoscopy, BAK
laparotomy sheet
Lapidus alternating air-pressure
   mattress
Lapidus bed
Lapidus bunionectomy
Laplacian montage
LaPorte total toe prosthesis
lapse of awareness
lapse of consciousness
large skull implant surgery
large vessel disease of diabetic foot
large vessel thrombosis
Lark scooter
Larmon forefoot procedure
Larmor equation
Larmor frequency
Larrey space
Larsen hip score
Larsen-Johansson disease
Larsen tendon-holding forceps
LARSI (lumbar anterior-root
   stimulator implants)
Lars Leksell Center for Gamma
   Surgery
Larson ligament reconstruction
larva, helminth
larval spike and slow wave
larva migrans, cutaneous
laryngeal dysarthria

laryngeal electromyography
laryngeal nerve, recurrent
laryngeal paralysis
laryngography, double-contrast
LA (ligament anchor) screw
LASE (laser-assisted spinal
 endoscopy)
Lasègue sign
laser
 argon
 ArthroProbe arthroscopic
 Candella SPTL
 CO_2 (carbon dioxide)
 cold
 Cr,TM,Ho:YAG crystal
 flashlamp pulsed dye
 gallium-arsenid (GaA) laser
 holmium (Ho)
 Ho:YAG
 KTP (potassium titanyl phosphate)
 KTP/532
 Lasermedic Microlight 830
 LaserPen
 LaserSonics Nd:YAG LaserBlade
 low energy lasers (LELs)
 low intensity laser therapy (LILT)
 low power
 Microlight 830
 Nd:YAG (neodymium: yttrium-
  aluminum-garnet)
 Opmilas CO_2 multipurpose
 red light neon (for acupressure
  points) (chiropractic)
 soft
 Surgilase CO_2
 VersaPulse
 VersaPulse holmium
 YAG (yttrium-aluminum-garnet)
laser-assisted capsular shift
laser-assisted capsulorrhaphy
laser-assisted spinal endoscopy
 (LASE)
laser chondroplasty
laser Doppler fluxmetry
laser Doppler velocimetry
Laserflo Doppler probe

laser image custom arthroplasty
 (LICA)
Lasermedic Microlight 830
laser nucleotomy
LaserPen
LaserScissors 390/20
Laserscope device
LaserSonics Nd:YAG LaserBlade
laser stylus profilometer
lashing of first and second metatarsals
lashing suture
lassitude
last
 bunion
 Keystone
LAT (left anterior temporal) EEG lead
lata, fascia
latah of Malaysia syndrome
Latarjet nerve
Latarjet procedure for recurrent
 shoulder instability
LATC (lateral talocalcaneal angle)
late maturers
latency
 absolute
 decline in
 distal motor
 interpeak (IPL)
 mean sleep
 motor
 short sleep
latent gout
latent nausea, in migraine
lateral acetabular shelf operation
lateral ampullar nerve
lateral antebrachial cutaneous nerve
lateral anterior thoracic nerve
lateral arcuate ligament
lateral atlantoaxial joint
lateral band rerouting
lateral bending views of spine
lateral buttress support
lateral cervical spine film
lateral column calcaneal fracture
lateral compartment liftoff
lateral condyle

lateral corticospinal tract
lateral costotransverse ligament
lateral cricoarytenoid muscle
lateral cutaneous nerve
lateral decubitus view
lateral dorsal cutaneous nerve
lateral entrapment
lateral epicondylitis
lateral femoral cutaneous nerve
lateral gaze center
lateral gaze mystagmus
lateral gaze palsy
lateral geniculate nucleus
lateral great muscle
lateral head of gastrocnemius
laterality
lateralization
lateralized activity
lateralized distribution
lateralized slowing
lateralizing deficit
lateralizing finding
lateralizing sign
lateral ligamentous sprain
lateral lumbosacral ligament
laterally displaced fracture
lateral malleolar ligament
lateral mamillary nucleus of Rose
lateral mass
lateral medullary syndrome
lateral motion racket sports
lateral occipital sulcus
lateral occipitotemporal gyrus
lateral opposed beam
lateral palpebral ligament
lateral pectoral nerve
lateral pinch testing
lateral plantar nerve
lateral popliteal nerve
lateral projection
lateral pterygoid muscle
lateral puboprostatic ligament
lateral recess
lateral rectus muscle
lateral sacrococcygeal ligament
lateral spinocerebellar tracts
lateral spinothalamic tract

lateral spring ligament of foot
lateral sulcus
lateral supraclavicular nerve
lateral sural cutaneous nerve
lateral talocalcaneal ligament
lateral temporomandibular ligament
lateral tensile force
lateral tension band of knee
lateral tomography
lateral translation force
lateral transverse thigh flap (LTTF)
lateral umbilical ligament
lateral vastus muscle
lateral ventricle
lateral view
lateral web
lateral wedge for sole or heel of foot
lateral wedge fracture
lateropulsion
late traumatic epilepsy
latissimus dorsi muscle
latissimus dorsi musculocutaneous
    free flap
lattice, fibrovascular
lattice relaxation time
latticework
Lauge-Hansen classification of ankle
    fracture
Lauge-Hansen stage II supination-
    eversion fracture
laughing and crying, pathologic
laughing seizures (gelastic epilepsy)
laughter, uncontrollable mirthless
Laugier sign
Laugier test
Laurence-Moon-Biedl-Bardet
    syndrome
Laurin lateral patellofemoral angle
Lausanne stereotactic robot
Lauth ligament
lavage
    angled showerhead
    bone
    CarboJet
    Exeter bone
    Hi Speed Pulse
    jet

lavage *(continued)*
  joint
  needle
  pulsatile jet
  pulsatile pressure
  Pulsavac
  Simpulse pulsing
  Simpulse S/I
law
  Bell-Magendie
  Heuter-Volkmann
  Rayleigh scattering
  Semon
  von Schwann
  Wolff
Lawson-Thornton plate
laxity
  joint
  ligament
  ligamentous
  varus stress
layer
  Bekhterev
  cambium
  parietal tendon sheath
  periosteal cambium
  tangential (of hand)
  visceral tendon sheath
Lazarus sign
"lazy eye" (amblyopia ex anopsia)
LB (longitudinal bipolar) montage
L/B (lesion-to-brain) ratio
L bars
LBP (low back pain)
LC-DCP (low contact dynamic
  compression plate)
LCL (lateral collateral ligament)
LCP (Legg-Calvé-Perthes disease)
LCR (ligamentous and capsular repair)
  system
LCS New Jersey knee prosthesis
LCS total knee system implant
LCT (liquid crystal contact thermog-
  raphy)
LDD (laser-assisted disk decompres-
  sion)

LDF (laser-Doppler flowmetry) probe
LDI-200
L-dopa-induced dyskinesia
LE (lower extremity)
Leach-Igou step-cut medial osteotomy
lead
  black EEG
  dual electrode
  EEG
  grid
  helical platinum
  left-sided EEG
  multi-electrode
  Retrox Fractal active fixation
  right-sided EEG
  sphenoidal fossae EEG
  white EEG
Leadbetter maneuver
lead encephalopathy (plumbism)
lead gout
leadpipe fracture
leadpipe rigidity
lead poisoning
lead wire
leaf
  dural
  inferior
  superior
leaflet, dural
leaflet of pachymeninges
leakage, cerebrospinal fluid (CSF)
leakage headache (of CSF)
leak, cerebrospinal fluid (CSF)
Leander chiropractic table
Leander motorized flexion table
Leander 790 Series distraction table
lean mass
LEAP (Lewis expandable adjustable
  prosthesis)
leather lacer gauntlet
Leatherman hook
Leber disease
Leber optic atrophy
Lebsche rongeur
Lebsche saw guide
Lebsche wire saw

lectins
  RCA (*Ricinus communis* agglutinin)
  UE (*Ulex europaeus*)
lectins antibody
Lectron II electrode gel
Ledderhose disease
Le Dentu suture
LED flash-point vertebrospinal naviga-
  tion system
Lee bone graft
leech
Leeds-Keio ligament prosthesis
Leeds spinal procedure
Lefferts rib shears
leflunomide (Arava)
Le Fort fibular fracture
Le Fort mandible fracture
Le Fort II fracture
LEFS (Lower Extremity Functional
  Scale)
left anterior oblique (LAO) projection
left anterior temporal (LAT) EEG lead
left-bearing nystagmus
left cervical vagus nerve trunk
left frontal (LF) EEG lead
left-hand dominant
left-handed patient
left hemiplegia
left motor (LM) EEG lead
left occipital (LO) EEG lead
left parietal (LP) EEG lead
left posterior oblique (LPO) position
left posterior temporal (LPT) EEG
  lead
left respiratory nerve (phrenic)
left-sided weakness
left superior vena cava ligament
left triangular ligament
left vena cava ligament
leg (pl. legs)
  badger
  baker
  bandy
  bayonet
  bow
  champagne-bottle
  flaccid

leg *(continued)*
  game
  gimpy
  lusty (of tabes dorsalis)
  nonpreferred
  paretic
  postphlebitic
  preferred
  restless
  rider's
  scissor
  scissoring of
  stork's
  tennis (plantaris rupture)
  unilateral spastic
Legasus Sport CPM (continuous
  passive-motion) device
leg drift
Legend ACL functional knee brace
Legend PCL functional knee brace
Leg Extension Power Rig
leg-foot-toe syndrome
Legg-Calvé-Perthes disease (LCP)
Legg-Calvé-Waldenström disease
Legg-Perthes shoe extension
Legg-Perthes sling
leg holder
leg length discrepancy
leg lengthening device
Lehman technique
Leibinger Micro Dynamic mesh
Leibinger microplate
Leibinger Micro Plus plate
Leibinger Micro Plus screw
Leibinger Micro System cranial
  fixation plate
Leibinger Micro System drill bit
Leibinger Micro System plate cutters
Leibinger Micro System plate-holding
  forceps
Leibinger Micro System pliers
Leibinger mini-Wurzbach
Leibinger Profyle system
Leica Aristoplan laser scanning micro-
  scope
Leichtenstern encephalitis
Leichtenstern sign

Leigh disease
Leigh necrotizing encephalopathy
Leigh subacute necrotizing
  encephalomyelitis
Leigh syndrome
Leinbach device
Leinbach femoral prosthesis
Leinbach osteotome
Leinbach screw
leiomyosarcoma
Leksell adapter to Mayfield device
Leksell cobalt-60 Gamma Knife
Leksell D-shaped stereotactic frame
Leksell-Elekta stereotactic frame
Leksell Gamma Knife
Leksell Gamma stereotactic frame
Leksell laminectomy rongeur
Leksell microstereotactic system
Leksell Model G stereotactic frame
Leksell posteroventral pallidotomy
Leksell rongeur forceps
Leksell stereotactic arc
Leksell stereotactic coordinate frame
Leksell-Stille thoracic rongeur
Lelièvre operation to block end-range
  pronation
LELs (low energy lasers)
LeMaitre Glow 'N Tell radiopaque
  tape
Lembert suture
Lemmon rib contractor
Lemmon sternal approximator
Lemmon sternal spreader
lemniscus
  lateral (in brain)
  medial
  spinal
lemon sign of spina bifida
Lempert bone curet
Lempert bone rongeur
Lempert periosteal elevator
Lempert rongeur forceps
LEMS (Lambert-Eaton myasthenic
  syndrome)
Lenart-Kullman technique

length
  axis
  hip axis
  limb
  radius
  stride
lengthening
  Achilles tendon
  Armistead ulnar
  gastrocnemius
  hamstring
  Ilizarov leg
  Lange tendon
  Silfverskiöld Achilles tendon
  Tachdjian hamstring
  tendon
  tendon Achilles (TAL)
  Vulpius
  Vulpius-Compere Z
  Z-slide lengthening
lengthening over nails (LON)
  procedure
lengthening reflex
LENI (lower extremity noninvasive)
Lennox-Gastaut syndrome
Lennox syndrome
Lenox Hill derotational knee brace
lenticular bone
lenticular nucleus
lenticulostriate artery
lentiform nucleus
Leon strain (type III poliomyelitis
  virus)
L-Episcopo-Zachary procedure
LE prep (lupus erythematosus
  preparation)
leptomeningeal carcinomatosis
leptomeningeal circulation
leptomeningeal cyst
leptomeningeal disease
leptomeningeal hemangioma
leptomeningeal metastases
leptomeningeal venous channel
leptomeningeal venous disruption
leptomeningeal venous drainage

leptomeninges
leptomeningitis
Lequesne Index
Léri pleonosteosis
Léri sign
Lerman cervical halo brace
Lerman multiligamentous knee control
   orthosis
LeRoy-Raney scalp clips
LeRoy scalp clip-applying forceps
LEs (lower extremities)
Lesch-Nyhan syndrome
lesion
   acute cerebellar hemispheric
   afferent nerve
   anterior parietal
   anterochiasmatic
   anteromedial humeral head
   atrophic
   Bankart shoulder
   Bennett
   bihemispheric
   biparietal
   bone surface
   brain stem
   Brown-Séquard
   bubbly bone
   callosal
   cartilaginous
   cavernous sinus
   cavitary
   central
   cerebral
   cervical cord
   chiasmal
   chiasmatic
   chondral delamination
   cleavage
   complete nerve
   conus medullaris
   cortical
   corticospinal pathway
   cyclops
   cystic
   deep
   deep-seated
   dendritic

lesion *(continued)*
   desmoid
   destructive
   disk
   dominant hemisphere
   dorsal root entry zone
   DREZ (dorsal root entry zone)
   Duret
   echogenic
   enhancing
   epicortical
   epileptogenic
   Essex-Lopresti
   excitatory
   expansile lytic
   extra-axial
   fibromuscular
   fibro-osseous
   fingertip
   focal
   focal hemispheric
   focal irritative
   focal ischemic
   frank
   frontal lobe
   HAGL (humeral avulsion of
     glenohumeral ligament)
   hamartomatous
   hemorrhagic
   high cervical spinal cord
   high-density
   high pontine
   high-signal
   Hill-Sachs shoulder
   homogeneous
   hyperintense
   hyperkeratotic
   hyperkeratotic plantar
   hyperostotic
   hypothalamic
   infranuclear
   intra-axial brain
   intracerebral
   intracranial vascular
   intramedullary
   intramedullary spinal
   intrasellar

lesion *(continued)*
  intraspinal
  invasive
  irregular-shaped
  irregularly shaped
  ischemic
  isointense
  keratotic
  Kidner
  kissing
  lateral temporal epileptogenic
  localized
  low density
  lower motor neuron
  Lynch and Crues type 2
  lytic
  lytic bone
  malignant
  mass
  MCRF (microfractured)
  medial longitudinal fasciculus
    (MLF)
  median nerve
  mesial temporal epileptogenic
  metabolic
  metaphyseal
  metastatic bone
  midbrain
  midline
  Monteggia
  multicentric brain
  multifocal
  multiple focal
  muscular
  nail bed
  neoplastic
  neurogenic
  nigrostriatal
  nondominant hemisphere
  nonenhancing
  noninvasive
  nucleus basalis
  obstructive (of the CSF pathways)
  occipital
  occult
  osseous
  osteoblastic

lesion *(continued)*
  osteocartilaginous
  osteochondral
  ostial
  outcropping of
  parasagittal
  parasellar
  parietal cortex
  parietal lobe
  parieto-occipital
  pedal hyperpigmented
  peripheral
  peripheral nerve
  periventricular
  Perthes-Bankart
  photon-deficient
  plaquelike
  polyostotic bone
  pontine
  posterior column
  posterior compartment
  posterior fossa
  posterior fossa-foramen magnum
  posterior language area
  posterior-superior humeral head
  pretectal
  primary
  radiofrequency
  radiopaque
  resectable
  reverse Hill-Sachs
  retrochiasmal
  retrochiasmatic
  ring-enhancing (on CT)
  root
  root entry-zone
  signal characteristics of
  skin
  SLAP (superior labrum anterior-
    posterior)
  slowly developing
  solitary
  sonolucent
  space-occupying
  spherical
  spinal cord
  Stener

lesion *(continued)*
 striatal
 structural
 subchondral
 subcortical intracranial
 subtentorial
 superficial
 supranuclear
 suprasellar
 supratentorial
 synchronous
 tectal
 temporal lobe
 thalamic
 thermolytic
 transfer
 transverse cord
 ulnar nerve
 uncommitted metaphyseal
 unresectable
 upper motor neuron
 wedge-shaped
 well-defined
 white matter
 Wolin meniscoid
lesion localization
lesion-to-background ratio
lesion-to-cerebrospinal fluid noise
lesion-to-muscle ratio
lesion-to-nonlesion count ratio
lesion-to-white matter noise
Lesquene Index of Severity of Osteoarthritis
lesser atrophy of disuse
lesser internal cutaneous nerve
lesser metatarsophalangeal joint
lesser multangular bone
lesser occipital nerve
lesser palatine nerve
lesser petrosal nerve
lesser rhomboid muscle
lesser sciatic notch
lesser splanchnic nerve
lesser superficial petrosal nerve
lesser toes
lesser trochanter
lesser zygomatic muscle

Lester muscle forceps
"let-down" migraine
leteprinim potassium (Neotrofin)
lethargic
lethargica, encephalitis
lethargy
lethica
Letournel guidelines
Letournel plate
Letterer-Siwe disease
letter reversals
leukemia, meningeal
leukemic infiltration of meninges
leukoaraiosis
leukocyte-endothelial adhesion
leukodystrophy
 Canavan
 globoid
 globoid cell
 hereditary cerebral
 Krabbe
 metachromatic (MLD)
 Pelizaeus-Merzbacher
 spongiform
 spongy degeneration
 sudanophilic
leukodystrophy with diffuse Rosenthal
 fiber formation
leukoencephalitis
 acute hemorrhagic
 acute necrotizing hemorrhagic
 necrotizing hemorrhagic
 postinfectious
 postvaccinial
 van Bogaert sclerosing
 viral
leukoencephalopathy
 multifocal
 necrotizing
 postinfectious
 progressive multifocal (PML)
 subacute sclerosing
leukoencephaly, metachromatic
leukomalacia, periventricular (PVL)
leukopenia, cerebral
leukosialin (CD43)
leukotome

leukotomy
leukotriene
LeukoVAX
Leung thumb loss classification
leuvectin
level
  automatic phrase
  engagement
  fat-fluid
  occipitocervical
  peak-and-trough
  pontine-medullary
  sensory
  trough-and-peak
leveling, joint
level of activity
level of alertness
level of consciousness (LOC)
level of demarcation in sensory testing
level of denervation
level of functioning, premorbid
level of sensory loss
lever, Lane bone
levering
Leveron doorknob turner device
levetiracetam
Levine orthopedic outcomes questionnaire
Levin thermocouple cordotomy
  electrode
Levis splint
levodopa, decarboxylation of
levodopa-induced dyskinesia
levodopa-induced psychosis
levorotatory
levoscoliosis
Levy & Rappel foot orthosis
Lewin baseball-finger splint
Lewin bone clamp
Lewin bone-holding forceps
Lewin bunion dissector
Lewin finger splint
Lewin-Gaenslen test
Lewin punch test
Lewin reverse Lasègue test
Lewin snuff test
Lewin spinal perforating forceps

Lewin standing test
Lewin-Stern thumb splint
Lewin supine test
Lewis-Chekofsky resection
Lewis expandable adjustable prosthesis
  (LEAP)
Lewis nail
Lewis periosteal elevator
Lewis rasp
Lewy body
Lexan jacket
Lexer chisel
Lexer gouge
Lexer osteotome
Lex-Ton spinal frame
Leyla bar
Leyla brain retractor
LF (left frontal) EEG lead
LFF (low filter frequency)
L-5 hydroxytryptophan (L-5HTP)
L5-S1 vertebral interspace
LFV (large field of view)
LGA (low grade astrocytoma)
LHB (long head of biceps)
Lhermitte-Duclos disease
Lhermitte sign
LH1000 arthroscopic leg holder
LIAD (low impact aerobic dance)
liberator elevator
Liberty CMC thumb brace
Liberty One splint
LICA (laser image custom
  arthroplasty)
Lichtheim aphasia
Lichtheim disease
Lichtman technique
licostinel (ACEA 1021)
lid flutter on EEG
Lidge cement gun
lid lag
Lido Active Multijoint System
Lidoback isokinetic dynamometry
  system
lidocaine and bupivacaine
lidocaine patch
lidocaine provocation test
Lidoderm (lidocaine patch 5%)

Lido Lift
Lido Passive Multijoint System
LIDO scale
Lido WorkSET (simulation,
    evaluation, and training)
Liebolt radioulnar technique
lienophrenic ligament
lienorenal ligament
Liepmann apraxia
LiF (lithium fluoride)
Life-Port drug delivery system
Life Satisfaction Index (LSI)
lifestyle, sedentary
Li-Fraumeni syndrome (LFS)
lift
    chiropractic laser nonsurgical face
    DiPalma shoe
    heel
    Hoyer
    Lido Lift
lifter, Yasargil tissue
lift-off of heel in walk
lift-off test
Ligaclip clip applier
Ligaclip hemostatic clip
ligament
    accessory
    accessory collateral
    accessory plantar
    accessory volar
    acromioclavicular
    acromiocoracoid
    alar
    alveolodental
    annular
    anococcygeal
    anterior calcaneoastragaloid
    anterior collateral (ACL)
    anterior costotransverse
    anterior costovertebral
    anterior costoxiphoid
    anterior cruciate
    anterior fibular
    anterior inferior tibiofibular
    anterior longitudinal (ALL)
    anterior medial
    anterior oblique

ligament *(continued)*
    anterior radioulnar
    anterior talofibular (ATF)
    anterior talotibial
    anterior tibiotalar
    apical
    Arantius
    arcuate popliteal
    arcuate pubic
    arterial
    atlantal
    attenuated
    auricular
    avulsed
    axis
    Bardinet
    Barkow
    beak
    Bellini
    Berry
    Bertin
    Bichat
    bifurcate
    bifurcated
    Bigelow
    Botallo
    Bourgery
    broad
    Brodie
    Burns
    calcaneoclavicular
    calcaneocuboid
    calcaneofibular (CF)
    calcaneonavicular
    calcaneotibial
    Caldani
    Campbell
    Camper
    capsular
    Carcassonne
    cardinal
    caroticoclinoid
    carpometacarpal
    Casser
    casserian
    caudal
    ceratocricoid

ligament *(continued)*
cervical
cervical mover
check
check rein
cholecystoduodenal
chondroxiphoid
ciliary
Civinini
Clado
Cleland
Cloquet
collateral
Colles
congenital laxity of
conjugate
conoid
conus
Cooper
coracoacromial
coracoclavicular
coracohumeral
corniculopharyngeal
coronary
costoclavicular
costocolic
costotransverse
costoxiphoid
cotyloid
Cowper
cricopharyngeal
cricosantorinian
cricothyroid
cricotracheal
cross
crucial
cruciate
cruciform
Cruveilhier
cuboideonavicular
cuneocuboid
cuneonavicular
cystoduodenal
deep collateral
deep dorsal sacrococcygeal
deep posterior sacrococcygeal
deep transverse metacarpal

ligament *(continued)*
deep transverse palmar
deltoid
Denonvilliers
dentate
denticulate
Denucé
diaphragmatic
dorsal calcaneocuboid
dorsal carpal
dorsal carpometacarpal
dorsal cuboideonavicular
dorsal cuneocuboid
dorsal cuneonavicular
dorsal metacarpal
dorsal metatarsal
dorsal radiocarpal
dorsal sacroiliac
dorsal talonavicular
dorsal wrist
Douglas
duodenal
duodenorenal
epihyal
external
external collateral
extracapsular
falciform
fallopian
femoral
Ferrein
fibular collateral
fibulotalar
fibulotalocalcaneal
flaval
floating
Flood
fundiform
gastrocolic
gastrodiaphragmatic
gastrohepatic
gastrolienal
gastropancreatic
gastrophrenic
gastrosplenic
genital
genitoinguinal

ligament *(continued)*
  Gerdy
  Gillette suspensory
  Gimbernat
  gingivodental
  glenohumeral
  glenoid
  glossoepiglottic
  Grayson
  Günz (Guenz)
  Günzberg (Guenzberg)
  Haines-McDougall medial
  hammock
  Helmholtz axis
  Henle
  Hensing
  hepatic
  hepatocolic
  hepatocystocolic
  hepatoduodenal
  hepatoesophageal
  hepatogastric
  hepatogastroduodenal
  hepatophrenic
  hepatorenal
  hepatoumbilical
  Hesselbach
  Hey
  Holl
  Hueck
  Humphry
  Hunter
  Huschke
  hyalocapsular
  hyoepiglottic
  hypsiloid
  iliofemoral
  iliolumbar
  iliopectineal
  iliotibial
  iliotrochanteric
  inferior calcaneonavicular
  inferior dorsal radioulnar
  inferior ilioischial
  inferior pubic
  inferior transverse scapular
  infrapatellar

ligament *(continued)*
  infundibulo-ovarian
  infundibulopelvic
  inguinal
  intercapital
  intercarpal
  interclavicular
  interclinoid
  intercornual
  intercostal
  intercuneiform
  interdigital
  interfoveolar
  intermetatarsal
  internal collateral
  interosseous
  interosseous cuneocuboid
  interosseous cuneometatarsal
  interosseous lunotriquetral
  interosseous metacarpal
  interosseous metatarsal
  interosseous sacroiliac
  interosseous talocalcaneal
  interosseous tibiofibular
  interosseous talocalcaneal
  intersesamoid
  interspinal
  interspinous
  intertransverse
  intervertebral
  intra-articular
  intra-articular sternocostal
  intrascapular
  ischiocapsular
  ischiofemoral
  Jarjavay
  jugal
  Krause
  laciniate
  lacunar
  Landsmeer
  Lannelongue
  lateral arcuate
  lateral collateral (LCL)
  lateral costotransverse
  lateral lumbosacral
  lateral malleolar

ligament *(continued)*
   lateral palpebral
   lateral puboprostatic
   lateral sacrococcygeal
   lateral "spring"
   lateral talocalcaneal (LTC)
   lateral temporomandibular
   lateral umbilical
   Lauth
   left superior vena cava
   left triangular
   left vena cava
   lienophrenic
   lienorenal
   limited proteoglycan matrix of
   Lisfranc
   Lockwood
   long fibers
   longitudinal
   long plantar
   lumbocostal
   lunotriquetral interosseous
   Luschka
   Mackenrodt
   macroscopic hemorrhage
   Maissiat
   Mauchart
   Meckel
   medial
   medial arcuate
   medial collateral (MCL)
   medial palpebral
   medial puboprostatic
   medial talocalcaneal
   medial ulnar collateral (MUCL)
   medial umbilical
   median arcuate
   meniscofemoral
   meniscotibial
   metacarpoglenoidal
   metacarpophalangeal
   microscopic hemorrhage of
   middle costotransverse
   middle umbilical
   mucosal suspensory
   natatory
   naviculocuneiform

ligament *(continued)*
   neocollateral
   nuchal
   oblique popliteal
   oblique retinacular
   occipital-atlas-axis
   occipitoaxial
   odontoid
   orbicular
   ovarian
   palmar
   palmar beak
   palmar carpal
   palmar carpometacarpal
   palmar metacarpal
   palmar oblique
   palmar radiocarpal
   palmar ulnocarpal
   patellar
   pectinate
   pectineal
   Petit
   Pétrequin
   petroclinoid
   phalangeal glenoidal
   phrenicocolic
   phrenicolienal
   phrenicosplenic
   phrenoesophageal
   phrenogastric
   phrenosplenic
   pisohamate
   pisometacarpal
   pisounciform
   pisouncinate
   plantar
   plantar cuboideonavicular
   plantar cuneocuboid
   plantar cuneonavicular
   plantar metatarsal
   posterior
   posterior costotransverse
   posterior cricoarytenoid
   posterior cruciate (PCL)
   posterior longitudinal (PLL)
   posterior medial
   posterior meniscofemoral

ligament *(continued)*
  posterior oblique (POL)
  posterior occipitoaxial
  posterior sacroiliac
  posterior sacrosciatic
  posterior sternoclavicular
  posterior talofibular (PTF)
  posterior tibiofibular
  posterior tibiotalar
  Poupart inguinal
  pterygomandibular
  pterygospinal
  pterygospinous
  pubocapsular
  pubocervical
  pubofemoral
  puboprostatic
  pubovesical
  pulmonary
  quadrate
  radial collateral
  radial metacarpal
  radiate
  radiate sternocostal
  radiocarpal
  radiolunotriquetral
  radioscaphocapitate
  radioscaphoid
  radioscapholunate
  reflected inguinal
  reflecting edge of
  reflex
  reflex inguinal
  retinacular
  Retzius
  rhomboid
  right triangular
  ring
  Robert
  round
  Rouviere
  sacrodural
  sacrospinous
  sacrotuberous
  Santorini
  Sappey
  scapholunate interosseous

ligament *(continued)*
  Scarpa
  Schlemm
  serous
  sesamoid
  sesamophalangeal
  sheath
  shelving edge of Poupart
  Simonart
  Soemmerring
  sphenomandibular
  spinoglenoid
  spiral
  splenocolic
  splenorenal
  spring
  Stanley cervical
  stellate
  sternoclavicular
  sternopericardial
  stretched out
  Struthers
  stylohyoid
  stylomandibular
  stylomaxillary
  superficial dorsal sacrococcygeal
  superficial posterior sacrococcygeal
  superficial transverse metacarpal
  superficial transverse metartarsal
  superior
  superior costotransverse
  superior pubic
  superior transverse scapular
  suprascapular
  supraspinous
  suspensory
  sutural
  syndesmotic
  synovial
  talocalcaneal
  talofibular
  talonavicular
  tarsal
  tarsometatarsal
  tectoral
  temporomandibular
  Testut

ligament *(continued)*
  Teutleben
  Thompson
  thoracic OPLL (ossification of the
    posterior longitudinal ligament)
  thyroepiglottic
  thyrohyoid
  tibial collateral
  tibial sesamoid
  tibiocalcaneal
  tibiofibular
  tibionavicular
  torn meniscotibial
  transverse atlantal
  transverse carpal
  transverse crural
  transverse genicular
  transverse humeral
  transverse intertarsal
  transverse metacarpal
  transverse metatarsal
  transverse perineal
  transverse tibiofibular
  trapezoid
  Treitz
  triangular
  triquetrohamate
  Tuffier inferior
  ulnar collateral (UCL)
  ulnocarpal
  ulnolunate
  ulnotriquetral
  urachal
  venous
  ventral sacrococcygeal
  ventral sacroiliac
  ventricular
  vertebropelvic
  vestibular
  volar carpal
  Walther oblique
  Weitbrecht
  Winslow
  Wrisberg
  xiphicostal
  xiphoid

ligament *(continued)*
  Y-shaped
  Zaglas
  Zinn
ligament anchor (LA) screw
ligament augmentation device
ligament avulsion
ligament laxity
ligament-membrane junction
ligamentomuscular protective reflex
ligament reconstruction
ligamentoplasty
ligamentotaxis
ligamentous and capsular repair (LCR)
ligamentous bouncing
ligamentous box
ligamentous complex
ligamentous disruption
ligamentous impingement, ankle
ligamentous insertion
ligamentous instability
ligamentous laxity
ligamentous luxation
ligamentous-muscular hypertrophy
ligamentous release
ligamentous sprain
ligamentous strain
ligamentous support
ligamentous thickening
ligament reconstruction/tendon
  interposition (LRTI)
ligament shrinkage by laser-induced
  heat
Ligamentus Ankle orthotic
ligand, neuroreceptor
ligation, clip
ligature carrier
ligature guide
ligature, stick tie
light
  excitation
  flashes of
  flashing
  intermittent flashes of
  Knifelight surgical
  patterned

light *(continued)*
  repetitive flashes of
  stroboscopic flashes of
  white
light-bulb sign of humeral head
light conductor
lightheaded
lightheadedness
lightning-like flexion spasm of head
light source, fiberoptic
Light Talker computerized communication device
Light-Veley headrest
LIH (Lars Ingvar Hansson) hook pin
Likert scale
Lilienthal rib spreader
Liliequist membrane
lilliputian disorder of visual perception
  in migraine
LILT (low intensity laser therapy)
limb
  amputated
  congenitally short
  ischemic
  nonischemic
  posture of
limb absence
  congenital intercalary
  congenital terminal
  ischemic
  nonischemic
limb apraxia, pure
limb asymmetry
limb ataxia
limb bud
limb-girdle dystrophy
limb-girdle-trunk paresis
limb hemodynamics
limb kinetic apraxia
limb length discrepancy (LLD)
limb-lengthening operation
limb-onset ALS (amyotrophic lateral
  sclerosis)
limb paresthesia
limb-salvage surgery
limbic cortex
limbic encephalitis

limbic encephalopathy
limbic input
limbic structures
limbic system
limitation of joint motion
limited compression
limited films
limited joint motion syndrome
limited proteoglycan matrix of
  ligaments
limited view
limit, torque
limitus
  hallux (HL)
  Z-slide lengthening in hallux
limp
  antalgic
  new-onset
LINAC (linear accelerator)
  Boston
  radiosurgery
  Siemens
  stereotactic radiosurgery
  University of Florida
  Varian
Linatrix suture
Lindau-von Hippel disease
Lindeman bur
Lindeman procedure
Linder sign
Lindgren oblique osteotomy
Lindholm open surgical tendon repair
Lindholm technique
Lindorf lag screws or position screws
Lindseth modified technique
Lindvall-Stille knife
line
  AC-PC (anterior commissure-
    posterior commissure)
  anterior humeral
  anterior spinal
  anterior-posterior intercommissural
  arterial
  Beau
  bisector
  Blumensaat
  central sacral (CSL)

line *(continued)*
  Chamberlain
  dentate
  divisionary
  epiphyseal
  equipotential
  Feiss
  Fränkel's white
  fracture
  Gennari
  George
  gluteal
  growth arrest
  Harris hip
  Hawkins
  heel bisector
  Heuter
  Hilgenreiner horizontal Y
  Hilgenreiner-Pauwels
  Hilgenreiner-Perkins (H-P)
  H-P (Hilgenreiner-Perkins)
  Hueter
  intercommissural
  isodose
  isoelectric
  isopotential
  joint
  Kaplan cardinal
  Kilian
  Klein
  Köhler
  Kjellberg 1% risk
  Langer
  large-bore intravenous
  lateral joint
  lead
  lucent
  McGregor
  medial joint
  metopic suture
  Meyer
  midscapular
  midspinal
  midsternal
  Moyer
  nipple
  Nélaton

line *(continued)*
  Ogston
  orbitomeatal
  parallel pitch
  Perkins
  photon therapy beam
  plumb
  popliteal
  posterior spinal
  pubococcygeal
  radiocapitellar
  Schoemaker
  Shenton
  soleal
  spinographic
  spinolaminar
  suture
  tidemark
  trough
  Ullman
  venous
  vertebral body
  Wagner
  Wineberger
  Zahn
  zero
linear accelerator (see *LINAC*)
linear accelerator radiosurgery
linear analog pain scale
linear and depressed skull fracture
linear array
  Acuson 5 MHz
  convex
  high-density
linear artifact
linear attenuation coefficient
linear band of maximal radiolucency
linear defect
linear density
linear fracture
linear infiltrate
linear lucency
linear markings
linear percussion machine
linear phased arrays
linear regression analysis
linear scanning

linear shadow
linear skull fracture
linear tomography
Linear total hip system and hip stem
linear skull fracture
linear translation force
linebacker's arm
line imaging
liner
　acetabular
　acetabular prosthetic
　cast
　DePuy acetabular
　Duraloc acetabular
　Enduron acetabular
　Gore-Tex cast
　grommet bone
　Hylamer acetabular
　polyethylene
　Polysorb
　Spenco
line scanning
line shadow
Ling hip prosthesis
lingual airway dysfunction
lingual bone
lingual dysarthria
lingual gyrus
lingual muscle
lingual nerve
lingula
lining cells, synovial
Link cementless reconstruction hip
　prosthesis
Link Endo-Model rotational knee
　prosthesis
Link Lubinus SP II hip replacement
　system
link, musculotendinous-osseous
Link Stack Split finger splint
Linvatec driver
Linvatec instruments
lion jaw tenaculum
Lioresal (baclofen)
lip
　acetabulum
　glenoid

lip (continued)
　lateral sulcus
　navicular
　osteophytic bone
　taenia
　tibia
lipid-coated microbubbles
lipid crystals, birefringent
lipid droplets
lipidosis (pl. lipidoses)
　cerebral
　cerebroside
　galactosylceramide
　neuronal
　sphingomyelin
　sulfatide
lipid peroxidation
lipid-sensitive MR
lipid storage disease
Lipiodol (iodized poppy seed oil)
　myelographic imaging agent
liplike projections of cartilage
lipoblastoma
lipoblastomatosis
lipochondrodystrophy
lipodermatosis
lipofibroma
lipofuscinosis, neuronal ceroid
lipohemarthrosis
lipoma
　holocord intradural
　intratentorial
lipomatous neuroectodermal tumor
lipomyelomeningocele
lipophilic contrast agents
lipopolysaccharide
liposarcoma
　myxoid-type
　pleomorphic
　round cell type
liposomes, antibody-conjugated para-
　magnetic (APCLs)
lipoxygenase pathway
lipping, osteophytic
Lippman hip prosthesis
Lippman test
Lipscomb modified McKeever
　arthrodesis

lip-smacking automatism
lip-smacking, repetitive
liquid crystal contact thermography
(LCT)
Liquipake contrast medium
Lisch nodule of the iris
Lisfranc amputation
Lisfranc articulation
Lisfranc below-knee prosthesis
Lisfranc dislocation
Lisfranc fracture
Lisfranc fracture-dislocation
Lisfranc injury
Lisfranc joint
Lisfranc ligament
LISREL questionnaire
Lissauer column
Lissauer paralysis
Lissauer tracts of spinal cord
lissencephaly, cobblestone
Lister scissors
Lister technique of pulley reconstruction
Lister tubercle
Listeria monocytogenes meningitis
listhesis
listing gait
Liston amputating knife
Liston bone-cutting forceps
Liston-Key bone-cutting forceps
Liston-Key-Horsley rib shears
Liston knife
Liston-Littauer bone-cutting forceps
Liston-Littauer rongeur
Liston phalangeal knife
Liston splint
Liston-Stille bone-cutting forceps
lists to the right (or left)
LiteNest portable seating system
literal (or phonemic) paraphasia
Littauer-Liston bone-cutting forceps
Littauer-West rongeur
litter, Neal-Robertson
Little disease
Little Leaguer's elbow
Little Leaguer's shoulder

Littler-Cooley transfer of abductor
digiti quinti
Littler opponensplasty
Littler pollicization
"live flesh" (hemifacial spasm)
liver blood deficiency (Chinese medicine term)
liver fire (Chinese medicine term)
liver heat (Chinese medicine term)
Liverpool prosthesis
liver qi stagnation (Chinese medicine term)
liver wind (Chinese medicine term)
liver yang deficiency (Chinese medicine term)
liver yin deficiency (Chinese medicine term)
living
    activities of daily (ADLs)
    normal activities of daily
Livingston intramedullary bar
LLC (long leg cast)
LLD (leg [or limb] length discrepancy)
LLE (left lower extremity)
Llorente dissecting forceps
Lloyd adapter for Smith-Petersen nail
Lloyd chiropractic table
Lloyd nail driver
Lloyd-Roberts fracture technique
LLWBC (long leg weightbearing cast)
LLWC (long leg walking cast)
LM (left motor) EEG lead
LMN (lower motor neuron)
LMR (localized magnetic resonance)
LNV (last normal vertebra)
load, loading
    axial
    carbohydrate
    cyclic
    Dilantin
    long axis compression
    posterior edge
    repetitive impulse
    rotatory (on spine)
    spinal axial
    torque

load and shift test
load-bearing structure
load-sharing classification
load-transmitting capability of knee
LOAF muscles of hand
  lumbricals
  opponens pollicis
  abductor pollicis brevis
  flexor pollicis brevis
Lo Bak spinal support
Loban adhesive drape
lobar atrophy of Pick
lobe
  cuneiform
  falciform
  flocculonodular
  frontal
  insular
  medial temporal
  mesiobasal temporal
  mesiotemporal
  occipital
  parietal
  temporal
  uncus of temporal
lobectomy
  anterior lobe
  anterior temporal (ATL)
  temporal
lobe signs, parietal
lobotomy, prefrontal
lobster claw deformity
lobule
  inferior parietal
  inferior temporal
  paracentral
  parietal
LOC (level of consciousness)
local compression fracture
local standby (anesthesia) technique
Localio procedure
localization
  electrophysiological nerve lesion
  intraoperative lesion
  lesion
  point
  target

localized delta activity
localized hypertrophic mononeuropathy
localized magnetic resonance (LMR)
localized mass effect
localized muscular atrophy
localizer
  Mayfield fiducial
  Risser
localizing neurologic signs
localizing neurologic symptoms
localizing or focal neurological signs
locator, Berman
lockable arthroscopic knot
Locke clamp
locked-in state
locked-in syndrome
locked intramedullary nailing
locked knee
Locke elevator
lock, heel
locking loop suture
locking of joint
locking pliers
locking-position test
lock-stitch
Lockwood ligament
locomotion, cadence
locomotor ataxia
locomotor mechanisms
locomotor pattern
locus
  genetic
  scanning
locus ceruleus of the pons
locus niger
Locus of Control, Recovery
Lodine (etodolac)
Lodine XL (etodolac extended-release)
LO (left occipital) EEG lead
Lofstrand crutch
Logan traction
logical memory (paragraph recall) test
log, motor activity
log-rolling of patient in bed
London unconstrained elbow prosthesis
L1-APo cephalometric measurement

L1-L5 (five lumbar vertebrae)
L1-L6 intervertebral disks
L1-NB cephalometric measurement
LON (lengthening over nails)
  procedure
long abductor muscle of thumb
long axial oblique view
long axis acquisition
long axis compression loading
long axis parasternal view
long axis slice
long axis traction chiropractic table
long axis view
Long Beach stereotactic robot
long bone fracture
long buccal nerve
long bone osteomyelitis
long ciliary nerve
longette, plaster
long extensor muscle
long fibers
long fibular muscle
long flexor muscle
longissimus muscle
longitudinal arch of foot
longitudinal arteriography
longitudinal blood supply
longitudinal B-mode
longitudinal epiphyseal bracket
longitudinal fasciculus, medial (MLF)
longitudinal fissure
longitudinal fracture
longitudinal ligament
longitudinal magnetization
longitudinal muscle
longitudinal narrowing
longitudinal nerves of Lancisi
longitudinal plantar arch
longitudinal relaxation
longitudinal taenia musculature
long leg weightbearing cast (LLWBC)
long-lived
long muscle
long palmar muscle
long peroneal muscle
long plantar ligament
long radial extensor muscle of wrist

long saphenous nerve
long-standing
long subscapular nerve
long-suffering
long-term memory
long thoracic nerve palsy
long tract signs
long TR/TE (T2-weighted image)
long TR, short TE
long tract signs
longus
  extensor hallucis
  flexor hallucis (FHL)
loop (cf. *loupe*)
  figure of 8 wire
  Meyer
  Meyer-Archambault
  peduncular
  Ransford
  vessel
  Vieussens
loop-lock cock-up splint
loose associations
loose bodies of knee
loose body, osteochondritic
loose fracture
loose joint body
loosening, aseptic
Loose procedure
Looser-Milkman syndrome
Looser zones in insufficiency fractures
Lo-Por vascular graft prosthesis
lorazepam (Ativan)
lordosis
  cervical
  compensatory lumbar
  lumbar
  occipitocervical
  reversal of cervical
  thoracic
lordotic curve
lordotic position
lordotic view
Lord total hip prosthesis
Lore suction tube and tip-holding
  forceps
Lorentzian line saturation

Lorenz cast
Lorenz cranial plate
Lorenz cranial screw
Lorenz hip reduction
Lorenzo screw
Lorenz osteosynthesis system
Lorenz sign
lorry driver's fracture
LOS (Lincoln-Ogeretzky Scale) test
Losee modification of MacIntosh
    technique
loss
    axonal
    central sensory
    complete visual
    contralateral
    cortical sensory
    dense sensory
    dissociated sensory
    estimated blood (EBL)
    functional
    hemi-field
    hemisensory
    hysterical visual
    ipsilateral
    level of sensory
    mechanical functional
    monocular visual
    motor
    neuronal
    partial visual
    peripheral sensory
    saddle area sensory
    sensory
    stocking-glove sensory
    visual
loss of consciousness
loss of motion
loss of resistance injection technique
loss of sphincter control
loss of spontaneity
loss of thoracic kyphosis
loss of vision
loss, periprosthetic bone
Lottes pin
Lottes triflanged medullary nail
Lou Gehrig disease

loud bruit
Louis-Bar syndrome
Louisiana State University (LSU)
    reciprocation-gait orthosis
loupe (cf. *loop*)
    binocular
    magnification
    magnifying
Loute wire tightener
Love-Adson periosteal elevator
Love-Gruenwald alligator forceps
Love-Gruenwald intervertebral disk
    forceps
Love-Gruenwald intervertebral disk
    rongeur
Love-Gruenwald pituitary forceps
Love-Gruenwald pituitary rongeur
Love-Kerrison cervical rongeur
Love-Kerrison laminectomy rongeur
Love-Kerrison rongeur forceps
Love nerve root hook
Love nerve root retractor
Lovell clubfoot cast
lovers' paralysis
Lovett clinical scale of strength
Lovibond angle
Loving Care/Springwall chiropractic
    mattress
LoVision playing cards
low angle scattering
low-angle shot (FLASH) technique
low back pain (LBP)
Low Back Pain Symptom Checklist
low back pathology
low back spinal support (see *Lo Bak*)
low bone mass
low CSF production
low density lesion
LowDye taping technique
Lowe-Breck cartilage knife
Lowe-Breck meniscectomy knife
Lowe-Miller unconstrained elbow
    prosthesis
Lowenberg sign
low energy lasers (LELs)
lower extremity (LE)
lower extremity arterial tree

Lower Extremity Functional Scale (LEFS)
lower extremity noninvasive (LENI)
lower lateral cutaneous nerve of arm
lower lumbar root compression
lower motor neuron (LMN)
lower motor neuron disease
lower motor neuron lesion, remote
lower motor neuron paralysis
lower motor neuron sign
lower pole of patella
lower radial palsy
lowest splanchnic nerve
Lowe syndrome
low field MR angiography
low field MR imaging
low field strength magnet
low field strength MR imaging
low grade astrocytoma
low grade malignant histiocytoma
low impact aerobic dance (LIAD)
low intensity pulsed ultrasound
Lowman bone-holding clamp
Lowman bone-holding forceps
Lowman chisel
Lowman-Gerster bone clamp
Lowman hand retractor
Lowman-Hoglund bone-holding clamp
Lowman-Hoglund chisel
Lowman retractor
Lowman shelf procedure
low molecular weight heparin
Low Profile leg holder
low-reading thermometer
low resolution thermography
low signal intensity
low surface reactive bioglass joint replacement material
low tide walking brace
low voltage fast activity
LP (left parietal) EEG lead
LP (lumbar puncture)
LP (lumboperitoneal) shunt
LPCh (lateral posterior choroidal) artery
L plate
LPPS (low pressure plasma spray)

LPPS hydroxyapatite adhesive
LPT (left posterior temporal) EEG lead
L rod, Luque
LRTI (ligament reconstruction/tendon interposition)
L-selectin
L-shaped incision
L-shaped rotator cuff tear
LSI (Life Satisfaction Index)
L spine (lumbar spine)
LSO (lumbosacral orthosis)
LS (lumbosacral) spine
LSU (Louisiana State University) reciprocation-gait orthosis
LSUMC (Louisiana State University Medical College)
LSUMC classification of motor and sensory function
LSUMC classification of nerve injury
LT (lunotriquetral) joint
LTC (lateral talocalcaneal) ligament
LTTF (lateral transverse thigh flap)
Lubben scale
Lubinus knee prosthesis
lubrication
    boundary
    elastohydrodynamic
Lucae bone mallet
Lucae nerve hook
Lucas chisel
Lucas-Cottrell osteotomy
Lucas gouge
Lucas-Murray knee arthrodesis
lucency, putaminal
lucent band
lucent defect
lucent line
lucid interval, in head trauma
Luck-Bishop bone saw
Luck procedure (of hand)
Ludington test
Ludloff incision
Ludloff sign
Ludloff technique
Ludwig nerve
LUE (left upper extremity)

Luer bone rongeur
Luer-Friedman bone rongeur
Luer-Hartmann rongeur
Luer rongeur forceps
Luer-Whiting rongeur forceps
lues (syphilis)
luetic (syphilitic)
Luhr Microfixation cranial plate
Luhr Microfixation System drill bit
Luhr Microfixation System plate cutters
Luhr Microfixation System plate-holding
    forceps
Luhr Microfixation System pliers
Luhr microplate
Luhr miniplate
Luhr pan plate
Luhr plate
Luhr screw
lumbago
lumbar anterior root stimulator
    implants (LARSI)
lumbar arachnoid peritoneal shunt
lumbar component of scoliosis
lumbar drainage
lumbar epidural abscess
lumbar iliocostal muscle
lumbar interspinal muscle
lumbarization
lumbarized spine
lumbar lordosis
lumbar nerve
lumbar plexus
lumbar pneumoencephalography
lumbar puncture (LP)
lumbar puncture test
lumbar puncture traumatic tap
lumbar quadrate muscle
lumbar root compression
lumbar rotator muscles
lumbar scoliosis
lumbar spine (L1 to L5 or L6)
lumbar spine stabilization training
lumbar spine view
lumbar splanchnic nerve
lumbar spondylosis
lumbar thecoperitoneal shunt syndrome
lumbar transverse process

lumbar vertebra
lumbocostal ligament
lumbodorsal fascia
lumboinguinal nerve
lumbopelvic dysfunction
lumboperitoneal shunt
lumbosacral chordoma
lumbosacral corset
lumbosacral fusion elevator
lumbosacral joint
lumbosacral kyphosis
lumbosacral plexopathy
lumbosacral plexus
lumbosacral radiculopathy
lumbosacral series
lumbosacral spine strain
lumbosacral traction
Lumbotrain lumbosacral support
lumbrical bar
lumbrical muscle flap
lumen, residual artery
Lumex Tub-Guard safety rail
Lumina telescope
Lunar DPX densitometer
Lunar Expert densitometer
Lunar Expert XL DXA scanner
Lunar scanner
lunate bone
lunate dislocation
lunate facet
lunate fracture
lunate-triquetral coalition
lunate wrist prosthesis
lunatomalacia
Lunceford-Pilliar-Engh hip prosthesis
Lunceford total hip replacement
Lundborg epilepsy
Lundholm plate
Lundholm screw
lung heat (Chinese medicine term)
lung yang deficiency (Chinese medi-
    cine term)
lung yin deficiency (Chinese medicine
    term)
lunocapitate bone
lunocapitate joint
lunotriquetral interosseous ligament

lunotriquetral (LT) joint
lunotriquetral ligament
lunotriquetral tear
Luongo hand retractor
lupus anticoagulant
lupus-associated chorea
lupus erythematosus preparation
  (LE prep)
Luque cerclage wire
Luque fixation device
Luque-Galveston rod
Luque II fixation system
Luque instrumentation
Luque L-rod
Luque loop fixation
Luque rectangle
Luque rod fixation for kyphosis
Luque segmental fixation
Luque sublaminar wire
Luque wire (wiring)
lurch
  abductor
  gluteal
Luschka (also von Luschka)
  bursa
  foramen of
  joint of
  ligament
  muscle of
  nerve of
lusty legs of tabes dorsalis
luxated bone
luxatio erecta shoulder dislocation
luxation
  ligamentous
  palmar
luxury collateral perfusion
luxury perfusion
Luys body
Luys, subthalamic nucleus of
Lyden-Lehman technique

Lyman-Smith brace
Lyman-Smith traction
Lyme arthritis
Lyme disease complex
LYMErix
lymphadenopathy
lymphangiography
lymphedema, familial
lymphocyte, B
lymphocytic choriomeningitis viral
  encephalitis
lymphocytic meningitis
lymphocytic pleocytosis (in CSF)
lymphoepithelioma
lymphogranuloma venereum viral
  encephalitis
lymphoma
  cerebral
  intracerebral
  intracerebral Hodgkin
  intracranial Hodgkin
  malignant
  primary brain
  primary CNS (central nervous
    system)
Lynch and Crues type 2 lesion
Lynco foot orthosis
Lynn technique
Lyofoam wound dressing
lyophilized dura
lyophilized spinal dural allograft
lyophilization (freeze-drying)
Lysholm-Gillquist score
Lysholm score for knee joint instability
Lysholm test
lysosomal absorption of cartilage
lysosomal enzymes
lysozymes
lytic bone lesion
Lytle splint

M, m

Mab-170 monoclonal antibody
MacAusland lumbar brace
MacAusland procedure
MacCarthy procedure
MAC (Miami Acute Care) cervical
  collar
MacDonald dissector
MacDougall diet
maceration
Macewen-Shands osteotomy
Macewen sign
MacGregor osteotome
machine (see *device*)
MacIntosh extra-articular tenodesis
MacIntosh knee prosthesis
MacIntosh over-the-top ACL
  reconstruction
Mackenrodt ligament
MacKenty periosteal elevator
MacKenzie exercises
MacKinnon-Dellon Diskriminator
  (two-point)
MacLean-Maxwell disease
MacNab-English shoulder prosthesis
MacNichol-Voutsinas classification
Macritonin
macroabscess, epidural
macroadenoma

macrocephaly
macrodactyly
Macrofit hip prosthesis
macrographia
macrogyria
macromolecular contrast-enhanced MR
  imaging
macromolecular drugs
macrophage adhesion molecule
macropsia
macroscopic hemorrhage
macroscopic magnetization moment
macroscopic magnetization vector
Macrotec imaging agent
macrovascular disease
MACTAR Questionnaire
macular fan
macular rash
macular sparing
macular star
maculoneural bundle
"mad cow disease" (bovine spongiform encephalopathy)
Maddacrawler Crawler crawling frame
Madden dynamic splint protocol
Maddox rod test
Madelung deformity
madness, myxedema

madreporic hip prosthesis
madura foot
maduromycosis
Maffucci syndrome
MAG (transcranial magnetic
  stimulation)
Magendie, foramen of
magenta ("beefy") tongue
Magerl hook-plate fixation
Magerl screw placement technique
Magerl transarticular screw fixation
Magilligan technique for measuring
  anteversion
Magna-Fx cannulated screw fixation
  system
MagnaPod pain relief magnets
Magnassager massager
Magna-SL scanner
Magnatherm diathermy unit
MagneCore magnetic therapy pads
Magnes 2500 WH (whole head)
  imager
magnet
  doughnut
  Dyonics Golden Retriever
  GE Signa 1.5T
  high field strength
  low field strength
  Magnex
  non-enclosed
  open
  Oxford
  pancake MRI
  passively shimmed superconducting
  resistive
  shim
  shimmed
  superconducting
  2T large bore
  tubular
magnetic controlled suturing (MCS)
magnetic dipole
magnetic field
magnetic field gradients (MFG)
magnetic field therapy
magnetic gradient
magnetic induction

magnetic moment
magnetic reaction (grasp reflex)
magnetic resonance angiography
  (MRA)
magnetic resonance arthrography
magnetic resonance imaging (MRI)
  (see *MRI terms*)
magnetic resonance myelography
magnetic resonance neurography
  (MRN)
magnetic resonance phase velocity
  mapping
magnetic resonance signal
magnetic resonance spectroscopy
  (MRS)
magnetic resonance spectrum
magnetic resonance velocity mapping
magnetic source imaging (MSI)
magnetic stimulation
Magnetic Support brace
magnetic susceptibility
magnetization
magnetization-prepared 3D gradient-
  echo (MP-RAGE) sequences
magnetization-prepared rapid gradient
  echo-water excitation
  (MRPRAGE-WE)
magnetoencephalogram (MEG)
magnetoencephalography (MEG)
Magnetom 1.5T scanner
Magnetom Open MRI
Magnetom SP MRI imager
Magnetom Vision MR system
Magnevist imaging agent
Magnex Alpha MR system
magnification, loupe
magnifying loupe
magnum, foramen
Magnum 800 bed
Magnuson-Stack shoulder arthrotomy
Ma-Griffith end-to-end anastomosis
Ma-Griffith repair of ruptured Achilles
  tendon
Ma-Griffith tendon anastomosis
main en griffe (clawhand)
maintenance of bone plate integrity
Maison retractor

Maisonneuve fibular fracture
Maisonneuve sign
Maissiat ligament
Maitland mobilization/manipulation
Majestro-Ruda-Frost tendon technique
major causalgia
major cystic malformation
major fracture fragment
major motor fit
major motor seizure
major sprain
Makar instruments/devices
Malacarne antrum
malacoplakia
malaise
malalignment syndrome
malangulation
malar bone
malar fracture
malaria
   cerebellar
   cerebral
Malawer excision technique
Malaysia, latah of
Malcolm-Lynn C-RXF cervical
   retractor frame
maldevelopment
maldirection
malformation
   angiographically occult vascular
      (AOVM)
   angiographically visualized vascular
      (AVVM)
   Arnold-Chiari
   arteriovenous (AVM)
   cavernous
   cerebral arteriovenous
   Chiari
   cryptic arteriovenous
   cryptic vascular (CVM)
   deep-seated arteriovenous
   dural arteriovenous
   dural venous
   familial arteriovenous
   glomus arteriovenous
   glomus-type arteriovenous
   infratentorial arteriovenous

malformation *(continued)*
   intermedullary cavernous
   intracranial
   juvenile arteriovenous
   major cystic
   medullary venous (MVM)
   retromedullary arteriovenous
   Spetzler-Martin classification of
      arteriovenous
   spinal vascular
   supratentorial arteriovenous
   venous
   Wyburn-Mason arteriovenous
malfunction, shunt
Malgaigne pelvic fracture
malignant acetabular osteolysis
malignant eccrine poroma
malignant glioma
malignant hyperthermia
malignant melanoma, plantar
malignant osteoid
malignant osteopetrosis
malignant perineuroma
malignant peripheral nerve sheath
   tumor (MPNST)
mal, impulsive petit
malingering
Malis angled-up bipolar forceps
Malis bipolar cautery forceps
Malis bipolar cautery scissors
Malis brain retractor
Malis CMC-II bipolar coagulator
Malis curet
Malis dissector
Malis elevator
Malis irrigation forceps
Malis-Jensen micro bipolar forceps
Malis jeweler bipolar forceps
Malis ligature passer
Malis needle holders
Malis nerve hook
Malis neurological scissors
Malis vessel supporter
malleable metal finger splints
malleable template
malleable thermal probe
malleolar torsion

Malleoloc ankle support
malleolus (pl. malleoli)
  collicular fracture of the medial
  fibular
  lateral
  medial
  tibial
Malleotrain supports and braces
mallet (see also *hammer*)
  Acufex
  Bergman
  bone
  boxwood
  cervical
  copper
  Cottle
  Crane
  Doyen bone
  Gerzog bone
  Hajek
  Heath
  Henning
  Hibbs
  Kirk
  lead-filled
  Lucae bone
  Mead
  Meyerding
  Miltex
  Ombredanne
  Ralks
  Richards
  Rush
  slotted
  Steinbach
  Surgical No Bounce
  Swanson
  Williger bone
  Wolfe-Boehler
mallet deformity
mallet finger
mallet fracture
mallet toes
malleus
Mallory-Head femoral stem
Mallory-Head rasp
Mallory-Head revision operation

Mallory-Head total hip prosthesis
Mally index
Malmö hip splint
mal perforant diabetic ulcer
malreduction of fracture
malrotation, axial
Maltz cartilage knife
Maltz rasp
malum coxae senile
malunion of fracture fragments
malunited
malversion
mamillary body
mamillary suture
mammalian cell product
management, pain
mandible (pl. mandibula)
mandibular angle
mandibular canal
mandibular fracture
mandibular nerve
mandibular notch
mandibulofacial dysostosis
maneuver (see also *reflex*; *sign*; *test*)
  Adson
  Adson modified
  alerting
  Allen
  Bárány-Nylen
  Barlow
  canalith repositioning
  circumduction
  closed manipulative
  costoclavicular
  Dandy
  Dix-Hallpike
  doll's head
  Epley
  eye opening and closing
  flexion-extension
  flexion-rotation-compression
  Foster-Kennedy
  Fowler
  Gowers
  Hippocratic
  hyperabduction
  Jendrassik

maneuver *(continued)*
   Kocher
   Lachman
   Leadbetter
   McMurray circumduction
   Meyn and Quigley
   Ortolani
   osteoclasis
   particle repositioning
   Parvin
   Phalen
   postural fixation back
   provocative
   rotation compression
   Schreiber
   Slocum
   Spurling
   Stimson
   tripoding
   Valsalva
   vestibulo-ocular
   Walton
manganese intoxication
manganese poisoning
Mangled Extremity Severity Score
   (MESS)
mania
   dancing (choreomania)
   epileptic
manifestation, clinical seizure
manipulate
manipulation
   back
   chiropractic joint
   fine
   gross
   Hippocrates
   Maitland
   medical (versus chiropractic)
   opening wedge
manipulation of articulations and
   adjacent tissues
manipulation under anesthesia (MUA)
manipulation with distraction, bifocal
manipulative procedures (adjustments)
Mankin scoring technique
Manktelow transfer procedure

Mann-Coughlin arthrodesis
Mann-Coughlin-DuVries cheilectomy
Mann-DuVries arthroplasty
mannerism, speech
Mann modified McKeever arthrodesis
Mann resection arthroplasty
Mann-Thompson-Coughlin arthrodesis
Mann-Whitney U test
manometer
manometric test
Manske technique
Mantel-Haenszel Chi-square test
mantle
   brain
   cement
   cerebral
   shunted
Mantoux test
manual dexterity
manual manipulation of spine,
   chiropractic
manual muscle test
manual percussion test
manual reduction
manual traction test for cervical
   radiculitis
manubriosternal joint
manubriosternal syndrome
manubrium
Manutrain active wrist support
map, mapping
   behavioral
   brain electrical activity (BEAM)
   cerebral sulci
   cortical
   Doppler color flow
   electrophysiologic
   evoked potential (EP)
   FMRI
   frequency domain
   functional
   language
   microelectrode
   motor cortex
   MRI
   MR velocity
   statistical

map *(continued)*
   time domain
   topographic
MAPF femoral stem
maple syrup urine disease (MSUD)
mapping of apraxia, cerebral
mapping of cortical function
mapping of language areas of brain
mapping the defect
Maquet procedure
marathoner's toe
marble bones
Marcacci muscle
Marcain
march
   epileptic
   focal motor sign with/without
      jacksonian (motor)
march foot
march fracture
march of cranial nerve palsy
march of scotoma
march of sensory deficit
Marchand-Waterhouse syndrome
Marchiafava-Bignami disease
Marchiafava-Bignami syndrome
marching band injury
Marcus-Balourdas-Heiple ankle fusion
   technique
Marcus grading scale for avascular
   necrosis
Marcus Gunn pupils
Marex MRI system
marfanoid hypermobility syndrome
Marfan syndrome
margin
   blurring of disk
   cortical
   disk
   orbital
   scapular
   tumor
marginal exostosis
marginal osteophyte formation
marginal sinus
marginal spur
margo

Marie ataxia
Marie-Bamberger disease
Marie-Charcot-Tooth disease
Marie-Foix sign
Marie hereditary spastic ataxia
Marie quadrilateral space
Marie sign
Marie-Strümpell disease
Marie-Strümpell spondylitis
Marie-Tooth disease
marimastat
Marin-Amat phenomenon
Marinesco-Sjögren syndrome
Marino transsphenoidal curet
Marino transsphenoidal dissector
Marino transsphenoidal enucleator
Marino transsphenoidal hook
Marin reamer
Marion screw
Markell Mobility Healing Clogs
Markell Mobility Shoes
Markell open-toe shoes
Markell tarso medius straight shoe
Markell tarso pronator outflare shoe
marker
   fiducial
   interspace width
   microsatellite
   osteolysis urine
   reflective
   Schoemaker-Burkart
   skin
   T cell surface
   tumor
Markham-Meyerding hemilaminectomy
   retractor
Marks-Bayne technique for thumb
   duplication
Mark VII cooling vest
Mark II CCMI (custom contour
   measuring instrument)
Mark II Chandler retractor
Mark II distal femur retractor
Mark II Kodros radiolucent awl
Mark II lateral collateral ligament
Mark II PCL retractor
Mark II S knee retractor

Mark II Sorrells hip arthroplasty
   retraction system
Mark II Stulberg hip positioner
Mark II Wixson hip positioner
Mark II Z knee retractor
Markwalder bone rongeur
Markwalder rib forceps
Markwort ankle support
Marmor modular knee prosthesis
Marmor replacement
marmoratus, status
Marn drill
Maroon-Jannetta dissector
Maroteaux-Lamy syndrome
Marquardt bone rongeur
marrow
   bone
   ectopic
   Graton bone matrix/marrow
      combination
   pluripotential
   red
   yellow
marrow cavity
marrow space, hyperintense
marrow stimulation technique
MARS (Modular Acetabular Revision
   System)
Marshall knee score
Marshall ligament repair technique
marshmallows
marsupialization
Martin cartilage chisel
Martin cartilage clamp
Martin cartilage forceps
Martin cartilage scissors
Martin diamond wire cutter
Martin disease
Martin-Gruber anastomosis
Martin-Gruber connection
Martini bone curet
Martin muscle clamp
Martin nerve root retractor
Martin patellar wiring technique
Martin retractor
Martin scissors

Martin Vigorimeter
Martorell aortic arch syndrome
Marval test
Marx protocol for treatment of osteoradionecrosis
Maryland Foot Score Profile
MAS (Motor Assessment scale)
masked facies of parkinsonism
masked gout
mask facies
mask, ISAH stereotactic immobilizing
Mason-Allen universal splint
Mason fracture classification system
Mason suction tube
mass (see also *lesion*)
   apperceptive
   cerebellar
   echogenic
   enhancing
   epidural
   expanding intracranial
   fat-free (body) (FFM)
   fibrin
   fluctuant
   focal
   hemispheral
   high density
   intermediate
   isodense
   lateral
   lean
   low density
   osteocartilaginous
   parasagittal intracranial
   parasellar
   paraspinal soft tissue
   posterior fossa brain
   presacral
   sellar
   signal lentiform
   soft tissue
   space-occupying
   suprasellar
   supratentorial
   well-demarcated
   well-encapsulated

massage
  deep
  effleurage
  ice
  Ohashiatsu
  Silhouette therapeutic
massager
  Body Sticks
  Equalizer Pro
  Flex-Node AcuVibe
  G5 Fleximatic massager/percussor
  G5 ProPower
  Infratonic electro-acoustical
  Intracell trigger point
  Ironman Triathlon Pro-Power
  Magnassager
  Morfam Quality Jeanie Rub
  Omni Roller
  Original Index Knobber II
  Original Jacknobber II trigger point
  Power Node AcuVibe
  Power Pillow cervical
  Reach Easy
  Scrip Muscle Master
  T-Bar trigger point
  Thera Cane trigger point
mass casualty accident (MCA)
mass effect of tumor
masseteric nerve
masseter muscle
masseter-temporalis stretch reflex
Massie sliding nail
mass lesion
mass limb reflex
mass motor reflex response
Masson fasciatome
Masson-Fontana stain
Masson-Goldner trichrome stain
Masson trichrome stain
Masson vegetant intravascular
  hemangioendothelioma
MAST (medical [or military] anti-
  shock trousers) pressure trousers
master knot of Henry
Masterstim chiropractic therapy
  system
Masterstim Micro therapy system

masticator nerve
masticatory attack
Mastin muscle clamp
mastocytosis, systemic
mastoid bone
mastoid notch
mat
  Harris and Beath footprint
  silicone
Matchett-Brown internal prosthesis
matchsticked
mater
  dura
  pia
material
  Adcon L Adhesion Control barrier
    gel
  alpha-BSM bone repair
  ArthroSorb solidifier
  bioceramic joint replacement
  Bio Skin
  bone replacement
  Collagraft bone graft matrix
  composite autologous
  DuraGen dural graft matrix
  Embarc bone repair
  Evazote foam
  extraneous
  flexible splinting
  Grafton demineralized bone matrix
    putty
  Hemaseel HMN tissue glue
  LactoSorb orthopedic wound
  Leibinger Micro Dynamic mesh
  nidus of embolic
  PerioGlas bone graft
  Plastazote foam
  Plasti-Pore prosthetic
  PLLA (poly L-lactic acid)
  poly L-lactic acid (PLLA) coating
  Polysplint A flexible splinting
  Porocoat prosthetic
  porous prosthetic
  Pro Osteon 500 bone graft
  Proplast prosthetic
  splinting
  Synergy flexible splinting

material *(continued)*
　SRS injectable cement
　Supazote foam
　SynMesh titanium mesh
　Tisseel fibrin sealant
　tophaceous
maternal CSF shunt dependency
Maternal Kradle support
Mathews drill points
Mathieu rasp
Mathys prosthesis
matricectomy, phenol
matrix (pl. matrices)
　bone
　cartilage
　chondroid
　collagen
　demineralized bone
　DuraGen dural graft
　extracellular
　germinal
　Graton bone matrix/marrow
　nail
　tumor
matrix injury
matrix integration
Matrix LR3300 laser imaging
matrix metalloproteinase-1 (MMP-1)
　to tissue inhibitor of metallo-
　proteinase-I (TIMP-1) ratio
Matroc femoral head
Matsen method
Matson-Alexander rib elevator
matter
　central gray
　cortical gray
　dorsal gray
　gray
　long spinal white
　midbrain
　periventricular white
　PVG (periventricular gray)
　subcortical white
　white
matte stem
Matthew cross-leg clamp
Matti-Russe technique

Mattis Dementia Rating Scale
mattress
　air
　Akros extended care
　Akros pressure
　alternating pressure
　chiropractic
　Clinisert
　Eggcrate
　eggcrate foam
　foam
　KinAir flotation
　Lapidus alternating air pressure
　Loving Care/Springwall chiro-
　　practic
　pressure
mattress suture
maturation
　disk
　electrographic
maturation index
maturers, late
maturity, skeletal
Mauchart ligament
Mauck procedure
Maxalt (rizatriptan benzoate)
MaxCast casting tape
Max FiberScan laser system
Maxicam (isoxicam)
Maxidriver
Maxilift Combi patient-lifting system
maxilla
maxillary fracture
maxillary nerve
maxillary sinus
maxillary spine
maximal assist
maximal cervical compression test
maximal effort key pinch stress
Maxima II TENS unit
Maxon suture
Max Plus MR scanner
Maxwell 3D Field Simulator
May anatomical bone plates
Mayfield/ACCISS stereotactic work-
　station
Mayfield three-pin skull clamp

Mayeda shelf
Mayer reflex
Mayer splint
Mayfield adaptor
Mayfield aneurysm clips
Mayfield brain spatula
Mayfield cranial aneurysm set
Mayfield curet
Mayfield fixation frame
Mayfield forceps
Mayfield head holder
Mayfield horseshoe headrest
Mayfield incision
Mayfield-Kees headrest
Mayfield-Larsen table
Mayfield miniature clip applier
Mayfield neurosurgical headrest
Mayfield neurosurgical skull clamp
Mayfield pinion
Mayfield rongeur
Mayfield skull clamp pin
Mayfield skull-pin head holder
Mayfield spinal curet
Mayfield temporary aneurysm clip
   applier
Mayfield tic headrest
Mayfield tongs
Mayo ankle arthroplasty
Mayo ankle prosthesis
Mayo block anesthesia
Mayo bunionectomy
Mayo classification of elbow fracture
Mayo Clinic stereotactic robot
Mayo-Collins retractor
Mayo Elbow Performance Index
   (MEPI)
Mayo hallux valgus operation
Mayo-Hegar needle holder
Mayo metatarsal head resection
Mayo resection arthroplasty
Mayo rigid cervical collar
Mayo scissors
Mayo semiconstrained elbow prosthesis
Mayo Thomas collar
Mayo wrist score
May-White syndrome

Mazas totally constrained elbow
   prosthesis
Mazet technique
mazindol (Sanorex)
Mazur ankle evaluation system
Mazur ankle fusion grading system
Mazur ankle rating system
MB&J knee positioner
MBK mobile-bearing knee implant
MBq (megabecquerel)
M-Brace knee brace
MCA (mass casualty accident)
MCA (middle cerebral artery)
MCA (motorcycle accident)
McArdle disease
McArdle syndrome
MCAT (modular coded aperture tech-
   nology) collimator
McAtee-Tharias-Blazina arthroplasty
McBride bunionectomy
McBride femoral prosthesis
McBride hallux valgus reduction
McCabe-Farrior rasp
McCain TMJ arthroscopic system
McCarroll-Baker procedure
McCash hand surgery
McCauley foot procedure
McClintoch brace
McCollough internal tibial torsion
   brace
McConnell capsular artery
McConnell taping of knee
McCune-Albright syndrome
McCutchen press-fit titanium femoral
   implant
McCutchen SLT hip prosthesis
McDavid ankle guard
McDavid hinged knee guard
McDermott-Scranton classification
   system
McDonald bone plates
McDowell Impairment Index (MII)
McElfresh-Dobyns-O'Brien technique
McElroy curet
McElroy instrumentation
McElvenny foot procedure

McFadden temporary aneurysm clips
McFarland-Osborne technique
McGee-Priest wire forceps
McGee splint
McGee wire-crimping forceps
McGill-Melzack scoring system
McGill neurological percussor
McGill Pain Questionnaire (MPQ)
McGlamry elevator
McGowan scale
McGregor line
McIndoe bone rongeur
McIndoe rongeur forceps
McIndoe scissors
McIntire splint
McIntosh test
McKay-Simons clubfoot operation
McKay-Simons CSR (complete subtalar release) operation
McKee-Farrar acetabular cup
McKee-Farrar cartilage knife
McKee-Farrar total hip arthroplasty
McKee totally constrained elbow prosthesis
McKeever arthrodesis for hallux limitus
McKeever-Buck elbow technique
McKeever cartilage knife
McKeever metatarsophalangeal fusion
McKeever Vitallium knee prosthesis
McKenzie brain clip forceps
McKenzie clip-applying forceps
McKenzie clip-bending forceps
McKenzie clip-introducing forceps
McKenzie enlarging bur
McKenzie exercises
McKenzie forceps
McKenzie hemostasis clip
McKenzie perforating twist drill
McKenzie reservoir
McKenzie silver clip
McKittrick transmetatarsal amputation
MCL (medial collateral ligament)
McLain-Weinstein classification of spinal tumors
McLaughlin-Hay technique
McLaughlin intertrochanteric plate

McLaughlin modification of Bunnell pullout suture
McLaughlin muscle to humeral defect transfer
McLaughlin nail
McLaughlin osteosynthesis apparatus
McLaughlin plate
McLaughlin screw
McLeod splint
McMaster bone graft
McMaster Health Index Questionnaire
McMurray maneuver
McMurray osteotomy
McMurray sign
McMurray test
McMurtry, kinematic indices of
McNaught keel
McNemar symmetry test
MCP (metacarpophalangeal) joint
MCR (midcarpal radial) portal
McReynolds driver-extractor
McReynolds open reduction technique
MCRF (microfractured) lesions
MCTC (metrizamide CT cisterno-gram)
MCTD (mixed connective tissue disease)
MCU (midcarpal ulnar) portal
MC walker brace
McWhorter shoulder approach
MD (muscular dystrophy)
MDA (Muscular Dystrophy Association)
MDAC (Muscular Dystrophy Association of Canada)
MDP ^{99m}Tc-methylene diphosphonate for bone scanning
Mead bone rongeur
Mead mallet
Mead periosteal elevator
Mead rongeur
mean flow velocity
mean maximal compression
Mears sacroiliac plate
Meary metatarsotalar angle
measles viral encephalitis

measure, measurement
  ANB cephalometric
  anthropometric
  APACHE II measure of disease
    severity
  attenuation
  Functional Independence (FIM)
  Canadian Occupational Perform-
    ance Measure
  cerebrospinal fluid flow
  FMA cephalometric
  foot-fall
  foot pressure
  F wave
  global m. of disability
  IMPA cephalometric
  impairment-based
  instrumental ADL
  interburst interval
  L1-APo cephalometric
  L1-NB cephalometric
  low energy photon attenuation
  minimum joint space (MJS)
  modified self-report measure of
    social adjustment
  motor
  NPo-FH cephalometric
  roof arc
  Schober
  SISI (short increments sensitivity
    index)
  skin fluorescence
  SNA cephalometric
  SNB cephalometric
  SN-MPA cephalometric
  SN tissue pressure
  torque
  true ratio
  U1-L1 cephalometric
  U1-NA cephalometric
  Wits cephalometric
  xenon washout technique
measurement of minimum joint space
  (MJS)
measurer
  Bunnell digital exertion
  digital exertion

measures of disability
mecaserim (Myotrophin)
mechanical disruption of thrombosis
mechanical distraction
mechanical functional loss
mechanical insult to spine
mechanics, body
mechanism
  Adjustable Leg and Ankle
    Repositioning
  antidromic vasodilator
  central extensor (CEM)
  concavity-compression
  extensor
  extensor hood
  flexor
  humeral
  locomotor
  Midas Rex (MB)
  pain
  plantar fascia as windlass
  quadriceps
  screw-home
  swallowing
  tendo Achillis
  terminal extensor (TEM)
  triggering
  video fluoroscopy of swallowing
  windlass
mechanism of injury (MOI)
mechanoreceptor
  Pacinian
  Ruffini
Meckel cave
Meckel cavity
Meckel ligament
Mecring acetabular prosthesis
MED (microendoscopic diskectomy)
Medasonics transcranial Doppler
Medasonic Vasculab photoplethysmograph
media (see *imaging agents*)
medial antebrachial cutaneous nerve
medial anterior thoracic nerve
medial arcuate ligament
medial brachial cutaneous nerve
medial calcaneal tubercle

medial collateral ligament
medial column calcaneal fracture
medial compartment
medial compartment loading
medial compressive force
medial cutaneous nerve
medial displacement calcaneal
 osteotomy
medial dorsal cutaneous nerve
medial eminence
medial facial spasm of Meige
medial faciotomy
medial femoral condyle
medial genuarthritis
medial gonarthrosis
medial great muscle
medial heel wedge shoe modification
medial intermuscular septum
medialization
medial joint line pain
medial ligament
medial lumbar intertransverse muscles
medially
medial longitudinal fasciculus (MLF)
 lesion
medial longitudinal fasciculus
 syndrome
medial malleolar fracture
medial malleolus
medial meniscus
medial metatarsal drift
medial nucleus, dorsal
medial occipitotemporal gyrus
medial palpebral ligament
medial pectoral nerve
medial physis
medial plantar nerve
medial popliteal nerve
medial pterygoid muscle
medial puboprostatic ligament
medial quadriceps advancement
medial rectus muscle
medial shelf
medial sole-wedge shoe modification
medial supraclavicular nerve
medial sural cutaneous nerve

medial talocalcaneal ligament
medial tibial stress syndrome (MTSS)
medial ulnar collateral ligment
 (MUCL)
medial umbilical ligament
medial vastus muscle
medial V-Y capsulotomy
median arcuate ligament
median atlantoaxial joint
median fissure, anterior
median nerve
median nerve compression
median nerve disorder
median nerve lesion
median nerve somatosensory evoked
 potential (M-SSEP)
median nucleus of Perlia
median parapatellar approach
median sacral artery
MedicAlert ID bracelets
medical linear accelerator
medical manipulation (versus
 chiropractic)
medical [or military] antishock
 trousers (MAST)
Medical Outcome Scale
Medical Research Council (MRC)
 classification of muscle function
Medicare
medications (see also *drugs; imaging
 agents*)
abciximab
ABLC (amphotericin B lipid
 complex)
Abrodil (methiodal sodium)
absolute alcohol
acecarbromal
acetaminophen
acetazolamide
acetazolamide sodium
acetic acid
acetylcarbromal (acecarbromal)
acetylcholine chloride
acetylcysteine
acetylcysteine sodium
acetyl-L-carnitine (Alcar)

medications *(continued)*

    acetylsalicylic acid (ASA; aspirin)
    ACTH (adrenocorticotropic
        hormone; corticotropin)
    Actonel (risedronate)
    Adalat (nifedipine)
    Adapin (doxepin HCl)
    adrenocorticotropic hormone
        (ACTH; corticotropin)
    Adriamycin (doxorubicin)
    Advil (ibuprofen)
    Aggrenox (dipyridamole/aspirin)
    A-hydroCort (hydrocortisone
        sodium succinate)
    AIT-082 (Neotrofin)
    Akineton (biperiden lactate)
    Alcar (acetyl-L-carnitine)
    alendronate (Fosamax)
    alfacalcidol (One-Alpha)
    alfa interferon
    alginate-collagen gel
    Alkphase-B
    allopurinol
    Alpha Chymar (chymotrypsin)
    alpha-chymotrypsin (chymotrypsin)
    alpha-galactosidase A
    alpha-BSM bone repair material
    alpha tocopherol
    alprazolam
    alteplase (Activase)
    aluminum chloride solution
    Alurate (aprobarbital)
    Alzene
    amantadine HCl
    ambenonium chloride
    Ambien (zolpidem tartrate)
    A-methaPred (methylprednisolone
        sodium succinate)
    Amicar (aminocaproic acid)
    Amigesic (salsalate)
    aminobenzoate sodium
    aminocaproic acid (Amicar)
    4-aminopyridine (4-AP)
    amiprilose hydrochloride
        (Therafectin)
    amitriptyline HCl (Elavil)
    AMI 227

medications *(continued)*

    amobarbital (Amytal)
    amobarbital sodium (Amytal
        Sodium)
    amoxapine
    amoxicillin
    ampakine CX-516
    Ampalex (CX516)
    amphetamine
    amphetamine aspartate
    amphetamine complex
    amphetamine sulfate
    amphotericin B lipid complex
        (ABLC)
    ampicillin
    Amytal (amobarbital)
    Amytal Sodium (amobarbital
        sodium)
    Anacin (aspirin, caffeine)
    Anacin-3 (acetaminophen)
    Anaprox DS (naproxen sodium)
    Ancef (cefazolin sodium)
    ancrod
    AnervaX
    Anexsia (hydrocodone bitartrate,
        acetaminophen)
    Anodynos (aspirin, salicylamide,
        caffeine)
    Anodynos DHC (hydrocodone
        bitartrate, acetaminophen)
    Ansaid (flurbiprofen)
    Antegren
    antiepilepsirine
    Antilirium (physostigmine
        salicylate)
    antipyrine
    antiresorptive
    Antivert (meclizine)
    Anturane (sulfinpyrazone)
    aprobarbital (Alurate)
    aprotinin
    Arava (leflunomide)
    Arduan (pipecuronium)
    arecholine hydrobromide
    Aredia (pamidronate disodium)
    Aricept (donepezil Hcl)
    Aristocort (triamcinolone acetonide)

medications *(continued)*

Aristospan (triamcinolone
  hexacetonide)
Armacodone
Artane (trihexyphenidyl HCl)
Artha-G (salsalate)
Arth-Aid (capsaicin/aloe)
Arthropan (choline salicylate)
Arthrotec (diclofenac sodium and
  misoprostol)
Arvin (ancrod)
ASA (acetylsalicylic acid; aspirin)
A.S.A. Enseals (aspirin)
ascorbic acid (vitamin C)
Ascriptin (buffered aspirin)
Ascriptin A/D (buffered aspirin)
ASD (azaspirodecanediones)
aspirin
Asproject (sodium thiosalicylate)
atenolol
Ativan (lorazepam)
atracurium besylate
Atromid (clofibrate)
atropine
atropine sulfate
auranofin
Aurorix (moclobemide)
aurothioglucose
Aurum
Avan (idebenone)
Aventyl (nortriptyline HCl)
Aviva (linopridine)
Avonex (interferon-1a)
Axotal (aspirin, butalbital)
azathioprine
Azdone (hydrocodone bitartrate,
  aspirin)
Azolid (phenylbutazone)
baclofen (Lioresal)
Bancap (acetaminophen caffeine,
  butalbital)
Bayer Aspirin
belladonna extract
Bellergal-S (belladonna extract,
  phenobarbital, ergotamine
  tartrate)

medications *(continued)*

Benadryl (diphenhydramine)
Benefen (ibuprofen topical gel)
BeneJoint (capsaicin, glucosamine,
  chondroitin sulfate)
Benemid (probenecid)
benztropine mesylate
besipirdine hydrochloride
Betadine (povidone-iodine)
beta interferon
betamethasone
Betaseron (interferon-1b)
Biofreeze with ILEX pain-relieving
  gel
Bioglass (calcium salts, phosphorus, sodium salts, silicon)
biperiden
biperiden lactate
Biphetamine (dextroamphetamine,
  amphetamine)
Blocadren (timolol maleate)
Bonefos (disodium clodronate
  tetrahydrate)
Botox (botulinum A toxin)
botulinum A toxin (Botox)
botulinum B toxin (Neurobloc)
bovine myelin (Myloral)
bromocriptine mesylate
bromodeoxyuridine
Brompton cocktail
Broxine (broxuridine)
broxuridine (Broxine)
buffered aspirin (Bufferin)
Bufferin (buffered aspirin)
bupivacaine HCl
Buprenex (buprenorphine HCl)
buprenorphine HCl
bupropion HCl
butabarbital (Butalan)
butabarbital sodium
Butalan (butabarbital sodium)
butalbital
Butazolidin (phenylbutazone)
Buticaps (butabarbital sodium)
Butisol Sodium (butabarbital sodium)
butorphanol tartrate

medications *(continued)*
  Cafergot (ergotamine tartrate,
    caffeine, belladonna extract,
    pentobarbital)
  caffeine
  Calan (verapamil HCl)
  Calcimar (calcitonin salmon)
  calcitonin salmon (Calcimar)
  calcitriol
  calcium gluconate
  calcium pyrophosphate
  Cama (buffered aspirin)
  cantharidin
  Cantharone (cantharidin)
  carbamazepine (Tegretol)
  carbidopa
  Cardizem (diltiazem HCl)
  carisoprodol
  carprofen
  Cataflam (diclofenac potassium)
  CCD 1042 (ganaxolone)
  cefazolin sodium
  cefotaxime (Claforan)
  ceftriaxone (Rocephin)
  Celebrex (celecoxib)
  celecoxib (Celebrex)
  Celestone (betamethisone)
  CellCept (mycophenolate, mofetil)
  Celontin Kapseals (methsuximide)
  Centrax (prazepam)
  cephalexin
  CerAxon (citicoline sodium)
  Cerebyx (fosphenytoin)
  Ceresine (CPC-211)
  Ceretec (technetium 99m)
  Cervene
  chloral hydrate
  chloramphenicol
  chlordiazepoxide
  chlordiazepoxide HCl
  chlorphenesin carbamate
  chlorpromazine
  chlorzoxazone
  choline magnesium trisalicylate
    (choline salicylate, magnesium
    salicylate)
  choline salicylate

medications *(continued)*
  chondroitin
  Chymodiactin (chymopapain)
  chymopapain
  chymotrypsin
  Cibacalcin (calcitonin)
  cisatracurium (Nimbex)
  citalopram
  citicoline sodium (CerAxon)
  Claforan (cefotaxime)
  clenoliximab
  clindamycin
  Clinoril (sulindac)
  clobazam
  clofibrate
  clomipramine HCl
  clonazepam
  clopidogrel bisulfate (Plavix)
  clorazepate dipotassium
  clorazepate monopotassium
  clotrimazole
  clozapine
  Clozaril (clozapine)
  Co-Gesic (hydrocodone bitartrate,
    acetaminophen)
  Codalan No. 1 (or 2 or 3) (codeine
    phosphate, acetaminophen,
    aspirin, caffeine)
  codeine
  codeine phosphate
  Cogentin (benztropine mesylate)
  Cognex (tacrine HCl)
  ColBenemid (probenecid,
    colchicine)
  colchicine
  collagen type 2 (Colloral)
  Colloral (collagen type 2)
  combretastatin A-4
  commercial dry ice
  Compassia (dronabinol)
  Compoz (diphenhydramine HCl)
  Comtan (entacapone)
  Contantokin-G (Con-G)
  Copaxone (glatiramer acetate)
  Cope (aspirin, caffeine, magnesium
    hydroxide, aluminum
    hydroxide)

medications *(continued)*
COP 1 (copolymer 1)
Cordase (injectable collagenase)
Cordox (CPC-111)
Corgard (nadolol)
Cortef (hydrocortisone)
corticosteroid
corticotropin
cortisone acetate
Cortone Acetate (cortisone acetate)
Cosamine DS (glucosamine, chondroitin, manganese)
COX-2 (cyclo-oxygenase-2) inhibitor
CPC-111 (Cordox)
CPC-211 (Ceresine)
Cuprimine (penicillamine)
curare (tubocurarine chloride)
cyclobenzaprine HCl
cyclophosphamide (Cytoxan)
cycloserine
cyclosporine
cytarabine liposomal injection (DepoCyt)
Cylert (pemoline)
cyproheptadine HCl
Cytotec (misoprostol)
Cytoxan (cyclophosphamide)
D-penicillamine
D.H.E. 45 (dihydroergotamine mesylate)
Dalgan (dezocine)
Dalmane (flurazepam HCl)
danaproid
Dantrium (dantrolene sodium)
dantrolene sodium
Darvon Compound-65 Pulvules (propoxyphene HCl, aspirin, caffeine)
Darvon Pulvules (propoxyphene HCl)
Darvon with A.S.A. Pulvules (propoxyphene HCl, aspirin)
Darvon-N (propoxyphene napsylate)
Dasin (aspirin, caffeine, atropine sulfate, ipecac)

medications *(continued)*
Datril (acetaminophen)
Daypro (oxaprozin)
DDAVP (deamino-D-arginine-vasopressin; desmopressin acetate)
Decadron (dexamethasone)
Delta-Cortef (prednisolone)
Deltasone (prednisone)
Demerol HCl (meperidine HCl)
Depacon (valproate sodium injection)
DepoCyt (cytarabine liposomal injection)
Depakene (valproic acid)
Depakote Sprinkles (divalproex sodium)
Depo-Medrol (methylprednisolone acetate)
deprenyl (selegiline HCl)
desipramine HCl
desmopressin acetate (DDAVP)
desflurane
Desoxyn (methamphetamine HCl)
desoxyribonuclease
Desyrel (trazodone)
dexamethasone
dexanabinol (HU-211)
Dexedrine (dextroamphetamine sulfate)
dextroamphetamine
dextroamphetamine saccharate
dextroamphetamine sulfate
dezocine
DHE (dihydroergotamine)
Diamox (acetazolamide sodium)
Diastat (diazepam rectal gel)
diazepam (Valium)
diaziquone
diclofenac (Pennsaid)
diclofenac potassium (Cataflam)
diclofenac sodium (Voltaren)
diclofenac sodium and misoprostol (Arthrotec)
dichloralphenazone (chloral hydrate, phenazone)
Didronel (etidronate disodium)

medications *(continued)*
diflunisal (Dolobid)
dihydrocodeine bitartrate
dihydroergotamine (DHE) mesylate
  nasal spray (Migranal)
dihydroxycholecalciferol
  (calcitonin)
dihydroxyphenylalanine (DOPA)
Dilantin (phenytoin sodium)
Dilantin Infatabs (phenytoin)
Dilaudid (hydromorphone HCl)
diltiazem HCl
diphenhydramine HCl (Benadryl)
dipyridamole
Disalcid (salsalate)
divalproex sodium
Doan's Pills (magnesium salicylate)
Dolacet (hydrocodone bitartrate,
  acetaminophen)
Dolene AP (propoxyphene HCl,
  acetaminophen)
Dolobid (diflunisal)
dopamine agonist
Dopar (levodopa)
Dopascan
Dopram (doxapram)
Doral (quazepam)
Doriden (glutethimide)
Dostinex (cabergoline)
dothiepin HCl (Prothiaden)
doxacurium chloride (Nuromax)
doxapram
doxepin (Sinequan)
doxorubicin (Adriamycin)
doxycycline (Vibramycin)
doxylamine succinate
dronabinol (Compassia)
Duocet (hydrocodone bitartrate,
  acetaminophen)
Duract (bromfenac sodium)
Duradyne (acetaminophen, aspirin,
  caffeine)
Duradyne DHC (hydrocodone
  bitartrate, acetaminophen)
Duragesic (fentanyl citrate)
Duramorph (morphine sulfate)
DuraPrep

medications *(continued)*
dynamine
Dynorphin A
EACA (epsilon aminocaproic acid)
Easprin (aspirin)
ebselen
Echovist (SHU 454)
Ecotrin (aspirin)
edrophonium chloride
Effexor XR (venlafaxine hydro-
  chloride) extended-release)
EHDP (etidronate disodium)
Elase (fibrinolysin, desoxyribo-
  nuclease)
Elase-Chloromycetin (fibrinolysin,
  desoxyribonuclease, chloram-
  phenicol)
Elavil (amitriptyline HCl)
Eldepryl (selegiline HCl)
eletriptan
elipridil
EMLA cream
Empirin with Codeine No. 2 (or 3
  or 4) (aspirin, codeine phos-
  phate)
ENA-713 (Exelon)
Enbrel (etanercept)
Endep (amitriptyline HCl)
Endostatin
Enlon-Plus (edrophonium chloride,
  atropine sulfate)
enoxaparin (Lovenox)
entacapone (Comtan)
ephedrine
epinephrine
epsilon aminocaproic acid (EACA)
Equagesic (meprobamate, aspirin)
Equizine M
ergoloid mesylates
Ergomar (ergotamine tartrate)
Ergostat (ergotamine tartrate)
ergotamine tartrate
erythromycin
Esgic (acetaminophen, aspirin,
  butalbital)
estazolam
Esterom

medications *(continued)*
etanercept (Enbrel)
etanidazole
ethchlorvynol
ethinamate
ethopropazine HCl
ethosuximide
ethotoin
ethyl chloride
etidronate (Didronel)
etodolac (Lodine, Ultradol)
etodolac extended-release
(Lodine XL)
etomidate
Eucalyptamint (menthol)
Eucalyptamint 2000 gel
EVAL (ethylene vinyl alcohol)
Excedrin (acetaminophen, aspirin,
caffeine)
Excedrin Migraine (acetaminophen,
aspirin, caffeine)
Exelon (rivastigmine tartrate)
Excedrin P.M. (acetaminophen,
diphenhydramine HCl)
FABRase (alpha-galactosidase A)
felbamate
Felbatol (felbamate)
Feldene (piroxicam)
fenoprofen (Nalfon)
fenoprofen calcium
fentanyl citrate
Fiblast (trafermin)
fibrinolysin (plasmin)
fibrin sealant
filgrastim (Neupogen)
Fioricet (acetaminophen, caffeine,
butalbital)
Fiorinal (aspirin, caffeine,
butalbital)
Fiorinal with Codeine No. 3
(aspirin, caffeine, butalbital,
codeine phosphate)
flesinoxan
Flex-all 454 (menthol, methyl
salicylate, trolamine)
Flexeril (cyclobenzaprine HCl)
Flexon (orphenadrine citrate)

medications *(continued)*
fluasterone (synthetic dehydroepiandrosterone)
fluconazole
flunarizine HCl
fluoxetine
fluoxetine HCl (Prozac)
flupirtine maleate
flurazepam HCl
flurbiprofen
fluvoxamine
FocalSeal-S neurosurgical sealant
Fortical (salmon calcitonin)
Fosamax (alendronate)
fosphenytoin (Cerebyx)
4-aminopyridine (4-AP)
fractionalized fish oil
Freedox (tirilazad mesylate)
fraxiparin (low molecular weight
heparin)
Frisium (clobazam)
frovatriptan (Miguard)
gabapentin (Neurontin)
Gabitril (tiagabine)
gadodiamide
gadopentetate dimeglumine
gadoteridol
gamma-hydroxybutyrate (GHB)
ganaxolone (CCD 1042)
ganglioside GM1
Gedocarnil
Gemnisyn (acetaminophen, aspirin)
Gemonil (metharbital)
Genagesic (propoxyphene HCl,
acetaminophen)
gepirone HCl
Gerimal (ergoloid mesylates)
Ginkgo biloba extract
glatiramer acetate
Gliadel implant
Gliadel wafer
glucosamine, chondroitin,
manganese (Cosamine DS)
glucosamine sulfate
glutethimide
GM-1 ganglioside (Sygen)
gold salts

medications *(continued)*
gold sodium thiomalate
Gramalil
Graton bone matrix/marrow
  combination injection
griseofulvin
guanethidine monosulfate
guanfacine (Tenex)
Haemophilus influenzae type B
  vaccine
halazepam
Halcion (triazolam)
Halfprin (aspirin)
haloperidol (Haldol)
Haltran (ibuprofen)
Hank buffered saline solution
HCl (hydrochloride)
Hedspa
hexachlorophene
Hexadrol (dexamethasone)
hirudin, recombinant
HU-211 (dexanabinol)
Hyalgan (hyaluronic acid)
Hydergine (ergoloid mesylates)
Hydrocet (hydrocodone bitartrate,
  acetaminophen)
hydrochloride (HCl)
hydrocodone and ibuprofen
  (Vicoprofen)
hydrocodone bitartrate
hydrocodone sodium succinate
hydrocortisone
hydrocortisone sodium succinate
Hydrocortone (hydrocortisone)
Hydrogesic (hydrocodone
  bitartrate, acetaminophen)
hydromorphone HCl
hydroxychloroquine sulfate
Hypericum perforatum herb
Hy-Phen (hydrocodone bitartrate,
  acetaminophen)
ibuprofen
idebenone
Ifex (ifosfamide)
ifosfamide
IGF-BP3 complex (SomatoKine)
IL (see *interleukin*)

medications *(continued)*
iloperidone (Zomaril)
imipramine (Tofranil)
Imitrex (sumatriptan succinate)
ImmTher
ImuLyme
Inderal (propranolol HCl)
Indocin SR (indomethacin)
indomethacin
infliximab (Remicade)
Infumorph (morphine sulfate)
injectable collagenase (Cordase)
injectable hyaluronic acid
  (Orthovisc)
inosine pranobex
insulin-like growth factor
interferon
interferon alfa
interferon beta-1b (Betaseron)
interferon tau
interferon-1a (Avonex)
interferon-1b (Betaseron)
interleukin-1 (IL-1)
interleukin-1 beta (IL-1b)
interleukin-1 receptor antagonist
  (IL-1Ra)
interleukin-2 (IL-2)
interleukin-4 (IL-4)
interleukin-6 (IL-6)
interleukin-8 (IL-8)
interleukin-10 (IL-10)
interleukin-12 (IL-12)
interleukin-15 (IL-15)
interleukin-17 (IL-17)
iodixanol (Visipaque)
iophendylate
IR501 immune therapy
Ismelin Sulfate (guanethidine
  monosulfate)
isocarboxazid
isoflurane
isometheptene mucate
Isoprinosine (inosine pranobex)
isopropyl alcohol
Isoptin (verapamil HCl)
isoxicam (Maxicam)
itraconazole

medications *(continued)*
izanidine hydrochloride (Zanaflex)
Janimine (imipramine HCl)
kanamycin sulfate
Kantrex (kanamycin sulfate)
Kefzol (cefazolin sodium)
Kemadrin (procyclidine HCl)
Kenacort (triamcinolone)
Kenalog (triamcinolone acetonide)
Kerasal
ketoconazole
ketoprofen
ketorolac tromethamine
Klonopin (clonazepam)
Lac-Hydrin (ammonium lactate)
Lamictal (lamotrigine)
lamotrigine
lanolin
Largon (propiomazine HCl)
Larodopa (levodopa)
L-baclofen
LDI-200
L-dopa (levodopa)
lecithin
leflunomide (Arava)
leteprinim potassium (Neotrofin)
LeukoVAX
leuvectin
levemopamil
levetiracetam
levodopa
Levo-Dromoran (levorphanol
    tartrate)
Levoprome (methotrimeprazine)
levorphanol tartrate
L-5-hydroxytryptophan (L-5HTP)
Librium (chlordiazepoxide HCl)
licostinel (ACEA 1021)
lidocaine and bupivacaine
lidocaine HCl
lidocaine patch 5%
Lidoderm (lidocaine patch 5%)
lidopridine
Life-Port drug delivery
lignocaine (lidocaine)
Lioresal (baclofen)
liquid nitrogen

medications *(continued)*
Liquiprin (acetaminophen)
lithium carbonate
Lodine (etodolac)
Lodine XL (etodolac extended-
    release)
Lodosyn (carbidopa)
Lopressor (metoprolol tartrate)
Lopurin (allopurinol)
lorazepam (Ativan)
Lorcet (hydrocodone bitartrate,
    acetaminophen)
Lortab (hydrocodone bitartrate,
    acetaminophen)
Lotusate (talbutal)
Lovenox (enoxaparin)
L-threonine
L-tryptophan
Luminal Sodium (phenobarbital
    sodium)
LYMErix (lipoprotein OspA,
    recombinant)
LY233053 neuroprotector
Macritonin (calcitonin [salmon])
Magan (magnesium salicylate)
magnesium salicylate
magnesium sulfate
Magnevist (gadopentetate
    dimeglumine)
Magsal (magnesium salicylate,
    phenyltoloxamine citrate)
MAOI (monoamine oxidase
    inhibitor)
Maolate (chlorphenesin carbamate)
maprotiline HCl
Marezine (cyclizine HCl)
Marcaine (bupivacaine HCl)
marimastat
Marplan (isocarboxazid)
Maxalt (rizatriptan benzoate)
Maxicam (isoxicam)
mazindol (Sanorex)
Mebaral (mephobarbital)
mecasermin (Myotrophin)
meclizine
meclofenamate sodium
Meclomen (meclofenamate sodium)

medications *(continued)*
MEDI-507
Medigesic (acetaminophen,
caffeine, butalbital)
Medihaler Ergotamine (ergotamine
tartrate)
Medipren (ibuprofen)
Medrol Dosepak (methyl-
prednisolone)
mefenamic acid (Ponstel)
memantine
Mentane (velnacrine)
menthol
Mepergan (meperidine HCl,
promethazine HCl)
meperidine HCl
mephenytoin
mephobarbital
meprobamate
merbromin
Mercurochrome (merbromin)
Mesantoin (mephenytoin)
Mestinon (pyridostigmine bromide)
Metastron (strontium-89)
metaxalone
methamphetamine HCl
metharbital
methiodal sodium
methocarbamol
methohexital
methotrexate (MTX)
methotrimeprazine
methsuximide
methyl-GAG (methylglyoxal-bis-
guanylhydrazone (MGBG)
Methylin (methylphenidate hydrochloride)
methylphenidate HCl (Methylin)
methylprednisolone (Solu-Medrol)
methylprednisolone acetate
methylprednisolone sodium
succinate (A-Methapred)
methylsalicylate
methylsergide maleate
methyprylon
methysergide maleate

medications *(continued)*
metoprolol tartrate
metrifonate (ProMem)
MGBG (methylglyoxal-bis-
guanylhydrazone)
Miacalcin (calcitonin salmon)
midazolam HCl
midazolam maleate
midodrine HCl
Midrin (isometheptene mucate,
dichloralphenazone, acetaminophen)
Migranal nasal spray (dihydroergotamine mesylate)
MigraSpray
Migratine (isometheptene mucate,
dichloralphenazone, acetaminophen)
Miguard (frovatriptan)
Mirapex (pramipexole dihydro-
chloride tablets)
Milontin Kapseals (phensuximide)
misoprostol
Mivacron (mivacurium chloride)
mivacurium chloride
Mobidin (magnesium salicylate)
Mobigesic (magnesium salicylate,
phenyltoloxamine citrate)
moclobemide
mofetil (CellCept)
Mogadon (nitrazepam)
molecusol-carbamazepine
Momentum (aspirin,
phenyltoloxamine citrate)
monoamine oxidase inhibitors
(MAOIs)
Mono-Gesic (salsalate)
morphine sulfate
Motrin IB (ibuprofen)
Movana
MS Contin (morphine sulfate)
MTX (methotrexate)
Mucomyst (acetylcysteine sodium)
mycophenolate (CellCept)
Myloral (bovine myelin)
Myochrysine (gold sodium
thiomalate)

medications *(continued)*

Myotrophin (insulin-like growth factor; mecasermin)
Mysoline (primidone)
Mytelase (ambenonium chloride)
nabumetone
nadolol (Corgard)
nadroparin (low molecular weight heparin)
nalbuphine HCl
Nalfon (fenoprofen calcium)
naloxone HCl
nambumetone
nandrolene decanoate
naphthylalkalones
Naprelan (naproxen sodium)
Naprosyn (naproxen)
naproxen (Aleve, Naprosyn, Naprelan)
Nardil (phenelzine sulfate)
Naropin (ropivacaine hydrochloride)
Natural Relief 1222
Nembutal (pentobarbital)
Neoral (cyclosporine for microemulsion)
Ne-Osteo
neostigmine bromide
neostigmine methylsulfate
Neotrofin (leteprinim potassium)
Nervine (diphenhydramine HCl)
Neuprex (rBPI-21)
Neurobloc (botulinum toxin type B)
NeuroCell
Neurontin (gabapentin)
nifedipine
Nimbex (cisatracurium)
nimodipine
Nimotop (nimodipine)
nitrofurazone
nitrous oxide
Noctec (chloral hydrate)
NoDoz (caffeine)
Noludar (methyprylon)
nomifensine maleate
nonsteroidal antiphlogistics

medications *(continued)*

Nootropil (piracetam)
Noradex (orphenadrine citrate)
Norcet (hydrocodone bitartrate, acetaminophen)
Norco (hydrocodone bitartrate and acetaminophen)
Norflex (orphenadrine citrate)
Norgesic (orphenadrine citrate, aspirin, caffeine)
Normiflo (low molecular weight heparin)
Norpramin (desipramine HCl)
nortriptyline (Pamelor)
Novocain (procaine HCl)
Nubain (nalbuphine HCl)
Numorphan (oxymorphone HCl)
Nuprin (ibuprofen)
NutraJoint gel
Nytol (diphenhydramine HCl)
Obetrol (dextroamphetamine sulfate, dextroamphetamine saccharate, amphetamine aspartate, amphetamine sulfate)
Oculinum (botulinum toxin type A)
oil of *Melaleuca alternifolia* (tea tree oil)
olanzapine (Zyprexa)
omega-3 fatty acids
omega-3 oils
Omniscan (gadodiamide)
Oncovin (vincristine)
One-Alpha (alfacalcidol)
1,25-dihydroxycholecalciferol (calcitonin)
opium
Orap (pimozide)
Orgaran (danaproid)
orphenadrine citrate
Ortholinum (botulinum toxin)
Orthovisc (injectable hyaluronic acid)
Orudis (ketoprofen)
osmic acid
Ossigel injectable bioengineered matrix

medications *(continued)*
Osteo-Bi-Flex
Osteomark monoclonal antibody-
based agent
Osteopatch
oxaprozin
oxazepam
oxcarbazepine
oxycodone HCl
oxycodone terephthalate
Oxycontin (oxycodone Hcl)
oxymorphone HCl
oxyphenbutazone
Pabalate (sodium salicylate,
aminobenzoate sodium)
Pamelor (nortriptyline)
Panadol (acetaminophen)
Pantopon (opium)
papaverine topical gel
Paradione (paramethadione)
Paraflex (chlorzoxazone)
Parafon Forte DSC (chlorzoxazone)
Paral (paraldehyde)
paraldehyde
paramethadione
Parlodel (bromocriptine mesylate)
paroxetine HCl extended
release
Parsidol (ethopropazine HCl)
Paxarel (acetylcarbromal)
Paxil CR extended release
(paroxetine HCl)
Paxipam (halazepam)
Peganone (ethotoin)
PEG-SOD (polyethylene glycol-
superoxide dismutase)
pemoline
penicillamine
Pennsaid (diclofenac)
pentazocine
pentazocine HCl
pentazocine lactate
pentobarbital
pentoxifylline
pentylenetetrazol
Percocet (oxycodone HCl,
acetaminophen)

medications *(continued)*
Percodan and Percodan-Demi
(oxycodone HCl, oxycodone
terephthalate, aspirin)
Percogesic (acetaminophen,
phenyltoloxamine citrate)
pergolide mesylate
Periactin (cyproheptadine HCl)
Permax (pergolide mesylate)
Pertofrane (desipramine HCl)
phenacemide
phenazone (antipyrine)
phenelzine sulfate
phenobarbital
phenobarbital sodium
phenol
phenoxymethylpenicillin
phensuximide
Phenurone (phenacemide)
phenylbutazone
phenytoin (Dilantin)
phenytoin sodium
PHNO (4-propyl-9-hydroxy-
naphthoxazine)
physostigmine
physostigmine salicylate
Phytodolor
pimozide (Orap)
piracetam
piroxicam
Placidyl (ethchlorvynol)
Plaquenil Sulfate (hydroxychloroquine sulfate)
plasmin (fibrinolysin)
Platinol
Plavix (clopidogrel bisulfate)
polyethylene glycol-superoxide
dismutase (PEG-SOD)
Ponstel (mefenamic acid)
porfiromycin (Promycin)
povidone-iodine
pramipexole (Mirapex)
Pravachol (pravastatin sodium)
pravastatin sodium (Pravachol)
prazepam
Predate S
Prednicen-M (prednisone)

medications *(continued)*
prednisolone
prednisone
pregabalin
Presalin (acetaminophen, aspirin,
    salicylamide, aluminum
    hydroxide)
Preservex
primidone (Mysoline)
probenecid (Benemid)
procaine HCl
Procardia (nifedipine)
procyclidine HCl
ProHance (gadoteridol)
ProMem (metrifonate)
promethazine HCl
Promycin (porfiromycin)
Propacet (propoxyphene napsylate,
    acetaminophen)
propentofylline
propiomazine HCl
propofol
propoxyphene HCl
propoxyphene napsylate
propranolol HCl (Inderal)
ProSom (estazolam)
Prosorba
ProstaScint imaging agent
Prostigmin (neostigmine
    methylsulfate)
protirelin
protriptyline HCl
Provigil (modafinil)
Prozac (fluoxetine hydrochloride)
pyridostigmine bromide
pyrilamine maleate
pyritinol
Quadramet (samarium Sm 153
    lexidronam)
quazepam (Doral)
quetiapine fumarate (Seroquel)
Quiet World (pyrilamine maleate,
    acetaminophen, aspirin)
quinupristin/dalfoprostin
radiopharmaceutical
rBPI-21 (Neuprex)

medications *(continued)*
Rebif (recombinant interferon
    beta-1a)
recombinant human bone morpho-
    genetic protein-2 (rhBMP-2)
recombinant human interferon-a2a
    (rhIFN-a2a)
recombinant interferon beta-1a
    (Rebif)
recombinant prourokinase
Relafen (nabumetone)
remacemide
Remeron (mirtazapine)
Remicade (infliximab)
Reminyl (galantamine)
ReoPro (abciximab)
Repan (butalbital, acetaminophen,
    caffeine)
Requip (ropinirole)
resiniferatoxin (RTX)
Restoril (temazepam)
Rexolate (sodium thiosalicylate)
rhBMP-2 (recombinant human
    bone morphogenetic protein)
rhIGF-1 (Myotrophin)
Rheumatrex Dose Pack
    (methotrexate sodium)
Ridaura (auranofin)
rifaximin
Rilutek (riluzole)
riluzole (Rilutek)
Rimadyl (carprofen)
risendronate (Actonel)
Risperdal (risperidone)
risperidone (Risperdal)
Ritalin-SR (methylphenidate HCl)
rivastigmine tartrate (Exelon)
rizatriptan benzoate (Maxalt)
Robaxacet (methocarbamol and
    acetaminophen)
Robaxin (methocarbamol)
Robaxisal (methocarbamol, aspirin)
Rocaltrol (calcitriol)
Rocephin (ceftriaxone)
rofecoxib (Vioxx)
Romazicon (flumazenil)

medications *(continued)*
 ropinirole HCl (Requip)
 ropivacaine hydrochloride
   (Naropin)
 Roxanol (morphine sulfate)
 Roxiam (remoxipride)
 Roxicet (oxycodone HCl,
   acetaminophen)
 Roxicodone Intensol (oxycodone
   HCl)
 Roxiprin (oxycodone HCl, oxy-
   codone terephthalate, aspirin)
 RTX (resiniferatoxin)
 Rufen (ibuprofen)
 sabeluzole
 Sabril (vigabatrin)
 St. John's wort (*Hypericum
   perforatum*)
 Saleto (acetaminophen, aspirin,
   salicylamide, caffeine)
 Salflex (salsalate)
 salicylamide
 salicylic acid liquid
 salicylic acid plaster
 salicylic acid tape
 saline
 salmon calcitonin nasal spray
 Salmonine (calcitonin salmon)
 samarium Sm lexidronam injection
   (Quadramet)
 salsalate
 Salsitab (salsalate)
 Sanorex (mazindol)
 Sansert (methylsergide maleate)
 scopolamine (Transderm-Scop)
 secobarbital
 secobarbital sodium
 Seconal Sodium (secobarbital
   sodium)
 selective serotonin reuptake
   inhibitor (SSRI)
 selegiline HCl (Zelapar)
 Serax (oxazepam)
 Serlect (sertindole)
 Seroquel (quetiapine fumarate)
 Serratia marcescens extract

medications *(continued)*
 sertindole (Serlect)
 sertraline HCl (Zoloft)
 Serzone (nefazodone)
 S-fluoxetine (racemic fluoxetine)
 Sibelium (flunarizine HCl)
 SIB-1508Y
 sibrafiban
 silver nitrate
 simvastatin (Zocor)
 Sinemet (carbidopa, levodopa)
 Sinequan (doxepin HCl)
 6-MNA
 Skelaxin (metaxalone)
 Skelid (tiludronate disodium)
 Sleep-Eze 3 (diphenhydramine
   HCl)
 SNX-111 (ziconotide)
 sodium hyaluronate (Hyalgan)
 sodium oxybate
 sodium salicylate
 sodium tetradecyl sulfate
 sodium thiosalicylate
 Solganal (aurothioglucose)
 Solu-Cortef (hydrocortisone sodium
   succinate)
 Solu-Medrol (methylprednisolone
   sodium succinate)
 Soma (carisoprodol)
 Soma Compound (carisoprodol,
   aspirin)
 SomatoKine (IGF-BP3 complex)
 Sominex (diphenhydramine HCl)
 Spartaject busulfan
 SSRI (selective serotonin reuptake
   inhibitor)
 SSZ (sulfasalazine)
 Stadol NS (butorphanol tartrate)
 Stelazine (trifluoperazine hydrochloride)
 St. John's wort (*Hypericum
   perforatum*)
 sulfasalazine (SSZ)
 sulfinpyrazone
 sulfinpyrazone
 sulindac

medications *(continued)*
sumatriptan succinate
Supac (acetaminophen, aspirin, caffeine, calcium gluconate)
suprofen
Suprol (suprofen)
Sygen (GM-1 ganglioside)
Symmetrel (amantadine HCl)
sympathomimetic stumulants
Synalgos (aspirin, caffeine)
Synalgos-DC (dihydrocodeine bitartrate, aspirin, caffeine)
Synapton (physostigmine)
Synchromed programmable drug pump
Synercid (quinupristin/dalfoprostin)
synthetic corticotropin-releasing factor (Xerecept)
Synvisc injection
tacrine HCl
tacrolimus
Talacen (pentazocine HCl, acetaminophen)
talbutal
Talwin (pentazocine lactate)
Talwin Compound (pentazocine HCl, aspirin)
Talwin NX (pentazocine HCl, naloxone HCl)
Tandearil (oxyphenbutazone)
Tasmar (tolcapone)
tea-tree oil (oil of *Melaleuca alternifolia*)
technetium 99m (Ceretec)
Tegretol (carbamazepine)
temazepam
Temodal (temozolomide)
temozolomide (Temodal)
Tempra (acetaminophen)
Tenex (guanfacine)
Tenormin (atenolol)
Tensilon (edrophonium chloride)
terbinafine
tetanus antitoxin
tetanus immune globulin
tetanus toxoid

medications *(continued)*
tetrahydroaminoacridine (THA, tacrine HCl)
T-Gesic (hydrocodone bitartrate, acetaminophen)
TGF-B (transforming growth factor-beta)
THA (tetrahydroaminoacridine, tacrine HCl)
thalidomide (Thalomid)
Thalomid (thalidomide)
Therafectin (amiprilose hydrochloride)
thiopental
Thorazine (chlorpromazine)
threonine
Threostat (threonine)
Thymone (protirelin)
tiagabine (Gabitril)
Ticlid (ticlopidine HCl)
ticlopidine HCl
tiludronate disodium (Skelid)
timolol maleate
Tirend (caffeine)
tirilazad mesylate
Tisseel fibrin sealant
tizanidine
TLC ABLC (amphotericin B lipid complex)
tocopherol (vitamin E)
Tofranil (imipramine HCl)
tolcapone (Tasmar)
Tolectin DS (tolmetin sodium)
tolmetin sodium
Topamax (topiramate)
topiramate
Toradol (ketorolac tromethamine)
Tracium (atracurium besylate)
trafermin (Fiblast)
Transderm-Scop (scopolamine)
transforming growth factor-beta (TGF-B)
Tranxene (clorazepate dipotassium)
tranylcypromine sulfate
trazodone HCl (Desyrel)
triamcinolone (Aristospan)

medications *(continued)*
triamcinolone acetonide
triamcinolone hexacetonide
Triapin (acetaminophen, caffeine,
    butalbital)
triazolam
trichloroacetic acid
Tridione (trimethadione)
trifluoperazine hydrochloride
    (Stelazine)
Trigesic (acetaminophen, aspirin,
    caffeine)
trihexyphenidyl (Artane)
Trilisate (choline salicylate,
    magnesium salicylate)
trimethadione
trimipramine maleate
trolamine
tromethamine
trypsin, crystallized
tubocurarine chloride
Tuinal (amobarbital sodium,
    secobarbital sodium)
Tusal (sodium thiosalicylate)
24,25-dihydroxycholecalciferol
Twilite (diphenhydramine HCl)
Tylenol (acetaminophen)
Tylenol with Codeine No. 1 (or 2,
    3, 4) (acetaminophen, codeine
    phosphate)
Tylox (oxycodone HCl, aceta-
    minophen)
Ultradol (etodolac)
Ultram (tramadol HCl)
Unisom (doxylamine succinate)
Valesin (acetaminophen, aspirin,
    salicylamide)
Valium (diazepam)
Valmid Pulvules (ethinamate)
valproate sodium injection
    (Depacon)
valproic acid
Valrelease (diazepam)
Vanquish (acetaminophen, aspirin,
    caffeine, magnesium hydroxide,
    aluminum hydroxide)
vasopressin (VP)

medications *(continued)*
velnacrine maleate
venlafaxine hydrochloride
    extended-release (Effexor XR)
verapamil
Versed (midazolam HCl)
Vibramycin (doxycycline)
Vicoprofen (hydrocodone and
    ibuprofen)
Vicodin (hydrocodone bitartrate,
    acetaminophen)
vigabatrin
viloxazine HCl
vincristine (Oncovin)
Vioxx (rofecoxib)
Visipaque (iodixanol)
vitamin C (ascorbic acid)
vitamin E (tocopherol)
Vivactil (protriptyline HCl)
Vivalan (viloxazine HCl)
Vivarin (caffeine)
Voltaren (diclofenac sodium)
VP (vasopressin)
Wellbutrin (bupropion HCl)
Wigraine (ergotamine tartrate,
    tartaric acid)
Wigrettes (ergotamine tartrate)
Wygesic (propoxyphene HCl,
    acetaminophen)
Xanax (alprazolam)
Xerecept (synthetic corticotropin-
    releasing factor)
Xubix (sibrafiban)
Xylocaine (lidocaine HCl)
Xyrem (gamma hydroxybutyrate)
Zanaflex (tizanidine hydrochloride)
Zarontin (ethosuximide)
Zebutal
Zelapar (selegiline hydrochloride)
Zeldox (ziprasidone hydrochloride)
ziconotide (SNX-111)
zinc oxide
ziprasidone hydrochloride (Zeldox)
Zocor (simvastatin)
zolmitriptan (Zomig)
Zoloft (sertraline HCl)
zolpidem tartrate

medications *(continued)*
  Zomaril (iloperidone)
  Zomig (zolmitriptan)
  Zonegran (zonisamide)
  zonisamide (Zonegran)
  Zyban (bupropion HCl)
  Zydone (hydrocodone and aceta-
    minophen)
  Zyloprim (allopurinol)
  Zyprexa (olanzapine)
medicine
  alternative
  Chinese
  photonic
  sports
Medicus bed
MEDI-507
Mediloy implant metal
MedImage scanner
mediolateral oblique view
mediolateral stress
mediopatellar
Medipedic Multicentric knee brace
Medi plaster scissors
Medi-Quet tourniquet
Medison scanner
medium (pl. media)
  contrast
  high osmolar (HOM)
  ionic contrast
  low osmolar (LOM)
  nonionic contrast
  radiopaque
medium voltage beta activity
Medmetric KT-1000 knee laxity
  arthrometer
Mednext bone dissecting system
Medoff sliding fracture plate
Medspec MR imaging system
Medtronic Activa tremor control
  therapy
Medtronic Delta pressure valve
Medtronic neuromuscular stimulator
Medtronic programmable drug pump
Medtronic spinal cord stimulator
Medtronic SynchroMed infusion
  device

Meduck anesthesia monitor
medulla (pl. medullas, medullae)
  dorsal
  postrema of
  rostral
  spinal
medulla oblongata syndrome
medullaris, conus
medullary canal
medullary grafting
medullary infarction
medullary syndrome, lateral
medullary tumor
medulloblast
medulloblastoma
  desmoplastic
  familial
  vermian
MEDX gamma camera
Meek clavicle strap
Meek pelvic traction belt
Mees lines
mefenamic acid (Ponstel)
MEG (magnetoencephalography)
Mega-Air bed
megacephaly
megahertz (MHz)
megalencephaly, benign familial
megalocephaly
Mega Tilt and Turn bed
megavolt (MV)
meglumine diatrizoate imaging agent
meglumine iodipamide imaging agent
meglumine iothalamate imaging agent
meglumine iotroxate imaging agent
megrim (migraine)
Meige, medial facial spasm of
Meige syndrome
Meissner corpuscle sensory receptor
Melaleuca alternifolia (tea tree) oil
melanin, leptomeningeal
melanocytoma, meningeal
melanoma
  intracortical
  iridocorneal
  leptomeningeal

melanoma *(continued)*
    plantar malignant
    subungual amelanotic
melanosis, parenchymal neurocuta-
    neous
melanotic schwannoma
melanotic whitlow
MELAS (mitochondrial encephalo-
    myopathy with lactic acidosis and
    strokelike) episodes
melena
Meleney infection
Meleney synergistic gangrene
Melkersson-Rosenthal syndrome
Melone classification of radius fracture
melon seeds in synovial fluid
melorheostosis of Leri
Memantine
membrane
    atlantoaxial (posterior)
    atlanto-occipital
    basement
    blood behind tympanic
    depolarization of neuronal
    discontinuous basement
    fibrin
    Gore-Tex surgical
    interosseous (IOM)
    Liliequist
    neuronal
    posterior (atlantoaxial)
    synovial
    thickened synovial
membrane irritability
membrane permeability
membrane potential
membrane receptors
memory
    declarative
    episodic
    figural
    gaps in
    immediate
    impaired
    long-term
    loss of
    procedural

memory *(continued)*
    recent
    recognition
    remote
    semantic
    sequence
    short-term
    verbal
    visual
    visual-spatial
Memory for Designs Test
memory for digits test
memory-impaired person
memory impairment
Memory Impairment Screen (MIS)
Mendel-Bekhterev reflex
Mendel-Bekhterev sign
Ménière syndrome
meningeal carcinomatosis
meningeal enhancement
meningeal fibrosis
meningeal hemorrhage
meningeal infiltrate
meningeal inflammation
meningeal irritation
meningeal leukemia
meningeal mesenchymal tissue
meningeal myelomatosis
meningeal nerve
meningeal sign
meningeal spread of tumor
meningeal streak
meningeal tumor
meninges (pl. of *meninx*)
meningioma
    angioplastic
    cavernous sinus
    cerebellopontine angle
    clival
    clivus
    convexity
    cranial base
    cutaneous
    cystic
    dermal
    endotheliomatous
    epidural

meningioma *(continued)*
  falcine
  falx
  fibroblastic
  fibrous
  intracranial
  intradural-extradural
  intraspinal
  malignant
  meningotheliomatous
  metastasizing
  multiple
  olfactory groove
  parasagittal
  petroclival
  posterior fossa
  psammomatous
  sphenoid ridge
  sporadic
  subdural
  subfrontal
  suprasellar
  tentorial
  transitional
  tuberculum sellae
meningioma en plaque
meningioma tumor
meningiosarcoma
meningism
meningismus
meningitic neurosyphilis
meningitic stria
meningitis (pl. meningitides)
  actinomycosis lymphocytic
  acute
  acute purulent
  Aerobacter aerogenes
  aseptic
  aseptic uremic
  bacterial
  Bacterium anitratum
  beta-hemolytic streptococcus
  beta strep
  Brucella abortus
  Brucella melitensis
  Brucella suis
  Candida

meningitis *(continued)*
  candidal
  carcinomatous
  cerebrospinal (CSM)
  chemical
  chronic
  chronic basal
  CMV (cytomegalovirus)
  Corynebacterium diphtheriae
  coxsackievirus
  cryptococcal
  diffuse syphilitic
  echinomycosis lymphocytic
  echovirus
  enterovirus
  Escherichia coli (E. coli)
  fungal
  group B streptococcal
  herpes simplex virus type 2
  Haemophilus influenzae
    (H. influenzae)
  Histoplasma
  Histoplasma capsulatum
  HIV (human immunodeficiency
    virus)
  Klebsiella pneumoniae
  leptospirosis lymphocytic
  Listeria monocytogenes
  lymphocytic
  lymphomatous
  meningococcal
  Meningococcus
  Mollaret
  mumps
  mycotic
  Naegleria
  Neisseria
  Neisseria catarrhalis
  Neisseria gonorrhoeae
  neonatal
  neoplastic
  Nocardia
  ornithosis lymphocytic
  otogenic
  paragonimiasis lymphocytic
  pneumococcal
  Pneumococcus

meningitis *(continued)*
   posterior basic
   Proteus vulgaris
   Pseudomonas aeruginosa
   purulent
   pyogenic
   rabies lymphocytic
   Rich theory of tuberculous
   Salmonella
   Salmonella choleraesuis
   sinogenic
   staphylococcal
   Staphylococcus aureus
   streptococcal
   Streptococcus agalactiae
   Streptococcus pneumoniae
   subacute
   subacute granulomatous
   syphilitic
   Toxoplasma
   toxoplasmosis lymphocytic
   Treponema pallidum
   trichinosis
   Trypanosoma gambiense
   tuberculous
   uremic aseptic
   Vibrio fetus
   viral
meningocele, sacral
meningococcal meningitis
meningoencephalitis (pl. meningo-
   encephalitides)
   arbomeningoencephalitis
   murine typhus
   Rocky Mountain spotted fever
   Trichinella spiralis
meningoencephalocele
   basal
   ethmoidal
   sphenoethmoidal
   spheno-orbital
   sphenopharyngeal
   stalk of
   transsphenoidal
meningoencephalocystocele
meningoencephalomyelitis
meningohypophyseal artery

meningomyelitis
meningomyelocele
meningomyelocystocele
meningothelioma
meningovascular neurosyphilis
meningovascular syphilis
meninx (pl. meninges)
meniscal arrow
meniscal autograft transplantation
meniscal injury
meniscal tear (see *tear*)
meniscal transplantation
meniscal trimmer blade
meniscectomy
   arthroscopic
   medial
   partial
   Patel medial
   subtotal
   subtotal lateral
   total
meniscectomy blade
meniscitis
meniscofemoral ligament
meniscorrhexis
meniscosynovial junction
meniscotibial ligament
meniscotome
   Bircher
   Bowen-Grover
   Grover
   Storz
meniscus (pl. menisci)
   acromioclavicular
   bridge of
   clefting of
   degenerative
   discoid
   frayed
   fraying of
   lateral
   medial
   menisci
   torn
Meniscus Arrow fixation device
Meniscus Mender II system
Menkes disease

Menkes kinky-hair syndrome
Menkes syndrome
Mennell sign
Mensor-Scheck technique
mental changes
mental deficiency
mental faculty
mental nerve
mentalis muscle
mental retardation
mental status changes
mental status examination
mental status questionnaire
mentation
    change in
    normal
Mentor tissue expander
Menzel olivopontocerebellar atrophy
Menzel olivopontocerebellar
    degeneration
MEP (motor evoked potential)
MEP (multimodality evoked potential)
MEPP (miniature endplate potential)
MERA (minor emergency room area)
MERAC (Musculoskeletal Evaluation,
    Rehabilitation and Conditioning)
    system
meralgia paresthetica (*not* myalgia)
Merchant angle
Merchant congruence angle
Merchant views
mercury poisoning
meridian therapy
meridian
    vertical visual
    yang
    yin
Meridian stem
Merkel disc sensory receptor
Merkel muscle
Merland classification of peri-
    medullary arteriovenous fistulas
Merle D'Aubigné pain and mobility
    rating scale
merlin/schwannomin (tumor suppres-
    sor NF2)
meroacrania

Merocel packing
MERRF (myoclonic epilepsy with
    ragged red fibers)
Merry Walker ambulation device
Mersilene suture
Mersilene tape
mesencephalic infarct
mesencephalic reticular formation
mesencephalon aqueduct
mesencephalon, embryonic
mesenchymal chondrosarcoma
mesenchymoma, pluripotential
mesh
    collagen-coated Vicryl
    Dumbach cranial titanium
    Leibinger Micro Dynamic
    metal
    polyglactin
    SynMesh titanium
    titanium
mesial aspect
mesial frontal lobe damage
mesial hemisphere
mesial hyperperfusion
mesial temporal sclerosis
mesialward
mesiotemporal lobe
mesoacromion
mesocephalic head shape
mesocuneiform bone
mesomelic dwarfism
mesothenar muscle
mesotenon (or mesotendon)
MESS (Mangled Extremity Severity
    Score)
messenger ribonucleic acid (mRNA)
metabolic bone disease
metabolic encephalopathy
metabolic lesion
metabolic myopathy
metabolic tremor
metabolism
    altered
    cerebral
    cortical
    fibroblast
    frontal lobe hypometabolism

metabolism *(continued)*
  global cerebral hypometabolism
  hypometabolism
  incremental ammonia
  muscle energy
  myelin
  neuronal
metabolite
  arachidonic acid
  washing out of accumulated
metabotropic glutamate receptor sub-
    type 5 (mGluR5)
metacarpal
  base of
  duplicated
metacarpal bones
metacarpal ligament, dorsal
metacarpal-phalangeal or metacarpo-
    phalangeal (MCP)
metacarpophalangeal arthroscopy
metacarpophalangeal articulation
metacarpophalangeal joint
metacarpoglenoidal ligament
metacarpophalangeal (MCP or MP)
    dislocation
metacarpophalangeal joint
metacarpus
metachromatic leukodystrophy
metaiodobenzylguanidine (MIBG)
  imaging agent
metal (see *implant metal*)
metallic foreign body
metal locator, Berman-Moorhead
metal-on-metal bearing surfaces
metamorphopsia of Amsler grid
metaphyseal chondrodysplasia
metaphyseal-diaphyseal junction
metaphyseal dysostosis
metaphyseal-epiphyseal angle
metaphyseal lesion
metaphyseal loading stem
metaphyseal lucent bands
metaphysis
metaplasia
  cartilaginous
  osteocartilaginous

metastasis (pl. metastases)
  bony
  brain
  cerebral
  distant
  extradural spinal
  intramedullary
  leptomeningeal
  osteoblastic
  osteolytic
  shunt-related
  spinal cord
metastatic bone survey
metastatic brain tumor
metastatic tumor to brain
metastatic tumor to cord
Metastron (strontium-89)
Metasul hip prosthesis
metatarsal bar shoe modification
metatarsal bone
metatarsalgia
  Morton
  secondary
metatarsal head
metatarsal head osteotomy
metatarsal lashing
metatarsal neck osteotomy
metatarsal overload syndromes
metatarsal pads
metatarsal parabola
metatarsal-phalangeal (MTP) joint
  space
metatarsocuboid joint
metatarsocuneiform (MC) arthrodesis
metatarsocuneiform joint
metatarsophalangeal (MTP) joint
  (MPJ) arthrodesis
metatarsotalar angle
metatarsus adductovarus deformity
metatarsus adductus (MTA)
metatarsus atavicus
metatarsus elevatus
metatarsus equinus
metatarsus internus
metatarsus latus
metatarsus primus adductus

metatarsus primus angle
metatarsus primus elevatus
metatarsus primus varus (MPV)
metatarsus supinatus
metatarsus valgus
metatarsus varus (MTV)
metatrophic dysplasia
Met Bar shoe modification
meter
  impedance
  Petrometer range-of-motion
  pinch
method
  Abbott
  Bleck
  Borggreve
  Budin-Chandler
  bundle-nailing
  Cobb
  Ferguson scoliosis measuring
  hydrogen washout
  Insall patella alta
  Kocher
  Matsen
  Mose
  Mosley anterior shoulder repair
  Prechtl
  proteinase-K extraction
  SANE (Single Assessment Numeric
    Evaluation)
  Stullberg
methotrexate (Rheumatrex)
methoxypolyethylene glycol-L-lysine-
  DTPA imaging agent
methyl alcohol poisoning
methylation-based clonality assay
methylation-specific polymerase chain
  reaction
methyl bromide
methylmethacrylate
  beads of
  centrifuged
methylmethacrylate cement
methylene blue dye
Methylin (methylphenidate hydrochloride)

methylmalonic aciduria
methylphenidate hydrochloride
  (Methylin)
methylprednisolone (Solu-Medrol)
methylprednisolone sodium succinate
  (A-Methapred)
metopic craniectomy
metopic suture
metopodynia
metopon
metrifonate (ProMem)
metrizamide cisternography
metrizamide computed tomographic
  cisternogram (MCTC)
metrizamide contrast material
metrizamide myelogram
metrizoate sodium contrast medium
metronomic eye movements
Mettler Autotherm diathermy
Mettler ultrasound
Metzenbaum chisel
Metzenbaum gouge
Metzenbaum scissors
Meuli arthroplasty
Meurig Williams spinal fusion plate
Meyer cervical orthosis
Meyerding bone skid
Meyerding chisel
Meyerding curved gouge
Meyerding finger retractor
Meyerding laminectomy blade
Meyerding laminectomy retractor
Meyerding mallet
Meyerding osteotome
Meyerding-Scoville blade
Meyerding self-retaining retractor
Meyerding spondylolisthesis
Meyerding-Van Demark technique
Meyer line
Meyer loop in brain
Meyer sublaminar wiring technique
Meyers-McKeever classification of
  tibial fracture
Meyhoefer bone curet
Meynert, nucleus basalis of
Meynet node

Meyn-Quigley maneuver
MFA (Musculoskeletal Function
Assessment)
MFD (monorhythmic frontal delta)
activity
MFD waves
MFG (magnetic field gradients)
MFG (manofluorography)
MG (myasthenia gravis) antibody
MGH osteotome
MG II prosthesis
mGluR5 (metabotropic glutamate
receptor subtype 5)
MGUS (monoclonal gammopathy of
uncertain significance)
mGy/MBq (milligray per megabec-
querel)
MHAQ (Modified Health Assessment
Questionnaire)
MHT (meningohypophyseal trunk)
artery
MHz (megahertz)
Miacalcin (calcitonin salmon)
Miami Acute Care (MAC) cervical
collar
Miami J cervical collar
Miami TLSO scoliosis brace
MIBG (metaiodobenzylguanidine)
imaging agent
MIBG scintigraphy
MIBG SPECT scan
mice, joint
Michael Reese articulated prosthesis
Michel clip
Michele vertebral biopsy
Michele vertebral body trephine
Michigan Bone Health Study
Michigan Hand Outcomes Question-
naire
microabscess
microadenoma
endocrine-inactive pituitary
pituitary
Micro-Aire blade
Micro-Aire debridement of bone
surfaces
Micro-Aire drill

Micro-Aire oscillating saw
Micro-Aire osteotome
Micro-Aire pulse lavage system
Micro-Aire reamer
microaneurysm, Charcot-Bouchard
microangiopathy
microatheroma
microballoon
embolization
Rand
microbipolar forceps
microbubbles, lipid-coated
microcatheter
Tracker 18
UltraLite flow-directed
microcavitation
Microcell-puff material
microcephalic
microcephaly
microcirculation, digital
microclip
microcuret
microcurrent interferential therapy
microdactylia
microdialysis, intracerebral
microdiskectomy (or microdiscec-
tomy), arthroscopic (AMD)
microdissector
FD-43
Rhoton
microdrill
microelectrode mapping
microelectrode recording guidance
microembolectomy
microembolus (pl. microemboli)
microendarterectomy, carotid
microendoscopic diskectomy (MED)
system
microfibrillar collagen hemostat
microfibrils of connective tissue
Microfoam dressing
microforceps
microfractured (MCRF) lesions
microfreer
microgeodic disease
microglioblastoma tumor
microgyria in parkinsonism

microgyrus
microhemorrhage
microinfarction
microinstability
microirrigation
micro-Kerrison rongeur
Microknit vascular graft prosthesis
Microlight 830 laser device
Microloc knee prosthesis
microlumbar diskectomy (MLD)
micromanipulator
micrometer device
MicroMite anchor suture
micromovement (wiggling and
    fidgeting)
micronerve hook
microneurography
microneurosurgery, endoscope-assisted
micronucleator
Micro-One dissecting forceps
Micro-One hook
Micro-One needle holder
Micro-One scissors
micro-pin, Pischel
microplate
    C-shaped
    H-shaped
    half-circle
    L-shaped
    Leibinger
    Luhr
    Storz Microsystem
    Synthes Microsystem
    T-shaped
    X-shaped
    Y-shaped
micropolygyria
microport
Micro-Probe tip
micropsia
Micro QuickAnchor
microradiograph
microreamer
microrecording-guided pallidotomy
microrongeur
microsatellite instability
microsatellite marker

microsaw
    oscillating
    Zimmer
microscissors
    Decker
    Yasargil
microscope
    double binocular operating
    Grenoble-Paris-Rennes (GPR) robot
    Leica Aristoplan laser-scanning
    operating
    robot neurosurgical
    stereotactic (or stereotaxic)
        operating
    Zeiss OPMI surgical
microscopic hemorrhage of ligaments
microscopy
    capillary
    confocal
    darkfield
    immuno-electron
    nail-fold
microsomia
    craniofacial
    hemifacial
microscrew, Barouk
Microscribe 3DX digitizer
Micro Series wire driver
microsphere
microstaple, Barouk
microsurgery
    computer-assisted
    guided
    stereotactic laser
    video-endoscope-assisted
microsurgical decompression
microsurgical dissection
microsurgical DREZ-otomy
microsurgical free flap
microsurgical free tissue transfer
microsuture
MicroTeq portable belt
Micro-Three microsurgery instruments
micro tear
Micro-Two forceps
Micro-Two needle holder
Micro-Two scissors

microtrauma
   cumulative
   repeated
microvascular decompression
microvascular disease
microvascular hemodynamics
microvasculature
microvolts (μV)
Micro-Z neuromusculator stimulator
micturition syncope
MID (multi-infarct dementia)
Midas Rex craniotomy bur
Midas Rex craniotomy saw
Midas Rex knife
Midas Rex mechanism
Midas Rex pneumatic instruments
Midas Rex saw
midaxillary line incision
midbody of vertebra
midbrain
   paramedian
   tegmentum of
midbrain aqueduct
midbrain compression, destruction
midbrain displacement syndrome
midbrain dysfunction
midbrain lesions
midbrain reticular formation (MRF)
midbrain stroke
midbrain subthalamic region
midbrain syndrome
midbrain tumor
midcalf
midcarpal joint
midcervical flexion myelopathy
Middeldorpf splint
Middeldorpf triangle
middle atlantoepistrophic joint
middle carpal joint
middle cerebellar peduncle
middle cerebral artery syndrome
middle cerebral artery territory stroke
middle cervical cardiac nerve
middle cluneal nerves
middle constrictor muscle of pharynx
middle costotransverse ligament
middle field strength MR imaging

middle frontal gyrus
middle medial palsy
middle meningeal nerve
middle-path regimen for spinal TB
middle radial palsy
middle scalene muscle
middle supraclavicular nerve
middle temporal gyrus
middle umbilical ligament
mid-dorsal back pain
midfacial fracture
midfemur
midfoot cavus
midfoot, swivel dislocation of
midget MRI scanner
midline cerebellum
midline shift on skull x-ray
midline tumors of the anterior lobe
midpalmar abscess
midpalmar space
midpatellar tendon
midpons
Midrin
midsagittal MR image
midshaft fracture
midshaft of femur
midshaft of humerus
midstance of gait
midsternum
midswing phase of gait
midtarsal joint
midthigh
MIE Deluxe Bubble inclinometer
migraine accompaniments
migraine aura
migraine diathesis
migraine equivalent
migraine headache
   abdominal
   acephalalgic
   acute confusional (ACM)
   aphasic
   basilar
   basilar artery
   Bickerstaff
   bilateral
   catamenial

migraine headache *(continued)*
  ciliary
  circumstantial
  classic
  classical
  classical abdominal
  cluster
  common
  complicated
  confusional
  facioplegic
  familial
  familial hemiplegic
  hemiparesthetic
  hemiplegic
  late-life
  let-down
  ocular
  ophthalmic
  ophthalmoplegic
  paroxysmal
  pectoralgic
  recurrent
  recurring
  red
  retinal
  seasonal
  syncopal
  unilateral
  vestibular
  white
migraine headache prodrome
migraine-like headache
migraine precipitated by:
  birth control pills
  coitus
  emotional tension
  exercise
  food
  menstruation
  nasal congestion
  pregnancy
  temperature changes
migraine precipitated premenstrually
migraine predisposition
migraine spectra
migraineur

migrainoid neuralgia
migrainous constitution
migrainous disorder
migrainous infarction
migrainous neuralgia
migrainous reaction
migrainous stroke
migrainous symptom
migrainous syncope
migrainous syndrome
migralepsy
Migranal (dihydroergotamine
  mesylate) nasal spray
migrans, erythema
MigraSpray
migration
  acetabular cup
  hallux
  humeral head
  prosthesis
  sesamoid
  staple
  stem cell
migration index, Reimer
migration, tilt, and motion
migratory arthralgia
Miguard (frovatriptan)
MII (McDowell Impairment Index)
Mik pad (slang for Mikulicz pad)
Mikhail bone block
Mikulicz angle
Mikulicz pad
Mikulicz sponge
Milch cuff resection of ulna technique
Milch fracture classification syndrome
Milch radioulnar joint repair
mild ataxia
Miles bone chisel
milestone
  delayed motor
  developmental of infants
Milgram test
miliary aneurysm
military [or medical] antishock
  trousers (MAST)
military missile head wound
milk-alkali disease

milk-alkali syndrome
milking of vessel
milk leg disease
Milkman syndrome
Millard-Gubler paralysis
Millard-Gubler syndrome
Millender-Nalebuff wrist arthrodesis
Millennium MLC-120
Miller-Fisher syndrome
Miller-Fisher test
Miller-Fisher variant of Guillain-Barré
    syndrome
Miller foot procedure
Miller Galante I condylar total knee
    system
Miller-Galante hip prosthesis
Miller-Galante knee arthroplasty
Miller-Gubler syndrome
Miller rasp
Miller-Senn retractor
Miller syndrome
Millesi modified technique
Millet neurological test instrument
milliampere (mA)
millicurie (mCi)
Milligan dissector
millijoule (mJ)
Milliknit vascular graft prosthesis
millimeter (mm)
millimeters of mercury (mmHg)
milling-cutter
milliroentgen
millisecond pulses per second
milliseconds (ms, msec)
millivolt (mV)
Mills dressing
Mills test
Milroy disease
Miltex cannulated pin and wire cutter
Miltex double-action pin cutter
Miltex-Kerrison cervical rongeur
Miltex mallet
Miltex pin puller
Miltex rib spreader
Miltex tendon-pulling forceps
Miltex tissue twist hook

Milwaukee cervicothoracolumbosacral
    orthosis
Milwaukee scoliosis brace
mimetic paralysis
mimocausalgia
Minaar classification of coalition
MindSet toe splint
miner's nystagmus
Miner osteotome
mineralization, bone
Minerva cast
Minerva fixation
Minerva jacket
Minerva neurosurgical robot
Minerva orthosis
Minerva vest
Mini-Acutrak small-bone fixation
    system
miniangiogram
miniblink on EEG
Mini C-arm device
minicatheter
minidriver
Mini GLS anchor
mini-Hoffmann external fixator
Mini-Hohmann podiatric retractor
mini-Kessler external fixator
minimal assist
minimal brain dysfunction
minimal-incision plantar fasciotomy
minimally displaced fracture
minimally invasive spinal surgery
    (MISS)
Mini-Mental State Examination
    (MMSE)
miniplate
    C-shaped
    H-shaped
    half-circle
    L-shaped
    Storz Microsystem
    T-shaped
    X-shaped
    Y-shaped
Miniport drug delivery system
Mini QuickAnchor

Mini-Ramp ramp
Mini-Revo Screw suture anchor
miniscrewdriver
minisponge
mini-squat
Minneapolis prosthesis
Minnesota Multiphasic Personality
Inventory (MMPI)
Minnesota Rate of Manipulation Test
Minnesota Test for Differential
Diagnosis of Aphasia (MTDDA)
Minnesota Test of Aphasia
minor causalgia
minor chorea
minor motor seizures
minor reflex dystrophy
minor reflex sympathetic dystrophies
Minor sign
minor sprain
minor syndrome, pectoralis
Mira cautery
Miralene suture
Mira Mark III cranial drill
Mira Mark V craniotome set
Mirapex (pramipexole dihydro-
chloride)
Mira reamer
Mirra classification
mirror
Apfelbaum
dental
mirror hand
mirror image aneurysms
mirroring
mirtazapine (Remeron)
MIS (Memory Impairment Screen)
MIS (minimum incision surgery)
misalign
Mishler flush valve
Miskimon cerebellar retractor
misplaced objects test
MISS (minimally invasive spinal
surgery)
misshapen
missiles, fully-jacketed (handgun)
missile wound

Mississippi Scale for Combat-Related
Post-traumatic Stress Disorder
Mital elbow release technique
Mitchell distal osteotomy to correct
hallux valgus
Mitchell osteotomy bunionectomy
Mitchell step-down osteotomy
Mitek bone anchor
Mitek GII suture anchor
Mitek knotless suture anchor
Mitek Mini GII suture
Mitek staples
Mitek Superanchor suture anchor
Mitek suture anchor
Mitek Vapr T electrode
mitigating factors
mitochondrial DNA
mitochondrial encephalomyopathy
mitochondrial myopathy
mitotic figures
Mitraflex SC sacral dressing
Mittlemeir broach
Mittlemeir ceramic hip prosthesis
Mittlemeir non-cemented femoral
prosthesis
Mitutoyo digital calipers
Mivacron (mivacurium)
mixed connective tissue disease
mixed nerve
mixed tumors
MixEvac bone-cement mixer
Mixter forceps
Mixter hemostat
Mixter ventricular needles
Miya hook ligament carrier
Miyakawa knee procedure
Mizuno technique
MKG knee support
MKM AutoPilot stereotactic system
MLD (metachromatic leukodystrophy)
MLD (microlumbar diskectomy)
MLF (medial longitudinal fasciculus)
MLF lesion
MLF syndrome
ml/min/100 g (milliliters per minute
per 100 grams)

MLS (mini lag-screw system)
MLSI (multiple line-scan imaging)
mm (millimeter)
MMCM (macromolecular contrast
  medium)
mmHg (millimeters of mercury)
mmol (millimoles)
mmol/kg (millimoles per kilogram)
mmol/L (millimoles per liter)
MMPI (Minnesota Multiphasic
  Personality Inventory)
MMP-1/TIMP-1 ratio
MMT (manual muscle test)
Mn (manganese)
$MnCl_2$ (manganese chloride 2)
  imaging agent
MNCV (motor nerve conduction
  velocity)
MND (motor neuron disease)
mnemonic retrieval of verbal information
mnemonics
MO (myositis ossificans)
MOAB, MoAb (monoclonal antibody), radiolabeled
Moberg arthrodesis
Moberg flap
Moberg-Gedda open reduction fracture
Moberg osteotome
Moberg pick-up stereognosis test
Mobetron electron beam system
mobile bearing knee implant
mobile magnetic resonance (MR)
  imager
Mobilimb CPM (continuous passive
  motion) device
mobility
  Duran passive
  fundamental aspects of
  independent in bed
  joint
  Maitland
  neural (physiotherapy)
  normal
  soft tissue
  spinal
  trigger point

mobility disability
mobility handicap
Mobility Healing Clogs
Mobility Shoes
mobilization
  Duran passive
  joint
  Maitland
  neural
  soft tissue
  spinal
  trigger point
Möbius (Moebius) syndrome
MOBS (Montefiore Organic Brain
  Scale)
modality
  passive treatment
  sensory
  therapeutic
model, Korr neurologic
modeling, regression
MODEMS (Musculoskeletal Outcomes
  Data Evaluation and Management
  System)
mode, press-fit
moderate ataxia
moderate dysarthria
Modic disk abnormality classification
Modic grade of inflammatory change
modification
  body mechanics
  Green-Laird m. of Reverdin
    osteotomy
  medial heel-wedge shoe
  metatarsal bar shoe
  Morrey
  shoe
modified Ashworth Scale for grading
  spasticity
modified birdcage coils
modified Dolenc procedure
modified dorsalis pedis myofascial flap
modified electron-beam CT scanner
modified extrabursal Chow technique
  of endoscopic carpal tunnel release
modified Harris Hip Score

Modified Health Assessment Questionnaire (MHAQ)
modified Isshiki type 4 thyroplasty
modified Lapidus arthrodesis
modified Mau bunionectomy
modified McBride bunionectomy
modified Oppenheimer splint
modified Rowe shoulder score
modified self-report measure of social adjustment
modified vessel image processor (mVIP) software
Modny pin
modular coded aperture technology (MCAT) collimator
modular socket
modulator, immune
Modulock posterior spinal fixation
modulus of elasticity
Moe bone curet
Moe distraction rod
Moe gouge
Moe impactor
Moe-Kettleson distribution of curves in scoliosis
Moe modified Cotrel cast
Moe osteotome
Moe spinal hook
Moe square-ended hook
Moe modified Harrington rod
Moebius (Möbius) syndrome
Moeltgen flexometer
mofetil (CellCept)
Mogadon (nitrazepam)
mogi postop shoe cover
Mohrenheim space
Mohr splint
Mohr syndrome
Mohtadi Quality of Life Assessment Score
MOI (mechanism of injury)
Moire topographic scoliosis screening assessment
moist heat
Molander-Olerud ankle scoring system
mold, Aufranc concentric hip
molding (or moulding) of skull

molecular genetics
molecule
   adhesion
   circulating intercelluluar adhesion molecule-1 (ICAM-1)
   circulating intercelluluar adhesion molecule-3 (ICAM-3)
   circulating vascular adhesion (VCAM)
   EC (endothelial cell) adhesion
   endothelial cell (EC) adhesion
   HLA-B27
   ICAM-1 (circulating intercelluluar adhesion molecule-1)
   ICAM-3 (circulating intercellular adhesion molecule-3)
   macrophage (mø) adhesion
   PECAM-1 (platelet and EC adhesion molecule-1)
   platelet and EC adhesion molecule-1 (PECAM-1)
   sialoadhesin (Sn)
   vascular cell adhesion molecule-1 (VCAM-1)
   VCAM (circulating vascular adhesion molecule)
   VCAM-1 (vascular cell adhesion molecule-1)
moleskin dressing
moleskin patch
moleskin strips
Molesworth-Campbell elbow approach
Mollaret meningitis
Mollaret triangle
Molt periosteal elevator
momentum, center-of-mass
Monarch knee brace
monarthric process
monarthritis
monarticular gout
Mönckeberg medial sclerosis
mongolian idiocy
monitor
   A-2000 BIS (Bispectral Index)
   Camino ICP
   eye movement (EM)
   ICP (intracranial pressure)

monitor *(continued)*
 intracranial
 Meduck anesthesia
 nerve integrity (Xomed NIM-2)
 Phoenix ICP
 Polar Vantage XL heart rate
 pressure
 Spiegelberg intracranial pressure
 subdural pressure
 submental EMG activity
 Tekscan in-shoe
 thoracic strain gauge
 Monitor-2, Nicolet Nerve Integrity
  (NIM-2)
monitoring
 fluorescein perfusion
 skinfold thickness
 thermocouple
Monk hip prosthesis
monoarticular
monoblock femoral stem prosthesis
monoclonal antibodies, human midkine
monoclonal antibody (MoAb) imaging
monoclonal gammopathy of uncertain
 significance (MGUS)
Monocryl suture
monocular acuity change
monocular blindness
monocular visual loss
monodactylism
monofilament nylon drain
Monofixateur external fixator
monolithic Al203 cup
monomalleolar ankle fracture
monomorphic wave
monomyoplegia
monomyositis multiplex
mononeural
mononeuritis multiplex
mononeuropathy
 cranial
 diabetic
 diabetic third nerve
 entrapment
 ischemic
 localized hypertrophic

mononeuropathy *(continued)*
 ocular
 sensory
mononeuropathy multiplex
monoparesis
monophasic anodal stimulus
monophasic cathodal stimulus
monophasic sharp wave
monoplegia, crural
monorhythmic frontal delta (MFD)
 activity
monorhythmic frontal delta (MFD)
 waves
monorhythmic frontal slowing
monorhythmic pattern
monorhythmic waves
monosodium urate crystal deposition
monostotic fibrous dysplasia
monosyllabic speech
monosynaptic reflex arc
Monro
 aqueduct of
 foramen of
Monro bursa
Monro-Kellie doctrine
montage
 bipolar
 circumferential bipolar
 common average reference
 common reference
 coronal bipolar
 Cz reference
 double-banana
 ear reference
 8-channel
 18-channel
 ipsilateral reference
 Laplacian
 LB (longitudinal bipolar)
 linked ear reference
 longitudinal bipolar (LB)
 noncephalic reference
 referential alternating
 referential block
 reformatting
 scalp-scalp

montage *(continued)*
  16-channel
  source derivation
  TB (transverse bipolar)
  transverse bipolar (TB)
  unipolar
Montefiore Organic Brain Scale
  (MOBS)
Monteggia fracture-dislocation of ulna
Monteggia lesion
Montenovesi rongeur
Montercaux fracture
Monticelli-Spinelli distractor
Monticelli-Spinelli fixator
Monticelli-Spinelli frame
Montreal hip positioner
Montreal pegboard
mood swing
Moon Boot brace
Mooney brace
Mooney cast
Moore bone elevator
Moore bone reamer
Moore-Darrach radioulnar joint repair
Moore fracture
Moore hand drill
Moore nail set
Moore osteotomy-osteoclasis
Moore pin
Moore plate
Moore stem
mooring
Morand spur
morbidity
  cognitive
  donor site
morcel (or morsel)
morcelize (or morselize)
morcellation, Robinson-Chung-
  Farahvar clavicular
Moreira bolt
Moreira plate
Moreland osteotome
Morel syndrome
Morfam Quality Jeanie Rub massager
Morgagni, hyperostosis of
Morgagni-Stewart-Morel syndrome

Morgan-Casscells meniscus suturing
  technique
Morgan disk pad
moribund appearance
moribund state
morning shakes
Moro reflex
morphology
  EEG complex
  fused alpha wave
  joint
  wave
morphometric data
morphometric evaluation
morphometry
  joint
  magnetic resonance imaging
Morquio sign
Morquio syndrome
Morrey arthritis grading system
Morrey-Bryan total elbow arthroplasty
Morrey modification of Boyd-
  Anderson biceps tendon repair
Morrey score
Morris biphase screw
Morris retractor
Morrison technique
Morrissy percutaneous fixation of
  slipped epiphysis
Morscher titanium cervical plate
morsel (or morcel)
morselize (or morcelize)
morselizer, graft
morselized bone graft
Morse sternal spreader
Morse tape
Morse tapered prosthetic post
Morse taper stem
mortise
  ankle
  axis of ankle
  cuneiform
  diaphyseal cortical
  joint
  mortised
  widening of the ankle, on x-ray
mortise cut

mortise joint
mortise view
mortising chisel
Morton foot
Morton-Horwitz nerve crossover sign
Morton metatarsalgia
Morton neuralgia
Morton neuroma
Morton sign
Morton syndrome
Morton test
Morton toe
Morvan chorea
Morvan disease
Morvan syndrome
mosaic arthroplasty
mosaic disorder of visual perception
  in migraine
mosaic plantar verruca
mosaic plantar wart
mosaicplasty, arthroscopic
MosaicPlasty system
Mose concentric rings
Mose method
Moseley bone age graph
Moseley fasciatome
Moseley straight line graph
Mosley method for anterior shoulder
  repair
Moss fixation system
Moss hook
Moss Miami load-sharing spinal
  implant system
Moss rod
Moss screw
moth-eaten appearance
mother-daughter-type plantar warts
Mother Jones dressing
motility
  extraocular
  ocular
motion
  active ankle joint complex range of
    (AAROM)
  active-assistive range of
  active integral range of (AIROM)

motion *(continued)*
  ankle dorsiflexion range of
    (ADROM)
  ankle inversion-eversion range of
  arc of
  continuous passive (CPM)
  end-range limitation of
  full range of (FROM)
  limitation of
  passive range of (PROM)
  plantarflexory
  protective limitation of range of
  range of
  scapulothoracic
  shear
  toe range of
  uninhibited ankle
motion capture system
motivation, patient
motor (EEG lead)
  left (LM)
  right (RM)
motor activity log
motor aphasia
motor apraxia
Motor Assessment scale (MAS)
Motor Club assessment of motor
  impairment
Motor Control Test (MCT)
motor cortex mapping
motor delay
motor disorder
motor dysphasia
motor evoked potential
motor fibers
motor function
motor hemiplegia, pure
motor impairment
  anterior horn cell level
  peripheral nerve level
  root level
  spinal nerve level
motor impersistence
motor jacksonian attack
motor loss
motor march, jacksonian

motor measures, to test sensory
    disturbance
motor negativism
motor nerve conduction study
motor nerve fibers
motor neurofibrils
motor neuron disease (MND)
motor nuclei
motor oil hygroma
motor output
motor paralytic bladder
motor paresis
motor performance
motor phenomena
motor potential
motor power
motor problem, high level
motor set-shifting
motor sign
motor skills
motor speech area of the brain, Broca
motor strip
motor symptoms
motor task activation
motor tic
motor transcortical aphasias
motor unit action potential
motor vehicle accident (MVA)
motor vehicle collision/crash (MVC)
motor vehicle injury (MVI)
motorcyclist's knee
Motoricity Index
motorized bur
motorized shaver
Mouchet paralysis of cubital nerve
Mouchet syndrome
moulage
Mount laminectomy rongeur
Mouradian rod
Mouradian screw
mouse, joint
mouthing phenomenon (pathological
    reflex)
mouth, tapir's (bouche de tapir)
movable joint
Movana

movement
adventitious
anomalous
arcuate
automatic hand
basal
bread-crumbling
choreic limb
choreiform
choreoathetoid
choreoathetotic
clonic
conjugate eye
decomposition of
dysconjugate eye
dysjunctive eye
dysmetric overshoot of eye
dyspractic
dysrhythmic
dystonic
fine finger
fly-catching m. of tongue
following
freezing of
functional
grades of
horizontal metronomic eye
hyperkinetic
Independent Living
initiation of
involuntary limb
irregular
jerking
jerky incoordinate
mouthing
nystagmoid
objective limited
organization of ocular
passive accessory intervertebral
    (PAIVMs)
passive physiological intervertebral
    (PPIVMs)
poverty of
prehensile hand
pseudoathetoid
purposeless

movement *(continued)*
  pursuit
  quasipurposive
  random
  rapid
  rapid-alternating (RAM)
  rapid eye (REM)
  reflex eye
  reflexive
  rhythmic slow eye
  roving eye
  roving ocular
  saccadic eye
  slow lateral eye (SEMs)
  smooth pursuit eye
  subjective limited
  supranuclear disorders of ocular
  symmetry of limb
  synkinetic motor
  tonic-clonic
  tremulous
  uncontrollable
  vermicular
  visual pursuit
  visual tracking
  volitional
  voluntary
  withdrawal
movement artifact
movement diagram
movement disorder
movers
  capital
  cervical
  prime
moving two-point discrimination
moxibustion
moyamoya disease
moyamoya vessel
Moynihan forceps
Moynihan towel clamp
MP (metatarsophalangeal or metacarpophalangeal) (MTP or MCP)
  joint
MPAP (multipurpose access port),
  Cordis

MPCh (medial posterior choroidal)
  artery
MPGR (multiplanar gradient-recalled)
  echo
MPJ (metatarsophalangeal joint)
MPNST (malignant peripheral nerve
  sheath tumor)
MPQ (McGill Pain Questionnaire)
MPR (multiplanar reformation)
MP-RAGE (magnetization prepared
  3D gradient-echo) sequences
MPS (myofascial pain syndrome)
MP35N implant metal prosthesis
MPV (metatarsus primus varus)
MRA (magnetic resonance
  angiography)
MRC (Medical Research Council)
  classification of muscle function
MRCAS ([Center for] Medical
  Robotics and Computer-Assisted
  Surgery)
MRF (midbrain reticular formation)
MRI (magnetic resonance imaging)
  acquisition time
  adiabatic fast passage
  analog-to-digital converter
  angular frequency
  angular momentum
  antenna
  array processor
  artifact
  Bloch equation
  Boltzmann distribution
  Carr-Purcell sequence
  Carr-Purcell-Meiboom-Gill
    sequence
  chemical shift
  circumferential dedicated knee coil
  coherence
  coil
  constructive interference in steady
    state (CISS)
  continuous wave
  contrast-to-noise ratio
  crossed coil
  cryomagnet

MRI *(continued)*
  cryostat
  demodulator
  detector
  diamagnetic
  diffusion
  digital-to-analog converter
  echo-planar imaging
  echo time (TE)
  echo (pl. echoes)
  eddy currents (pl. eddies)
  excitation
  Faraday shield
  fast-Fourier transform
  fast spoiled gradient echo
    acquisition
  fat suppression technique
  fat-suppressed proton-density fast
    spin-echo imaging
  fat-suppressed 3D spoiled gradient-
    echo imaging
  fat-suppressed T2-weighted fast
    spin-echo imaging
  ferromagnetic
  FID (free induction decay)
  field gradient
  field lock
  filling factor
  filtered-back projection
  flip angle
  Fourier transform
  free induction decay (FID)
  free induction signal
  frequency
  frequency encoding
  functional (fMRI)
  gadolinium enhancement
  gauss
  Golay coil
  gradient coil
  gradient magnetic field
  gyromagnetic ratio
  heavily T2-weighted
  Helmholtz coil
  hertz (Hz)
  homogeneity
  image acquisition time

MRI *(continued)*
  inductance
  inhomogeneity
  interface
  interpulse time
  intraoperative
  inversion
  inversion recovery
  inversion time (TI)
  kilohertz (kHz)
  Larmor equation
  Larmor frequency
  lattice
  line imaging
  line scanning
  line width
  LMR (localized magnetic resonance)
  longitudinal magnetization
  longitudinal relaxation
  Lorentzian line
  macroscopic magnetization moment
  macroscopic magnetization vector
  magnetic dipole
  magnetic field
  magnetic gradient
  magnetic induction
  magnetic moment
  magnetic resonance
  magnetic resonance signal
  magnetic susceptibility
  magnetization
  Magnetom Open
  multiple line-scan imaging (MLSI)
  multiple plane imaging
  multiple sensitive point
  nuclear magnetic resonance
  nuclear signal
  nuclear spin
  nuclear spin quantum number
  nucleon
  nutation
  open
  optimized pulse sequence
  orientation: coronal; sagittal;
    transverse
  paramagnetic
  partial saturation

MRI *(continued)*

permanent magnet
permeability
phantom
phase
phased-array surface coil
phase-sensitive detector
pixel (picture element)
planar spin imaging
point imaging
point scanning
precession
precessional frequency
PRESS-CSI sequence
proton
pulse length
pulse sequences
pulse width
pulse, radiofrequency
pulsed gradients
quadrature detector
quality factor
quenching
radian
radiofrequency (RF)
radiofrequency coil
radiofrequency pulse
readout delay
receiver
receiver coil
reconstruction
relaxation rate
relaxation time
repeated FID (free induction decay)
repetition time (TR)
rephasing gradient
resistive magnet
resolution, spatial
resonance
resonant frequency
RF (radiofrequency)
RF coil
RF pulse
rotating frame of reference
S/N ratio (signal-to-noise)
saddle coil
saturation recovery

MRI *(continued)*

saturation transfer
selective excitation
selective irradiation
sensitive plane
sensitive point
sensitive volume
sequence time
sequential plane imaging
sequential point imaging
shim coil
shimming
Signa Special Procedures (SP)
signal-to-noise ratio (SNR or
   S/N ratio)
simultaneous volume imaging
skin depth
SNR (signal-to-noise ratio)
solenoid coil
spectrometer
spectrum
spin
spin density
spin echo
spin-echo imaging
spin-lattice relaxation time
spin-spin relaxation time
spin-warp imaging
steady state free precession (SSFP)
stereotactic
superconducting magnet
surface coil MR
T1 (spin-lattice or longitudinal
   relaxation time)
T2 (spin-spin or transverse
   relaxation time)
TE (echo time)
tesla (T)
3D Fourier transformation MRI
   (3DFT MRI)
3D Fourier transform imaging
TI (inversion time)
TR (repetition time)
transverse magnetization
tuning
tunnel
2D Fourier transform imaging

MRI *(continued)*
   vector
   volume imaging
   voxel (volume element)
   zeugmatography, Fourier
      transformation
MRI bone bruise
MRI-derived target coordinates
MRI with gadolinium enhancement
MRM (magnetic resonance myelo-
   gram)
MRN (magnetic resonance neurog-
   raphy)
mRNA (messenger ribonucleic acid)
MRP (multidrug resistance protein)
MRS (magnetic resonance spec-
   troscopy)
MRU (molecular recognition unit)
ms (milliseconds)
MS (multiple sclerosis) plaquing
MSA (multiple system atrophy)
   syndrome
MSAD (multiple scan average dose)
MSC cold pack
MSD (midsagittal diameter)
msec (millisecond)
MSI (magnetic source imaging)
MSLT (multiple sleep latency test)
MST (multifocal sharp transient)
MST-6A1-4V implant metal prosthesis
MS-325 imaging agent
MSTS/ISOLS questionnaire
MSTS score
MSUD (maple syrup urine disease)
MT (or MTP) joint (metatarso-
   phalangeal)
MTA (metatarsus adductus)
MTDDA (Minnesota Test for Differ-
   ential Diagnosis of Aphasia)
MTM 2 bur
MTP (metatarsophalangeal)
   MTP capsule
   MTP joint
MTR (magnetization transfer ratio)
MTS servo-hydraulic testing machine
MTSS (medial tibial stress syndrome)
MTV (metatarsus varus)

MUA (manipulation under anesthesia)
MUAP (motor unit action potential)
Mubarak-Hargens decompression
   technique
MUCL (medial ulnar collateral
   ligament)
mucocele, intracranial
mucocutaneous muscle
mucocyst
mucolipidosis III (pseudo-Hurler
   deformity)
mucoperiosteal thickening
mucopolysaccharides
mucopolysaccharidosis
mucopurulent drainage
mucormycosis, rhinocerebral
mucosal suspensory ligament
mud pack bath
Mueli wrist prosthesis
Mueller ATF ankle brace
Mueller back brace
Mueller Duo-Lock hip prosthesis
Mueller hinged knee brace
Mueller Lite ankle brace
Mueller muscle
Mueller orthopedic shoulder brace
Mueller wrap-around knee brace
Muhlberger orbital implant prosthesis
Mulder sign
Mulholland and Gunn criteria
Müller (Mueller)
Müller arthrodesis
Müller classification of humerus
   fractures
Müller muscle
Müller knee procedure
Müller saw
multiangle multislice acquisition
   magnetic resonance imaging
multangular bone, accessory
multangular, greater (or lesser)
multangular ridge fracture
multiaxial joint
MultiBoot orthosis
multicentric lesion
multicomponent pheresis
multicrystal gamma camera

Multidex hydrophilic powder wound
dressing
multidirectional shoulder instability
multidrug resistance protein (MRP)
multiecho axial
multiecho coronal image
multiecho image
multiecho sequence
multifield beam
multifidus muscle
Multifire VersaTack
multifocal lesions
multifocal leukoencephalopathy,
progressive (PML)
multifocal myoclonus
multifocal seizures
multiforme, glioblastoma
multi-infarct dementia (MID)
multi-item indices in rehabilitation
testing
Multileaf Collimator
multilinear regression analysis
Multilingual Aphasia Examination
Controlled Oral Word Association
Test
Multi-Lock hip prosthesis
Multi-Lock knee brace
Multilok hand operating table
multimodal image fusion technique
multimodality evoked potential (MEP)
multimodality imaging
multinuclear magnetic resonance
imaging
Multipaks, Ortho-Ice
multipennate muscle
multiphasic multislice magnetic
resonance imaging technique
multiplanar compression
multiplanar fluoroscopic stress view
multiplanar gradient-recalled (MPGR)
echo
multiplanar ligamentotaxis
multiplanar magnetic resonance
imaging
multiplanar reformatted radiographic
and digitally reconstructed images
multiple cartilaginous exostoses

multiple cortical infarcts
multiple enchondromatosis (Ollier
disease)
multiple exposure volumetric
holography (MEVH)
multiple focal lesions
multiple fractures
multiple hereditary osteochondromatosis
multiple line-scan imaging (MLSI)
multiple meningiomas
multiple neuroma
multiple plane imaging
multiple sclerosis (MS)
benign form
chronic progressive
chronic relapsing
exacerbating-remitting
graying of vision in
Ishihara color plate test for
primary progressive
relapsing-remitting
secondary progressive
multiple sclerosis plaquing
multiple sclerosis plateau
multiple sensitive point
multiple sleep latency test (MSLT)
multiple slice acquisition
multiple small strokes (état lacunaire)
multiple symphalangism
multiple system atrophy (MSA)
multiple strand suture method
multiple suture synostosis
multiple trauma
multiplex
mononeuritis
paramyoclonus
Multi Podus boot system
Multipoise headrest
MultiPolar bipolar cup
multipulse nuclear magnetic resonance
(NMR) imaging
multipulse stimulation
multishot echo planar imaging
multislice FLASH 2D
multislice multiphase spin-echo
imaging technique

multislice spin-echo sequence
multisystem disease
Multitak SS suture anchor
Multitak suture system
mumbling automatism
Mumford-Gurd arthroplasty
Mumford-Gurd procedure
mumps encephalitis
mumps viral encephalitis
Münchmeyer disease
Mundinger-Reichert stereotactic frame
murine typhus meningoencephalitis
"murmuring a perpetual litany"
murmurs (thrills)
Murphy gouge
Murphy heel cord advancement
Murphy-Lane bone skid
Murphy osteotome
Murphy punch test
Murray-Jones splint
Murray-Thomas splint
Murray Valley (Australian X) viral
    encephalitis
muscle (see Table of Muscles in the
    Appendix)
    abdominis rectus
    abductor
    abductor hallucis
    adductor
    adductor pollicis
    ADQ (abductor digiti quinti)
    anconeus
    antagonistic
    anterior papillary
    antigravity
    antistriated
    APB (abductor pollicis brevis)
    APL (abductor pollicis longus)
    appendicular
    articular
    aryepiglotticus
    ascending oblique
    atrophied
    BBC (biceps, brachialis,
        coracobrachialis)
    belly of
    biarthrodial

muscle *(continued)*
    biceps brachii
    biceps femoris
    biopsy
    bipennate
    bipenniform
    brachial
    brachialis
    brachioradialis
    broad
    bronchoesophageal
    calf
    cardiac
    Casser
    casserian
    cervical interspinal
    cervical rotator
    Chassaignac
    cheek
    ciliary
    circumpennate
    coccygeal
    compressor
    coracobrachial
    corrugator
    cowl
    cremaster
    cricothyroid
    cruciate
    cucullaris
    cutaneomucous
    cutaneous
    degeneration of muscle
    deltoid
    denervated
    denervation of
    depressor
    digastric
    dilator
    dorsal interosseous
    DRAM (de-epithelialized rectus
        abdominis)
    ECRB (extensor carpi radialis
        brevis)
    ECRL (extensor carpi radialis
        longus)
    ECU (extensor carpi ulnaris)

muscle *(continued)*

   EDB (extensor digitorum brevis)
   EDC (extensor digitorum communis)
   EDL (extensor digitorum longus)
   EDQ (extensor digitorum quinti)
   EHL (extensor hallucis longus)
   EIP (extensor indicis proprius)
   enlarged calf
   EPB (extensor pollicis brevis)
   epicranial
   EPL (extensor pollicis longus)
   EQP (extensor quinti proprius)
   erector
   eustachian
   extensor
   external oblique
   external obturator
   external pterygoid
   extraocular
   extrinsic
   eyeball
   facial
   fan-shaped
   fasciculations of
   fast
   fauces
   FCR (flexor carpi radialis)
   FCU (flexor carpi ulnaris)
   FDC (flexor digitorum communis)
   FDI (first digital interosseous)
   FDL (flexor digitorum longus)
   FDP (flexor digitorum profundus)
   FDQ (flexor digiti quinti)
   FDS (flexor digitorum sublimis)
   FDS (flexor digitorum superficialis)
   femoral
   FHB (flexor hallucis brevis)
   FHL (flexor hallucis longus)
   fibrosed
   fibular
   finger flexor
   fixation
   fixator
   flat
   flat abdominal
   flexor
   Folius

muscle *(continued)*

   FPB (flexor pollicis brevis)
   FPL (flexor pollicis longus)
   fusiform
   Gantzer
   gastrocnemius
   Gavard
   gemellus
   genioglossal
   geniohyoid
   ghost
   glossopalatine
   glossopharyngeal
   gluteal
   gluteus
   gluteus maximus
   gluteus medius
   gluteus minimus
   gracilis
   greater posterior rectus
   greater psoas
   Guthrie
   hamstring
   Hilton
   Horner
   Houston
   humeroperoneal
   hyoglossal
   hypothenar
   iliac
   iliocostal
   iliopsoas
   incisive
   index extensor
   inferior constrictor
   inferior gemellus
   inferior longitudinal
   inferior oblique
   inferior posterior serratus
   inferior rectus
   inferior tarsal
   infrahyoid
   infraspinatus
   infraspinous
   innermost intercostal
   inspiratory
   intercostal

muscle *(continued)*
interfoveolar
intermediate great
internal oblique
internal obturator
internal pterygoid
interosseous
interspinal
intertransverse
intra-auricular
intraocular
intraspinous
intrinsic
involuntary
ischiocavernosus
isometric
Jarjavay
Jung pyramidal auricular
Klein cutaneomucous
Kohlrausch
Koyter
Landströn
Langer axillary arch
larynx
lateral cricoarytenoid
lateral great
lateral lumbar intertransverse
lateral pterygoid
lateral rectus
lateral vastus
latissimus dorsi
lesser rhomboid
lesser zygomatic
levator
levator ani
ligamentum interfoveolare
ligamentum mallei laterale
lingual
LOAF (lumbricals, opponens
   pollicis, abductor pollicis brevis,
   flexor pollicis brevis)
long
long abductor
long extensor
long fibular
long flexor
longissimus

muscle *(continued)*
longitudinal
long palmar
long peroneal
long radial extensor
lumbar iliocostal
lumbar interspinal
lumbar quadrate
lumbar rotator
lumbrical
Luschka
major
Marcacci
masseter
medial great
medial lumbar intertransverse
medial pterygoid
medial rectus
medial vastus
mentalis
Merkel
mesothenar
middle constrictor
middle scalene
motor point of
mucocutaneous
Müller (Mueller)
multifidus
multipennate
mylohyoid
nasal
nonstriated
notch
oblique arytenoid
oblique auricular
obturator
occipitofrontal
Ochsner
Oddi
ODQ (opponens digiti quinti)
Oehl
omohyoid
opponens pollicis
opposing
orbicular
orbital
organic

muscle *(continued)*
overpull of
palate
palatine
palatoglossus
palatopharyngeal
palmar interosseous
papillary
paraspinal
paravertebral
pectinate
pectineal
pectoral
pectoralis major
pectoralis minor
pectorodorsalis
pennate
penniform
peroneal
pharyngopalatine
Phillips
piriform
plantar
plantar interosseous
plantaris
platysma
pleuroesophageal
popliteal
posterior
posterior auricular
posterior cervical intertransverse
posterior cricoarytenoid
posterior scalene
posterior tibial
postvertebral
Pozzi
procerus
profundus
progressive neuropathic
pronator
psoas
pubococcygeal
quadrate
quadriceps
radial flexor
rectococcygeus
rectourethral

muscle *(continued)*
rectouterine
rectovesical
rectus abdominis
rectus femoris
red
Reisseisen
retronuchal
rider's
rotator
Rouget
round pronator
Ruysch
sacrococcygeal
sacrospinalis
Santorini
sartorius
scalene
scalp
Sebileau
second tibial
semimembranous
semispinal
semitendinosus
septal papillary
serratus anterior
serratus posterior
shawl
short
short adductor
short extensor
short fibular
short flexor
short palmar
short peroneal
short radial extensor
Sibson
skeletal
skeletal striated
slow
smaller helix
smaller pectoral
smaller posterior rectus
smaller psoas
smallest scalene
smooth
Soemmerring

muscle *(continued)*
  soleus
  somatic
  sphincter
  spinal
  spindle-shaped
  splenius
  stapedius
  sternal
  sternochondroscapular
  sternoclavicular
  sternocleidomastoid
  sternocostal
  sternohyoid
  sternothyroid
  strap
  straplike
  stretching of
  striated
  striated cardiac
  subcostal
  subscapularis
  subvertebral
  superficial back
  superficial flexor
  superior tarsal
  supinator
  supraspinatus
  suspensory
  synergistic
  tailor's
  temporal
  temporoparietal
  tensor
  teres major
  teres minor
  thenar
  thigh
  thoracic interspinal
  thoracic longissimus
  thoracic rotator
  tibial
  tibialis anterior
  tibialis posterior
  toe extensor
  toe flexor

muscle *(continued)*
  TRAM (transverse rectus abdominis
    myocutaneous)
  transverse arytenoid
  transversospinal
  transversus abdominis
  trapezius
  triangular
  triceps
  trigonal
  true back
  trunk
  twigs to the piriformis
  two-bellied
  ulnar extensor
  ulnar flexor
  unipennate
  urogenital diaphragmatic
  unstriated
  uvula
  Valsalva
  vastus intermedius
  vastus lateralis
  vastus medialis
  vastus medialis obliquus (VMO)
  ventral sacrococcygeal
  vertical
  visceral
  VMO (vastus medialis obliquus)
  vocal
  voluntary
  white
  Wilson
  wrinkler
  yoked
  zygomatic
muscle action in arthritis
muscle-action potential
muscle anatomy
muscle artifact
muscle atrophy
muscle attachment
muscle belly
muscle biopsy
muscle bulk
muscle clamp

muscle contractility
muscle contraction
muscle contracture
muscle coordination
muscle cramp
muscle denervation
muscle disorder
muscle dissection
muscle dysmorphia
muscle dystrophy
muscle energy metabolism
muscle fascicle
muscle fiber action potential
muscle fiber conduction velocity
muscle fiber wasting
muscle-firing patterns
muscle flap transposition
muscle forceps
muscle function
muscle glycogen supersaturation
muscle group
muscle guarding
muscle hook
muscle imbalance
muscle insufficiency
muscle interference pattern
muscle irritability
muscle ischemia
MuscleMax electrical muscle
    stimulator
muscle origin
muscle palsy, extraocular
muscle-paretic nystagmus
muscle-pedicle bone graft
muscleplasty
muscle potential
muscle power
muscle pump (anatomical)
muscle relaxant
MuscleSense electrical muscle
    stimulator
muscle-setting exercises
muscle sheath
muscle soreness
muscle spasm
muscle-splitting incision
muscle sprain

muscle stimulator, Back Hammer
muscle strain
muscle strength
muscle stretch
muscle-tendon injury
muscle tissue
muscle tone
muscle training
    concentric
    eccentric
muscle transfer
muscle wasting
muscle-wasting fasciculations
muscular atrophy
    scapuloperoneal
    Vulpian-Bernhardt spinal
    Welander distal
    Werdnig-Hoffmann spinal
muscular bridging
muscular dystrophy (MD)
    Becker
    benign X-linked recessive
    Duchenne
    Erb
    fascioscapulohumeral
    Gowers
    Kiloh-Nevin ocular form of
        progressive
    oculopharyngeal
Muscular Dystrophy Association
    (MDA)
Muscular Dystrophy Association of
    Canada (MDAC)
muscular lesion
muscular spondylitis
muscular tonus
musculature
    axial
    cervical
    paraspinal
    paraspinous
    paretic
    scalene
musculocutaneous free flaps
musculocutaneous nerve
Musculoskeletal Function Assessment
    (MFA)

Musculoskeletal Outcomes Data
   Evaluation and Management
   System (MODEMS)
musculoskeletal trauma
Musculoskeletal Tumor Society
musculospiral nerve (radial)
musculospiral paralysis
musculotendinous cuff
musculotendinous junction
musculotendinous-osseous link
Musgrave footprint pedobarograph
musicogenic epilepsy
muslin sling
Mustard iliopsoas transfer
MUSTPAC (medical ultrasound 3D
   portable with advanced communications) imaging
mutated exon
mutation
   de novo
   germline
   heterozygote point
   inherited splice
   nonsense
   single-basepair insertion
   Y-box
mutational analysis
mutation screening
mute, akinetically
mute toe signs
mutism
   akinetic
   elective
   hyperpathic akinetic
   hysterical
   postictal
muzzle velocity (in handgun injury)
MV (megavolt)
mV (millivolt)
MVA (motor vehicle accident)
MVC (motor vehicle collision/crash)
MVD (microvascular decompression)
MVI (motor vehicle injury)
MVM (medullary venous malformation)
MVR blade
MWD (microwave diathermy)
myalgia

myasthenia
   congenital
   ocular
myasthenia gravis (MG)
   familial infantile
   transient neonatal
myasthenic crisis
myasthenic ptosis
myasthenic symptom
myasthenic syndrome
mycobacterium
Mycobacterium malmoense
Mycobacterium terrae
mycetoma
mycophenolate (CellCept)
Mycoplasma pneumoniae encephalitis
mycosis fungoides palmaris et
   plantaris
mycotic aneurysm
mycotic infections of bones and joints
mycotic intracranial aneurysm
mycotic meningitis
myectomy
myelalgia
myelanalosis
myelapoplexy
myelasthenia
myelatelia
myelatrophy
myelauxe
myelencephalon
myelenic neuroma
myeleterosis
myelin
   subcortical
   subependymal
myelinated nerve fiber
myelin basic protein
myelin bleb
myelin damage
myelin metabolism
myelination
myelinoclasis, acute perivascular
myelinolysis
   central pontine
   extrapontine
   pontine

myelin sheath
myelitis
  acute transverse
  ascending
  herpes simplex
  herpes zoster
  postinfectious
  subacute necrotizing
  transverse
myeloablation
myeloblastoma
myelocele
myelocystocele
myelocystomeningocele
myelocytoma
myelodiastasis
myelodysplasia
myelofibrosis
myelogram
  cervical
  corduroy cloth pattern on
  magnetic resonance
  metrizamide
myelographic block
myelographic contrast medium
myelography with (or without)
    contrast
  air
  cervical
  complete
  Hypaque
  lumbar
  lumbosacral
  magnetic resonance (MRM)
  metrizamide
  Pantopaque
  positive contrast
  thoracic
myelography dye
myelolipoma
myeloma
  indolent
  localized
  multiple
  plasma cell
  sclerosing
  solitary

myelomalacia
myelomeningitis
myelomeningocele
myelomere
myeloneuritis
myelo-opticoneuropathy, subacute
  (SMON)
myeloparalysis
myelopathy
  AIDS
  cervical
  cervical spondylotic (CSM)
  CMV (cytomegalovirus)
  compression
  midcervical flexion
  necrotizing
  noncompressive
  progressive subacute
  radiation
  radiation-induced
  spinal stenotic
  spondylitic
  spondylotic
  subacute necrotizing
  transverse
  vacuolar
myelopathy of the spinal cord
myelophthisis
myeloplegia
myeloradiculitis
myeloradiculopathy
myelorrhagia
myelorrhaphy, commissural
myeloschisis, dorsal
myelosclerosis
myelosyphilis
myelosyringosis
myelotomy, midline
Myers-Briggs Personality Inventory
Myers-Briggs Type Indicator (MBTI)
  test
Myers knee retractor
Myerson sign
mylohyoid muscle
mylohyoid nerve
Myloral (bovine myelin)
myoasthenia

myoblast
myoblastoma, granular cell
Myobock artificial hand
myobradia
myocele
myocelialgia
myocelitis
myocellulitis
myocerosis
myocervical rigid collar
myoclasis
myoclonia
   eyelid
   facial
   Ramsey Hunt dyssynergia
     cerebellaris
myoclonic epilepsy
myoclonic jerk
myoclonic seizure
myoclonic spells
myoclonic triangle
myoclonus
   action
   Baltic
   benign
   branchial
   cherry red spot
   epileptic
   essential
   familial essential
   focal
   generalized
   hereditary essential
   infantile
   intention
   Mediterranean
   multifocal
   nocturnal (NM)
   nonepileptic
   nonprogressive
   ocular
   palatal
   palate
   palatopharyngolaryngo-oculo-
     diaphragmatic
   partial
   postanoxic intention

myoclonus *(continued)*
   postaxonic
   posthypoxic
   progressive
   rhythmical
   segmental
   spinal
   spiral
   spontaneous generalized
   startle
   static
   stimulus-induced
   stimulus-sensitive
   subcortical segmental
   symptomatic
   transient
myoclonus epilepsy associated with
   ragged-red fibers (MERRF)
Myo/Cr (myoinositol/creatine ratio)
myocutaneous flap
myocutaneous graft
myocytoma
myodegeneration
myodemia
myodesis, suture
myodiastasis
myodynia
myodystonia
myoedema
myoelectric control for upper arm
   prosthesis
myofascial flap
myofascial muscular tissues
myofascial pain syndrome (MPS)
myofascial periosteal juncture
myofascial release
myofascial stretching exercises
myofasciitis, interstitial
myofibril
   disorganized
   striated
myofibroma
myofibrosis
myofibrositis
MyoForce test
myofusio-periostitis
myogelosis

myoglobinuria, march
myohypertrophia
myoinositol/creatine (Myo/Cr) ratio
myointimal proliferation
myoischemia
myokerosis
myokymia
  exercise-induced
  facial
  limb
  superior oblique
myokymic discharge
myolipoma
myolysis
myoma
myomalacia
myomatosis
myomectomy (myomatectomy)
myomelanosis
myonecrosis
myoneural ischemia
myoneural junction
myoneural necrosis
myoneuralgia
myoneurasthenia
myoneurectomy
myoneuroma
myoneurosis
myopachynsis
myopalmus
myoparalysis
myoparesis
myopathic dystrophy
myopathic scoliosis
myopathic weakness
myopathy (pl. myopathies)
  acquired
  alcoholic
  centronuclear
  congenital
  dystrophic
  endocrine
  entrapment
  fingerprint body
  hereditary
  idiopathic polymyositis
  Kiloh-Nevin ocular

myopathy *(continued)*
  metabolic
  mitochondrial
  myotubular
  nemaline rod
  ocular
  polymyositis
  postinfectious
  primary
  reducing body
  sarcoid
  sarcotubular
  steroid
  storage
  subclinical
  thyroid
  thyrotoxic
  zebra body
  zidovudine-induced
myophagism
myoplasty
myopsychopathy
myorrhaphy
myorrhexis
myosalgia
myosarcoma
Myoscint (monoclonal antibody Fab to
  myosin labeled with indium-111)
myosclerosis
myoseism
myositis
  clostridial
  focal nodular
  granulomatous
  inclusion body (IBM)
  inflammatory
  ischemic
  myositides
  ossificans
  proliferative
  streptococcal
  tension
  viral
myositis fibrosa
myositis ossificans (MO)
myospasm
myospasmia

myostasis
myostatic contracture
myosteoma
myosynizesis
myotendinous junction
myotenontoplasty
myotenositis
myotenotomy
myotomal diagram of pain
myotomal distribution
myotomal muscular pain
myotomal pattern
myotome
myotomy
myotonia
    chondrodystrophic
    congenital
myotonic discharge
myotonic dystrophy

myotonic facies
myotonic pupil
myotonic syndrome
MyoTrac and MyoTrac 2 EMG
    monitoring
Myotrophin (mecasermin)
myotube
myotubular myopathy
Myoview imaging agent
Mysoline (primidone)
myxedema coma
myxedema madness
myxofibroma
myxoid neurothekeoma
myxoma
    nerve sheath
    soft tissue
myxomatous degeneration
myxosarcoma

N, n

NA (neuropathic arthropathy)
NAA (N-acetylaspartate)
NAAP (National Arthritis Action
Plan)
nabumetone (Relafen)
N-acetylaspartate (NAA)
Naden-Rieth hip prosthesis
nadolol (Corgard)
nadroparin
Naegleria meningitis
Naffziger sign
Naffziger syndrome
nail, nailing
adjustable
Ainsworth modification of Massie
antegrade femoral ·
AO slotted medullary
AP
Augustine boat
Bailey-Dubow
Barr
Bickel intramedullary
blind medullary
boat
Brooker femoral
Brooker-Wills
cannulated
Chick

nail, nailing *(continued)*
Christensen interlocking
closed
closed Küntscher
closed unlocked
cloverleaf intramedullary
cloverleaf Küntscher
condylocephalic
crutch-and-belt femoral closed
Curry hip
Derby
Deyerle pin
diamond-shaped medullary
Dooley
double-ended
double-hollow
dynamic locking
elastic stable intramedullary (ESIN)
Ender
Ender flexible medullary
Engel-May
extension
femoral neck
fixator-augmented
fluted titanium
four-flanged
gamma locking
Grosse-Kempf

nail, nailing *(continued)*
   Grosse-Kempf interlocking
      medullary
   Hagie pin
   Hahn bone
   half-and-half
   hallux
   Hansen-Street
   Harris condylocephalic
   Harris hip
   Harris medullary
   Holt
   hooked intramedullary
   hooked medullary
   Huckstep
   INRO surgical
   intramedullary (IM)
   ingrown (onychocryptosis)
   interlocking
   interlocking intramedullary
   intramedullary
   Inyo
   Jewett
   Johannson hip
   Kaessmann
   Ken sliding
   Knowles
   Küntscher medullary
   left-sided
   Lewis
   locked intramedullary
   locking
   Lottes triflanged medullary
   Massie II
   Massie sliding
   McKee tri-fin
   McLaughlin
   medullary
   Moore
   nested
   Neufeld
   noncannulated
   Nylok self-locking
   open
   OrthoSorb pin
   Palmer bone
   PGP

nail, nailing *(continued)*
   Pidcock
   prebent
   Pugh sliding
   reconstruction
   retrograde femoral
   Richards reconstruction
   right-sided
   Rush flexible medullary
   Rush pin
   Russell-Taylor interlocking
      medullary
   Rydell
   Sage triangular
   Sampson medullary
   Sarmiento
   Schneider medullary
   Seidel humeral locking
   self-broaching
   self-locking
   Slocum
   Smillie
   Smith-Petersen femoral neck
   Smith-Petersen transarticular
   spring-loaded
   static locking
   Steinmann extension
   Street
   Sven-Johansson femoral neck
   telescoping
   Temple University
   Terry nails
   Thatcher
   Thornton
   Tiemann
   titanium
   triangular medullary
   triflange
   triflanged Lottes
   Uniflex intramedullary
   V-medullary
   Venable-Stuck
   Vesely-Street split
   Vitallium Küntscher
   Watson-Jones
   Webb
   Z fixation

nail, nailing *(continued)*
   Zickel intramedullary
   Zickel subtrochanteric
   Zickel supracondylar medullary
nail assembly, Massie
nail base
nail bed
nail bed lesion
nail-fold microscopy
nail matrix
nail starter, Ritchie
nail sulcus
NAIP (neuronal apoptosis inhibitory protein)
Nalebuff arthrodesis
Nalebuff classification
Nalebuff-Millender technique
Namaqualand hip dysplasia
nambumetone
nandrolene decanoate
nanoparticulate contrast agent
NAP (nerve-action potential)
naphthylalkalones
Naprelan (naproxen sodium)
Naprosyn (naproxen)
naproxen (Aleve, Naprosyn, Naprelan)
narcolepsy cataplexy syndrome
narcoleptic
Naropin (ropivacaine hydrochloride)
narrowed joint space
narrowing
   diffuse
   disk space
   focal
   foraminal
   joint space
   neural foramina
   segmental
   thecal sac
nasal bone
nasal fracture
nasal muscle
nasal nerve
nasal notch
nasal septum hematoma
nasal thermistor
Nashold biopsy needle

Nashold TC electrode
nasion
nasociliary nerve
nasociliary neuralgia
nasoethmoidal encephalocele
nasofrontal encephalocele
nasolabial fold, flat
nasopalatine nerve
nasopharyngeal craniopharyngioma
nasopharyngeal EEG leads
nasopharyngeal electrode
NASS (North American Spine Society)
natatory ligament
National Ankylosing Spondylitis Society
National Arthritis Action Plan (NAAP)
National Arthritis Data Workgroup
National Association for Mental Health
National Association for the Deaf
National Association for the Visually Handicapped
National Collegiate Athletic Association (NCAA)
National Fibromyalgia Research Association (NFRA)
National Institute of Arthritis and Musculoskeletal and Skin Diseases (NIAMS)
National Institute of Mental Health (NIMH)
National Institute of Neurological and Communicative Disorders and Stroke (NINCDS)
National Institute of Neurological Communicative Disease and Stroke, Alzheimer Disease and Related Disorders Association (NINCDSADRDA)
National Institute of Neurological Disorders and Stroke (NINDS)
National Institute on Aging (NIA)
National Institute on Mental Health (NIMH)
National Institutes of Health (NIH)

National Institutes of Health Stroke
Scale
National Multiple Sclerosis Society
(NMSS)
National Neurofibromatosis Founda-
tion (NNFF)
National Operating Committee on
Standards for Athletic Equipment
(NOCSAE)
National Society for the Prevention of
Blindness
National Special Olympics
National Spinal Cord Injury Associa-
tion (NSCIA)
National Technical Institute for the
Deaf (NTID)
native tissue harmonic imaging
(NTHI)
Natural-Hip system
Natural-Knee II prosthesis
Natural Relief 1222
Naughton-Dunn triple arthrodesis
Nauth traction apparatus
Nautilus machine
navicular bone
  accessory
  carpal
  cartilaginous
  lip of
  tarsal
navicular body fracture
  dorsal cortical avulsion
  medial tuberosity
navicular cookie in shoe
navicular drift
navicular drop
navicular view
naviculectomy
naviculocapitate fracture syndrome
naviculocuneiform joint
naviculocuneiform ligament
navigation, frameless
Navigator virtual endoscopic visualization system
NCAA (National Collegiate Athletic
Association)
NC/AT (normocephalic, atraumatic)

NCCU (neurological critical care unit)
NCL-Arp monoclonal antibody
imaging agent
NCL-ER-LHZ monoclonal antibody
imaging agent
NCL-PGR monoclonal antibody
imaging agent
NCP (NeuroCybernetic Prosthesis)
system
NCS (nerve conduction study)
NC-stat nerve conduction system
NCV (nerve conduction velocity)
NDT (neurodevelopmental techniques)
Nd:YAG (neodymium: yttrium-
aluminum-garnet) laser
Neal-Robertson litter
near-anatomic position of joint
near-infrared spectroscopy
near reflex
near-resonance spin-lock contrast
NEB (New England Baptist) hip
prosthesis
neck
  aneurysmal
  basal
  bone
  crick in the
  femoral
  metatarsal
  muscles of
  stiff
  supple
  surgical
  swan
  talar
  webbed
  wry
neck ache
neck compression test
neck fracture
Neck-Huggar cervical support pillow
neck reflex, tonic
neck school
neck-shaft angle (NSA) of femur
neck stiffness
NECKSYS home neck care system
Neck-Trac passive motion system

Nec Loc cervical collar
necrosis
  aseptic
  avascular (AVN)
  bridging
  cerebral radiation (CRN)
  diffuse
  embolic
  epiphyseal ischemic
  femoral head
  fibrinoid
  gangrenous
  hemorrhagic
  ischemic needle of femoral head
    (INFH)
  Marcus grading scale for avascular
  muscle
  myoneural
  neuronal
  Paget quiet
  postreduction ischemic
  pressure
  radiation
  septic
  skin
  soft tissue
  thermal
necrotic bone
necrotizing encephalitis
necrotizing fasciitis
NED (no evidence of disease)
needle
  Adson aneurysm
  Adson scalp
  aneurysm
  Arthrotek RC
  Backlund biopsy
  band circling
  Beath
  Bier lumbar puncture
  biopsy
  bone biopsy
  bone round
  bore
  Bouge
  Bunnell tendon
  Colorado microdissection

needle *(continued)*
  cone biopsy
  cone ventricular
  Cournand arteriogram
  Cournand-Grino arteriogram
  Craig biopsy
  Cushing ventricular
  D'Errico ventricular
  Dandy ventricular
  dural
  EMG (electromyogram)
  Estridge biopsy
  eye
  Feild-Lee brain biopsy
  Framer tendon-passing
  Frazier ventricular
  Gallie
  Hawkeye suture
  Hemo-Drain
  Hoen ventricular
  hubbed
  Huber
  Intracath
  Jamshidi
  Keith
  Kronecker aneurysm
  lumbar puncture
  micro
  Mixter ventricular
  Nashold biopsy
  nonferromagnetic
  Pace ventricular
  Parhad-Poppen arteriogram
  Parham band circling
  P-4
  PMT biopsy
  Poppen ventricular
  pressure (teishein)
  Protect Point
  Quincke lumbar puncture
  Reichert-Mundinger biopsy
  Retter aneurysm
  Rhoton
  SafeTap tapered spinal
  scalp
  Scoville ventricular
  Shaw aneurysm

needle *(continued)*
    Sheldon-Spatz vertebral arteriogram
    side-aspirating biopsy
    Smiley-Williams arteriogram
    spinal
    stereotactic biopsy
    teishein
    tendon-passing
    TruCut
    Tuohy lumbar puncture
    ventricular
    ventriculostomy
    Verbrugge
    Whitacre spinal
    wire circling
needle biopsy, CT-scan directed
needle electrode
needle electromyography
needle holder (also see *holder*)
    Adson dural
    Ayers
    Donaghy angled suture
    Dubecq-Princeteau angulating
    Micro-One
    teishein
    titanium microsurgical
    Vickers
    Wangensteen
    Webster
needle lavage
needle manometer technique
needlescope
Neer acromioplasty
Neer classification of shoulder fractures
    (I-III)
Neer hemiarthroplasty
Neer-Horowitz fracture classification
Neer impingement sign
Neer lateral view
Neer shoulder replacement prosthesis
Neer trans-scapular view
Neer-Vitallium humeral prosthesis
Neff meniscus knife
negative impression cast
negative scotoma
negativism, motor (gegenhalten)

neglect
    auditory
    left/right side of body
    organic unilateral
    polymodal
    spatial
    supervised
    tactile
    unilateral
    unilateral organic
    unilateral visual
    visual
neglect syndrome
Negri bodies
Negro sign
Neiguan acupressure point P6
Neisseria meningitidis meningitis
Neivert osteotome
Nélaton dislocation of the ankle
Nélaton line
Nélaton rubber tube drain
N_z electrode
Nelson finger exerciser
Nelson rib retractor
Nelson rib spreader
Nelson scissors
Nelson sign
Nelson syndrome
nemaline body
nemaline myopathy
neoadjuvant chemotherapy
neocerebellum
neocollateral ligament
neocortex
neodymium: yttrium-aluminum-garnet
    laser (Nd:YAG laser)
neoformans, Cryptococcus
neointimal thickening
neologisms (nonsensical words)
neologistic paraphasia
neonatal EEG recording
neonatal flatfoot
neonatal Horner syndrome
neonatal meningitis
neonatal neurological syndrome
neonatal reflex

neonatal seizures
neonatal tyrosinemia
neonatal withdrawal seizures
neopallium
neoplasm
   CNS
   frontal
   interdigital
   intracranial
   malignant
   temporal horn
   spinal cord
neoplasm of the spinal cord
neoplastic cord damage
neoplastic destruction of spinal
   elements
neoplastic disorder
   benign
   malignant
neoplastic fracture
neoplastic meningitis
neoplastic invasion of meninges
neoplastic invasion of roots
neoplastic process of the superior
   orbital fissure
neoprene RocketSoc ankle brace
neoprene support brace
Neoral (cyclosporine microemulsion)
Neotrofin (leteprinim potassium)
Ne-Osteo bone morphogenic protein
neotendon
neovascularitization, postoperative
nephritis, systemic lupus erythematosus (SLE)
nephritogenic
Neri bowing sign
nerve (see Table of Nerves in the
     Appendix)
   abdominopelvic splanchnic
   abducens
   accelerator
   accessory
   accessory phrenic
   accessory vagal
   acoustic
   afferent digital
   alveolar

nerve *(continued)*
   ampullar
   anal
   Andersch
   anal
   anococcygeal
   antebrachial
   aortic
   Arnold
   articular
   atrophy of optic
   auditory
   augmentor
   auricular
   auriculotemporal
   autonomic
   axillary
   baroreceptor
   Bell long thoracic
   Bock
   buccal
   buccinator
   calcaneal
   cardiac
   cardiopulmonary splanchnic
   caroticotympanic
   carotid sinus
   cavernous
   celiac
   centrifugal
   centripetal
   cerebral
   cervical
   cervical splanchnic
   chorda tympani
   ciliary
   circumflex
   cluneal
   coccygeal
   cochlear
   compression of
   common fibular
   common palmar digital
   common peroneal
   common plantar digital
   corticopontocerebellar
   course of

nerve *(continued)*
  cranial, I-XII (see *cranial nerves*)
  crural interosseous
  cubital
  cutaneous
  Cyon
  deep fibular
  deep peroneal
  deep petrosal
  deep temporal
  demyelinated
  dental
  depressor Ludwig
  diaphragmatic
  digastric
  digital
  dorsal interosseous
  dorsal lateral cutaneous
  dorsal medial cutaneous
  dorsal scapular
  efferent digital
  eighth cranial
  eleventh cranial
  encephalic
  entrapped
  esodic
  ethmoidal
  excitor
  excitoreflex
  exodic
  external acoustic
  external respiratory Bell
  external saphenous
  external spermatic
  facial
  femoral cutaneous
  fibular
  fifth cranial
  first cranial
  fourth cranial
  frontal
  furcal
  fusimotor
  Galen
  gangliated
  gastric
  genitocrural

nerve *(continued)*
  glossopharyngeal
  gluteal
  gustatory
  hemorrhoidal
  Hering sinus
  hypoglossal
  iliohypogastric
  ilioinguinal
  infraoccipital
  infraorbital
  infratrochlear
  inhibitory
  intercarotid
  intercostal
  intercostobrachial
  intercostohumeral
  intermediary
  intermediate Wrisberg
  Jacobson
  jugular
  labial
  lacrimal
  Lancisi
  Langley
  laryngeal
  Latarjet
  levator ani
  lingual
  longitudinal Lancisi
  Ludwig
  lumbar
  lumboinguinal
  Luschka (also von Luschka)
  mandibular
  masseteric
  masticator
  maxillary
  medial cutaneous
  median
  meningeal
  mental
  mixed
  motor
  musculocutaneous
  musculospiral
  myelinated

nerve *(continued)*
- mylohyoid
- nasal
- nasociliary
- nasopalatine
- neurofibroma of interdigital
- ninth cranial
- obturator
- oculomotor
- olfactory
- olivocerebellar
- ophthalmic
- optic
- orbital
- palatine
- palmar digital
- parasympathetic
- parolfactory
- parotid
- pectoral
- percutaneous interosseous (PIN)
- perineal
- peripheral
- peripheral third
- periradicular
- peroneal
- phrenic
- pinched
- plantar digital
- pneumogastric
- popliteal
- presacral
- preservation of
- pressor
- proper digital
- pterygoid canal
- pterygopalatine
- pudendal
- quadrate
- radial
- rectal
- respiratory
- root of
- rootlets of
- rostral cervical
- saccular
- sacral

nerve *(continued)*
- saphenous
- sartorius
- Scarpa
- sciatic
- second cranial
- secretomotor
- secretory
- sensory branch of radial (SBRN)
- seventh cranial
- sinus Hering
- sinuvertebral
- sixth cranial
- somatic
- spinal accessory
- spinocerebellar
- splanchnic
- statoacoustic
- subclavian
- subcostal
- sublingual
- suboccipital
- subscapular
- sudomotor
- superficial peroneal
- supraclavicular
- supraorbital
- suprascapular
- supraspinatus
- supratrochlear
- sural
- sympathetic
- tectocerebellar
- temporomandibular
- tenth cranial
- tentorial
- terminal
- tethering of
- third cranial
- thoracoabdominal
- thoracodorsal
- tibial communicating
- tibial
- Tiedemann
- tonsillar
- trifacial
- transection of

nerve *(continued)*
  transverse
  trigeminal
  trigeminocerebellar
  trochlear
  twelfth cranial
  tympanic
  ulnar
  ulnar digital
  unmyelinated
  unroofing of
  utricular
  utriculoampullar
  vagus
  Valentin
  vascular
  vasoconstrictor
  vasodilator
  vasomotor
  vasosensory
  vertebral
  vesical
  vestibular
  vestibulocerebellar
  vidian
  visceral
  volar interosseous
  Willis
  Wrisberg
  zygomatic
  zygomaticotemporal
nerve ablation
nerve-action potential (NAP)
nerve biopsy
nerve conduction study (NCS)
nerve conduction velocity (NCV)
nerve disorder, vestibular
nerve entrapment
nerve entrapment syndrome
nerve fascicle
nerve fiber membrane depolarization
nerve growth factor (NGF)
nerve head, ischemia of the
nerve hook
  Dandy
  Lahey Clinic
  Malis

nerve hook *(continued)*
  Scoville
  Smithwick
nerve injury
nerve of Wrisberg
nerve pain from cervical or brachial
  plexus injury ("stinger")
NervePace nerve conduction monitor
nerve palsy, tardive ulnar
nerve paralysis
nerve plexus
nerve root
  extrathecal
  intradural
nerve root compression
nerve root cutoff
nerve root dissector
nerve root edema
nerve root embarrassment
nerve root fila
nerve root gutter
nerve root injection
nerve root injury
nerve root irritation
nerve root retractor
nerve root sheath
nerve root sheath effacement
nerve root sleeve
nerve root syndrome
nerve separator-spatula
nerve sheath myxoma
nerve sheath tumor
nerve tape
nerve terminal
nerve transfer
nerve trunk
nerve twig
nervous system
  parasympathetic
  sympathetic
nervous system integrity
nervousness
nervus intermedius neuralgia
nests of tumor cells
network, neural
Neubeiser splint
Neufeld cast

Neufeld nail
Neufeld traction
NeuFlex metacarpophalangeal joint
    implant
NEUGAT (neutron/gamma transmis-
    sion) method
Neuprex (rBPI-21)
Neurairtome
neural arch
neural arch resection technique
neural compromise
neural crest origin
neural deficit
    peripheral
    radicular
    spinal
    thalamic
neural foramen (pl foramina)
    narrowing of
    widely patent
neuralgia
    abdominal
    ciliary
    cranial
    geniculate
    glossopharyngeal
    Hunt
    hypoglossal
    intercostal
    intractable
    migrainous
    migrainous cranial
    Morton
    nasociliary
    nerve entrapment
    nervus intermedius
    occipital
    paratrigeminal
    petrosal
    postherpetic
    pterygopalatine
    Sluder
    sphenopalatine
    Trélat-Charlin
    trigeminal (tic douloureux)
    trigger point
    vagoglossopharyngeal

neuralgia *(continued)*
    vestibular
    vidian
neuralgic amyotrophy
neuralgic pain
neural mobilization
neural network
neural progenitor cells
neural regeneration
neural-tube defect
neural reorganization
neural stem cells
neural tension
neurapraxia
neurasthenia
neuraxis, spinal
neurectomy
    chemical
    obturator
    vestibular
neurenteric cyst
neurilemmoma, hourglass-type of
neurilemmoma tumor
neurinoma, acoustic
neuritic plaque (plaquing)
neuritic senile plaques
neuritis (see also *polyneuritis*)
    axial
    brachial
    brachial plexus
    heavy metal
    idiopathic plexus
    interdigital
    ischemic
    ischemic optic
    lumbosacral plexus
    multiple
    optic
    relapsing hypertrophic
    retrobulbar
    traction
    vestibular
neuroablative surgery
neuroacanthocytosis
neuroanatomic correlate
neuroanatomy
neuroanesthesia

neuroangiography
neuroarthropathy
  atrophic
  diabetic
neuroastrocytoma
neuroaxis radiotherapy
neuroaxonal dystrophy
neurobehavioral syndrome
Neurobehavioral Cognitive Status
  Examination
Neurobehavioral Rating Scale
neuroblastoma
  dumbbell-type
  Hutchinson type
  intra-abdominal
  occipital
  olfactory
  Pepper
Neurobloc (botulinum toxin type B)
neuroblockage
neuroborreliosis, tertiary
NeuroCell (Genzyme tissue repair)
NeuroCell-HD
NeuroCell-PD
neurocentral joint
neurochemical
neurocirculatory check
neurocirculatory status
NeuroCol neurosurgical sponge
neurocranium
neurocutaneous island flap
neurocutaneous syndrome
NeuroCybernetic Prosthesis (NCP)
  pulse generator
neurocysticercosis
neurocytoma
  central
  intraventricular
neurodegenerative disease
neurodevelopment
neurodevelopmental techniques (NDT)
neurodiagnostic imaging
neurodissector, Penfield
NeuroDrape surgical drape
neuroectodermal tumor, primitive
neuroendocrine abnormality
neuroendocrine carcinoma

neuroendocrine dysfunction
neuroendoscope, rigid
neurofibrillary degeneration
neurofibrillary tangle
neurofibrils, motor
neurofibroma
  dermal
  diffuse
  discrete
  dumbbell
  epithelioid
  intraparotid facial
  nodular
  nonplexiform cutaneous
  orbital
  pacinian
  plexiform
  solitary
neurofibroma of interdigital nerve
neurofibromatosis, cranio-orbital-
  temporal
neurofibromatosis type 1 (NF1) (Von
  Recklinghausen disease)
neurofibromatosis type 2 (NF2)
neurofibroma tumor
neurofibromin
neurofilament
neurofunctional surgery
neurogenic bladder
  refluxing spastic
  spastic
neurogenic bowel
neurogenic disorder
neurogenic dysfunction
neurogenic fracture
neurogenic hypertension
neurogenic hyperventilation, central
neurogenic lesion
neurogenic motor evoked potentials
  (NMEP)
neurogenic pulmonary edema
neurogenic sarcoma
neurogenic tumor
neuroglia
neurography, magnetic resonance
  (MRN)
neuroholography

neurohormone
neurohypophyseal germinoma
neurohypophysectomy
neurohypophysial
neurohypophysis
neuroimaging procedure
neuroimmune dysfunction
neurointerventional radiology
neuroleptic, atypical
neuroleptic malignant syndrome
neuroleptic medication
neuroleptics
NeuroLink II EEG data acquisition
   system
Neurolite (technetium-99m bicisate)
   imaging agent
Neuro Lobe software
neurologic (or neurological)
neurological critical care unit (NCCU)
neurological deficit
neurological deterioration
neurological examination
neurological impairment
neurological improvement
neurologically intact
neurological rehabilitation
neurological scissors, Strully
neurologic deficit
neurologic deterioration
neurologic disease, emotional lability
   following infectious
neurologic dysfunction
neurologic exam, physiologic
neurologic integrity
neurologic paraneoplastic syndrome
neurologic signs, focal
neurologic substrate
neurologic symptom
neurologist
neurology, behavioral
neurolysis
   external
   interfascicular
   internal
   intramuscular

neuroma
   acoustic
   amputation
   false
   gasserian ganglion
   incisional
   interdigital
   intermetatarsal
   Morton
   multicystic acoustic
   multiple
   myelenic
   neuromata
   nevoid
   palisaded encapsulated
   peripheral nerve
   plexiform
   posttraumatic
   solitary circumscribed
   traumatic
   trigeminal
   true
   Verneuil
NeuroMap system
neuromechanical spinal chiropractic
   management
Neuromed Octrode implantable device
Neuromed stimulator
Neuromeet nerve approximator
neuromotor dysfunction
neuromuscular blockade
neuromuscular disease
neuromuscular electrical stimulation
   (NMES)
neuromuscular facilitation, proprioceptive (PNF)
neuromuscular junction
neuromuscular re-education
neuromuscular transmission
neuromyasthenia, epidemic
neuromyelitis optica
neuromyopathy
   carcinomatous
   uremic
neuromyotonia

neuron (pl. neurons)
  abnormal epileptic
  afferent
  alpha motor
  collateral sprouting
  cortical
  corticobulbar motor
  corticospinal motor
  dopamine energy
  epileptic
  firing of
  foci of abnormal epileptic
  gamma motor
  giant
  lower motor
  motor
  pedunculopontine
  presynaptic
  pyramidal
  secreting
  striatal
  thalamocortical relay (TCR)
  upper motor
neuronal activity
neuronal aggregate
neuronal apoptosis inhibitory protein
  (NAIP)
neuronal dropout
neuronal dysfunction
  cortical
  subcortical
neuronal loss
neuronal membrane
neuronal membrane depolarization
neuronal metabolism
neuronal migration
neuronal necrosis
neuronal precursors
neuronavigational system
neuronavigator attachment to Mayfield
  head holder
neuronitis, vestibular
neuronopathy, subacute motor
neuronophagy
neuron-specific enolase (NSE)
  antibody
neuron-specific protein

Neurontin (gabapentin)
neuro-ophthalmic
neuro-ophthalmologic function
neuro-ophthalmological test
neuro-ophthalmology
neuro-otologist
neuro-otology
neuropathic ankle
neuropathic arthritis
neuropathic arthropathy (NA)
neuropathic bladder
neuropathic joint
neuropathic spinal arthropathy
neuropathic tarsal-metatarsal joint
neuropathic ulceration
neuropathology
neuropathophysiology
neuropathy (see also *peripheral*
  neuropathy)
  acquired demyelinative
  acute autonomic
  AIDP (acute inflammatory
    demyelinating polyradicular)
  AIDS
  alcoholic
  amyloid
  anterograde fast component
  autonomic
  axonal
  brachial plexus
  B vitamin deficiency
  carcinomatous
  chronic alcoholism
  compression
  compressive
  congenital hypomyelination
  cranial
  demyelinating
  Denny-Brown
  diabetic
  diabetic autonomic
  diabetic ischemic
  diabetic peripheral
  diabetic sensory
  diabetic thoracoabdominal
  distal
  dying-back

neuropathy *(continued)*
  entrapment
  familial
  familial amyloid
  familial sensory radicular
  familial visceral
  femoral
  focal
  giant axonal
  handcuff
  heavy metal
  hereditary motor and sensory
    (HMSN)
  hereditary peripheral
  hereditary sensorimotor (HSMN)
  hereditary sensory (HSN)
  hereditary sensory radicular
  heredofamilial
  hypertrophic interstitial
  immunoglobulin M paraproteinemic
  inflammatory demyelinating
  ischemic
  ischemic optic
  isoniazid-induced
  lead
  metachromatic leukodystrophy
  multifocal
  nonprogressive
  nutritional
  occupational
  onion-bulb formation of
  optic
  paraproteinemic
  peripheral
  progressive
  progressive hypertrophic
  progressive hypertrophic interstitial
  pure sensory
  radicular
  relapsing
  retrograde fast component
  rheumatoid
  sensorimotor
  sensorimotor peripheral
  sensory
  sensory-motor-autonomic

neuropathy *(continued)*
  Shy-Drager
  slow component
  steroid-sensitive
  subclinical
  suprascapular
  symmetrical diffuse
  traumatic
  Wegener granulomatosis-associated
    peripheral
neuropeptide K
neuroperfusion pump
neuropharmacology
neurophysiologic
neurophysiology
NeuroPlan system
neuroplasticity
neuroplasty fat graft
neuropore, rostral
NeuroPro rigid fixation system
neuroprotective agent
neuroprotective therapy
neuropsychiatric syndrome
neuropsychological evaluation
neuropsychological impairment
neuropsychological testing
neuropsychologic battery of tests
neuropsychology, clinical
neuropsychometric test
neuropsychopharmacology
neuroradiologic examination
neuroradiology, interventional
neuroreceptor ligand
neurorrhaphy
  epineurial
  perineurial
neurosarcoidosis
neurosarcoma
NeuroScan 3D imager
NeuroSector ultrasound system
neurosheet
neurosis, traumatic
neurosonogram
neurosonography
neurosonology
Neuro SPGR software

neurosurgery
  endoscopic
  keyhole
  image-guided functional
  pediatric
  stereotaxic
neurosurgical evaluation
neurosurgical skull clamp, Gardner
neurosyphilis
  Argyll Robertson pupils of tabetic
  meningitic
  meningovascular
  parenchymatous
  paretic
  tabetic
neurotensin
neurothekeoma
  cellular
  myxoid
neurotmesis
neurotologic surgery
neurotomy, Spiller-Frazier
neurotoxic drugs
neurotoxic effect
neurotoxicity
Neuro-Trace
neurotransmission, adrenergic
neurotransmitter
neurotransplantation
neurotraumatic evolution of Charcot
  joint disease
Neurotrend probe
Neurotrend system
neurotripsy
neurotropic MR imaging contrast
  agents
neurotropism
neurotuberculosis
  intracranial tuberculous subdural
    empyema
  tuberculoma
  tuberculous meningitis
neurovascular bundle
neurovascular compression
neurovascular corn
neurovascular impairment
neurovascular island pedicle flaps

neurovascular status
neurovascular structures
neuroworsening
neutral and load drill guide
neutral body mechanics
neutral calcaneal stance position
neutral hip position
neutralizing antibody
neutral positioning
neutral spine position
neutron/gamma transmission (NEU-
  GAT) method
neutropenia
Neviaser acromioclavicular technique
Neviaser classification of frozen
  shoulder
Neviaser-Wilson-Gardner transfer
Neville tracheal and tracheobronchial
  prosthesis
Nevin-Jones subacute spongiform
  encephalopathy
nevoid neuroma
nevus (pl. nevi), pedal intradermal
new bone formation (incorporation)
New England Baptist (NEB)
  acetabular cup
New England Baptist arthroplasty
Newington brace
New Jersey LCS knee prosthesis
Newman classification of radial
  fracture
new-onset limp
New Orleans endarterectomy stripper
Newport MC hip orthosis brace
Newton ankle prosthesis
newtons of force (SI units)
Newvicon vacuum chamber
  pickupNew Mind Set toe splint
New York criteria for anklylosing
  spondylitis
New York diagnostic criteria for
  rheumatoid arthritis
New York Glass suction tubes
New York Orthopedic front-opening
  orthosis
New York University insert for orthosis
NEX (number of excitations)

NexGen complete knee replacement components
Nextep knee brace
Nexus hip prosthesis
Nexus implant
N fiducial localization stereotactic system
NF1 (neurofibromatosis type 1)
NF1-associated malignancy
NF1 gene expression
NF2 (neurofibromatosis type 2)
NF2 gene mutation
NFRA (National Fibromyalgia Research Association)
NGF (nerve growth factor)
NHP (Nottingham Health Profile)
NHPT (Nine Hole Peg Test)
NIA (National Institute on Aging)
NIAMS (National Institute of Arthritis and Musculoskeletal and Skin Diseases)
Nicholas five-in-one reconstruction technique
Nicholas ligament technique
Nicky knot
Nicola forceps
Nicola pituitary rongeur
Nicola shoulder procedure
Nicola rasp
Nicola scissors
Nicolet Nerve Integrity Monitor-2 (NIM-2)
Nicoll bone replacement material
Nicoll cancellous bone graft
Nicoll plate
NICU (neurological intensive care unit)
nidus
    diameter of
    volume of
nidus obliteration
nidus of embolic material
nidus of osteoid osteoma
Niebauer-King technique
Niebauer metacarpophalangeal joint Silastic prosthesis
Niebauer prosthesis
Niemann-Pick disease

Niemann-Pick syndrome
Nievergelt syndrome
niger, Aspergillus
night cramps
night nurse's paralysis
NightOwl pocket polygraph system
Night Splint support
nightstick fracture
night terror (pavor nocturnus)
nigral cells
nigrostriatal lesion
nigrostriatal pathway
NIH (National Institutes of Health) Stroke Scale
Nimbex (cisatracurium)
NIMH (National Institute of Mental Health)
Nimotop (nimodipine)
NIM-2 (Nicolet Nerve Integrity Monitor-2)
NINCDS (National Institute of Neurological and Communicative Disorders and Stroke)
NINCDSADRDA (National Institute of Neurological Communicative Disease and Stroke, Alzheimer Disease and Related Disorders Association)
NINDS (National Institute of Neurological Disorders and Stroke)
Nine Hole Peg Test (NHPT)
ninety-ninety (90/90) intraosseous wiring
91-41 MeV proton
Ninhydrin print test
ninth cranial nerve (glossopharyngeal nerve)
Niopam contrast medium
nipper
    House-Dieter malleus
    nail
nipple-like osteophyte formation
NIPS (noninvasive programmed stimulation)
Niro bone-cutting forceps
Niro wire-twisting forceps
NIRS (near-infrared spectroscopy)
Nirschl technique

Nishimoto Sangyo scanner
Nissl degeneration
Nitinol flexible guide wire
nitrite, headaches from
nitrogen
  compressed
  direct pour of liquid
NK hand evaluation system
N-K 330 BRQ exercise tables
NM (nocturnal myoclonus)
NMEP (neurogenic motor evoked
  potentials)
NMES (neuromuscular electrical
  stimulation)
NMR (nuclear magnetic resonance)
NMS unit
NMSS (National Multiple Sclerosis
  Society)
NNFF (National Neurofibromatosis
  Foundation)
no-angulation view
Nocardia abscess of choroid plexus
Nocardia asteroides
Nocardiaform madurae
nocardiosis, cerebral
nociception
nociceptive afferent system
nociceptive reflexes
nociceptive tissues
nociceptor agents
nociceptor irritation
nociceptor sites
nociperception
NOCSAE (National Operating Committee on Standard for Athletic
  Equipment)
nocturnal epilepsy
nocturnal leg muscle spasticity
nocturnal paresthesia
nocturnus, pavor (night terror)
nodding, head
node (pl. nodes)
  Bouchard
  Flack
  gouty
  Haygarth
  Heberden

node *(continued)*
  Meynet
  Osler
  Parrot
  Ranvier
  Schmorl
no discernible findings
nodular fasciitis
nodular neurofibroma
nodule (pl. nodules)
  cutaneous
  glial
  Lisch
  ossific
  rheumatoid
  Schmorl
  surfer's
  synovial
  tendon
nodulus
Noiles fully constrained tricompartmental knee prosthesis
Noiles posterior stabilized knee
  prosthesis
Noiles rotating-hinge total knee
  prosthesis
noise
  lesion-to-cerebrospinal fluid
  lesion-to-white matter
  startling
NoLok screw
Nomad electromyogram
no man's land area of hand
nominal aphasia
Nomos pin-free attachment stereotactic
  system
nonabsorbable synthetic cerclage
nonacoustic cerebellopontine angle
  tumor
nonambulant individual
nonambulatory patient
"no-name, no-fame" bursa of knee
nonarticular radial head fracture
nonatherosclerotic aneurysm
  dissecting
  fusiform
nonbeveled

non-coma, in head injury
noncommunicating hydrocephalus
nonconvulsive status epilepticus
noncovalent collagen bonding
nondisplaced fracture
nondominant hemisphere lesion
nondominant putaminal hemorrhage
nondystrophic spinal deformity
nonelaborative speech
nonembolic cerebral infarction
nonenclosed magnet
nonenhanced CAT scan
nonepileptic myoclonic contraction
nonepileptiform activity
nonepileptiform sharp transient
nonfenestrated stem
nonfluent aphasic speech
nonfocal neurologic exam
nonfunctioning
nongerminomatous germ-cell tumor
nonglial tumor
nonglycosylated bacterial cell product
nonhinged linked prosthesis
nonhomonymous field defect
nonicteric sclerae
noninvasive brain tests
noninvasive imaging study
noninvasive soft tissue evaluation
nonionic contrast medium
nonionic paramagnetic contrast
    medium
nonketotic hyperglycemia
nonlamellar bone
non-neoplastic tumors
nonoperative orthopedic management:
    traction, weights, bedrest
nonossified tarsal navicular cartilage
nonossifying fibroma
nonosteoconductive bone-void filler
nonosteogenic fibroma
nonparalytic poliomyelitis
nonphasic forms of nystagmus
nonradiopaque foreign body
nonresponsive
nonresponsiveness
nonresponsive state
nonsecreting pituitary adenoma

nonsense mutation
nonsensical words (neologisms)
nonseptic cardioembolic cerebral
    infarction
nonspecific activating thalamic nuclei
nonsteroidal anti-inflammatory drug
    (NSAID)
nonstriated muscle
nonsubtraction images
nonsuppurative osteomyelitis
nonsyndromic bicoronal synostosis
nonsyndromic unicoronal synostosis
nontender
nontraumatic dislocation
nonunion
    diaphyseal
    elephant foot
    fibrous
    horse-hoof
    oligotrophic
    torsion wedge
nonunion of fracture fragments
nonunion of fracture site
nonweightbearing (NWB) brace
nonweightbearing view
Norco (hydrocodone bitartrate and
    acetaminophen)
NordiCare Back Therapy System
    (BTS)
NordiCare Enabler exerciser
NordiCare Strider exerciser
Nordt knot tightener
norepinephrine
Norian SRS (skeletal repair system)
Norland bone densitometry
Norland pQCT XCT2000 scanner
Norland XR26 bone densitometer
normal affect
normal, cosmetically and functionally
normalization of EEG
normalization of sleep habit
Normalize hip prosthesis
normal last shoes
normal mechanical tension (in hand)
normal mobility
normal motor potentials on EMG
normal pressure hydrocephalus (NPH)

normal, upper limits of
Normiflo (low molecular weight
  heparin)
normocephalic, atraumatic (NC/AT)
normothermia
Norris Scale
North American Spine Society
  (NASS)
North Coast reacher device
Northern hybridization technique
North-South retractor
Northwick Park Index of Independence in ADLs (activities of daily
  living)
Norton ball reamer
nortriptyline (Pamelor)
Norwood tenodesis
NOS (not otherwise specified)
nosebleed (epistaxis)
no-stretch RocketSoc ankle brace
notch
  acetabular
  cerebellar
  clavicular
  coracoid
  costal
  cotyloid
  craniofacial
  ethmoidal
  fibular
  frontal
  greater sciatic
  helix
  interclavicular
  intercondylar
  interpeduncular
  intervertebral
  ischial
  jugular
  Kernohan
  lesser sciatic
  mandibular
  mastoid
  nasal
  palatine
  parietal
  parotid

notch *(continued)*
  popliteal
  preoccipital
  presternal
  pterygoid
  radial
  radial sigmoid
  sacrosciatic
  scapular
  sciatic
  semilunar
  sigmoid
  sphenopalatine
  spinoglenoid
  sternal
  supraorbital
  suprasternal
  tentorial
  thyroid
  trigeminal
  trochlear
  ulnar
  vertebral
notchplasty blade
Nothnagel syndrome
notochord
notochordal remnants
Nottingham Extended ADL Index
  (domestic, kitchen, leisure, mobility)
Nottingham Health Profile (NHP)
  score for quality of life
Nottingham Ten-Point ADL Scale
Novafil suture
Novopaque contrast medium
Novus LC threaded interbody fusion
  cage
Novus LT titanium interbody fusion
  cage
NOX (number of excitations)
noxious stimulus
Noyes flexion-rotation drawer test
Noyes function questionnaire
Noyes knee rating scale
NPH (normal pressure hydrocephalus)
NPo-FH cephalometric measurement
NREM (nonrapid eye movement)
  sleep

NSA (neck-shaft angle) of femur
NSAID (nonsteroidal anti-inflammatory
drug)
NSCIA (National Spinal Cord Injury
Association)
NSE (neuron-specific enolase) antibody
N-telopeptide test
NTHI (native tissue harmonic
imaging)
NTID (National Technical Institute for
the Deaf)
nubbin sign
nuchal aching
nuchal ligament
nuchal rigidity
nuchal stiffness
nuchocephalic reflex
nuclear arrangement, string of pearls
nuclear bone imaging scan
nuclear cisternography
nuclear magnetic resonance (NMR)
nuclear paralysis
nuclear signal
nuclear spin quantum number
nuclear weakness
nuclectomy, percutaneous
nuclei, ventrolateral thalamic sensory
nucleoli, eosinophilic
nucleon
Nucleotome aspiration probe
Nucleotome Endoflex instrument
Nucleotome Flex II flexible cutting
probe
Nucleotome system for lumbar
diskectomy
nucleotomy, laser
nucleus (pl. nuclei)
abducens (or abducent)
accessory oculomotor
ambiguous
amygdaloid
arcuate
autonomic oculomotor
Cajal interstitial
caudate
centromedian
cochlear

nucleus (continued)
contralateral dentate
Darkshevitch (Darkschewitsch)
Deiter
dentate
dorsal cochlear
dorsal medial
Edinger-Westphal
facial
fastigial
geniculate
habenular
head of caudate
inferior olivary
interstitial
intralaminar thalamic
lateral geniculate
lateral mamillary
lenticular
lentiform
median
motor
motor
nonspecific activating
nonspecific thalamic
oculomotor-trochlear
olivary
ossific
Perlia medial
PF (parafascicular)
pigmentary
pontine
pontis
prerubral field
pretectal
prominent
raphe
red
Schwalbe
septal
specific thalamic
subthalamic
suprachiasmatic
tractus solitarius
ventral
ventral cochlear
ventral intermedius (VIM)

nucleus *(continued)*
    vestibular
    vestibulocochlear
    Westphal-Edinger
nucleus basalis of Meynert
nucleus caudalis dorsal root entry zone
    operation
nucleus gracilis
nucleus lateralis of Le Gros Clark
nucleus of Cajal
nucleus of cerebellum, Deiter
nucleus of Darkschewitsch
nucleus of Gudden
nucleus of tractus solitarius
nucleus of trigeminal nerve
nucleus of vagus, dorsal
nucleus pulposus, herniated (HNP)
nucleus, subthalamic
nudge control for prosthesis
Nu Gauze dressing
Nu Gauze sterile gauze bandage
NuKO knee orthosis
null cell adenoma
null position nystagmus
number of excitations (NEX) on MRI
numbness
    circumoral
    transient
Nurick classification of spondylosis
Nurolon suture
nurse, circulating
nursemaid's elbow
nut
    conical tapered
    hex
    jam
    Kirschner traction bow
    lock
    ring
    traction bow
    umbrella
    VDS (ventral derotating spinal) hex
Nu-Tip disposable scissor tip with
    reusable handle and shaft
NutraJoint gel
nutrient flap
NWB (nonweightbearing)

Nycomed contrast
Nylatex nylon-latex wrap
Nylen-Bárány maneuver
Nylok self-locking nail
nylon suture
nylon threads as drains
Nymox urinary test
nystagmogram
nystagmoid beating
nystagmoid jerk
nystagmoid movement
nystagmoid quaver
nystagmologist
nystagmus
    abduction
    acquired
    ageotropic
    alternating
    apogeotropic
    asymmetric
    Bruns
    caloric
    central
    central vestibular
    centrally caused
    cerebellar
    circular
    coarse
    congenital
    congenital idiopathic
    congenital latent
    conjugate
    contralateral monocular
    convergence-evoked
    convergence-retraction
    diagonal
    dissociated (ataxic)
    downbeat
    downbeating
    drug-induced
    dysjunctive
    elliptical
    end-gaze jerk
    end-point (physiologic)
    fast component of
    fine rapid
    fixation

nystagmus *(continued)*
    gaze-evoked
    gaze-paretic
    geotropic
    irregular
    jelly
    jerk (rhythmic)
    lateral-gaze
    left-bearing
    lid
    manifest latent
    miner's
    muscle-paretic
    nonphasic forms of
    null position
    oblique
    ocular
    optokinetic (OKN)
    palatal
    party
    pendular (nonphasic) forms of
    periodic
    periodic alternating
    phasic
    physiologic (end-point)
    physiologic (railway)
    positional
    positional (of central origin)

nystagmus *(continued)*
    positional (of peripheral origin)
    postrotational
    railway (physiological)
    rapid
    rebound
    retraction-convergence
    retractory
    reversed optokinetic
    rhythmic (jerk)
    right-bearing
    rotary
    rotatory
    see-saw
    sensory-deprivation
    torsional
    toxic
    transient
    true
    unidirectional
    upbeat
    upbeating
    vertical
    vestibular
    vestibular end-organ
    voluntary
NYU (New York University) orthosis

O, o

OA (osteoarthritis)
OAK (Orthopädische Arbeitsgruppe
    Knie) score
O&M (orientation and mobility)
OAR (Ottawa Ankle Rule)
oarsman's wrist
oasthouse urine disease
OAsys knee brace
oath hand
OATS (osteochondral autograft
    transfer system)
OAV (oculoauriculovertebral) dysplasia
OAWO (opening abductory wedge
    osteotomy)
OBD (organic brain disease)
Ober-Barr procedure for brachio-
    radialis transfer
Oberhill laminectomy retractor
Ober tendon technique
Ober test
obese knee osteoarthritis
obesity belt
object agnosia
objective limited movement
objective symptoms of impairment
objective vertigo
oblique displacement osteotomy
oblique muscle

oblique arytenoid muscle
oblique auricular muscle
oblique axial MR imaging
oblique fracture
oblique ligament
oblique metaphyseal osteotomy
oblique muscle
oblique popliteal ligament
oblique radiograms
oblique retinacular ligament
oblique slide osteotomy
oblique view
oblique wiring technique
obliquity, pelvic
obliteration
    frontal sinus
    nidus
    sphenoid sinus
    sulcal
    surgical
obliterative response
OBL RC5 soft tissue anchor
O'Brien classification of radial fracture
O'Brien cross-arm test
O'Brien needle test
O'Brien rib hook
O'Brien test for diagnosis of SLAP
    lesion

obscuration of vision
obsessive-compulsive disorder (OCD)
obstetric brachial plexus palsy
obstetrician's hand
obstetric paralysis
obstructing embolus
obstruction
  cerebrospinal fluid
  hydrocephalic
obstructive hydrocephalus
obstructive lesion of the CSF pathways
OBT stereotactic frame
obtundation
obtunded
obturator
  conical
  core biopsy
  Endotrac
  Keene
obturator muscle
obturator nerve
obturator neurectomy
obturator sheath
obturator sign
ObusForme back support
Obwegeser-Dalpont internal screw
  fixation
Obwegeser sagittal mandibular
  osteotomy technique
occipital (EEG lead)
  left (LO)
  right (RO)
occipital-atlas-axis ligaments
occipital-axis joint
occipital bone
occipital condyle
occipital fissure
occipital fracture
occipital gyrus
occipital lesion
occipital lobe contusion
occipital lobe tumor
occipital negative sharp transient on
  EEG
occipital neuralgia
occipital neuroblastoma
occipital pole

occipital-temporal sulcus
occipital tip
occipital vault remodeling
occipital vessel
occipital view of skull
occipitoanterior
occipitoatlantoaxial fusion
occipitoaxial ligament
occipitocervical articulation
occipitocervical level
occipitofrontal circumference
occipitofrontal muscle
occipitomastoid suture
occipitoparietal suture
occipitoposterior
occipitosphenoid suture
occipitotemporal gyrus
occipitotemporal, medial
occipitotemporal sulcus
occipitotemporopontine tract
occiput
occluding spring emboli
occluding thrombus
occlusal plane
occlusal segment
occlusion
  aqueductal
  arterial
  balloon
  basilar
  bilateral carotid artery
  carotid artery
  carotid cavernous fistula
  common carotid artery
  deep venous
  embolic
  infrapopliteal artery
  intracranial vascular
  subclavian artery
  unilateral carotid artery
  vascular
  vertebral artery
  vertebrobasilar
occlusion of artery
occlusive arterial thrombus
occlusive cerebrovascular insult
occlusive lesion

occult cerebral vascular malformation
    (OCVM)
occult fracture
occult hydrocephalus
occult lesion
occult, roentgenographically
occult scapholunate ganglion
occult seizure
occult spinal dysraphism
occult subluxation
occulta, spina bifida (SBO)
occupational therapist, registered
    (OTR)
occupational therapy (OT)
OCD (obsessive-compulsive disorder)
OCD (osteochondral defect) of the
    glenoid fossa
ochronosis
Ochsner muscles
OCI (osteitis condensans ilii)
OCL (Orthopedic Casting Lab) splint
O'Connor finger dexterity test
OCT (optical coherence tomography)
    surgical imaging probe
OctreoScan (indium-111 pentetreotide)
Octreotide scintigraphy
ocular bobbing
ocular flutter
ocular globe topography
ocular mononeuropathy
ocular motility
ocular motor nucleus
ocular movements, roving
ocular muscle paresis
ocular myasthenia
ocular myoclonus
ocular myopathy
ocular nystagmus
ocular pneumoplethysmography (OPG)
ocular vertigo
oculoauriculovertebral (OAV)
oculocephalic reflex
oculocephalic response
oculocerebrorenal syndrome
oculogyric crisis
oculomotor apparatus
oculomotor apraxia

oculomotor disturbance
oculomotor dysfunction
oculomotor nerve (third cranial nerve)
oculomotor nucleus
oculomotor paresis
oculomotor sign
oculomotor-trochlear nucleus
oculopharyngeal dystrophy
oculopharyngeal muscular dystrophy
oculoplethysmography (OPG)
oculoplethysmography/carotid
    phonoangiography (OPG/CPA)
oculopneumoplethysmography
oculosubcutaneous syndrome of Yuge
oculovestibular reflex
OCVM (occult cerebral vascular
    malfornation)
OD (osteochondritis dissecans)
Oddi muscle
Oden classification of peroneal tendon
    subluxation
Odland ankle prostheses
ODN (ophthalmodynamometry)
odontoid bone
odontoid fracture
odontoid ligament
odontoid peg
odontoid (dens) process
    fractured
    pannus deformity of
odontoid synchondrosis
odontoid view
O'Donoghue facetectomy
O'Donoghue splint
O'Donoghue Unhappy Triad (OUT)
odontogenic fibromyxoma
odontoma
ODQ (opponens digiti quinti) muscle
OEC knee immobilizer
OEC popliteal pad
OEC wrist/forearm support
Oehl muscles
OEIS (omphalocele, cloacal exstrophy,
    imperforate anus, spinal deformity)
    complex
O electrode (occipital) (O_1, O_2, O_z)
off-center cut

Office of Vocational Rehabilitation
(OVR)
offloading knee brace
offset, head-stem
Ogden anchor
Ogden classification of epiphyseal
fracture
Ogden plate
Ogston line
Ogstron-Verebelyi decancellation
procedure
Ohashiatsu massage
Oh hip prosthesis
ohm (pl. ohms)
ohmmeter
ohms impedance
OIF (Osteogenesis Imperfecta
Foundation)
oil
Melaleuca alternifolia
tea-tree
ointment
Pickles
Whitfield
OIRDA (occipital dominant intermit-
tent rhythmic delta activity)
Oklahoma ankle joint orthosis
OKN (optokinetic nystagmus)
OKQ (Osteoporosis Knowledge
Questionnaire)
OKT3 monoclonal antibody
OKT4 monoclonal antibody imaging
agent
OKT8 monoclonal antibody imaging
agent
olanzapine (Zyprexa)
Oldberg brain retractor
Oldberg dissector
Oldberg intervertebral disk rongeur
Oldberg pituitary forceps
Oldberg pituitary rongeur
Olds pin
olecranon bursitis
olecranonectomy
olecranon fossa
olecranon process
olecranon tip fracture

Olerud internal fixator
Olerud-Molander ankle scoring system
Olerud-Molander fracture classification
Olerud PSF fixation system
Olerud PSF rod
Olerud PSF screw
olfaction
olfactory aura
olfactory bulb
olfactory groove, meningioma of the
olfactory hallucination
olfactory nerve (first cranial nerve)
olfactory neuroblastoma
olfactory psychomotor seizure
olfactory seizure
olfactory symptoms
oligoarthritis, undifferentiated
oligoarticular arthritis
oligoastrocytoma
oligoclonal IgG bands in cerebrospinal
fluid
oligodendrocyte cell
oligodendroglial cell
oligodendroglioma, anaplastic
oligodendroglioma-astrocytoma
oligodendroglioma tumor
oligodendroma
oligohydramnios
oligonucleosoma
olisthesis
olisthetic vertebra, wedging of
olisthy
olivary hypertrophy
olivary nucleus
olive
inferior
posterior (in brain)
superior (in brain)
Olivecrona aneurysm clips
Olivecrona brain spatula
Olivecrona clip-applying and removing
forceps
Olivecrona dural dissector
Olivecrona dural scissors
Olivecrona-Gigli saw
Olivecrona rasp
Olivecrona rongeur

Olivecrona saw
Olivecrona scissors
Olivecrona-Toennis clip-applying forceps
Olivecrona trigeminal knife
Olivecrona trigeminal scissors
Olivecrona wire saw
olive ring
olive wire
Olivier-Bertrand-Talairach stereotactic
head frame
olivopontocerebellar atrophy
olivopontocerebellar degeneration
Ollier approach to hips, modified
Ollier disease
Ollier rake retractor
Ollier-Thiersch skin graft
Olympia VACPAC back support
Olympics, National Special
Olympus digital camera
omagra
omalgia
omarthritis
Ombredanne mallet
OMC (short orientation-memory-
concentration) test
Omega compression hip screw system
Omega hand surgery splinting material
omega-3 oils
Omer-Capen technique
omitis
Ommaya ventriculoperitoneal shunt
Ommaya ventriculostomy reservoir
Omnifit-HA stem for total hip arthro-
plasty
Omnifit knee prosthesis
Omnifit Plus hip system
Omni-Flexor wrist exerciser
Omnipaque (iohexol) nonionic imaging
agent
Omni Prep electrolyte gel for EEG
Omni retractor
Omni Roller massager
Omniscan (gadodiamide) nonionic
contrast medium
omoclavicular
omodynia
omohyoid

omoplata
omosternum
Omotrain active shoulder support
OMT (osteomanipulative therapy)
oncocytoma
oncoprotein
Oncovin (vincristine)
Ondine curse
one-bar external fixator
one-bone forearm
one-dimensional chemical shift
imaging (1D-CSI)
one-handed kitchen utensils
one-legged hop test
one-part fracture
one-shot echo planar imaging
ONI (old nerve injury)
onion bulb appearance of myelin
sheaths
onion bulb changes on biopsy
onion bulb formation of neuropathy
onion peel appearance on x-ray
onionskin configuration of collagenous
fibers
onionskin distribution of sensation
onlay cancellous iliac graft
onlay posterior cruciate ligament
reconstruction technique
on-off effect of L-dopa in parkinsonism
on-off phenomenon
onset
adult
juvenile
latency of
pauciarticular
polyarticular
short latency to sleep
sleep
systemic
onset of sleep
Ontario Cohort Study of Running-
Related Injuries
ontogenetic
onychectomy
onychocryptosis (ingrown nail)
onychogryphosis
onychomycosis

onycho-osteodysplasia
onychotomy
OPAL knee brace
opaque wire suture
OPD4 monoclonal antibody imaging
  agent
open-bowl cement mix technique
open-break fracture
open-configuration magnetic resonance
  system
open dislocation
open fontanelle
open fracture
opening-base wedge osteotomy
opening osteotomy
opening pressure on lumbar puncture
  (spinal tap)
opening wedge manipulation and
  reapplication of plaster
open-lip (type II) schizencephaly
open magnet
open magnetic resonance imaging
open-mouth odontoid x-ray view
open MRI
open neural tube defect
open plantar fasciotomy
open reduction and internal fixation
  (ORIF)
open tendon repair
opera glass hand
Operating Arm system
operations (also *approach*; *procedure*;
    repair; *technique*)
  Abbott-Fischer-Lucas hip arthrodesis
  Abbott-Gill osteotomy
  Abbott knee approach
  Abbott-Lucas shoulder
  abduction osteotomy
  ablation
  ablative arthroplasty
  ablative surgery
  abrasion arthroplasty
  ACF (anterior cervical fusion)
  Achilles tendon lengthening
  ACL (anterior cruciate ligament)
    repair

operations *(continued)*
  acromioclavicular arthroplasty
  Adams arthrodesis
  Adams hip
  adduction osteotomy
  adductor tenotomy
  Adkins spinal fusion
  adrenal medulla transplantation
  Akin phalangeal osteotomy
  Albee-Delbert
  Albee spinal fusion
  Albert procedure
  Allen open reduction of calcaneal
    fracture
  Allman modification of Evans
    ankle reconstruction
  allogenic transplantation
  AMBI fixation
  Amspacher-Messenbaugh
  Amstutz resurfacing
  Amstutz total hip replacement
  Amstutz-Wilson osteotomy
  AMTR (anteromedial temporal lobe
    resection)
  amygdalohippocampectomy
  Anderson-Fowler procedure
  Anderson-Hutchins
  Andrews iliotibial band
    reconstruction
  aneurysmal clipping
  ankle-level arteriotomy
  anterior capsular shift
  anterior capsulolabral reconstruction
    (ACLR)
  anterior cervical fusion (ACF)
  anterior corpectomy
  anterior cruciate ligament (ACL)
    repair
  anterior lobectomy
  anterior retropharyngeal approach
  anterior transcallosal approach
  anteromedial temporal lobe
    resection (AMTR)
  AO/ASIF compression
  AO group shoulder arthrodesis
  APR cement fixation

operations *(continued)*
Arafiles elbow arthrodesis
Arana-Iniquez intracranial cyst
    removal
Armistead ulnar lengthening
arthrodesis
arthrorisis (arthroereisis)
arthroplasty
arthroscopic acromioplasty
arthroscopic bioabsorbable tack
    repair of shoulder
arthroscopic coplaning
arthroscopic debridement
arthroscopic glenohumeral release
arthroscopic labrectomy
arthroscopic microdiskectomy
arthroscopic mini open rotator cuff
    repair
arthroscopic mosaicplasty
arthroscopic resection
arthroscopic screw fixation
arthroscopic suture anchor repair of
    shoulder
arthroscopic synovectomy
arthroscopic transacromial repair of
    coracoacromial ligament
arthroscopic transglenoid suture
    repair of shoulder
arthroscopic transhumeral recon-
    struction of rotator cuff tear
arthroscopic wafer
arthroscopy
arthrotomy
articular reconstruction
Ashworth hand arthroplasty
ASIF screw fixation
Aston cartilage reduction
Atasoy V-Y
atlanto-occipital fusion
Aufranc cup arthroplasty
Austin-Akin bunionectomy
Austin Moore arthroplasty
Austin Moore hemiarthroplasty
autoadrenal transplantation for
    Parkinson disease
autogenous bone graft

operations *(continued)*
autogenous peroneus longus free
    graft
autograft of adrenal medulla tissue
autograft replacement
Auto-Implant
automated percutaneous lumbar
    diskectomy (APLD)
Averill total hip replacement
Avila
avulsion
Axer-Clark procedure
Axer varus derotational osteotomy
axial percutaneous pinning (hand)
Baciu-Filibiu dowel ankle
    arthrodesis
Badgley iliac wing resection
Bailey-Badgley anterior cervical
    approach
Bailey-Badgley cervical spine
    fusion
Bailey-Dubow osteotomy
Baker-Hill osteotomy
Baker patellar advancement
Baker translocation
BAK laparoscopic
Balacescu-Golden
Baldwin Bowers radioulnar joint
balloon embolization
balloon occlusion
Bandi
Bankart-Putti-Platt
Bankart shoulder repair
Banks-Laufman
Barnhart repair
Barrasso-Wile-Gage arthrodesis
Barr open reduction and internal
    fixation
Barr-Record arthrodesis
Barr tendon transfer
Barr tibial fracture fixation
Barsky
Bartlett nail fold
basal osteotomy
base wedge osteotomy
basilar crescentic osteotomy

operations *(continued)*
   Batchelor-Brown arthrodesis
   Batch-Spittler-McFaddin
   Bateman hemiarthroplasty
   Bateman modification of Mayer
      transfer
   Bateman shoulder
   Bauer-Tondra-Trusler
   Baumgard-Schwartz tennis elbow
   Beall-Webel-Bailey
   Bechtol arthroplasty
   Beckenbaugh
   Becker tendon repair
   Becton
   Bellemore-Barrett-Middleton-
      Scougall-Whiteway
   Bell-Tawse open reduction
   Bennett posterior shoulder approach
   Bennett quadriceps plastic
   BERG (balloon-assisted, endo-
      scopic, retroperitoneal, gasless)
      lumbar interbody fusion
   Berman-Gartland metatarsal
      osteotomy
   Bernese periacetabular osteotomy
   B.H. Moore
   biceps tendon tenodesis
   Bickel-Moe
   Bilhaut-Cloquet
   bimalleolar approach to ankle
      arthrodesis
   biocompartmental replacement of
      knee
   bioelectrical repair of delayed
      union or nonunion
   Bircher-Weber
   Black-Bröstrom staple
   Blair ankle fusion
   Blair-Morris-Dunn-Hand ankle
      arthrodesis
   Blair tibiotalar arthrodesis
   Bleck recession
   Bloom-Raney modification
   Blount displacement osteotomy
   Blount tracing
   Blundell-Jones

operations *(continued)*
   Bohlman cervical fusion
   bone-blocking
   bone graft repair
   Bonfiglio modification
   Booth wire osteotomy
   Bora
   Borggreve limb rotation
   Bose nail fold excision
   Bosworth bone peg insertion
   Bosworth shelf
   Bosworth spinal fusion
   Bowers radial arthroplasty
   Boyd amputation
   Boyd-Anderson biceps tendon
      repair
   Boyd approach
   Boyd-Bosworth
   Boyd-McLeod tennis elbow
   Boyd-Sisk posterior capsulorrhaphy
   Boyes brachioradialis transfer
   Brackett-Osgood knee approach
   Brackett-Osgood-Putti-Abbott
   Brady-Jewett
   Bragg-peak radiosurgery
   Brahms foot
   Brain arthroplasty
   brain biopsy
   Brand tendon transfer
   Brannon-Wickstrom
   Brantigan-Voshell
   Braun
   Brett-Campbell tibial osteotomy
   bridle posterior tibial tendon transfer
   Bristow-Helfet
   Bristow-May
   Bristow shoulder reconstruction
   Brittain arthrodesis
   Brockman foot
   Brooker-Jones tendon transfer
   Brooks cervical fusion
   Brooks-Gallie cervical
   Brooks-Jenkins atlantoaxial fusion
   Brooks-Jenkins cervical
   Brooks-Seddon transfer
   Broomhead approach

operations *(continued)*
  Brostrom
  Brostrom-Gould lateral ankle
    instability
  Brown knee approach
  Brown knee joint reconstruction
  Bruser knee approach
  Bryan arthroplasty
  Bryan-Morrey elbow approach
  Buck-Gramcko
  Bugg-Boyd
  Buncke
  bunionectomy, tricorrectional
  bunionette excision
  Bunnell posterior tibial tendon
    transfer
  Bunnell tendon repair
  Burgess
  Burkhalter transfer
  Burow skin flap
  Butler fifth toe
  Calandriello hip reduction
  Calandruccio fixation
  calcaneal resection
  calcanectomy
  calcaneocuboid arthrodesis
  calcaneonavicular bar resection
  calcaneotibial fusion
  Caldwell-Coleman flatfoot
  Caldwell-Durham tendon
  Callahan approach
  Callahan fusion
  Camitz opponensplasty
  Campbell-Akbarnia arthrodesis
  Campbell elbow approach
  Campbell-Goldthwait
  Campbell posterior bone block
  Campbell posterior shoulder
    approach
  Canale osteotomy
  Capello total hip replacement
  Capener lateral rachitomy
  capitellocondylar arthroplasty
  capsular release
  capsular-shift reconstruction
  capsulolabral
  capsulotomy

operations *(continued)*
  Carceau-Brahms ankle arthrodesis
  Carnesale hip approach
  carotid artery ligation
  carotid bifurcation endarterectomy
  carotid ligation
  Carrell fibular substitution
  Caspari repair
  Castle
  Cave hip approach
  Cave knee approach
  Cave-Rowe shoulder dislocation
  cementless surface replacement
    arthroplasty
  cementless total hip replacement
  central commissurotomy
  centralization of radius
  cervical sympathectomy
  cervico-occipital fusion
  Chandler arthrodesis
  Chandler hip fusion
  Chapchal knee arthrodesis
  Charcot hip arthrodesis
  charged-particle radiosurgery
  Charnley ankle arthrodesis
  Charnley compression-type knee
    fusion
  Charnley hip replacement
  Charnley-Houston arthrodesis
  Chaves-Rapp muscle transfer
  cheilectomy
  cheilotomy
  chemical rhizotomy
  chemonucleolysis
  chevron osteotomy
  Chiari innominate osteotomy
  Childress ankle fixation
  Cho cruciate ligament reconstruction
  chondrocyte transplant
  Chopart amputation with tendon
    balancing
  Chow endoscopic carpal tunnel
    release
  Chrisman-Snook reconstruction of
    ankle ligaments
  Chuinard autogenous bone graft
  Chuinard-Petersen ankle arthrodesis

operations *(continued)*
  cingulotomy
  Clancy-Andrews reconstruction
  Clancy ligament
  Clark transfer
  Clayton-Fowler
  Clayton resection arthroplasty
  CLB (conjoined lateral band)
    rerouting
  Cleveland-Bosworth-Thompson
  clip ligation of aneurysm
  clipping of aneurysm
  closed base wedge osteotomy
    (CBWO)
  closed manipulative
  closing wedge high tibial osteotomy
    (CWHTO)
  Cloward back fusion
  Cloward cervical arthrodesis
  Cloward cervical disk approach
  clubfoot release
  coating of aneurysm
  Cobb scoliosis measuring
  coccygeal
  Cocklin toe
  Codivilla tendon lengthening
  Codman saber-cut shoulder
    approach
  Coleman flatfoot
  Cole tendon fixation
  Collis broken femoral stem
  Colonna-Ralston ankle approach
  Colonna shelf
  Colonna trochanteric arthroplasty
  Coltart fracture
  Compere-Thompson arthrodesis
  compression screw arthrodesis
  computed tomography-guided
    percutaneous trigeminal
    tractotomy-nucleotomy
  computerized dynamic
    posturography
  computer-assisted microsurgery
  condylectomy
  cone arthrodesis

operations *(continued)*
  conjoined lateral band (CLB)
    rerouting (in swan-neck hand
    deformities)
  Contour DF-80 total hip
  contoured loop fixation
  Coonrad total elbow arthroplasty
  Coonse-Adam knee approach
  Copeland-Howard shoulder
  cordotomy
  corrective lengthening osteotomy
  corrective osteotomy
  corticotomy
  costotransversectomy
  Cotrel-Dubousset derotation
  Couch-Derosa-Throop transfer
  countersinking osteotomy
  Coventry vagus osteotomy
  Cozen-Brockway
  Cracchiolo forefoot arthroplasty
  Cracchiolo-Sculco implant
  cranial base reconstruction
  cranial synostosis surgical repair
  craniocervical decompression
  craniofacial reconstruction
  cranioplasty
  craniotomy
  Crawford-Adams cup arthroplasty
  Crego hip reduction
  Crego tendon transfer
  crescentic base wedge osteotomy
  cruciate ligament reconstruction
  cryohypophysectomy
  CSR (complete subtalar release)
  CT-assisted stereotactic craniotomy
  CT-guided stereotactic
  Cubbins arthroplasty
  Cubbins shoulder approach
  cup-on-cup arthroplasty of the hip
  Curtin plantar fibromatosis excision
  Curtis-Fisher knee
  Curtis PIP joint capsulotomy
  Darrach extensor carpi ulnaris
    tenodesis
  Darrach-McLaughlin
  Das Gupta
  D'Aubigné femoral reconstruction

operations *(continued)*
Davey-Rorabeck-Fowler decompression
Davis drainage
De Andrade-MacNab occipitocervical arthrodesis
Debeyre-Patte-Elmelik rotator cuff
decompression carpectomy
decompression craniectomy
decompression craniotomy
decompression fasciotomy
decompression laminectomy
degloving
deltoid-splitting shoulder approach
Dennyson-Fulford extra-articular subtalar arthrodesis
Dewar-Barrington arthroplasty
Dewar cervical
Dewar-Harris shoulder
Deyerle femoral fracture
Diamond-Gould syndactyly
diaphyseal osteotomy
diaphysectomy
Dias-Giegerich fracture
Dickinson-Coutts-Woodward-Handler osteotomy
Dickson-Diveley foot
Dickson transplant
digital nerve repair
Dimon-Hughston fracture fixation
diskectomy (or discectomy)
distal metatarsal osteotomy
distal oblique osteotomy
distraction-compression bone graft arthrodesis
distraction lengthening
division of corpus callosum
Dockery
Doll trochanteric reattachment
Domen laminoplasty
dome proximal tibial osteotomy
Dorrance
dorsal pedal bypass
double arthrodesis
dowel arthrodesis
dowel graft
doweling spondylolisthesis

operations *(continued)*
Dowling intracranial cyst removal
DREZ (dorsal root entry zone) modification of Eriksson
Drummond wire
DST&G (doubled semitendinosus and gracilis) autograft
Dunn-Brittain foot stabilization
Dunn-Hess trochanteric osteotomy
Dunn hip
Durham flatfoot
duToit-Roux arthroplasty
duToit-Roux staple capsulorrhaphy
DuVries arthroplasty
DuVries hammer toe repair
DuVries modified McBride hallux valgus
DuVries phalangeal condylectomy
DuVries reconstruction
DuVries technique for overlapping toe
Dwyer clawfoot
Eaton arthroplasty
Eaton-Littler
Eaton-Malerich fracture-dislocation
Eberle contracture release
Ecker-Lotke-Glazer tendon reconstruction
ECT (European compression technique) fixation
ECTR (endoscopic carpal tunnel release)
Eden-Hybbinette arthroplasty
Eden-Lange
Edward
Eftekhar broken femoral stem
Eggers tendon transfer
Elizabethtown osteotomy
Ellis Jones peroneal tendon
Ellison lateral knee reconstruction
Elmslie-Cholmeley foot
Elmslie peroneal tendon
Elmslie-Trillat patellar
Elmslie-Trillat transplant
Elmslie triple arthrodesis
Emmon osteotomy
en bloc laminectomy

operations *(continued)*
  en bloc resection
  endarterectomy
  Ender rod fixation of fracture
  endoscopic carpal tunnel release
    (ECTR)
  endoscopic division of incompetent
    perforating veins
  endoscopic endonasal trans-
    sphenoidal
  endoscopic neurosurgery
  endoscopic plantar fasciotomy
  endoscopic retrocalcaneal decom-
    pression
  endoscopic strip craniectomy
  endovascular coil embolization
  Engh total hip replacement
  Enneking knee arthrodesis
  epicondylectomy
  epiduroscopy
  epineural repair
  epineurotomy
  epiphysiodesis
  Eppright dial osteotomy
  Erickson-Leider-Brown
  Eriksson cruciate ligament
    reconstruction
  escharotomy
  Essex-Lopresti axial fixation
  Essex-Lopresti fixation of calcaneal
    fracture
  European compression technique
    (ECT) fixation
  evacuation of blood clot
  Evans ankle joint instability
  Evans ankle reconstruction
  Evans calcaneal distraction wedge
    osteotomy
  Evans calcaneal lengthening
  Evans lateral ankle reconstruction
  Evans osteotomy
  Evans tenodesis
  Eve
  eversion endarterectomy
  Ewald total elbow replacement
  Ewald-Walker knee arthroplasty
  Exact-Fit ATH hip replacement

operations *(continued)*
  excision arthroplasty
  extended tibial in situ bypass
  extensor brevis arthroplasty
  extensor tenotomy
  extracranial sectioning of cranial
    nerves
  extracranial-to-intracranial bypass
  Eyler flexorplasty
  facet fusion
  facetectomy
  Fahey approach
  Fahey-O'Brien
  failed joint replacement
  Fairbanks technique with Sever
    modification
  Farmer
  fascial release
  fascicular repair
  fasciectomy
  femorodistal bypass
  Ferciot-Thomson excision
  Ferguson hip reduction
  Ferguson-Thompson-King
    two-stage osteotomy
  Ferkel torticollis
  Fernandez osteotomy
  fetal pig cell transplantation
  fetal substantia nigra transplantation
  fetal ventral mesencephalic tissue
    transplantation
  fibular head resection
  Ficat
  first rib resection
  first-toe Jones repair
  Fish cuneiform osteotomy
  five-in-one knee ligament repair
  flexor tendon graft
  flexor tendon transfer
  flexor tenotomy
  Flynn
  forage
  foraminotomy
  Forbes modification of Phemister
    graft
  forefoot arthroplasty
  four-bar external fixation

operations *(continued)*
  Fowler tendon transfer
  Fowles dislocation
  Fox-Blazina knee
  fracture repair
  free body fusion
  French supracondylar fracture
  Fried-Green foot
  Fried-Hendel tendon
  Froimson-Oh arm
  frontal craniotomy
  frontotemporal craniotomy
  Frost foot
  Frost posterior tibialis tendon
    lengthening
  Fulkerson oblique tibial tubercle
    osteotomy
  functional posterior rhizotomy
  Furnas-Haq-Somers
  fusion
  Gaenslen
  Galeazzi patellar
  Gallie ankle arthrodesis
  Gallie cervical fusion
  Gallie subtalar fusion
  Gallis foot
  Galveston sacral fixation
  gangliolysis
  Ganley modification of Keller
    arthroplasty
  Gant osteotomy
  Garceau-Brahms arthrodesis
  Gardner
  Gartland
  gasless retroperitoneal video-
    assisted spine
  gastrocnemius recession
  Gatellier-Chastang ankle approach
  Gelman foot
  Gerard resurfacing
  Getty decompression
  Ghormley arthrodesis
  Ghormley shelf
  Giannestras metatarsal oblique
    osteotomy
  Giannestras step-down modified
    osteotomy

operations *(continued)*
  Gibson approach
  Gibson-Piggott osteotomy
  Gigli saw osteotomy
  Gilbert-Tamai-Weiland
  Gillies-Millard cocked-hat
  Gill-Manning-White spondylolisthesis
  Gill modification of Campbell
    ankle
  Gill shelf
  Gill-Stein arthrodesis
  Girdlestone pseudarthrosis
  Girdlestone-Taylor
  Girdlestone tendon transfer
  Glynn-Neibauer
  Goldner-Clippinger
  Goldstein spinal fusion
  Goldthwait-Hauser
  Gordon-Brostrom
  Gordon-Taylor
  Gouffon fixation
  Graber-Devernay hip
  greater tuberosity osteotomy
  Green-Banks
  Greenfield osteotomy
  Greulich-Pyle
  Grice-Green extra-articular subtalar
    arthrodesis
  Gristina-Webb shoulder arthroplasty
  Gritti-Stokes distal thigh
  Grosse-Kempf tibial
  grouped fascicular repair
  Groves-Goldner
  Gruca lower leg
  Guleke-Stookey approach
  Guller resection
  Gustilo-Kyle cementless total hip
    arthroplasty
  guttering
  Guttmann subtalar arthrodesis
  Guyon tunnel release
  Haddad-Riordan arthrodesis
  Hall facet fusion
  hallux interphalangeal joint
    arthrodesis
  hammer toe correction with
    interphalangeal fusion

operations *(continued)*
Hammon foot
hamstring lengthening
hamstring release
Hamus wrist arthroplasty
hanging toe
Hardinge femoral approach
Hardinge vastus lateralis
Hark foot
Harmon cervical approach
Harmon shoulder approach
Harmon transfer
Harrington rod fixation
Harrington total hip arthroplasty
Harris-Beath arthrodesis
Harris-Smith cervical fusion
Hass
Hassmann-Brunn-Neer elbow
Hastings bipolar hemiarthroplasty
Hauser bunionectomy
Hauser heel cord
Hauser patellar
Hay-Groves shelf
heel cord advancement
helmet-molding therapy
hemiarthroplasty
hemicallotasis
hemicraniectomy
hemicraniotomy
hemilaminectomy
hemiphalangectomy
hemisacrectomy with hemi-
  pelvectomy
Hendel correction of scaphocephaly
Henderson approach
Henderson arthrodesis
Henry-Geist spinal fusion
Henry radial approach
Herbert screw fixation
Hermodsson internal rotation
Herndon-Heyman foot
Hey-Groves-Kirk
Heyman-Herndon clubfoot
Heyman-Herndon-Strong
Hibbs-Jones spinal fusion
high tibial osteotomy
Hill-Nahai-Vasconez-Mathes

operations *(continued)*
hindfoot arthrodesis
hip pinning
Hirschhorn compression approach
His-Haas
Hitchcock arm
Hitchcock tendon
Hoffer ankle
Hoffmann-Clayton
Hoffman-Mohr unicoronal cranial
  synostosis repair
Hohmann-Thomasen metatarsal
  osteotomy
Hoke Achilles tendon lengthening
Hoke arthrodesis
Hoke tibial palsy
holistic approach
hook pin fixation
Hoppenfeld-Deboer
Horwitz-Adams ankle fusion
Houghton-Akroyd
Hovnanian transfer
Howard
Howorth approach
Howse total hip replacement
Huber opponensplasty
Hughston-Degenhardt reconstruction
Hughston-Hauser
Hughston-Jacobson
Hungerford-Krackow-Kenna knee
  arthroplasty
hunterian ligation of aneurysm
Huntington tibial
I-beam hemiarthroplasty
I-beam hip
ICLH double-cup arthroplasty
IDET (intradiscal electrothermal)
  annuloplasty
Ilizarov ankle arthrodesis
Ilizarov corticotomy
Ilizarov limb lengthening
implant arthroplasty
Inclan modification of Campbell
  ankle
Inclan-Ober
infratemporal approach
infratentorial approach

operations *(continued)*
Inglis-Cooper
Inglis-Ranawat-Straub
Ingram bony bridge resection
Insall-Burstein-Freeman knee
 arthroplasty
inside-out Bankart shoulder instability
inside-out meniscal repair
in situ vein bypass to ankle
interbody arthrodesis
interbody fusion
interhemispheric approach
intermetatarsal angle-reducing
internal fixation compression
 arthrodesis of ankle
interphalangeal fusion
interpositional arthroplasty of foot
interpositional elbow arthroplasty
interstitial radiosurgery
intertransverse fusion
intertransverse process arthrodesis
intra-articular knee fusion
intracranial arterial bypass
intracranial glossopharyngeal
 rhizotomy
intradiscal electrothermal
 annuloplasty
intraforaminal approach
ipsilateral approach
Irvine ankle arthroplasty
Isseis-Aussies scoliosis
Jackson rod insertion
Jaffe
Janecki-Nelson shoulder
Jansey
Japas osteotomy
Jeffery
John Barnes myofascial release
John C. Wilson arthrodesis
Johnson hemiphalangectomy
Johnson pelvic fracture
Johnson-Spiegl hallux varus
 correction
joint fluid aspiration
Jones-Brackett
Jones cock-up toe
Jones-Ellison ACL reconstruction

operations *(continued)*
J.R. Moore
Juvara foot
Kapandji-Sauvé radioulnar joint
 repair
Kapel elbow dislocation
Kaplan
Karakousis-Vezeridis
Kashiwagi
Kates forefoot arthroplasty
Kates-Kessel-Kay
Kaufer tendon
Kelikian-Clayton-Loseff
Kelikian-McFarland
Kelikian modified Z osteotomy
Kelikian-Riashi-Gleason
Keller arthroplasty
Keller-Brandes
Keller bunionectomy
Keller foot
Keller hallux valgus
Keller resection arthroplasty
Kellogg-Speed fusion
Kendrick-Sharma-Hassler-Herndon
Kennedy ligament
Kessel-Bonney extension osteotomy
Kessler posterior tibial tendon
 transfer
keyhole craniotomy
keyhold tenodesis
Key intra-articular knee arthrodesis
Kickaldy-Willis arthrodesis
Kidner foot
King-Richards dislocation
King-Steelquist
Kirk distal thigh
Kirschner wire (K wire) fixation
Klein approach
Kleinert repair
Klisic-Jankovic
Knobby-Clark
Kocher-Langenbeck ilioinguinal
 repair of acetabular fracture
Kocher lateral J approach
Kocher-McFarland hip arthroplasty
Koenig arthroplasty
Koenig-Schaefer approach

operations *(continued)*
  Kortzeborn hand
  Koutsogiannis-Fowler-Anderson
    osteotomy
  Kramer-Craig-Noel osteotomy
  Krempen-Silver-Sotelo nonunion
  Kronner external fixation
  Krukenberg hand
  Kumar-Cowell-Ramsey
  Kumar spica cast
  labyrinthectomy
  Lamb muscle transfer
  Lambrinudi dropfoot
  laminectomy
  laminoplasty
  laminotomy
  Lange Achilles tendon reconstruction
  Lange hip reduction
  Lange tendon lengthening and
    repair
  Lapidus hammertoe
  Larmon forefoot
  Larson ligament reconstruction
  laser-assisted capsulorrhaphy
  laser-assisted spinal endoscopy
    (LASE)
  laser image custom arthroplasty
    (LICA)
  laser microsurgery
  Latarjet
  lateral acetabular shelf
  lateral approach
  lateral band rerouting
  lateral cerebellopontine angle
    approach
  lateral extracavitary approach
  Leach-Igou step-cut medial
    osteotomy
  Leeds spine
  leg compartment release
  Lehman
  Lelièvre (to block end-range
    pronation)
  Lenart-Kullman
  lengthening over nails (LON)
  L'Episcopo-Zachary
  Lewis-Chekofsky resection

operations *(continued)*
  LICA (laser image custom
    arthroplasty)
  Lichtman
  Liebolt radioulnar
  ligamentous release
  ligament reconstruction
  limb lengthening
  limb salvage
  limb sparing
  LINAC (linear accelerator)
    radiosurgery
  Lindeman
  Lindgren oblique osteotomy
  Lindholm open surgical tendon
    repair
  Lindseth modified
  Lipscomb modified McKeever
    arthrodesis
  Littler-Cooley
  Lloyd-Roberts fracture
  Localio
  LON (lengthening over nails)
  Loose
  Lorenz hip reduction
  Losee modification of MacIntosh
  Lowman shelf
  L-shaped capsulotomy
  Lucas-Murray knee arthrodesis
  Luck hand
  Ludloff approach
  Lunceford total hip replacement
  Luque rod fixation
  MacAusland
  MacCarthy
  MacEwen-Shands osteotomy
  MacIntosh over-the-top repair
  MacIntosh tenodesis
  MacNab shoulder repair
  Magilligan measuring
  Magnuson-Stack shoulder
    arthrotomy
  Ma-Griffith ruptured Achilles
    tendon repair
  Ma-Griffith tendon anastomosis
  Majestro-Ruda-Frost tendon

operations *(continued)*
Malawer excision
Mallory-Head total hip revision
Mankin
Manktelow transfer
Mann-Coughlin arthrodesis
Mann-DuVries arthroplasty
Mann modified McKeever
arthrodesis
Mann resection arthroplasty
Mann-Thompson-Coughlin
arthrodesis
Manske
Maquet
Marcus-Balourdas-Heiple ankle
fusion
Marks-Bayne thumb duplication
Marmor replacement
Marshall ligament repair
Martin osteotomy
Matchett-Brown hip arthroplasty
Matti-Russe
Mauck (reverse) knee
Mayo bunionectomy
Mayo hallux valgus modified
Mayo metatarsal head resection
Mayo total elbow arthroplasty
Mazet
McBride bunionectomy
McBride hallux abductovalgus
reduction
McCarroll-Baker
McCarty hip
McCash hand
McCauley foot
McConnell
McElfresh-Dobyns-O'Brien
McElvenny foot
McFarland-Osborne
McKay-Simons clubfoot
McKay-Simons CSR (complete
subtalar release)
McKeever arthrodesis for hallux
limitus
McKeever-Buck elbow
McKeever medullary clavicle
fixation

operations *(continued)*
McKeever metatarsophalangeal
fusion
McKittrick transmetatarsal
amputation
McLaughlin-Hay
McLaughlin muscle transfer into
humeral defect
McReynolds open reduction
McWhorter posterior shoulder
approach
medial displacement calcaneal
osteotomy
medial parapatellar arthrotomy
medial quadriceps advancement
medial V-Y capsulotomy
meniscal transplantation
Mensor-Scheck
metatarsal neck osteotomy
metatarsocuneiform joint fusion
metatarsophalangeal joint fusion
Meuli arthroplasty
Meyerding-Van Demark
microdiskectomy
microendoscopic diskectomy
microfracture of eburnated bone
surfaces
microlumbar diskectomy (MLD)
microsurgery
microsurgical diskectomy
middle fossa transtentorial translabyrinthine approach
Milch cuff resection
Milch elbow
Milch radioulnar joint repair
Millender-Nalebuff wrist arthrodesis
Miller flatfoot
Miller-Galante arthroplasty
Millesi modified
mini-fragment plate fixation
minimal incision
Mital elbow release
Mitchell bunionectomy
Mitchell distal osteotomy to correct
hallux valgus
Miyakawa knee
Mizuno

operations *(continued)*
MLD (microlumbar diskectomy)
Moberg-Gedda open reduction
modified Bristow
modified Brostrom lateral ankle
instability
modified Hoke-Miller flatfoot
modified Kessler
modified Lapidus arthrodesis
modified McBride bunionectomy
modified mold and surface
replacement arthroplasty
modified Watson-Jones ankle
tenodesis
modified Wilson osteotomy
Moe scoliosis
Molesworth-Campbell elbow
approach
monofilament wire fixation
monospherical shoulder arthroplasty
Monticelli-Spinelli distraction
Moore-Darrach radioulnar joint
repair
Morgan-Casscells meniscus suturing
Morrey-Bryan elbow arthroplasty
Morrey modification of Boyd-
Anderson biceps tendon repair
Morrison
Morrissy percutaneous slipped
epiphysis fixation
mosaicplasty
Mosley method for anterior
shoulder repair
Mubarak-Hargens decompression
Mueller (Müller) hip arthroplasty
Mueller knee
multiarc LINAC radiosurgery
multilevel laminectomy
Mumford-Gurd acromioclavicular
Mumford-Gurd arthroplasty
Murphy heel cord advancement
muscle shortening
Nalebuff-Millender
Naughton-Dunn triple arthrodesis
Neer unconstrained shoulder
arthroplasty
neural arch resection

operations *(continued)*
neurectomy
neurolysis
neurotransplantation
Neviaser-Wilson-Gardner
New England Baptist hip
arthroplasty
Nicholas five-in-one reconstruction
Nicola shoulder
Nicoll fracture repair
Niebauer-King
Nirschl
nucleus caudalis dorsal root entry
zone operation
Ober-Barr transfer
oblique osteotomy
O'Brien pelvic halo
obturator neurectomy
Obwegeser-Dalpont internal screw
fixation
Obwegeser sagittal mandibular
osteotomy
occipital interhemispheric approach
occipitoatlantoaxial fusion
occipitocervical arthrodesis
occipitocervical fusion
O'Donoghue ACL reconstruction
Ogstron-Verebelyi decancellation
Ollier arthrodesis approach
Omer-Capen
onlay posterior cruciate ligament
reconstruction
open-door laminoplasty
opening base wedge osteotomy
open tendon repair
opercular cortex
Oriental flap
ORIF (open reduction, internal
fixation)
Osborne-Cotterill elbow dislocation
Osgood rotational osteotomy
Osmone-Clarke foot
osteoarticular autologous tissue
transfer
osteochondral autograft transfer
osteochondral transplantation
osteoclasis

operations *(continued)*
osteoplastic craniotomy
osteoplastic laminectomy
Ostrup
over-the-top knee
Pack
Paddu knee
pallidal brain stimulation
pallidotomy guided by microelectrode recording
Palmer-Widen shoulder
Paltrinieri-Trentani resurfacing
panmetatarsal head resection
pantalar arthrodesis
pantalar fusion
pants-over-vest
Papineau
parapatellar arthrotomy
parietal cortectomy
Patel medial meniscectomy
patellar tendon substitution
patellar tendon transfer (PTT)
Paterson
Paulos ligament
Pauwel proximal osteotomy
Pauwel Y osteotomy
Peacock transposition
pedicle screw fixation
Pemberton acetabuloplasty
Pemberton pericapsular osteotomy
PENS (percutaneous electrical nerve stimulation)
percutaneous corticotomy
percutaneous heel cord lengthening
percutaneous high frequency rhizotomy
percutaneous lengthening of Achilles tendon
percutaneous nuclectomy
percutaneous osteotomy
percutaneous pin insertion
percutaneous pinning
percutaneous radiofrequency coagulation
percutaneous repair
percutaneous tenotomy
percutaneous thermal rhizotomy

operations *(continued)*
percutaneous trigeminal tractotomy-nucleotomy
Perry-Nickel
Perry-O'Brien-Hodgson
Perry-Robinson cervical
phalangeal condylectomy
Pheasant elbow
Phemister onlay bone graft
Pilliar total hip replacement
plantar fasciotomy
plantar flexor proximal metatarsal
platform posturography
Platou osteotomy
PMR (posteromedial release) for clubfoot
polyethylene femoral buck plug
porous-coated total hip replacement
portmanteau
posterior fossa exploration
posterior GPi pallidotomy
posterior lumbar interbody fusion (PLIF)
posterior tibialis tendon lengthening
posterolateral interbody fusion (PLIF)
posteromedial release (PMR) for clubfoot
posteroventral pallidotomy
Post shoulder arthroplasty
Potts eversion osteotomy
primary repair
proximal metatarsal approach
proximal phalanx osteotomy
pseudarthrosis
pterional approach
PTT (posterior tibialis tendon transfer)
pulp-plasty
pulsed electromagnetic therapy
pulsed-field gel electrophoresis
Putti knee arthrodesis
Putti-Platt arthroplasty
radialization of club hand
radial recession osteotomy
radical nail bed ablation of ingrowing toenail

operations *(continued)*
    radiosurgery
    radiosurgical corpus callostomy
    Radley-Liebig-Brown resection
    ray resection
    reefing
    reefing of the medial retinaculum
      of the knee
    refixation of chondral fragments
    Regnauld free phalangeal base
      autograft for hallux limitus
    Regnauld modification of Keller
      arthroplasty
    Reichenheim-King
    release of abductor hallucis muscle
    resection arthroplasty
    resection of epileptogenic focus
    resection of iliopsoas tendon
    resurfacing
    retrogeniculate hamstring release
    retromastoid craniotomy
    retrosigmoid transmeatal approach
    Reverdin-Green foot
    Reverdin-Green osteotomy
    reverse Mauck knee
    revision acromioplasty
    revision arthroplasty
    revision total hip
    rhachotomy
    rhizotomy
    Ridlon hip reduction
    Ring UPM knee or hip replace-
      ment
    Riordan opponensplasty
    Robinson anterior cervical
      diskectomy
    Robinson anterior cervical fusion
    Robinson-Chung-Farahvar
      morcellation
    Robinson-Riley cervical arthrodesis
    Robinson-Southwick fusion
    Rockwood-Green
    Rogers cervical fusion
    Roos approach
    Root-Siegal osteotomy
    Rose foot
    Rosomoff cordotomy

operations *(continued)*
    rotational osteotomy
    rotational scarf bunionectomy
    rotator cuff repair
    Roux-duToit staple capsulorrhaphy
    Roux-Goldthwait
    Rowe posterior shoulder approach
    Rowe-Zarins shoulder
      immobilization
    Ruiz-Mora
    Russe approach
    Ryerson triple arthrodesis
    saber-cut approach
    sacral nerve stimulation (SNS)
      therapy
    sacrospinous ligament suspension
    SAF hip (self-articulating femoral)
      replacement
    Sage-Clark
    sagittal band reconstruction
    Saha transfer
    saline-enhanced MR arthrography
      of shoulder
    Salter pelvic osteotomy
    salvage
    Salzer resurfacing
    Samilson osteotomy
    saphenous vein extracranial-
      intracranial bypass graft
    Sargent knee
    Sarmiento trochanteric fracture
    Sauvé-Kapandji (S-K) reconstruc-
      tion of distal radioulnar joint
    Scaglietti closed reduction
    scaphotrapeziotrapezoid (STT)
      arthrodesis
    Scarborough total hip replacement
    scarf bunionectomy, rotational
    Schaberg-Harper-Allen
    Schanz angulation osteotomy
    Schauwecker patellar wiring
    Schlein elbow arthroplasty
    Schneider hip arthrodesis
    Schnute wedge resection
    Schrock
    Scott glenoplasty
    screw fixation

operations *(continued)*

Scuderi
SDR (selective dorsal rhizotomy)
Seddon modification
segmental epidural nerve block
  with local anesthesia
segmental spinal fixation
selective dorsal rhizotomy (SDR)
self-articulating femoral (SAF) hip
  replacement
self-bearing ceramic total hip
  replacement
Selig hip
Sell-Frank-Johnson extensor shift
semitendinosus tenodesis
Senegas hip approach
sesamoidectomy
Sever-L'Episcopo shoulder repair
SFA (subclavian flap aortoplasty)
Sharrard transfer
shelf
Shepherd internal screw fixation
Sherk-Probst
shish kebab
shoelace fasciotomy
shortening collectomy
shortening osteotomy
short-rod/two-claw
Shriver-Johnson arthrodesis
Shuffors internal screw fixation
Siffert-Forster-Nachamie arthrodesis
Siffert-Storen intraepiphyseal
  osteotomy
Silfverskiöld Achilles tendon
  reconstruction
silhouette capsulectomy
silicone implant arthroplasty
Silver bunionectomy
Simmonds-Menelaus metatarsal
  osteotomy
Simmons cervical spine fusion
Simmons keystone
single pedicle subtraction
  osteotomy
sinus tarsi peg
S-K (Sauvé-Kapandji) reconstruction of distal radioulnar joint

operations *(continued)*

Skoog
skull base reconstruction
Slocum fusion
Slocum knee
Smith-Petersen cup arthroplasty
Smith-Petersen sacroiliac joint
  fusion
Smith-Robinson cervical fusion
Smith-Robinson diskectomy
SNS (sacral nerve stimulation)
  therapy
Sofield femoral deficiency
soft tissue reconstruction
somatectomy
Somerville
Souter hip
Southwick slide
Southwick-Robinson cervical
  approach
Speed arthroplasty
Speed-Boyd radioulnar
Spencer tendon lengthening
Spier elbow arthrodesis
Spiessel internal screw fixation
Spiller-Frazier neurotomy
spinal canal endoscopy
Spira
Spittler
SPLATT (split anterior tibial
  tendon transfer)
split biceps tendon tenodesis
split patellar approach
split posterior tibial tendon transfer
split-thickness skin excision (STSE)
spondylectomy
Sponsel oblique osteotomy
SRS (stereotactic radiosurgery)
Stack shoulder
Staheli shelf
Stamm
Stanmore knee replacement
Stanmore shoulder arthroplasty
Stanmore total hip replacement
staple fixation
Staples-Black-Brostrom ligament
  repair

operations *(continued)*
  Staples elbow arthrodesis
  Stark-Moore-Ashworth-Boyes
  Steel shelf
  Steel triple innominate osteotomy
  Steindler flexorplasty
  Steindler stripping
  Steinhauser internal screw fixation
  Stener-Gunterberg hip
  step-cut osteotomy
  stereotactic biopsy
  stereotactic implantation of
    ventriculoperitoneal shunt
  stereotactic laser microsurgery
  stereotactic pallidotomy
  stereotactic percutaneous lumbar
    diskectomy
  stereotactic placement of depth
    electrodes
  stereotactic radiosurgery
  stereotactic thalamotomy
  stereotactic tractotomy
  stereotactic ventral pallidotomy
  STT (scaphotrapeziotrapezoid)
    arthrodesis
  sternal-splitting approach
  Stewart arm
  Stewart-Harley ankle arthrodesis
  Stiles-Bunnell transfer
  Stone bunionectomy
  Strayer tendon
  Strickland tendon repair
  subclavian flap aortoplasty (SFA)
  subcutaneous palmar fasciotomy
  subfrontal transbasal approach
  suboccipital craniotomy
  suboccipital muscle release
  suboccipital posterior fossa
    approach
  suboccipital transmeatal craniotomy
  subperiosteal corticotomy
  subtalar arthrodesis
  subtalar arthrotomy
  subtalar capsulotomy
  subtalar distraction bone block
    fusion
  subtalar release

operations *(continued)*
  subtalar stabilization
  subtemporal approach
  subtotal vertebrectomy
  subtraction osteotomy
  Sugioka transtrochanteric osteotomy
  Sundaresan approach
  Suppan foot
  supracerebellar approach
  supracondylar femoral derotational
    osteotomy
  supramalleolar osteotomy
  suprasyndesmotic screw fixation
  supratentorial approach
  surface replacement
  surgical decompression
  suspension laminotomy
  Sutherland-Greenfield osteotomy
  Sutherland hip
  suturectomy
  Swanson Convex condylar
    arthroplasty
  Swanson interpositional wrist
    arthroplasty
  Swanson metatarsophalangeal joint
    arthroplasty
  Swanson silicone wrist arthroplasty
  Swedish approach
  Syme amputation
  symmetric vertebral fusion
  sympathectomy
  syndactylization
  synovectomy
  synovial biopsy
  Tachdjian hamstring lengthening
  TAL (tendo Achillis lengthening)
  talonavicular arthrodesis
  talonavicular capsulotomy
  talonavicular cuneiform arthrodesis
  tarsal tunnel release (TTR)
  Taylor-Daniel-Weiland
  TCR (tethered cord release)
  temporo-occipital approach
  tendon interposition arthroplasty
  tendon lengthening
  tendonplasty
  tendon transfer

operations *(continued)*
tendon transplant
tenectomy
tenodesis of the heel cord
tenoplastic reconstruction
tenorrhaphy
tenotomy
tension band fixation
terminal Syme
Teuffer
THA (total hip arthroplasty)
Thackray low friction arthroplasty
thalamectomy
thalamotomy
Tharies hip replacement
thermal capsulorrhaphy
Thomas-Thompson-Straub transfer
Thompson-Henry
Thompson posterior radial
    approach
Thompson telescoping V osteotomy
tibial tubercle transfer
tibiocalcaneal arthrodesis
tibiocalcaneal fusion
tibiotalar arthrodesis
tibiotalar fusion
tibiotalar salvage
tibiotalocalcaneal fusion
Tikhoff-Linberg radical arm
Tikhoff-Linberg shoulder resection
TKA (total knee arthroplasty)
TLIF (transforaminal lumbar
    interbody fusion)
Tohen tendon
tongue and trough
Torgerson-Leach modified
Torg knee reconstruction
Torkildsen shunt
total articular resurfacing
    arthroplasty (TARA)
total hip arthroplasty (THA)
total hip replacement (THR)
total knee arthroplasty (TKA)
total synovectomy
T-plasty modification of Bankart
    shoulder
TPL-6 total hip replacement

operations *(continued)*
transcallosal approach
transcerebellar approach
transchoroidal approach
transclival approach
transcranial approach
transfibular approach for arthrodesis
transfibular fusion
transforaminal lumbar interbody
    fusion (TLIF)
transfrontal approach
transfrontal-naso-orbital approach
translabyrinthine approach
translational osteotomy
transmalleolar ankle arthrodesis
transmaxillosphenoidal approach
transmetatarsal amputation
transnaso-orbital approach
transoral approach
transpedal multiplanar wedge
    osteotomy/fusion
transpedicular approach
transpetrosal approach
transplantation of autologous adrenal
    medullary tissue
transsphenoidal approach
transsternal approach
transsylvian-transventricular
    approach
transsyndesmotic screw fixation
transtemporal approach
transtentorial approach
transthoracic approach
transtrochanteric approach
transverse chevron osteotomy
transzygomatic approach
trephination
trephine craniotomy
Trethowan-Stamm-Simmonds-
    Menelaus-Haddad triangulation
triad knee repair
triangular external ankle fixation
triaxial total elbow arthroplasty
trigeminal neuroma extirpation
trigger thumb release
Trillat osteotomy
triple tarsal fusion

operations *(continued)*
    TR-28 total hip replacement
    Trumble arthrodesis
    Tsuge tendon repair
    tunnel posterior cruciate ligament reconstruction
    Turco clubfoot release
    Turco posteromedial release
    Turco repair of talipes equinovarus
    "turn-up" plasty
    Turvy internal screw fixation
    twist drill craniostomy
    two-sleeve
    two-stage hip fusion
    two-strut tibial graft
    Uematsu shoulder arthrodesis
    ulnocarpal arthrodesis
    ultrasound-guided echo biopsy
    ultrasound-guided stereotactic biopsy
    unicompartmental joint arthroplasty
    unilateral posteroventral pallidotomy
    U osteotomy
    vagal rhizotomy
    Valenti arthroplasty
    valgus-extension osteotomy
    Vandenbos and Bowers
    variable screw placement fixation (VSP)
    VASS (video-assisted spine surgery)
    Vastamaki
    vastus medialis advancement
    Veleanu-Rosianu-Ionescu
    ventrolateral thalamotomy
    Verdan
    Verebelyi-Ogston decancellation
    vertebrectomy
    vertical sagittal split osteotomy (VSO)
    vestibular neurectomy
    vest-over-pants
    veterinary approach
    Vidal-Adrey fracture
    Vitallium cup arthroplasty
    volar plate repair

operations *(continued)*
    volumetric stereotactic surgical resection
    Volz total wrist arthroplasty
    Volz-Turner reattachment
    V osteotomy
    VSP (variable screw placement) fixation
    Vulpius Achilles tendon reconstruction
    Vulpius-Compere tendon
    Vulpius equinus deformity
    V-Y plasty correction of varus toes
    Wadsworth elbow approach
    wafer distal ulna resection
    Wagner multiple K-wire osteosynthesis
    Wagner open reduction
    Wagoner cervical
    Warner-Farber ankle fixation
    Warren White Achilles tendon lengthening
    Watkins fusion
    Watson-Cheyne
    Watson-Jones ankle tenodesis
    Watson-Jones arthrodesis
    Weaver-Dunn acromioclavicular
    Weber-Brunner-Freuler-Boitzy
    Weber-Vasey traction-absorption
    wedge excision of ingrowing toe nail
    Weil osteotomy with modified Ronconi
    West and Soto-Hall patella
    White arthrodesis
    Whitecloud-LaRocca arthrodesis
    Whitesides-Kelly cervical
    Whitman osteotomy
    Williams-Haddad
    Wilson double oblique osteotomy
    Wilson-Jacobs tibial fixation
    Wilson-Johansson-Barrington arthrodesis
    Wilson-McKeever arthroplasty
    Wiltberger anterior cervical approach

operations *(continued)*
  Wiltse ankle osteotomy
  Winograd ingrown nail
  Winston-Lutz LINAC-based
    radiosurgery
  Winter spondylolisthesis
  wire fixation
  Wirth-Jager tendon
  Wisconsin wire fixation
  Woodward
  wrap-around toe transfer
  wrapping of aneurysm
  Wu bunionectomy
  Yee posterior shoulder approach
  Yoke transposition
  Yount
  Zadik foot
  Zadik total nail-bed ablation
  Zancolli capsuloplasty
  Zancolli rerouting
  Zaricznyj ligament
  Zarins-Rowe ligament
  Zazepen-Gamidov
  Zeier transfer
  Zickel nail fixation
  Zickel subtrochanteric fracture
  Z-lengthening of tendon
  Z-plasty
  Z-plasty release
  Z-slide lengthening
opercular epilepsy
operculum
  cerebral
  frontal
  frontoparietal
  insula
  medial
  occipital
  sylvian
  temporal
OPG (ophthalmoplethysmography)
OPG/CPA (oculoplethysmography/
  carotid phonoangiography)
ophthalmic migraine
ophthalmic nerve
ophthalmodynamometry (ODN)

ophthalmoplegia
  internuclear (INO)
  progressive external
  pseudo-internuclear
  supranuclear
ophthalmoplegic migraine
ophthalmoplethysmography (OPG)
ophthalmoscopic examination
opisthotonic position
opisthotonic posture (posturing)
opisthotonos
OPLL (opacification of posterior
  longitudinal ligament)
Opmilas CO_2 multipurpose laser
Opmilas 144 Plus laser system
Opmi microscope drape
OP-1 (osteogenic protein-1) implant/
  bone graft
Oppenheim brace
Oppenheim disease
Oppenheimer knuckle-bender splint
Oppenheimer splint, modified
Oppenheim gait
Oppenheim reflex
Oppenheim sign
opponens bar
opponensplasty
  Camitz
  Goldmar
  Groves
  Huber
  Littler
  Phalen-Miller
  Riordan finger
opposable thumb
opposed GRE images
opposed loop-pair quadrature MR coil
opposed-phase GRE imaging
opposing muscle
opposite foot-strike phase of gait
opposite toe-off phase of gait
opposition, finger
opposition of hand or thumb muscles
  hard
  soft
Opraflex incise drape

Op-Site dressing
opsoclonia (opsoclonus; dancing eyes)
opsoclonus-myoclonus syndrome
Opteform 100HT bone graft
optical back-scatter
optical coherence tomography (OCT)
optical digitizer, StealthStation
optical imaging
optical isomer
optical localization fiber
optical surface imaging (OSI)
Optical Tracking System (OTS)
optical triangulation
optic atrophy, Leber
optic chiasm tumors
optic disk
    edema of
    pallor of the
optic encephalitis
optic glioma tumor
optic globe
optic nerve (second cranial nerve)
optic nerve atrophy
optic nerve compression
optic nerve defect
optic nerve head, ischemia of the
optic neuritis
optic neuropathy
optic pathway glioma
optic pathway tumor
optic radiation of Gratiolet
optic recess
optic strut
optic tract
optic-type spongiform encephalopathy
optico-chiasmatic cistern, arachnoiditis
    of the
Opti-Curve therapeutic pillow
Opti-Fix II acetabular cup
optimal extensor function
optimal imaging planes
Optimark MRI contrast agent
optimized pulse sequence (MRI)
Option hip system
Optiray (ioversol) nonionic contrast
    medium
optoelectronic motion analysis

optokinetic nystagmus (OKN)
optokinetic response
optokinetic testing
Orabilex contrast medium
O'Rahilly classification of limb
    deficiency
oral apraxia
oral-buccal-lingual dyskinesia
Oralex ultrasound imaging agent
oral petit mal
oral thermistor (used during EEG)
Orap (pimozide)
Oratec cautery probe
orbicular ligament
orbicular muscle
Orbis-Sigma cerebrospinal fluid shunt
    valve
orbit
    angular process of
    bony
orbital apex
orbital bone
orbital mass compression
orbital muscle
orbital nerve
orbital neurofibroma
orbital pseudotumor
orbital rim stepoff
orbitofrontal region
orbitosphenoid bone
orbitotomy, open sky
orbitozygomatic approach
Orca fluoroscopic C-arm
Oregon ankle prosthesis
Oregon Digit Recognition test
Oregon Poly II ankle prosthesis
Oretorp arthroscopy knife
Orfit splints
Orfizip wrist cast
organ
    Corti
    Golgi
    proprioceptive end
organic brain disease (OBD)
organic brain syndrome with psychosis
organic denial
organic headache

organic inattention
organic mental syndrome
organic muscle (visceral muscle)
organic signs (of brain damage)
organic unilateral neglect
organization of ocular movements
organization, somatotopic
organoaxial
organomegaly
organophosphorus insecticide poisoning
Orgaran (danaparoid sodium)
Oriental flap
orientation
    coronal
    disk to magnetic field
    disturbed
    sagittal
    spatial
    temporal
    transverse
orientation and mobility (O&M)
orientation-memory-contraction
    (OMC) test
orientation to person, place, and time
oriented, fully
oriented in all spheres
oriented x 3 (times 3) (to person,
    place, and time)
oriented x 4 (times 4) (to person,
    place, time, and future plans)
ORIF (open reduction and internal
    fixation)
Original Index Knobber II massager
Original Jacknobber II trigger-point
    massager
origin, muscle
Origin Tacker staples
Orion anterior cervical plate
Oris pin
ORLAU (Orthotic Research and
    Locomotor Assessment Unit)
ORLAU swivel walker orthosis
Orozco cervical plate
Orr-Buck traction
OrthAbility KAF orthosis
Orthacor material
Orthair oscillating saw

Orthairtome wire driver
Orthawear antiembolism stockings
Orth-evac autotransfusion system
Orthion traction machine
Ortho-Cel padding
orthocephalic
Orthochrome implant metal
Orthoclone
Orthocomp cement
Ortho Development instruments/
    devices
Orthodoc presurgical planning system
orthodromic sensory study
orthodromic velocity
Ortho Dx electrotherapy system
OrthoDyn bone substitute material
Orthofix Cervical-Stim bone growth
    stimulator
Orthofix external fixator
Orthofix intramedullary nail
Orthofix M-100 distractor
Orthofix miniature fixator
Orthofix prosthesis
Orthofix screw
Ortho-Foam elbow/heel pad
Ortho-Foam protector
OrthoGen implantable stimulator for
    nonunion of fracture
OrthoGen/OsteoGen stimulator
Ortho-Glass splint material
orthogonal plane
Ortho-Grip silicone rubber handle
Ortho-Ice Multipaks
Ortholav jet lavage
Ortholoc Advantim knee revision
    system
Ortholoc implant metal
OrthoLogic 1000 bone-growth
    stimulator
Orthomedics cervical support
Orthomet
Ortho-Mold lumbar body jacket
OrthoNail intramedullary fixation
    device
orthopaedic or orthopedic
orthopaedic oxford
OrthoPak II bone growth stimulator

orthopantogram
OrthoPAT perioperative autotransfusion system
orthopedic *or* orthopaedic
orthopedic bed
orthopedic evaluation
orthopedic hardware
orthopedic propeller
Orthopedic Trauma Association
  (OTA) fracture classification
orthophoria
orthoplast jacket
orthopod
orthoposer device
orthoptic evaluation
orthoroentgenogram
OrthoSearch Internet search engine
Orthoset radiopaque bone cement
orthosis (see also *prosthesis*; *splint*)
  abduction hip
  accommodative
  ADS (anterior dynamized system)
  A-frame
  airplane splint
  Alden CDI
  ankle-foot (AFO)
  ankle-foot plastic
  articulated AFO
  Atlanta brace
  bail-lock knee joint
  balance padding
  bar and shoe
  Biothotic foot
  Boston brace thoracolumbosacral
  cable twister
  calcaneal spur cookie
  caliper
  CASH thoracolumbosacral
  C-bar
  cervical
  cervicothoracic
  cervicothoracolumbosacral (CTLSO)
  chairback
  cock-up splint
  copolymer ankle-foot
  custom
  custom-fabricated

orthosis *(continued)*
  Denis Browne bar foot
  dermoplast/plastizote
  Diabetic D-Sole foot
  dial lock
  elastic knee cage
  elastic twister
  elbow-wrist-hand (EWHO)
  Engen palmar finger
  figure of 8 thoracic
  Fillauer bar foot
  FirmFlex custom
  flexion-extension control cervical
  floor-reaction ankle-foot
  foot (FO)
  Foot Levelers
  four-poster cervical
  Frejka pillow
  Gaffney joint
  gator plastic
  Gilette modification of ankle-foot
  Gillette joint
  GunSlinger shoulder
  G/W Heel Lift, Inc.
  halo cervical
  halo extension
  halo traction
  halo-vest
  heat-molded petroplastic ankle-foot
  heel lift
  HGO (hip guidance)
  hip-knee-ankle-foot (HKAFO)
  Hyperex
  Ilfield splint
  J-24 cervical
  J-35 hyperextension
  J-45 contraflexion
  J-55 postfusion
  Jewett-Benjamin cervical
  Jewett contraflexion
  Jewett hyperextension
  Jewett postfusion
  Jewett thoracolumbosacral
  Klenzak
  knee extension
  knee-ankle-foot (KAFO)
  Knight-Taylor thoracolumbosacral

orthosis *(continued)*
    lateral heel wedge
    Legg-Perthes disease
    Lenox Hill knee
    Lerman
    Lerman multiligamentous knee
        control
    Levy & Rappel foot
    Ligamentus Ankle
    long leg
    long opponens
    LSU reciprocation-gait (Louisiana
        State University)
    Lynco foot
    Malleoloc ankle
    medial heel wedge
    medial sole wedge
    metatarsal bar
    metatarsal pads
    Meyer cervical
    Milwaukee cervicothoraco-
        lumbosacral
    Minerva
    molded AFO
    molded ankle-foot
    MultiBoot
    Newport MC (maximum control)
        hip
    New York Orthopedic front-
        opening
    New York University insert for
    Newington
    NuKO knee
    Oklahoma ankle joint
    ORLAU swivel walker
    OrthAbility KAF
    orthotic coiled spring twisters
    outrigger upper limb
    parapodium
    Parawalker
    Phelps
    plantar arch support
    plastic floor reaction ankle-foot
    Plastizote arch support
    Plastizote collar cervical
    Pneu-Trac
    polypropylene

orthosis *(continued)*
    polypropylene ankle-foot
    posterior leaf spring
    posterior leaf spring ankle-foot
    pressure-relieving
    PSA thermoplastic
    PTB (patellar tendon bearing)
        ankle-foot
    PTB plastic
    PTS (patellar tendon stabilization)
    Rebel knee
    reciprocating gait (RGO)
    RGO II
    rib belt
    Rochester HKAFO (hip-knee-ankle-
        foot)
    rubber ischial lift
    safety pin
    Scottish Rite hip
    Seattle
    Select joint
    semirigid
    semirigid polypropylene ankle-foot
    Shaeffer rigid
    short opponens
    shoulder-elbow-wrist-hand
        (SEWHO)
    SMO (supramalleolar)
    Sof Sole motion control
    soft collar cervical
    SOMI (sternal occipital mandibular
        immobilization)
    SportsFit thumb
    spring-loaded lock
    spring-wire ankle-foot
    standard shell ankle-foot (AFO)
    standing frame
    steel sole plate
    supramalleolar (SMO)
    Swedish knee cage
    Tachdhian
    Taylor thoracolumbosacral
    Thera-Band Resistive Therapy
        System
    Thera-Soft hand/wrist
    thermoplastic ankle-foot
    Thomas collar cervical

orthosis *(continued)*
  Thomas heel
  thoracolumbosacral (TLSO)
  thumb
  TIRR foot-ankle
  TLSO (thoracolumbosacral)
  tone-reducing ankle-foot (TRAFO)
  Toronto
  Toronto parapodium
  total contact (TCO)
  TPE ankle-foot
  TPE biomechanical foot orthosis
  trilateral knee-ankle-foot
  trimlines for ankle-foot
  twister cable brace
  two-poster cervical
  UCB foot
  UCBL (University of California
    Berkeley Laboratory)
  UCBL (University of California
    Biomechanics Lab)
  Ultrabrace
  underarm
  Viscoheel K
  Viscoheel N
  Viscoheel SofSpot
  Viscolas
  Von Rosen splint hip
  Whitman arch support
  Williams
  wrist-driven flexor hinge
  Zinco ankle
OrthoSorb absorbable fixation pin
orthostatic dizziness
orthostatic intolerance
orthostatic syncope
orthostatic tremor
Orthotech Controller knee brace
orthotic plate
Orthotic Research and Locomotor
  Assessment Unit (ORLAU)
orthotic twisters to treat internal or
  external rotation
orthotics, half-shoe
orthotist
orthotome resector
OrthoTrac adhesive bandage

OrthoTrac pneumatic vest
Orthotron exerciser machine
Ortho-Vent nonadhesive bandage
Ortho-Vent traction
Orthovisc (injectable hyaluronic acid)
OrthoVision orthopedic table
Ortolani click
Ortolani maneuver
Ortolani sign
Ortolani test for diagnosis of posterior
  shoulder instability
os (pl. ossa)
  os acetabuli
  os acromiale
  os basilare
  os calcis
  os capitatum
  os coccygis
  os coxae
  os cuboideum
  os cuneiforme
  os frontale
  os hamatum
  os ilium
  os ischii
  os lacrimale
  os lunatum
  os naviculare
  os occipitale
  os pedis
  os pisiforme
  os pubis
  os sacrum
  os scaphoideum
  os sphenoidale
  os temporale
  os trapezoideum
  os trigonum
  os triquetrum
  os zygomaticum
Osborne-Cotterill elbow technique
OSCAR ultrasonic bone cement
  removal system
oscillating hollow saw
oscillating magnetic field
Oscillating Techniques for Isometric
  Stabilization (OTIS)

oscillating tremor
oscillation, macro saccadic
oscillograph
oscillopsia, torsional monocular
OS-5/Plus 2 knee brace
Osgood-Schlatter disease
OSI Arthroscopic Leg Holder
OSI Extremity Elevator
OSI Well Leg Support
Osler nodes
Osm (osmole)
Osmone-Clarke foot procedure
osmotic blood-brain barrier disruption
osmotic demyelination syndrome
osseointegrated prosthesis
osseous bridge
osseous destructive process
osseous dysplasia
osseous graft
osseous metastases
osseous outgrowth
osseous remodeling
osseous spiral lamina
osseous structure
osseous survey
osseous union
ossicle
   accessory
   Riolan
ossiferous
ossific nodule
ossific nucleus of navicular
ossification
   abnormal
   enchondral
   endochondral
   heterotopic
   intracartilaginous
   irregular enchondral
   muscle
   periarticular heterotopic (PHO)
   peripheral
   primary center of
   secondary center of
   soft tissue
ossification center
ossification of soft tissue (on x-ray)

ossification variant
ossified body
ossifying fibroma of long bone
ossifying fibromyxoid tumor
Ossigel injectable bioengineered
   matrix
ossimeter
Ossotome bur
osteal
ostealgia
osteal stenoses
ostectomy, fibular
osteitis
   condensing (of clavicle)
   phalangeal tuberculous
   sclerosing nonsuppurative
osteitis condensans ilii (OCI)
osteitis deformans
osteitis fibrosa cystica
osteitis fragilitans
osteitis ossificans
osteitis pubis
ostemia
ostempyesis
OsteoAnalyzer device
osteoaneurysm
osteoarthritic change
osteoarthritic chondrocyte transduction
osteoarthritic spur
osteoarthritis (OA)
   degenerative
   dysplastic
   erosive
   generalized
   obese knee
   post-traumatic
   traumatic
osteoarthritis padded night-sleeve
   brace
osteoarthropathy
osteoarthrosis
osteoarthrotomy
osteoarticular autologous tissue
   transfer
osteoarticular graft
osteoarticular transplant
osteoarticular tuberculosis

Osteo-Bi-Flex
osteoblastic bone regeneration
osteoblastic metastasis
osteoblastic tumor
osteoblastoma
osteoblast-related gene
Osteobond cement
osteocachexia
osteocalcin
OsteoCap hip prosthesis
osteocartilaginous graft
osteocartilaginous lesion
osteocartilaginous mass
osteocartilaginous metaplasia
osteochondral autograft transfer system
   (OATS)
osteochondral defect (OCD)
osteochondral fracture
osteochondral graft
osteochondral lesion of talus
osteochondral shell autograft
osteochondral transplantation
osteochondritic loose body
osteochondritic separation of epiphyses
osteochondritis
   crushing
   epiphyseal
   juvenile
   puncture wound
osteochondritis deformans juvenilis
osteochondritis dissecans (OD)
osteochondritis ischiopubica
osteochondritis juvenilis
osteochondritis necroticans
osteochondrofibroma
osteochondrolysis
osteochondroma
   epiphyseal
   soft tissue
osteochondromatosis
   multiple
   multiple hereditary
   synovial
osteochondromatous dysplasia,
   epiarticular
osteochondropathy
osteochondrophyte

osteochondrosarcoma
osteochondrosis dissecans
Osteo-Clage cable system
osteoclasis
osteoclast
osteoclastic erosion
osteoclastic giant cell
osteoclast-mediated bone resorption
osteoclastoma
osteocondensation
osteocope
osteocystoma
osteocyte
osteodiastasis
osteodynia
osteodystrophy
   auriculo-osteodystrophy
   azotemic
   renal
   uremic
osteoenchondroma
osteofibrochondrosarcoma
osteofibromatosis
osteofibrous dysplasia
osteogenesis, distraction
Osteogenesis Imperfecta Foundation
   (OIF)
osteogenic protein-1 (OP-1)
osteogenic sarcoma
Osteogenics BoneSource bone replacement material
OsteoGen implantable bone growth
   stimulator
OsteoGram bone density test
OsteoGram 2000 densitometer
osteohalisteresis
osteoid osteoma, juxta-articular
osteoinduction
osteolipochondroma
osteolipoma
Osteolock femoral prosthesis
Osteolock hip prosthesis
Osteolock, Precision
osteology
osteolysis
   acromioclavicular
   periprosthetic

osteolysis *(continued)*
    progressive
    scalloping
    transient phalangeal
osteolysis of distal clavicle
osteolysis urine marker
osteolytic metastases
osteoma
    ivory
    juxta-articular osteoid
    osteoid
    parosteal
    spongy
osteomalacia
    hematogeneous
    senile
osteomanipulative therapy
    (chiropractic)
Osteomark bone loss urine test
Osteomark monoclonal antibody-based
    agent
Osteomark test (NTx Assay)
osteomatosis
Osteomed instruments/devices
osteomesopyknosis
osteomized
osteomyelitic sinus
osteomyelitis
    Ackerman criteria for
    acute hematogenous (AHO)
    blastomycotic
    Brucella
    chronic pyogenic
    conchiolin
    diffuse sclerosing
    focal sclerosing
    Garré sclerosing
    hematogenous
    iatrogenic
    long bone
    nonsuppurative
    nonunion
    pedal
    pin-track
    postfracture
    post-traumatic chronic
    Pseudomonas aeruginosa

osteomyelitis *(continued)*
    salmonella
    sclerosing nonsuppurative
    secondary or acute hematogenous
    Staphylococcus aureus spinal
    tuberculous
    typhoid
osteomyelitis variolosa
osteomyelodysplasia
osteon
osteonal bone
osteonecrosis
    dysbaric
    Ficat classification of femoral head
osteoneuralgia
Osteonics-HA coated implant
Osteonics hip prosthesis
Osteonics Omnifit-HA hip stem
Osteonics Scorpio posterior-cruciate-
    retaining total knee system
Osteopatch transdermal skin patch
osteopathic manipulative therapy
    (OMT)
osteopathic scoliosis
osteopathy, doctor of (D.O.)
osteopenia, generalized
osteopenic bone stock
osteoperiosteal graft
osteoperiostitis
osteopetrosis
osteophyte
    acromioclavicular joint
    bony
    bridging
    cervical
    fringe of
    horseshoe
    jagged
    marginal
osteophytectomy
osteophyte formation
    beaklike
    hooklike
    marginal
    nipple-like
osteophytic bone lip
osteophytic lipping

osteophytic proliferation
osteophytosis
osteoplastica
osteoplasty
osteopoikilosis
osteoporosis
  corticosteroid-induced
  disuse
  juvenile
  post-traumatic
  postmenopausal
  senile
Osteoporosis Knowledge Questionnaire
  (OKQ)
osteoporotic bone
osteopsathyrosis idiopathica
osteoradionecrosis
Osteosal test to measure osteoporosis
osteosarcoma
  cardiac
  classical
  extraosseous
  fibroblastic
  intracortical
  intraosseous
  juxtacortical
  osteoblastic
  parosteal
  periosteal
  telangiectatic
osteosclerosis
Osteoset bone graft substitute
osteosis
osteospongioma
Osteo Stim implantable bone growth
  stimulator
osteosynovitis
osteosynthesis
  biological
  plate
  Wagner multiple K-wire
osteotelangiectasia
osteothrombophlebitis
osteothrombosis
osteotome (also periosteotome)
  Acufex
  Albee

osteotome *(continued)*
  Alexander costal
  Alexander-Farabeuf periosteotome
  Anderson-Neivert
  Andrews
  Army
  Aufranc
  Ballender periosteotome
  bayonet
  Blount
  Bowen
  box
  Brown periosteotome
  Campbell
  Carroll-Legg
  Carroll-Smith-Petersen
  Cavin
  Cebetome
  Cherry
  Cinelli
  Clayton
  Cloward spinal fusion
  Cobb
  Compere
  costal periosteotome
  Cottle
  Crane
  curved
  Dautery
  Dawson-Yuhl
  Dingman
  fine
  Fomon periosteotome
  Furnas bayonet
  grooving
  guarded
  guided
  Hardt-Delima
  Hendel guided
  Hibbs curved
  Hibbs straight
  Hoke
  Joseph
  Joseph periosteotome
  Lambotte curved
  Lambotte straight
  Leinbach

osteotome *(continued)*
    Lexer
    MacGregor
    Meyerding curved
    Meyerding straight
    MGH
    Micro-Aire
    Miner
    mini-Lambotte
    mini-Lexer
    Mitchell
    Moberg
    Moe
    Moreland
    Murphy
    Neivert
    Padgett
    Parkes
    Peck
    Rhoton
    Rish
    rotary
    Sheehan
    Silver
    Simmons
    Smith-Petersen curved
    Smith-Petersen straight
    Stille
    straight
    Swanson
    Swiss pattern
    thin
    U.S. Army
    unguarded
    Weck
    West
osteotomized
osteotomy (see also *operations*)
    Abbott-Gill
    abduction hip
    adduction hip
    Akin phalangeal
    Amstutz-Wilson
    angulation
    arcuate
    Austin
    Axer varus derotational

osteotomy *(continued)*
    Bailey-Dubow
    Baker-Hill
    ball-and-socket
    basal
    base wedge
    basilar crescentic
    basilar metatarsal
    basilar wedge
    Berman-Gartland metatarsal
    Bernese periacetabular
    bicorrectional Austin
    bifurcation
    biplane trochanteric
    biplaning of
    block
    Blount displacement
    Blundell-Jones hip
    Bonney-Kessel dorsiflexionary
        tilt-up
    Booth wire
    Borden-Spencer-Herman
    Brackett
    Brett-Campbell tibial
    calcaneal
    calcaneus dome
    Campbell tibial
    Canale
    chevron metatarsal
    Chiari innominate
    closing abductory wedge (CAWO)
    closing base wedge (CBWO)
    closing wedge high tibial
        (CWHTO)
    Cole
    corrective lengthening
    countersinking
    Coventry vagus
    crescent-shaped
    crescentic base wedge
    cuneiform
    cup-and-ball
    curved
    cutting jig for chevron
    decompressive
    delayed femoral
    derotational

osteotomy *(continued)*
  dial pelvic
  diaphyseal
  Dickinson-Coutts-Woodward-
    Handler
  Dickson
  Dimon
  displacement
  distal Akin phalangeal
  distal first metatarsal
  distal L
  distal metatarsal
  distal oblique
  dome
  dome proximal tibial
  dome-shaped
  dorsal closing wedge metatarsal
  double
  Dunn-Hess trochanteric
  Dwyer
  Elizabethtown
  Emmon
  Eppright dial
  Evans calcaneal distraction wedge
  extension
  femoral derotation
  Ferguson-Thompson-King
    two-stage
  Fernandez
  fibular
  Fish cuneiform
  flexion
  free-floating
  Fulkerson oblique tibial tubercle
  Gant
  geometric extension
  Giannestras metatarsal oblique
  Giannestras step-down modified
  Gibson-Piggott
  Gigli saw
  greater tuberosity
  Greenfield
  Green-Laird modification of
    Reverdin procedure
  Haas
  Helal
  high tibial

osteotomy *(continued)*
  Hohmann
  Hohmann-Thomasen metatarsal
  Ingram
  innominate
  intertrochanteric
  intracapsular
  Irwin
  Japas
  Kalamchi
  Kalish
  Keck and Kelly
  Kelikian modified Z
  Kessel-Bonney extension
  Koutsogiannis-Fowler-Anderson
  Kramer modification of Hohmann
  lateral acetabular shelf
  lateral closing wedge
  Leach-Igou step-cut medial
  Lindgren oblique
  Lucas-Cottrell
  MacEwen-Shands
  malleolar
  Martin
  McMurray
  medial displacement calcaneal
  medial opening wedge
  metatarsal
  metatarsal head
  metatarsal neck
  Mitchell distal
  Mitchell posterior displacement
  Mitchell step-down
  modified Mau
  modified Wilson
  oblique displacement
  oblique metaphyseal
  oblique slide
  oblique, with derotation
  Obwegeser sagittal mandibular
  open base wedge
  open wedge
  opening
  opening abductory wedge (OAWO)
  opening wedge
  Osgood rotational
  Pauwel proximal

osteotomy *(continued)*
- Pauwel Y
- peg-in-hole
- pelvic
- Pemberton circumacetabular
- Pemberton pericapsular
- percutaneous
- periacetabular
- plantarflexory proximal metatarsal
- Platou
- posterior displacement
- Potts eversion
- Potts tibial
- proximal first metatarsal
- proximal phalangeal
- radial recession
- reduction
- Reverdin-Green
- Root-Siegal
- rotational
- rotational scarf
- Salter innominate
- Salter pelvic
- Samilson
- sandwich
- scarf
- Schanz angulation
- Schede hip
- shortening
- Siffert-Storen intraepiphyseal
- Simmonds-Menelaus metatarsal
- single pedicle subtraction
- Sofield
- Southwick
- spike
- Sponsel oblique
- Steel triple innominate
- step
- step-cut
- subtalar posterior displacement
- subtraction
- Sugioka transtrochanteric
- supracondylar femoral derotational
- supracondylar varus
- supramalleolar
- supratubercular wedge
- Sutherland-Greenfield

osteotomy *(continued)*
- Swanson
- talar
- talar neck
- talocalcaneal
- tarsal wedge
- Thompson telescoping V
- through-and-through V-shaped horizontal
- tibial
- translational
- transverse
- transverse chevron
- trapezoidal
- Trillat
- triplane
- trochanteric
- U
- V
- valgus
- valgus-extension
- varus derotational
- vertical sagittal split (VSSO)
- visor/sandwich
- Waterman
- wedge-shaped
- Weil modified Ronconi
- Whitman
- Wilson double oblique
- Wiltse ankle

osteotomy-osteoclasis
osteotomy, sigmoid cavity of radius
osteotribe (rasp)
osteotripsy
OsteoView digital bone densitometer
OsteoView 2000 digital imaging
ostia (pl. of ostium)
os trigonum syndrome
Ostrup technique
Oswestry Disability Score
Oswestry Low Back Pain Disability Questionnaire
OT (occupational therapy)
OTA (Orthopedic Trauma Association)
OTA/AO classification
otic ganglion

OTI instruments/devices
OTIS (Oscillating Techniques for
    Isometric Stabilization)
otocerebritis
otocranial
otocranium
otoencephalitis
otogenic meningitis
otolithic crisis of Tumarkin
otoneurologic
otoneurology
otorrhea, cerebrospinal fluid (CSF)
ototoxicity
OTR (occupational therapist,
    registered)
OTR (ocular tilt reaction)
Ottawa Ankle Rules (OARs)
Otto Bock modular PTB prosthesis
Otto pelvis dislocation
OUT (O'Donoghue's Unhappy Triad)
outburst, aggressive
outcome, clinical
outcomes (see *index, questionnaire,
    scale, score, survey*)
Outerbridge ridge for joint or articular
    surface damage in chondromalacia
Outerbridge staging of degenerative
    arthritis
outer table
outflow cannula
outflow of ventricle
outgrowth, osseous patellar
outlet
    pelvic
    thoracic
    ventricular
    widened thoracic
outlet radiographs
outlet view
out-of-cast ankle brace
out-of-phase GRE images
out-of-phase signal on EEG
outpatient communication/cognition
    treatment
outpatient physical therapy
output, motor
outrigger, Harrington distraction

outrigger upper limb orthosis
outrigger with splint
out-toeing
Ovadia-Beals classification of tibial
    plafond fracture
ovale, foramen
overactivity, sympathetic
overbreathing, voluntary hysterical
overcorrection of hallux valgus
over-dependent attitude
overdrilled
Overdyke hip prosthesis
overextension
overgrowth
    bony
    edge
overhead film
overhead oblique view
overhead suspension
overhead-throwing athlete
Overholt clip-applying forceps
overlap
    talocalcaneal
    tibiofibular
overlapped uprights in orthosis
overlapping of toes
overlay, functional
overlying attenuation artifact
overpronator
overpull of muscle
overreading of EEG
overriding of fracture fragments
overriding toes
oversampling on EEG
oversewn
over-the-top position
Overton dowel graft
overtraining
overuse injury
overuse syndrome of the foot and
    lower leg in athletes
overuse syndrome of the wrist
overwhelming of extensor muscles
ovoids, terminal axonal
OVR (oculovestibular reflex)
OVR (Office of Vocational Rehabil-
    itation)

Owen gauze dressing
Owen silk
Owen suture
Owestry staple
oxalic gout
oxaprozin
"ox-eye" (buphthalmos)
Oxford fixator
Oxford magnet
Oxford scale measuring muscle
   strength
oxford shoe, orthopaedic
Oxford unicompartmental devices

oxidative injury
oxidative stress
Oxilan (ioxilan) imaging agent
oximetry, transcranial cerebral
Oxo kitchen scissors
oxycephaly
Oxycontin (oxycodone HCl)
oxygen
   hyperbaric (for osteomyelitis)
   transcutaneous (PtcO$_2$)
oxygen cisternography
oxyphenbutazone
oyster-shell brace

P, p

P (posterior)
PA (posteroanterior or posterior-anterior)
PA and lateral views
pacchionian bodies
pacchionian granulations
Paced Auditory Serial Addition Test (PASAT)
pacemaker
  subcortical
  thalamic
pacemaker theory, facultative
Pace ventricular needle
pachygyria
pachymeningeal feeding artery
pachymeninges, leaflets of
pachymeningitis cervicalis hypertrophica
pachyonychia
pacinian corpuscle
pacinian mechanoreceptor
pacinian nerve endings of hand
pacinian neurofibroma
pack, packing
  Adaptic
  Avitene
  cold
  Gelfoam
  hot

pack *(continued)*
  Hydrocollator
  Kool Kit cold therapy
  Merocel
  MSC cold
  steam
  vaginal
packaging, Relay
packer, Woodson dura
Pack technique
PACs (picture archive and communication system) for x-rays
PACU (postanesthesia care unit)
pad, padding
  ABD (abdominal) lap
  Aquatech cast
  Arthopor
  balance
  buttock
  calcaneal fat
  cast
  Charnley foam suture
  contoured felt
  cotton cast
  digital
  fat
  fatty heel
  felt

pad *(continued)*
   fibrocartilaginous
   finger
   fingertip
   Hapad heel
   Hapad medial arch
   heel ("cookies")
   horseshoe heel
   horseshoe-shaped felt
   Hydrocollator
   J
   Kerlix cast
   knee-control orthosis
   knuckle
   lamb's wool
   MagneCore magnetic therapy
   metatarsal (shoe modification)
   Mik
   Mikulicz
   Morgan disk
   navicular shoe
   OEC popliteal
   Ortho-Cel
   Ortho-Foam elbow/heel
   painful heel
   patellar orthosis
   Pedifix hammertoe
   plantar fat
   proximal
   pubic
   Redigrip knee
   reticulated polyurethane
   retropatellar fat
   scalene fat
   scaphoid shoe
   Scholl
   shock-absorbent heel
   shoe heel
   Silopad friction
   Sof-Rol cast
   spur
   thickness of heel
   Vac-Pac
   velvet foam
   Zimfoam
padded bolsters
paddie (or patty), cottonoid

paddle bip coagulator
Paddu knee procedure
Padgett baseline pinch gauge
Padgett hydraulic hand dynamometer
Padgett osteotome
pad/protector, Decubinex
Paget-associated osteogenic sarcoma
Paget disease
pagetoid bone
Paget osteitis deformans
pagodone
pain
   aching
   acute
   atypical
   band-like
   boring
   bright
   burning
   calcaneal
   causalgic
   central
   chronic
   chronic low back (CLBP)
   chronic subtalar joint
   continuous
   contralateral
   cramping
   deafferentation
   dermatomal distribution of
   diffuse
   diskogenic
   dull
   dull aching
   dystonic
   electric shock-like
   endogenous
   exacerbation of
   fibromyalgia joint
   fibromyalgic
   gouty
   intense
   intermittent
   intractable
   jabbing
   joint line
   kinetic foot

pain *(continued)*
  lancinating
  low back (LBP)
  machine gun-like
  medial joint line
  mid-dorsal back
  myofascial
  myotomal muscular
  nerve root
  neuralgic
  perimalleolar
  periscapulitis shoulder
  persistent
  phantom
  phantom-limb
  plantar
  postherpetic
  postherpetic facial
  post-traumatic neck
  pounding
  pricking
  prickling
  pulsating
  radiation of
  radicular
  recalcitrant
  referred
  referred neuritic
  residual
  responded purposefully to
  Roland index of low back
  sclerotomal
  searing
  shooting
  splint-like
  stabbing
  static foot
  steady
  stinging
  tearing
  throbbing
  ticlike
  vise-like
  volleys of
pain amplification syndromes
pain and temperature pathways
pain at rest

pain behaviors
PainBuster infusion pain management
  kit
Pain Disability Index
painful-arc syndrome
painful heel pad
painful obstruction (Chinese medicine
  term)
pain mechanism
pain score
pain syndrome
painter's encephalopathy
pain threshold
pain with weightbearing
Pais fracture
PAIVMs (passive accessory intervertebral movements)
Palacos bone cement
palatal myoclonus
palatal nystagmus
palatine bone
palatine muscle
palatine nerve
palatine notch
palatoglossus muscle
palatopharyngeal muscle
palatopharyngo-oculodiaphragmatic
  myoclonus
palatopharyngolaryngo-oculo-
  diaphragmatic myoclonus
pale disk
pale infarct
paleencephalon
paleocerebellar
paleocortex
paleokinetic
Paley classification of complications
paliacusis
palilalia
palindromic rheumatism
palinopsia
palipraxia
palisaded encapsulated neuroma
palisade formation
Palister-Hall syndrome
pallesthesia (vibratory sense)
pallidal brain stimulation

pallidal magnetic resonance signal
    hyperintensity
pallidal syndrome
pallidotomy
    Leksell posteroventral
    microrecording-guided
    posteroventral
    stereotaxic ventral
    unilateral posteroventral
pallidus, globus
pallium
palmar advancement flap
palmar aponeurosis
palmar beak ligament
palmar carpal ligament
palmar carpometacarpal ligament
palmar crease
palmar erythema
palmar fascia
palmar fasciotomy
palmar fibromatosis
palmar fibrous fasciculi
palmar ganglion
palmar interosseous muscle
palmaris longus tendon
palmar ligament
palmar luxation
palmar metacarpal ligament
"palmar migraine"
palmar muscle
palmar oblique ligament
palmar plate
palmar radiocarpal ligament
palmar space
palmar tilt
palmar ulnocarpal ligament
Palmaz-Schatz
Palmaz stent
Palmer bone nail
Palmer classification of cartilage tear
Palmer-Widen shoulder technique
palmomental reflex
palpation
palsy
    abducens nerve
    ataxic cerebral
    backpack

palsy *(continued)*
    Bell
    bilateral gaze
    bridegroom's
    bulbar
    cerebral (CP)
    common peroneal nerve
    complete ulnar nerve
    cranial nerve
    crossed-leg
    Dejerine-Klumpke
    diabetic third-nerve
    Duchenne-Erb
    dyskinetic cerebral
    Erb
    Erb-Duchenne
    extraocular muscle
    facial nerve
    fourth nerve
    gaze
    handlebar
    Hoke procedure for tibial
    honeymoon
    horizontal gaze
    hypotonic cerebral
    idiopathic facial nerve
    ipsilateral
    ipsilateral facial
    ipsilateral gaze
    juvenile progressive bulbar
    Klumpke
    labioglossolaryngeal
    lateral gaze
    long thoracic nerve
    lower radial
    march of cranial nerve
    median nerve
    middle medial
    middle radial
    obstetric brachial plexus
    peripheral seventh nerve
    peroneal
    persistent facial
    postganglionic oculosympathetic
    progressive
    progressive bulbar
    progressive supranuclear (PSP)

palsy *(continued)*
  pseudobulbar
  pure athetoid
  pure spastic
  pursuit
  radial nerve
  saccadic
  "Saturday night" radial
  sciatic
  shaking
  sixth nerve
  spastic cerebral
  supranuclear
  supranuclear gaze
  tardive median nerve
  tardive ulnar nerve
  third nerve
  Todd
  turnip planter's
  ulnar nerve
  upper median
  vertical gaze
Paltrinieri-Trentani resurfacing
  procedure
Palumbo knee brace
Palumbo stabilizing brace
Pamelor (nortriptyline)
Panalok RC absorbable soft tissue
  anchor
Panalok suture anchor
pancarpal destructive arthritis
pancerebellar involvement
Pancoast (thoracic inlet) syndrome
pancytokeratin immunostain
pandiculation
P&O (prosthetics and orthotics)
pandysautonomia
Pandy test
panencephalitis
  rubella
  subacute sclerosing (SSPE)
panfacial fracture
panhypopituitarism
Panje voice button prosthesis
panmetatarsal head resection
Panner disease
pannus deformity of odontoid

pannus of synovium
pantalar arthrodesis
pantalar fusion
Panthers, Gray
Pantopaque myelography
pantrapezial arthritis
panty girdle, Cadenza
papaverine intra-arterial infusion
papaverine topical gel
paper
  Shutrack carbon
  tracing
Papez circuit
papillary muscle
papilledema
  high grade
  long-standing
  marked
papilloma, choroid plexus
papilloma of fourth ventricle
Papineau grafting
PAR (postanesthesia recovery) room
para-articular bone remodeling
para-articular calcification
parabola, metatarsal
paracentral lobule
paracentral scotoma (pl. scotomata)
paracervical region
Parachute Corkscrew suture anchor
Parachutist ankle brace
paracusis
paradoxical ipsilateral hemiparesis
paradoxical sleep (REM sleep)
paraepilepsy
parafascicular nucleus
parafascicular thalamotomy (PFT)
parafascicularis of thalamus
paraffin oil bath
paraganglioma
paragrammatism
paragraphias
paragraph recall test (after head
  injury)
parahippocampal gyrus
parahippocampus
paralexic errors
parallel bars

parallelism of articular surface
parallel squat exercise
paralysis
  acute ascending motor
  ascending
  backpack
  Bell palsy
  Benedikt's ipsilateral oculomotor
  bilateral
  birth
  Brown-Séquard
  cerebral
  Chaves-Rapp
  compression
  conjugate
  contralateral facial
  convergence
  cranial nerve
  crutch
  Cruveilhier
  decubitus
  deglutition
  Dejerine-Klumpke
  Dewar-Harris
  Dickson
  diver
  equinovarus of spastic
  Erb
  Erb-Duchenne
  facial
  familial hypokalemic periodic
  familial periodic
  flaccid
  frank
  functional
  gaze
  Gubler
  Haas
  Henry
  Hunt
  hyperkalemic periodic
  hypokalemic periodic
  hysterical
  infantile
  infranuclear
  ipsilateral
  ipsilateral facial

paralysis *(continued)*
  jake (Jamaica ginger)
  juvenile
  Klumpke
  Klumpke-Dejerine
  labioglossolaryngeal
  labioglossopharyngeal
  Landry ascending
  laryngeal
  Lissauer
  lovers'
  lower motor neuron
  Millard-Gubler
  mimetic
  musculospiral
  nerve
  "night nurse's"
  normokalemic familial periodic
  nuclear
  obstetric
  periodic
  peripheral nerve
  peroneal
  postepileptic
  postdormital sleep
  postictal
  Pott
  predormital sleep
  pseudobulbar
  Ramsay Hunt
  reflex
  Remak
  rucksack
  Saturday night
  sensory
  sleep
  spastic
  supranuclear
  thyrotoxic periodic
  tick
  Todd motor postepileptic
  transient
  trigeminal
  ulnar nerve
  unilateral
  upper motor neuron
  Vastamaki

paralysis *(continued)*
  vesical
  Volkmann ischemic
  Weber
  Wernicke-Mann predilection
  Whitman
paralysis agitans
  Hunt juvenile
  juvenile
paralysis in an extremity
paralytic calcaneus
paralytic scoliosis
paramagnetic
paramalleolar arteries
Paramax angled driver
paramedian sagittal plane
parameningeal
parameters, Denavit-Hartenberg
paramyoclonus multiplex
paraneoplastic cerebellar degeneration
paraneoplastic encephalomyelitis
  (PEM)
paraneoplastic syndrome
paranoia
paraparesis
  flaccid
  spastic
parapatellar plica
paraphasia *(not* paraphrasia)
  formal verbal
  literal
  neologistic
  phonemic (or literal)
  semantic
  verbal
paraphasic error
paraphasic speech, fluent
paraphrasia *(not* paraphasia)
paraphyseal cysts
paraplegia
  alcoholic
  ataxic
  cerebral
  congenital spastic
  Erb spastic
  familial amyotrophic dystonic

paraplegia *(continued)*
  familial spastic
  flaccid
  hereditary spastic
  infantile spastic
  Pott
  senile
  spastic
  spinal
  toxic
paraplegic
parapodium orthosis
parapodium, Toronto
parapraxia
pararthrosis
parasagittal head region
parasagittal intracranial mass
parasagittal lesion
parasagittal meningioma
parasagittal region
parasagittal scar
parasagittal tumor
parascapular flap
parasellar mass
parasellar tumor
Parasmillie double-bladed knife
parasomniac conscious state
paraspinal abnormality
paraspinal infection
paraspinal muscle
paraspinal musculature
paraspinal soft tissue mass
paraspinal soft tissue shadowing
paraspinous musculature
parasternal bulge
parasternal heave
parasternal long-axis view
parasthesia, facial
parastriate cortex
parasympathetic innervation
parasympathetic nerve
parasympathetic nervous system
parasympathetic pupillary constrictor
  fibers
parasympathin
paratendinitis, Achilles

paratenon
P:A ratio (peroneal to anterior
    compartment)
paratonia
Paratrend 7 and 7+ blood gas
    sensor
paratrigeminal syndrome of Raeder
paratrooper fracture
paravermian region
paravertebral gutter
paravertebral musculature
paravertebral nerve plexus
paravertebral venous plexus
Parawaker orthosis
paraxial hemimelia (complete and
    incomplete)
parenchyma
    cerebral
    spinal cord
parenchymal brain cysticercosis
parenchymal brain stem syndrome
parenchymal hemorrhage
parenchymatous atrophy
parenchymatous cerebellar
    degeneration
parenchymatous hemorrhage
parenchymatous neurosyphilis
parent circulation
parent vessel sacrifice
paresis
    abducens nerve
    canal
    central facial
    complete ptosis of third nerve
    cranial nerve
    crural
    early ulnar nerve
    extraocular muscle
    gaze
    general
    ipsilateral facial
    limb-girdle-trunk
    motor
    ocular muscle
    oculomotor
    partial ptosis of third nerve
    radial nerve

paresis *(continued)*
    spastic
    "watershed" area
paresis of gaze
paresis of up gaze
paresthesia
    bandlike
    circumoral
    digital
    facial
    intermittent
    limb
    nocturnal
    transient
paresthesia steering
paresthetica
    cheiralgia
    meralgia
paretic jerks
paretic leg
paretic musculature
paretic neurosyphilis
Parhad-Poppen arteriogram needle
Parham band
Parham band circling needle
Parham band tightener
Parham-Martin bone clamp
Parham-Martin fracture apparatus
Parham metal band
parietal association areas
parietal bone
parietal cephalohematoma
parietal cortex lesion
parietal cortex, postrolandic
parietal EEG lead (P)
    left (LP)
    right (RP)
parietal gyrus
parietal lesion
parietal lobe contusion
parietal lobe disease
parietal lobe lesion
parietal lobe sign
parietal lobe tumor
parietal notch
parietal pleura
parietal signs

parietal suture
parietal tendon sheath layer
parietomastoid suture
parieto-occipital aphasia
parieto-occipital lesion
parieto-occipital sulcus
parieto-occipital suture
parietotemporal area
Parinaud syndrome
Paris ultrasound system
park bench position
Parkes osteotome
Parkinson disease
parkinsonian hypokinesia
parkinsonian symptoms
parkinsonian tremor
parkinsonism
    drug-induced
    en bloc turning in
    encephalopathic
    familial
    masked facies of
    postencephalitic
    sporadic
parkinsonism-dementia complex of
    Guam
parolfactory nerve (callosal area)
Parona space (subtendinous)
paronychia
parosmia
parosteal chondrosarcoma
parosteal osteogenic sarcoma
parosteal osteosarcoma
parosteal osteoma tumor
parosteal sarcoma tumor
parotid nerve
parotid notch
parotitis
paroxetine hydrochloride (Paxil CR)
    extended-release
paroxysmal changes
paroxysmal choreoathetosis seizure
paroxysmal convulsions
paroxysmal discharge
paroxysmal migraine
paroxysmal patterns of epilepsy
paroxysm of a seizure

Parquetry Block Test
Parrish-Mann hammertoe technique
parrot-beak meniscus tear
Parrot node
Parrot sign
parry fracture
pars interarticularis
pars interarticularis fenestration
pars planitis
Parsonage-Turner disease
Parsonage-Turner syndrome
Parsons knob
Parsons third intercondylar tubercle
Parsons tubercle
partial amnesia
partial closure
partial complex seizure
partial elementary seizures with motor
    symptoms
partial obliteration of lateral ventricle
    (on scan)
partial ossicular replacement prosthesis
    (PORP)
partial pressure of oxygen of brain
    tissue (P[ti]O_2)
partial ptosis of third nerve paresis
partial sacrectomy
partial saturation technique
partial-thickness tear
partial tonic seizure
particle
    Ivalon
    polyvinyl alcohol
particle of bone
particle repositioning maneuver
particulate debris
particulate embolizate
particulate graft
Partridge band
Partsch chisel
Partsch gouge
Parvin maneuver
PASA (proximal articular set angle)
PASAT (Paced Auditory Serial
    Addition Test)
pascals of force (SI units)
passage, adiabatic fast

passer
Batzdorf cervical wire
Brand tendon
Bunnell tendon
Charnley wire
curved
Framer tendon
Hewson suture
ligature
Malis ligature
suture
tendon
passing out
passive accessory intervertebral movements (PAIVMs)
passive dorsiflexion
passive elastic stiffness
passive head rotation
passive physiological intervertebral movements (PPIVMs)
passive range of motion (PROM) exercise
passive traction table
passive treatment modalities
Passow chisel
PASTA (polarity-altered spectral selective acquisition imaging)
paste
bone
conductive EEG
EEG electrolyte
electrode
Unna
past-pointing
patch
ash leaf
blood
epidural blood
Osteopatch transdermal skin
periosteal
postsynaptic neuronal membrane
shagreen p. in tuberous sclerosis
St. John's transdermal
vein
patella
apex of head of
bipartite

patella *(continued)*
chondromalacia
dislocated
floating
Hedrocel revision
high-riding
lower pole of
minima
skyline x-ray view of
subluxing
undersurface of
patella alta
patella baja
patella cup
patellae OUT (O'Donoghue's Unhappy Triad)
patellapexy
patellaplasty
Patella Pusher
patellar advancement
patellar aligner
patellar apprehension test
patellar bursitis
patellar button
patellar chondromalacia
patellar contour
patellar dislocation
patellar edge
patellar entrapment
patellar fat pad
patellar fossa
patellar groove
patellar inhibition test
patellar instability
patellar jerk
patellar ligament
patellar orthosis pad
patellar pole
patellar reflex (quadriceps stretch reflex)
patellar retraction test
patellar shaving
patellar stabilization brace
patellar subluxation
patellar tendinosis
patellar tendon avulsion
patellar tendon-bearing cast (PTB)

patellar tendon bone block
patellar tendon rupture
patellar tracking
patellectomy
patellofemoral arthritis
patellofemoral articular cartilage
patellofemoral brace
patellofemoral crepitation
patellofemoral interaction
patellofemoral joint space
patellofemoral pain syndrome
patellofemoral realignment
patelloquadriceps tendon
Patel medial meniscectomy
paternal haplotype
Paterson procedure
pathetic nerve
pathoanatomy
pathogen
    Actinomadura madurae
    actinomycetoma
    Clostridium tetani
    Cryptococcus neoformans
    eumycetoma
    Myobacterium bovis
    Mycobacterium malmoense
    Neisseria meningitidis
    Nocardiaform madurae
    peptostreptococcus
    Plasmodium falciparum
    Streptococcus agalactiae
    Streptococcus viridans
pathogenesis
pathognomonic sign
pathologic dislocation
pathologic flatfoot
pathologic fracture
pathologic fracture dislocation
pathologic hyperreflexia
pathologic laughing and crying
pathologic reflexes
    Babinski
    frontal lobe
    grasp
    root
    snout
    suck

pathologic spondylolisthesis
pathologist, speech
pathomechanical process
pathomechanics
    gait
    juvenile flatfoot
pathway
    adenosine diphosphate
    amygdalofugal
    cerebellar
    corticifugal
    corticobulbar
    corticospinal motor
    CSF (cerebrospinal fluid)
    CSF outflow
    dentato-olivary
    descending motor
    developmental
    frontopontocerebellar
    geniculocortical
    lipoxygenase
    neural
    nigrostriatal
    pain and temperature
    perforant
    pyramidal
    reticulocortical
    retinal
    retrochiasmal visual
    retrogeniculate
    retrovestibular neural
    stretch reflex
    subcortical
    synaptic
    thalamocortical
    visual
patient
    agitated
    ambulatory
    apallic
    aphasic
    arousable
    brain-dead
    comatose
    combative
    disoriented
    distractible

patient *(continued)*
    docile
    floppy (infant)
    fully conscious
    head-injured
    hydrocephalic
    hypotonic
    incoherent
    labile
    left-handed
    lethargic
    moribund
    nonambulatory
    nonresponsive
    obtunded
    posturing
    rapidly deteriorating
    right-handed
    spinal cord-injured
    stuporous
    unresponsive
    vegetative
patient motivation
Patil stereotactic head frame
Patil stereotactic head holder
Patrick fabere sign
Patrick test
Patte score
pattern
    alpha blocking
    alpha coma
    AO fracture
    beta coma
    bilateral benign epileptiform
    burst suppression
    checkerboard
    Collimator plugging
    continuous slow wave
    corduroy cloth
    cytokine secretion
    delta brush
    dermatomal
    desynchronized
    diffuse delta
    diffusely low voltage
    dimple-dimple hand
    discontinuous

pattern *(continued)*
    DISI collapse
    disorganized
    EMG incomplete interference
    epileptiform
    focal periodic
    full recruitment
    gait
    generalized periodic
    graft loading
    gyral
    high voltage slow
    hypsarrhythmic
    ictal epileptiform
    infantile
    interictal epileptiform
    intermixed focal and multifocal
    intermixed spike
    invariant EEG
    isoelectric
    knuckle-knuckle hand
    locomotor
    low voltage
    monorhythmic
    myotomal
    occipital delta
    paroxysmal
    phantom spike and wave
    pneumoencephalographic
    polyclonal
    polyspike and wave paroxysmal
    pseudoepileptiform
    reciprocal loading
    recruitment
    rhythmic theta
    scoliosis curve
    seizure
    sigmoid hair
    sigmoid scalp hair
    sleep
    slow spike and wave
    spindle coma
    storiform
    subclinical seizure
    suppression burst
    surface convexity
    temporal sawtooth

pattern *(continued)*
   theta coma
   triphasic wave
   vertebral body picture frame
pattern-induced epilepsy
patterning
pattern reversal visual evoked response
pattie or patty
   cement
   cotton
   cottonoid
pattie tray
patting automatism
patulous
pauciarticular onset
paucity
Paufique blade
Paulos ligament technique
Paulson knee retractor
Paulus plate
Paulus trocar
Pauwel angle of femoral neck fracture
Pauwel fracture classification
Pauwel Y osteotomy
Pavlik bandage
Pavlik harness
Pavlik sling
Pavlik splint
pavor nocturnus (night terror)
Paxil CR (paroxetine hydrochloride)
   extended-release
Payr sign
PB (paraffin bath)
p-boronophenylalanine (BPA)
PC (posterior commissure)
PCA (patient-controlled analgesia)
PCA (porous-coated anatomic)
   prosthesis
PCA (posterior cerebral artery)
PCA (posterior communicating artery)
PCA E-Series femoral prosthesis
PCA knee prosthesis
PCF (posterior cervical fusion)
PCL (posterior cruciate ligament)
PCL Pro device
PCoA (posterior communicating
   artery)

PCR (polymerase chain reaction)
PCReflex infrared tracking system
PDA (polymorphic delta activity)
pDEXA bone densitometer
PDLs (physical daily living skills)
PDN (prosthetic disk nucleus) device
PDS (polydioxanone) suture
PE (pulmonary embolism)
PEA (pulseless electrical activity)
Peabody Developmental Motor Scale
Peabody splint
Peacock transposing technique
PEAK anterior compression plate
   system
PEAK channeled plate system
peak height velocity
peak of wave on EEG
peak torque
Pean clamp
Pean forceps
peapod intervertebral disk rongeur
pearl-and-string sign
"pearls, string of," nuclear arrangement
Pearson attachment to Thomas frame
   or splint
Pearson correlation coefficients
Pearson-Spearman correlation
Pease bone drill
Pease-Thomson traction
PeBA suture anchor
PECAM-1 (platelet and EC adhesion
   molecule-1)
Peck osteotome
Pecquet, cistern of
pectinate ligament
pectinate muscle
pectineal ligament
pectineal muscle
pectoralgic migraine
pectoral girdle
pectoralis major muscle
pectoralis major syndrome
pectoralis minor muscle
pectoralis minor syndromepectoral
   muscle
pectoral nerve

pectoral reflex
pectorodorsalis muscle
pectus carinatum
pectus excavatum deformity
pedal disability
pedal hyperpigmented lesions
pedal intradermal nevi
pedal osteomyelitis
Pedestal, IMP Surgical Leg
Pediatric Rheumatology Disease
   Registry
Pediatric Ultrasound Bone Analyzer
pedicle
   congenital skin tube
   spinal
   subaxial cervical
   vascular
   vertebral
pedicle bone graft
pedicle cover
pedicle erosion
pedicle finder
pedicle finger
pedicle of vertebra
pedicle probe
pedicle sclerosis
pedicle screw, TSRH (Texas Scottish
   Rite Hospital)
Pedifix hammertoe pad
pedis
   dorsalis
   tinea
Pedlar portable stationary bicycle
pedobarography
   Biokinetics
   dynamic
   foil
   Musgrave footprint
pedobarographic technique
pedorthic
pedorthist
pedorthotist
peduncle
   cerebellar
   cerebral
   inferior cerebellar
   middle cerebellar

peduncular segment of superior
   cerebellar artery
pedunculated
pedunculopontine neuron
pedunculopontine nucleus pars
   compacta
PEG (pneumoencephalogram)
peg
   beef bone intramedullary
   bone
   fixation
   Harrison-Nicolle polypropylene
peg and socket bone
pegboard
   Montreal
   Purdue
pegged tibial prosthesis
pegging
peg graft or grafting
peg test of arm disability
Peiper-Beyer laminectomy rongeur
P electrode (parietal) (P_1-P_{10} and P_z)
Pelite shoe liner
Pelizaeus-Merzbacher disease
   adult form
   infantile form
Pelizaeus-Merzbacher leukodystrophy
Pellegrini-Stieda disease
Pelorus stereotactic system
Peltier thermode
pelvic bone
pelvic brim
pelvic fracture frame
pelvic girdle
pelvic girdle joints
pelvic inlet
pelvic obliquity
pelvic outlet
pelvic rim fracture
pelvic ring fracture
pelvic rock test
pelvic sling
pelvic splanchnic nerve
pelvic tilt, bent-knee
pelvic traction
pelvic ultrasound CT scan
pelvic unleveling

pelvic view
pelviectasis
pelvimetry, Mengert index in
pelvis
  android
  anthropoid
  assimilation
  beaked
  bony
  brachypellic
  contracted
  cordate
  cordiform
  Deventer
  dolichopellic
  dwarf
  false
  female
  flat
  frozen
  funnel-shaped
  greater
  gynecoid
  hardened
  heart-shaped
  inverted
  juvenile
  Kilian
  kyphoscoliotic
  kyphotic
  lesser
  longitudinal oval
  lordotic
  male
  masculine
  mesatipellic
  Nägele
  osteomalacic
  Otto
  platypelloid
  portable film of
  Prague
  pseudo-osteomalacic
  rachitic
  scoliotic
  small
  spider

pelvis *(continued)*
  spondylolisthetic
  transverse oval
  true
PEM (paraneoplastic encephalomyelitis)
Pemberton acetabuloplasty
Pemberton pericapsular osteotomy
Pemberton spur-crushing clamp
PEMF (pulsed electromagnetic field)
  therapy
pencil
  electrosurgical
  grease
  skin
penciling of ribs
pencil test
pendactyly
pendular nystagmus
penetrating injury
Penfield elevator
Penfield neurodissector
Penfield retractor
pen galvanometer
Penn fingernail drill
penniform muscle
Pennig dynamic wrist fixator
Pennig minifixator
Pennsaid (diclofenac)
Pennsylvania bimanual work sample
Penn wire-cutting scissors
Penrose drain
PENS (percutaneous electrical nerve
  stimulation)
PENS (percutaneous epidural neurostimulator)
pen, skin-marking
penta-acetic acid
People-Finder
Pepper neuroblastoma
peptide
  cross-linked N-telopeptides (NTx)
  procollagen I aminoterminal
    propeptide (PINP)
  procollagen I carboxyterminal
    propeptide (PICP)
peptostreptococcus

perarticulation
Perceived Therapeutic Efficacy Scale
percent of total disability
perception
   constant touch
   light touch
   threshold
   vibratory
Perception 5000 PC-based ultrasound
   scanner
PercScope percutaneous diskectomy
   system
perceptual disturbance, high level
percussion sign
Percuss-O-Matic "jackhammer"
   reflexology device
percussor
   G5 Fleximatic massager/percussor
   McGill neurological
percutaneous autogenous dowel bone
   graft
percutaneous automated diskectomy
   under fluoroscopy
percutaneous cordotomy
percutaneous diskoscope
percutaneous electrical nerve stimulation (PENS)
percutaneous epidural neurostimulator
   (PENS)
percutaneous interosseous nerve (PIN)
percutaneous Kirschner (K) wire
percutaneous nuclectomy
percutaneous pinning
percutaneous radiofrequency trigeminal rhizolysis
percutaneous repair
percutaneous retrogasserian glycerol
   rhizolysis (PRGR)
percutaneous thermal rhizotomy
percutaneous trigeminal tractotomy-
   nucleotomy (TR-NC)
percutaneous vertebroplasty
Percy amputating saw
Percy amputation retractor
perencephaly
Perfecta hip prosthesis
PerFixation interference screw

perforating cutaneous nerve
perforating fracture
perforator
   Acra-Cut cranial
   cranial
   Cushing cranial
   D'Errico
   DGR cranial
   Heifetz cranial
   McKenzie
perforator bur, Adson
perforator vessel
performance, ball skill
Performance knee prosthesis
Performance Wrap knee support
perfusate solution
perfusion
   luxury
   misery
   regional cerebral
perfusion abnormality
perfusion of brain
perfusion pressure
periacetabular osteotomy
periaqueductal gray matter
periaqueductal region
periaqueductal structures
periarteritis nodosa
periarthritis
periarticular calcification
periarticular fibrositis
periarticular fracture
periarticular heterotopic ossification
   (PHO)
periarticular ossification
periaxial space
pericallosal artery
pericapsulitis
perichondral bone
pericranial flap
pericranium, autologous
pericyte, Zimmerman
peridural fibrosis
perikaryon
perilesional bone
perilesional edema
perilunate carpal dislocation

perilunate fracture dislocation (PLFD)
perilunate instability
perimalleolar pain
perimedullary arachnoiditis
perimetry test
perimysiitis
perimysium
perineural
perineurial fibroblastoma tumor
perineurial neurorrhaphy
perineurioma
 intraventricular
 malignant
perineurium
period
 apneic
 apneustic
 ictal
 interictal
 non-REM
 postictal
 REM (rapid eye movements)
 sleep-onset REM
 sleep-onset REM (SOREMP)
period between complexes
periodic alternating nystagmus
periodic debridement
periodic lateralized epileptiform
 discharges (PLEDs)
periodicity, internal transverse
periodic paralysis
PerioGlas bone graft material
perioperative antibiotic therapy
perioral tremor
periorbital Doppler study
periorbital ecchymosis
periosteal bone formation
periosteal button
periosteal chondroma
periosteal cover
periosteal creep
periosteal elevator
periosteal fibroma
periosteal new bone formation
periosteal osteosarcoma
periosteal reaction
periosteal reflex

periosteal sarcoma
periosteal stripping
periosteal transplantation
periosteotome (see *osteotome*)
periosteotomy
periosteum
periostitis
 florid reactive
 suppurative
 traumatic
periostomy
peripheral blood mononuclear cells
peripheral facial spasm
peripheral fields of vision
peripheral fracture
peripheral gangrene
peripheral lesion
peripheral nerve function deficits
peripheral nerve injury
peripheral nerve lesion
peripheral nerve level motor impairment
peripheral nerve regeneration conduit
peripheral nerve sheath tumor (PNST)
peripheral neural deficit
peripheral neuritis
peripheral neuropathy (see also
 neuropathy)
 acrylamide
 alcohol
 amyloidosis
 arsenic
 avitaminosis B_1
 avitaminosis B_6
 avitaminosis B_{12}
 bacterial
 barbiturates
 Bassen-Kornzweig
 botulism
 brucellosis
 carcinoma
 chronic hepatitic failure
 chronic ischemia due to
  atherosclerosis
 Dejerine-Sottas
 diabetes mellitus
 dinitrophenol

peripheral neuropathy *(continued)*
 diphtheria
 emetine
 ethyl alcohol
 gastrointestinal shunts
 gold
 griseofulvin
 Guillain-Barré postinfectious
 hypoglycemia
 infectious hepatitis
 insecticides
 isonicotinic acid
 leprosy
 lupus erythematosus (LE)
 macrocryoglobulinemia
 macroglobulinemia
 malabsorption syndrome
 measles
 mercury
 methyl alcohol
 mononucleosis
 multiple myeloma
 mumps
 myxedema
 pantothenic acid deficiency
 polyarteritis nodosa
 porphyria
 Refsum
 sarcoidosis
 serum sickness
 sprue
 sulfonamides
 Tangier
 thallium
 tricresyl phosphate
 tuberculosis
 typhoid
 uremia
 vaccination
 vincristine
 Whipple disease
peripheral neuropathy tremor
peripheral origin weakness
peripheral ossification
peripheral pulses symmetrical and
 intact

peripheral quantitative computed
 tomography (pQCT)
peripheral sensory deficit
peripheral sensory loss
peripheral seventh nerve palsy
periprosthetic bone loss
periprosthetic bone resorption
periprosthetic fracture
periprosthetic leak
periprosthetic osteolysis
periradicular nerve
periradicular sheath
perirhinal cortex
perirolandic cortex
periscapulitis shoulder pain
peristriate cortex
peritendinitis
peritenon
peritoneal catheter, Raimondi
peritoneal ligament
peritonitis, CSF-induced
peritrapezial arthritis
peritumoral brain edema
periulcer venous channels in venous
 stasis ulcers
periungual
perivascular plane
periventricular density
periventricular gray (PVG) matter
periventricular lesion
periventricular leukomalacia
periventricular white matter
Perkins line
Perkins test
Perkins traction
Perlia medial nucleus
Perma-Hand braided silk suture
Perman cartilage forceps
permanent magnet
permeability, membrane
peroneal bone
peroneal island flap
peroneal muscular atrophy
peroneal nerve
peroneal nerve palsy, common
peroneal obliterative thrombus

peroneal paralysis
peroneal post
peroneal spastic flatfoot
peroneal tendon dislocation
peroneal-tibial trunk
peroneal vein
peroneus brevis
peroneus longus
peroneus tertius
peroxidation, lipid
peroxide flush
peroxisomal disorder
perpendicular sign
per primam healing
Perry-Nickel technique
Perry-O'Brien-Hodgson technique
Perry-Robinson cervical technique
perseveration of action
perseveration of drawing
perseveration of speech
perseverative disorder
persistence of rhythm
persistent facial palsy
persistent trigeminal artery
persistent vegetative state
personality
    frontal lobe
    interictal epileptic
personality disorder
person, memory-impaired
person years at risk (PYR)
Perthes-Bankart lesion
Perthes disease
Perthes epiphysis
Perthes reamer
Perthes test
pertrochanteric fracture
perturbers
pes abductus
pes anserine bursitis
pes anserinus
pes arcuatus
pes calcaneocavus
pes calcaneovalgus
pes calcaneus
pes cavovalgus
pes cavovarus

pes cavus
pes cavus-type deformity
pes contortus
pes equinovalgus
pes equinovarus
pes equinus
pes excavatus
pes malleus valgus
pes planovalgus
pes plantigrade planus
pes planus
pes planus deformity
pes pronation
pes supinatus
pes valgus
pes varus
PET (positron emission tomography)
    scan
PET with 3D SSP test
petaling edges of cast
petechia (pl. petechiae)
Petit ligament
petit mal 3-per-second spike and wave
    complexes
petit mal epilepsy
petit mal, oral
petit mal seizure
petit mal status
petit mal variant
petit pas gait
Petit triangle
Petren gait
Pétrequin ligament
Petrie spica cast
petrissage
petrobasilar suture
petroccipital
petroclinoid ligament
petroclival meningioma
petroclival region
petromastoid
Petrometer range-of-motion meter
petro-occipital joint
petro-occipital synchondrosis
petrosal bone
petrosal ganglion
petrosal nerve

petrosal neuralgia
petrosal sinus
petrosal vein
petrosectomy
petrositis
petrosomastoid
petrosphenobasilar suture
petrosphenoid
petrospheno-occipital suture
petrosquamosal
petrosquamous suture
petrous bone
petrous carotid canal stenosis
petrous portion of temporal bone
petrous pyramid
petrous region
petrous ridge
petrous segment of carotid artery
Peyronie disease
Peyton brain spatula
PFC femoral prosthesis
PFC total hip system
PFD (polyurethane foam dressing)
Pfeiffer syndrome
PFFD (proximal focal femoral
    deficiency)
P450 2D6 gene
p53 accumulation
p53 gene
PF Night splint
PF nucleus (parafascicular)
PFS (primary fibromyalgia syndrome)
PFT (parafascicular thalamotomy)
PFT (postop flexor tendon) traction
    brace
PGA synthetic absorbable suture
PGK (Panos G. Koutrouvelis, M.D.)
    stereotactic device
p-glycoprotein
PGP nail
phaeohyphomycosis, cerebral
phakomatoses
phalangeal bones
phalangeal branches
phalangeal glenoidal ligament of hand
phalangeal herniation
phalangeal tuberculous osteitis

phalangectomy, partial proximal
phalanx (pl. phalanges)
    base of
    distal
    middle
    proximal
    waist of
Phalen maneuver
Phalen-Miller opponensplasty
Phalen position
Phalen sign
Phalen test
phantom limb pain
phantom pain
phantom sensation
phantom spike and wave pattern
pharyngeal dysarthria
pharyngomaxillary space
pharyngopalatine muscle
phase
    burst
    corticomedullary (CP)
    heel contact
    heel-off
    in
    midswing
    out of
    toe-off
phase angle
phased-array surface coil
phase difference
phase lag
phase relation
phase reversal
phase reversing slow wave
phase sensitive detector
phase shift of sleep-wake cycle
phase spike
phasic nystagmus
plate and screw system
    MRI-compatible
    titanium
Pheasant elbow technique
Phelps brace
Phelps orthosis
Phelps scapulectomy
Phemister-Bonfiglio technique

Phemister elevator
Phemister onlay bone graft technique
Phemister rasp
phenol matricectomy
phenol nerve blocks
phenolization
phenomenon (pl. phenomena)
  A
  baked-brain
  Bancaud
  Bell
  Burner
  combined-flexion
  crus
  delay
  doll's eye (oculocephalic reflex)
  extinction
  freezing
  gelling
  "glued to the floor"
  Gordon knee
  Gowers
  Kernohan notch
  kindling
  Koebner
  Marin-Amat
  mouthing (pathological reflex)
  on-off
  paroxysmal
  Piltz-Westphal
  psychomotor
  Raynaud
  Robin Hood (steal syndrome)
  Schiff-Sherrington
  setting-sun
  steal
  Uhthoff
  unilateral Raynaud
  V
  vertebral steal
  zone
phenotype, PiMZ
phenotype variation
phenylketonuria (PKU)
phenoxymethylpenicillin
phenytoin (Dilantin)
phenytoin-induced choreoathetosis

pheresis, multicomponent
Philadelphia collar cervical support
Philadelphia halo
Philadelphia neck stabilizer
Philadelphia Plastizote cervical brace
Philips CT scanner
Philips linear accelerator (LINAC)
Philips toe force gauge
Phillips muscle
Phillips screwdriver
phlebogram
phleborheography (PRG)
phlebothrombosis
phlegm (Chinese medicine term)
phlegm damp (Chinese medicine term)
phlegm heat (Chinese medicine term)
PHN (postherpetic neuralgia)
PHNO (4-propyl-9-hydroxynaphthox-
    azine)
PHO (periarticular heterotopic ossifi-
    cation)
phocomelia
  complete
  distal
  proximal
Phoenix cranial drill
Phoenix hip prosthesis
Phoenix ICP monitor
Phoenix ventriculostomy catheter
phonatory seizure
phonemic (or literal) paraphasia
phonophobia in migraine
phonophoresis
Phoresor drug delivery system
Phoresor II iontophoretic drug
    delivery system
phosphenes
phospholipids
phosphoproteins
phosphorus nuclear magnetic
    resonance spectroscopy (P-MRS)
phosphorus-32 therapy
phosphorylase deficiency
photic driving with EEG
photic epilepsy
photic pattern-evoked responses
photic response

photic stimulation
photobleaching of porphyrins
photocell plethysmography
photoconvulsive response
photometrazol test
photomotogram
photomyoclonic jerking
photomyoclonic response
photon densitometry
Photon radiosurgery system (PRS)
photoparoxysmal response
photophobia in migraine
photoplethysmograph, Medasonic
   Vasculab
photoplethysmographic digit
photoplethysmography (PPG)
photoreceptor degeneration
photopsia
   Christmas-tree
   kaleidoscope
photosensitivity
photothermolysis
phrase-completion difficulties
phrase level, automatic
phrenic nerve
phrenicocolic ligament
phrenicolienal ligament
phrenicosplenic ligament
phrenoesophageal ligament
phrenogastric ligament
phrenosplenic ligament
phrenovertebral junction
phylogenetic
physeal anatomy
physeal arrest of growth
physeal bar formation
physeal cartilage
physeal closure
physeal damage
physeal distraction
physeal fracture
physeal injury
physeal plate fracture
physeal separation
physes (see *physis*)
physiatrist
physiatry

physical daily living skills (PDLs)
physical dependence
physical medicine and rehabilitation
   (PM&R)
physical therapist
physical therapy (PT)
physiologic flatfoot
physiologic neurologic exam
physiologic nystagmus
   end-point
   railway
physiologic tremor
physiology, cyber
Physio-Stim Lite bone growth
   stimulator
physiotherapist
physiotherapy
physis (pl. physes)
   distal tibial
   fibular
   fused
   medial
   unfused
physocephaly
physostigmine
phytanic acid storage disease
Phytodolor
phytosis
pia arachnoid
pia mater
pial vessels
piano key sign
piano wire dorsiflexion brace
PICA (Porch Index of Communicative
   Ability)
PICA (posterior inferior cerebellar
   artery) syndrome
Pick body
Pick chisel
Pick dementia
Pick disease
Picker Magnascanner for bone
   metastases
Picket Fence fiducial localization
   stereotactic system
Picket Fence leg positioner
Pickles ointment

pickup, Newvicon vacuum chamber
pickwickian syndrome
PICP (procollagen I carboxyterminal
  propeptide)
picture archive and communication
  system (PACs) for x-rays
picture, complex thematic
picture element (pixel)
picture-frame pattern of vertebral
  bodies
Pidcock check pin
piece, chin-occiput
piecemeal, removed
Piedmont fracture
Pierce forceps
piercer, triangular bone
Pierrot-Murphy tendon technique
piezoelectric potentials
piezoelectric stimulator
"pigeon-toeing" gait
pigmentary degeneration of the globus
  pallidus
pigmented villonodular synovitis (PVS)
pigmentosa, retinitis
Pilates method of exercise
Pillay syndrome
Pillet hand prosthesis
Pilliar total hip replacement
Pilling-Liston rongeur
pillion fracture
Pillo-Pedic cervical traction pillow
pillow (cushion)
  abduction
  Bio-Gel decubitus
  Carter elevation
  Carter foam
  cervical
  cervical support
  D-Core support
  Econo-Wave cervical
  elevate on
  foam
  Frejka
  immobilization
  Neck-Huggar cervical support
  Opti-Curve therapeutic
  Pillo-Pedic cervical traction

pillow *(continued)*
  PRN
  Sacro-ease (HMR)
  Tri-Core cervical
  wedge
pillow fracture
pillow orthosis for hip
pill-rolling tremor of parkinsonism
piloerection prior to seizure
pilonidal cyst
pilonidal dimple
pilonidal sinus
Pilot drill
Piltz-Westphal phenomenon
pimozide (Orap)
PiMZ phenotype
pin, pinning
  absorbable
  absorbable polyparadioxanone
  Acufex distractor
  alignment
  Allofix freeze-dried cortical bone
  Austin Moore
  ball guide
  ball-point guide
  ball-tip guide
  beaded hip
  beaded reamer guide
  Beath
  Bilos
  biodegradable
  Biofix system
  Böhler (Boehler)
  Bohlman
  breakaway
  Breck
  calcaneal
  calibrated
  Canakis
  Charnley
  clavicle
  closed
  collapsible
  Compere threaded
  Compton clavicle
  Conley
  Crego-McCarroll

pin *(continued)*
   cross
   Crowe pilot point on Steinmann
   Davis
   Day
   Denham
   DePuy
   Deyerle II
   distractor
   drawing
   drill
   Ender
   Fahey-Compere
   femoral guide
   Fischer transfixing
   Fisher half
   fixation
   Gardner skull clamp
   Gingrass and Messer pins
   Gouffon hip
   guide
   Hagie
   Hagie hip
   half
   halo
   Hansen-Street
   Hare
   Hatcher
   Haynes
   Hessel-Nystrom
   hip
   hook
   hook-end intramedullary
   hydroxyapatite-coated
   in situ
   Intraflex intramedullary
   intramedullary
   Jones compression
   Knowles
   Krankendonk
   Küntscher
   LIH (Lars Ingvar Hansson) hook
   locating
   Lottes
   marble bone
   Mayfield skull clamp
   McBride

pin *(continued)*
   metallic
   Modny
   Moore
   Olds
   open
   Oris
   OrthoSorb absorbable fixation
   partially threaded
   PDS (poly-p-dioxanone)
   percutaneous
   Pidcock check
   polyparadioxanone, absorbable
   poly-p-dioxanone (PDS)
   precurved ball-tipped guide
   Pritchard Mark II
   rasp
   resorbable
   Rhinelander
   Riordan
   Roger Anderson
   Rush
   Schanz
   Schneider
   Schweitzer
   self-broaching
   Serrato forearm
   Shriner
   skeletal traction
   skull
   Smith-Petersen
   smooth Steinmann
   socket
   Sofield
   Stader
   Steinmann
   Street medullary
   strut-type
   tapered
   threaded
   threaded Steinmann
   tibial drill
   titanium half
   traction
   transarticular
   transfixing
   transfixion

pin *(continued)*
   Turner
   Tutofix cortical
   Varney
   Venable-Stuck
   Vom Saal
   Wagner closed
   wrench
   Zimmer
pin care
pin extraction torque
pin fixation
PIN (percutaneous interosseous nerve)
PIN (posterior interosseous nerve)
   entrapment
pinch-band forceps
pinched nerve
pinch, key
pinch power, thumb-
pinch strength
PinchTrack Commander strength tester
pineal apoplexy
pineal body, calcified
pineal calcification
pineal gland, calcified
pineal gland tumor
pinealoma, ectopic
pinealoma tumor
pineoblastoma
pineocytoma
pin fixation
ping-pong bone
ping-pong fracture
pin headrest
pinhole, bone
pinion, Mayfield
pin length
Pinn.ACL guide system
pinning, intrafocal
pinning, Kapandji
pinocytotic vesicle
PINP (procollagen I aminoterminal
   propeptide)
pinpoint pupils
pinprick sensation
pinprick test of sensation
   absent

pinprick *(continued)*
   impaired
   normal
pins and needles sensation
pin-site infection
pin-skin interface
Pinto distractor
pin-tract infection
pin traction
pin-tract sepsis
pinwheel
   Cleanwheel neurological
   Safe-T-Wheel
   Wartenberg neurological
pinwheel testing
PION (posterior interosseous nerve)
   syndrome
Piotrowski sign
PIP (proximal interphalangeal)
PIP articulation
PIP flexion crease
PIP joint
pipe bone
pipe stemming of ankle-brachial index
PIPJ (proximal interphalangeal joint)
Pipkin classification of femoral fracture
pi plate
Pirie bone
piriform cortex
piriformis syndrome
piriform muscle
piriform sinus
Pirogoff amputation
Pisces spinal cord stimulation system
Pischel micropin
pisiform bone of wrist
pisohamate ligament
pisometacarpal ligament
pisotriquetral joint
pisounciform ligament
pisouncinate ligament
pistol grip
piston, cannulated expulsion
pistoning of drill
piston sign
pitch angle
pitch, calcaneal

pitchfork retractor
pitch of threads on screw
Pittsburgh collimator helmet
Pittsburgh Gamma Knife unit
Pittsburgh pelvic frame
pituitary ablation, total
pituitary adenoma
  ACTH-producing
  chromophobe
  nonsecreting
pituitary apoplexy
pituitary cachexia
pituitary curet
pituitary fossa
pituitary gland
pituitary "incidentaloma"
pituitary microadenoma
pituitary rongeur
pituitary stalk distortion (PSD)
pituitary tumor
pivot, Accu-Line dual
pivoting sports
pivot of calcar
Pivot Pole walking device
pivot-shift sign
pivot-shift test
pivot synovial joint
pivot transfers
pixel (picture element)
PIXI peripheral densitometer
Pixsys Flashpoint
PKG (protective knee guard)
PKU (phenylketonuria)
placebo response
placement, EEG electrode
placode, neural
plafond fracture
plafond, tibial
plagiocephalic
plagiocephaly
plain tomograms
plain x-ray films
planar spin imaging
plane
  anatomic
  areolar
  axial

plane *(continued)*
  capsular
  coronal
  E
  extrapial
  fascial
  flexion-extension
  frontal
  gonion-gnathion
  Hensen
  Hodge
  horizontal
  intercommissural axial
  internervous
  intertubercular
  Ludwig
  median sagittal
  mesiodistal
  midsagittal
  orthogonal
  paramedian sagittal
  pelvic
  perivascular
  sagittal
  sella-nasion
  spinous
  sternoxiphoid
  subcostal
  subgaleal
  subpial
  suprasternal
  thoracic
  transverse
  tumor cleavage
  varus-valgus
  vertical
plane of cleavage of tumor
plane joint
plane/planing, visiospatial
planer
  calcar
  Rubin bone
  Rubin cartilage
plane synovial joint
planigrams
planigraphy
planning, rehabilitation

planovalgus
  pes
  talipes
planovalgus foot deformity
plantar aponeurosis
plantar arterial arch
plantar axial view
plantar calcaneal spur
plantar calcaneocuboid ligament
plantar calcaneonavicular ligament
plantar callosities
plantar cuboideonavicular ligament
plantar cuneocuboid ligament
plantar cuneonavicular ligament
plantar fascia as windlass mechanism
plantar fasciitis
plantar fasciotomy
plantar flexed
plantar flexion, forced
plantar flexion-inversion deformity
plantar flexor motion
plantar flexor proximal metatarsal
  osteotomy
plantar interosseous muscle
plantar keratosis
plantar ligament
plantar malignant melanoma
plantar metatarsal ligament
plantar muscle
plantar pain
plantar puncture wound
plantar quadrate muscle
plantar reflex, equivocal
plantar response
plantar spur
plantar tuberosity
plantar vault
plantaris muscle
plantaris rupture
plantarward
plantar wart
  mother-daughter type
  mosaic
  satellite
  single
plantigrade foot

planus
  fixed bony
  talipes
plaque
  MS (multiple sclerosis)
  neuritic
  neuritic senile
  senile
plaquing
plasma cell myeloma tumor
plasmacytoma, extramedullary
plasmapheresis
plasmatoma, solitary
Plasmodium falciparum
Plastalume finger splint
Plastazote foam
plaster
  corn removal
  Hapset hydroxyapatite bone graft
  salicylic acid
  Velpeau
  Zoroc
plaster of Paris (POP) bandage
plaster of Paris cast
plaster slab splint
plaster splint
plaster toe cap
plastic bowing fracture
plasticity, cross-modal
plastic, thermolabile
Plastiport TORP prosthesis
Plastizote arch support
Plastizote cervical collar orthosis
Plastizote material
plasty, trans-bone
plate
  acetabular reconstruction
  AcroMed VSP
  Aesculap ABC cervical
  alar
  anchor
  AO blade
  AO condylar blade
  AO contoured T
  AO hook
  AOI blade

plate *(continued)*
  AO reconstruction
  AO semitubular
  AO small fragment
  Armstrong
  ASIF right-angle blade
  axial
  Badgley
  Bagby angled compression
  basal
  Batchelor
  biodegradable
  blade
  Blount blade
  bone
  bone flap fixation
  bony
  Bosworth spine
  Burns
  buttress
  C-shaped
  Calandruccio side
  cap-and-anchor
  cartilaginous growth
  CASP (contoured anterior spinal)
  Caspar cervical
  cervical locking
  cloverleaf
  coaptation
  cobra-head
  Collison
  compression
  condylar
  conical tectal
  connecting
  Continuum total knee base
  contoured T-plate
  cortical
  cranial bone fixation
  cribriform
  DCP (dynamic compression)
  deck
  DePuy
  Deyerle
  dorsal
  double-H
  Driessen hinged

plate *(continued)*
  dual
  Duopress
  Dwyer-Hall
  dynamic compression (DCP)
  eccentric dynamic compression
    (EDCP)
  Eggers bone
  11-hole
  Elliott femoral condyle blade
  end
  epiphyseal cartilage
  ethmovomerine
  E-Z Flap cranial bone
  femoral
  fibrocartilaginous
  fiducial
  five-hole (5-hole)
  fixed-angle blade
  flat
  flexor palmar
  foot
  Forte distal radius
  four-hole (4-hole)
  frontal
  fusion
  gait
  Gallannaugh bone
  growth
  Hagie sliding nail
  Haid cervical
  half-circle
  Hansen-Street
  Harlow
  Harm posterior cervical
  Harris
  heavy side
  heavy-duty femur
  Hicks lugged
  Hoen skull
  Holt nail
  Howmedica Microfixation cranial
  H-shaped
  Hubbard
  I plate of Yuan
  interfragmentary
  intertrochanteric

plate *(continued)*
- Jergesen I-beam
- Jergesen tapered
- Jewett nail overlay
- Jones compression
- Kaneda
- Kessel
- L-shaped
- Laing
- Lane
- Lawson-Thornton
- LC-DCP
- Leibinger 3-D
- Leibinger Micro Plus
- Leibinger Micro System cranial fixation
- Letournel
- localization-compression grid
- Lorenz cranial
- Louis
- low contact dynamic compression (LC-DCP)
- L-shaped
- Luhr micro
- Luhr Microfixation cranial
- Luhr mini
- Luhr pan
- Lundholm
- Luque-Galveston
- Luque II
- malleable
- Massie
- McBride
- McLaughlin intertrochanteric
- Mears sacroiliac
- Medoff sliding
- meningioma of the cribriform
- Meurig Williams
- microfixation
- Milch
- minifragment
- Moe intertrochanteric
- Moore sliding nail
- Moreira
- Morscher cervical
- Müller (Mueller) compression blade nail

plate *(continued)*
- Neufeld
- neutralization
- Newman
- Nicoll
- occipitocervical
- Ogden
- orbital
- Orozco cervical
- orthotic
- Osborne
- overlay
- palmar
- Paulus
- PEAK channeled
- pedicle
- peg-base
- pi
- plain pattern
- planar
- plantar
- pterygoid
- Pugh
- pylon attachment
- quadrangular positioning
- quadrigeminal
- reconstruction
- resorbable
- Richards side
- Richards-Hirschhorn
- roof
- Rotator Cuff Buttress (RCB)
- Roy-Camille cervical
- Roy-Camille occipitocervical
- Roy-Camille pedicle
- Schweitzer spring
- semitubular compression
- Senn
- serpentine
- seven-hole (7-hole)
- 17-hole
- Sherman bone
- side
- Simmons
- six-hole (6-hole)
- skull
- slide

plate *(continued)*
  slotted femur
  Smith-Petersen
  Smith-Petersen intertrochanteric
  SMO (supramalleolar orthosis)
  spoon
  stabilization
  stainless steel
  stainless steel preformed skull
  steel sole
  Steffee
  Steffee pedicle
  Steffee screw
  stem base
  Storz Microsystems cranial fixation
  subchondral bone
  supracondylar
  Synthes cervical
  Synthes dorsal distal radius
  Synthes Microsystem cranial fixation
  Syracuse I
  T
  tantalum preformed skull
  tarsal
  T buttress
  tectal
  Temple University
  tendon
  Thornton nail
  3-D (three-dimensional)
  three-hole (3-hole)
  titanium
  toe
  Townley tibial plateau
  Townsend-Gilfillan
  trial base
  T-shaped
  T-shaped AO
  tubular
  Tupman
  twisted
  two-hole (2-hole)
  UCP compression
  Uslenghi
  V blade
  V nail
  Venable

plate *(continued)*
  vertebral body
  Vitallium
  volar
  VSP (variable screw placement)
  Wainwright
  Wenger
  Whitman
  Wilson
  wing
  Wright
  Wurzburg
  X-shaped
  Y bone
  Y-shaped
  Zimmer femoral condyle blade
  Zimmer side
  Zimmer Y
  Z-shaped
  Zuelzer hook
plate and screw system
plateau
  multiple sclerosis
  tibial
plateau fracture
plate bender
platelet amyloid precursor protein
  (APP)
platelet and EC adhesion molecule-1
  (PECAM-1)
platelet anti-aggregant
platelet-derived growth factor
platelet membrane fluidity
plate osteosynthesis
platform
  ceiling-mounted robotic
  echospeed
  force
platform posturography
plating technique
Platinol
platinum coil
Platou osteotomy
platybasia
platycephaly
platypellic pelvis
platypelloid pelvis

platypodia
platysma muscle
platyspondylosis
platyspondyly
Plavix (clopidogrel bisulfate)
play, excessive joint
Playmaker functional knee brace
PlayTuf knee brace
PLC (posterolateral corner) of knee
pleating of ligamentum flavum
PLED (periodic lateralized epilepti-
    form discharge) syndrome
pledget, Betadine-soaked
pledget of gauze
Plenk-Matson rasp
pleocytosis
    CSF
    lymphocytic
pleomorphic
pleomorphic hyalinized angiectatic
    tumor
pleomorphism, nuclear
pleonosteosis, Léri's
plerocephalic edema (or papilledema)
plethysmography
    air
    digital
    impedance
    photocell
pleuroesophageal muscle
plexiform neurofibromas
plexiform neuroma
Plexiglas splint
plexitis, brachial
plexopathy
    brachial
    idiopathic
    lumbar
    lumbosacral
    neoplastic
    radiation
    radiation-induced
plexus
    Batson
    brachial
    calcification of choroid
    carotid

plexus *(continued)*
    choroid
    clinoid venous
    lumbar
    lumbosacral
    nerve
    paravertebral nerve
    paravertebral venous
    sciatic
    spinal nerve
    subdermal
    venous
plexus hypogastricus superior
plexus injury
plexus of Santorini
plexus papilloma, choroid
PLF (posterior lumbar fusion)
PLFD (perilunate fracture dislocation)
pliable stent
plica (pl. plicae)
    medial
    parapatellar
    suprapatellar
    synovial
plicated dural sheath
plication
    disk
    soft tissue
    thermal capsular
plication suture
plicectomy
pliers
    Compaction
    flat-nose
    Howmedica Microfixation System
    Leibinger Micro System
    locking
    Luhr Microfixation System
    needle-nose
    pair of
    Power-Grip
    Storz Microsystems
    Synthes Microsystem
    taper-nose
    wire-cutting
PLIF (posterior lumbar interbody
    fusion)

PLIF (posterolateral interbody fusion)
PLL (posterior longitudinal ligament)
PLLA (poly L-lactic acid) coating
   material
plombage, bone
PLSA (posterolateral spinal artery)
plug
   bone
   bone-graft
   Buck
   cement
   Exeter intramedullary bone
   patellar
Plum-Blossom acupunture needle
plumbism (lead poisoning)
plumb line
Plummer sign
pluripotential marrow
pluripotential stem cells
PM&R (physical medicine and
   rehabilitation)
PMH (pure motor hemiparesis)
PMI-6A1-4V implant metal
PML (progressive multifocal leukoencephalopathy) viral encephalitis
PMMA (antibiotic-impregnated
   polymethylmethacrylate) beads
PMMA (polymethylmethacrylate) bone
   cement
PMMA rod
PMR (posteromedial release) for
   clubfoot
P-MRS (phosphorus nuclear magnetic
   resonance spectroscopy)
PMS (periodic movements [of the
   legs] syndrome)
PMT biopsy needle
PMT halo system cervical collar or
   support
PNET (primitive neuroectodermal
   tumor)
Pneu Knee Airprene inflatable knee
   brace
pneumatic bone
pneumatic compression therapy
pneumatic drill
pneumatic foot pump (mechanical)

pneumatic tourniquet cuff
pneumoarthrogram
pneumoencephalitis
pneumoencephalogram (PEG)
pneumoencephalographic pattern
pneumoencephalography, lumbar
pneumoencephalomyelogram
pneumoencephalomyelography
pneumocephalus
   epidural
   intracranial
   spontaneous
   tension
pneumogastric nerve
pneumogram, impedance
PNF (proprioceptive neuromuscular
   facilitation) exercise
PNST (peripheral nerve sheath tumor)
P(ti)O$_2$ (partial pressure of oxygen of
   brain tissue)
POAH (posterior occipitoatlantal
   hypermobility)
pocket, subfascial
podagra
podiatrist
podiatry
Podiatry Institute
podocyte
PodoFlex reflexology device
podogeriatrics
podopediatrics
PO electrode (parieto-occipital)
   (P$_3$, P$_4$, P$_7$, P$_8$, P$_z$)
Pogan buggy
poikilothermia
point
   bleeding
   Crowe pilot
   dorsal
   drill
   electrode insertion
   end
   entry
   Erb
   frontopolar
   glenoid
   Krackow

point *(continued)*
  Mathews drill
  Neiguan acupressure P6
  Pauly
  preauricular
  pressure
  Raney-Crutchfield drill
  target
  trigger
  twist drill
  Universal drill
pointer
  hip
  shoulder
point imaging
point localization
point scanning
point-search acupuncture instruments
point tenderness
Poirier, space of
poisoning
  barbiturate
  carbon tetrachloride
  Jamaica ginger
  lead
  manganese
  mercury
  methyl alcohol
  organophosphorus insecticide
Poisson ratio
POL (posterior oblique ligament)
Poland classification of epiphyseal
  fracture
Poland syndrome
polar bearing
Polar Care ice therapy device
Polaris adjustable spinal cage
polarity-altered spectral selective
  acquisition (PASTA) MRI imaging
polarity
  EEG wave
  electrical
  negative
  opposite signal
  positive
  reversal of

polarity *(continued)*
  simultaneous opposite
  stimulus
polarization, electrode
Polar-Mate coagulator
Polar-Med postop shoe cover
polar moment of inertia
polarographic P(ti)O$_2$ catheter probe
Polarus Plus humeral fixation system
Polar Vantage XL heart rate monitor
Polar Wrap cold therapy
pole
  frontal
  patellar
  temporal
pole of scaphoid
poliodystrophy, progressive cerebral
polioencephalitis hemorrhagica
  superior
polioencephalopathy
poliomyelitis
  nonparalytic
  pseudo-Babinski sign in
poliomyelitis encephalitis
poliomyelitis viral encephalitis
polished stem
Polk finger goniometer
pollex pedis
Polley-Bickel biopsy trephine
pollicization
  Buck-Gramcko
  Gillies
  Littler
  Riordan finger
pollicization of finger
polyacetal resin
polyarteritis
  alcoholic
  nonalcoholic
polyarteritis nodosa
polyarthritis
polyarthropathy
polyarticular gout
polyarticular juvenile rheumatoid
  arthritis
polyarticular symmetric tophaceous
  joint inflammation

polyaxial joint
polybutester suture
polycarbonate eyeguards
Polycentric and Wide-Track knee
   system
polyclonal pattern
polydactyly
   postaxial
   preaxial
   radial
   rudimentary postaxial
   thumb
Polydek suture
Polyderm hydrophilic polyurethane
   foam dressing
Poly-Dial acetabular cup prosthesis
Poly-Dial insert
polyester tow
polyester tripled hamstring graft
polyethylene
   compression-molded
   cross-linked
   high density
   ultrahigh molecular weight
polyethylene button
polyethylene failure
polyethylene femoral buck-plug
   procedure
polyethylene liner
polyethylene proximal brims in quadrilateral contour
polyethylene tibial component
polyethylene wear
polygenic
polyglacine suture
polyglactin mesh dural graft
polyglactin rods
polyglactin sutures
polyglycolide rods, self-reinforced
polygyria
polyimages, visual
polylactide screw
poly L-lactic acid (PLLA) coating
   material
polymer
   cold-curing
   self-curing

polymerase chain reaction (PCR)
polymer deformation
polymerized
polymethylmethacrylate (PMMA) rod
polymicrogyria
polymodal neglect
polymorphic activity
polymorphic waves
polymorphism, APOE
polymyalgia rheumatica
polymyopathy (see also *myopathy*)
   alcoholic
   centronuclear
   rod body
polymyositis, idiopathic
polymyositis myopathy
polyneuritiformis, heredopathia
   atactica
polyneuritis (see also *neuritis*)
   acute febrile
   acute infectious
   chronic relapsing
   idiopathic
   infectious (Guillain-Barré syndrome)
polyneuritis cranialis
polyneuropathy (see also *neuropathy*)
   acute inflammatory
   chronic inflammatory demyelinating
     (CIDPN)
   chronic relapsing
   diabetic sensorimotor
   distal
   dying-back
   dysimmune
   gestational
   idiopathic
   peripheral
   recurrent
   sarcoid
   sensorimotor
   sensorimotor axonal
   subacute
   symmetric
   symmetrical
   thallium
   uremic
polyopsia of cerebral origin

polyostotic bone lesion
polyostotic fibrous dysplasia
polyparadioxanone pin, absorbable
poly-p-dioxanone (PDS) pin fixation
polyphasic sharp wave
Polypin biodegradable implant
polypropylene insert
polypropylene orthosis
polyradiculoneuropathy
   chronic inflammatory (CIP)
   demyelinating
   inflammatory
   inflammatory demyelinating
polyradiculopathy
   acute inflammatory
   acute inflammatory demyelinating
     (AIDP)
   chronic inflammatory demyelinating
     (CIDP)
   diabetic
polyradioculoneuropathy
polyrhythmic activity
polyrhythmic waves
Polysar splint
Polysit drug delivery system
polysomnogram, 48-hour
polysomnographic sleep study
polysomnography
Polysorb liner
Polysorb suture
polyspike and slow wave complex
polyspike and wave paroxysmal
   pattern
Polysplint A flexible splinting material
polysynaptic
Polytechnic foot-pressure measuring
   plate
polytetrafluoroethylene graft (PTFE)
polytomography
polytrauma
polyurethane cast
polyurethane foam dressing (PFD)
polyurethane foam embolus
polyvinyl alcohol (PVA) particles
polyvinyl alcohol splinting material
polyvinyl alcohol sponge
Pompe disease

Pond adjustable splint
Pond fracture
P_1-P_4 segments of posterior cerebral
   artery (PCA)
pongid posture
pons (pl. pontes)
   caudal
   infarctions of the
pons and midbrain, tegmentum of
Ponseti splint
pontine angle
pontine contusion
pontine gaze center
pontine glioma tumor
pontine hemorrhage
pontine infarct(ion)
pontine lateral gaze center
pontine lesion, high
pontine-medullary levels
pontine myelinolysis
pontine parareticular formation
   (PPRF)
pontis, nucleus
pontocerebellar fiber
pontocerebellar glioma
pontomedullary junction
pontomedullary region
pontomesencephalic junction
pontotegmental syndromes
pool, hydrotherapy
pool therapy
poorly differentiated tumor
pop, popping
POP (plaster of Paris) bandage
popeye arm
popliteal cyst
popliteal fossa
popliteal muscle
popliteal nerve
popliteal notch
popliteal recess
Poppen-Blalock carotid clamp
Poppen forceps
Poppen-Gelpi laminectomy retractor
Poppen Gigli saw guide
Poppen intervertebral disk rongeur
Poppen Ridge Sensitometer

Poppen ventricular needle
popping of joint
popping sensation
pop rivet
Porch Index of Communicative Ability
  (PICA)
porcine heterografts
porencephalia
porencephalic cyst
porencephalous
porencephaly, cystic
porfiromycin (Promycin)
Porocoat AML noncemented prosthesis
porocoating
Porocoat prosthetic material
poroid hidradenoma
poroma, malignant eccrine
Porometal noncemented femoral
  prosthesis
Poron insole
poroplastic splint
porosis
  cerebral
  epiphyseal
porosity, volumetric
porous apatite ceramics
porous-coated acetabular cup implant
porous-coated anatomic (PCA) knee
  prosthesis
porous coated total hip replacement
porous ingrowth
porphyrins, fluorescent
PORP (partial ossicular replacement)
  prosthesis
Port-A-Cath
portable C-arm image intensifier
  fluoroscopy
portable commode
Porta-Deck ramp
portal
  anterior aspect of ankle
  anterocentral arthroscopic
  anterolateral
  anteromedial arthroscopic
  arthroscopic entry
  arthroscopy
  Caspari arthroscopic

portal *(continued)*
  distal radioulnar joint
  MCR (midcarpal radial)
  MCU (midcarpal ulnar)
  midcarpal radial (MCR)
  midcarpal ulnar (MCU)
  midlateral
  patellar
  port of Wilmington
  posterior aspect of ankle
  posterolateral arthroscopic
  posteromedial arthroscopic
  radiocarpal
  subacromial arthroscopic
  superolateral
  superomedial
  Swedish
  trans-Achilles arthroscopic
  transmalleolar arthroscopic
  Wilmington arthroscopic
Porter-Richardson-Vainio technique
Porteus Maze Test
porthole
portion
  accessory
  cord
portmanteau procedure
Portnoy ventricular cannula
Portnoy ventricular catheter
Porzett splint
Posey belt
Posey grip
Posey restraint
POSI (position of safe immobilization)
POSICAM PET system
position
  abdominal brace
  barber chair
  bayonet fracture
  beach chair
  Bonner
  Brickner
  calcaneal stance
  conjugate forward gaze
  decubitus
  dorsal
  dorsal lithotomy

position *(continued)*
  dorsal recumbent
  figure 4 (figure of 4)
  Fowler
  frogleg
  full lateral
  Gaynor-Hart
  hook-lying
  horizontal
  intrinsic plus
  jackknife
  jet pilot
  Jones
  jumper's knee
  kneeling
  Kraske
  lateral decubitus
  lateral park bench
  lithotomy
  lotus
  medial genicular
  near-anatomic
  neutral calcaneal stance
  neutral hip
  neutral spine
  normal anatomic
  opisthotonic
  over-the-top
  park bench
  Phalen
  prayer
  prone
  proximal bow
  rectus
  resting calcaneal stance
  reverse Trendelenburg
  scissor leg
  semi-Fowler
  semisitting
  side-lying
  Sims
  spinal fusion
  static
  stress tolerant
  supine
  three-quarters prone

position *(continued)*
  Trendelenburg
  W-sitting
positional nystagmus of central origin
positional nystagmus of peripheral
  origin
positional tremor
positioner (holder)
  acetabular cup
  Allen
  Allen arthroscopic
  arm
  Bareskin knee
  cup
  Hold-and-Hold
  knee
  leg
  Mark II Stulberg hip
  Mark II Wixson hip
  MB&J knee
  Montreal hip
  Picket Fence leg
  Prep-Assist
  Profex arthroscopic leg
  Stulberg hip
  Stulberg Mark II leg
  Surg-Assist leg
  Wixson hip
position of function, splinted in
position of safe immobilization (POSI)
position sense
positive abilities
positive bottle sign
positron emission tomography scan
  (PET)
post
  Morse tapered prosthetic
  perineal
  peroneal
  status
  thumb
postactivation exhaustion on
  electromyogram
postactivation increment on
  electromyogram
postanesthesia recovery (PAR)

postanoxic coma
postanoxic encephalopathy
postauricular ecchymosis
postaxonic myoclonus
postcalcaneal bursitis
postcast compression reflex sympathetic dystrophy
postcasting syndrome
postcentral sensory gyrus
postcentral sulcus
postconcussion syndrome
postdialysis seizure
postdiuresis seizure
postdormital sleep paralysis
Postel hip status system
postencephalitic parkinsonism
postepileptic paralysis
posterior ampullar nerve
posterior antebrachial cutaneous nerve
posterior-anterior (PA) view
posterior aorta transposition of great
 arteries
posterior arch of atlas (C1)
posterior atlantoaxial membrane
posterior auricular muscle
posterior auricular nerve
posterior brachial cutaneous nerve
posterior calcaneal bursitis
posterior cervical fusion (PCF)
posterior cervical intertransverse
 muscle
posterior cervical triangle
posterior circulation aneurysm
posterior circulation stroke
posterior colliculus
posterior column deficits of spine
posterior column disease
posterior column lesions
posterior commissure
posterior communicating artery (PCA)
posterior compartment lesion
posterior costotransverse ligament
posterior cricoarytenoid ligament
posterior cricoarytenoid muscle
posterior cruciate ligament
posterior cutaneous nerve

posterior displacement osteotomy
 of calcaneus
posterior drawer test
posterior edge loading
posterior ethmoidal nerve
posterior femoral cutaneous nerve
posterior fossa
posterior fossa brain mass
posterior fossa brain tumor
posterior fossa decompression
posterior fossa endoscopy
posterior fossa epidermoid tumor
posterior fossa lesion
posterior fossa stare
posterior fossa tumor
posterior fracture-dislocation
posterior GPi pallidotomy for
 Parkinson disease
posterior gray column of cord
posterior gray horns of the spinal
 canal
posterior inferior cerebellar artery
 (PICA)
posterior inferior communicating
 artery (PICA)
posterior interosseous nerve syndrome
posterior intraoccipital joint
posterior joint syndrome
posterior labial nerves
posterior language area lesion
posterior-lateral (posterolateral) view
posterior leaf spring orthosis
posterior ligament
posterior lobe tumors
posterior longitudinal ligament
posterior lumbar fusion (PLF)
posterior lumbar interbody fusion
 (PLIF)
posterior medial ankle ligaments
posterior medial ligament
posterior median septum of cord
posterior mediastinum
posterior meniscofemoral ligament
posterior metatarsal arch
posterior occipitoatlantal hypermobility
 (POAH)

posterior occipitoaxial ligament
posterior olive in brain
posterior root ganglia
posterior sacroiliac ligament
posterior sacrosciatic ligament
posterior scalene muscle
posterior scapular nerve
posterior scrotal nerve
posterior shin splint
posterior skull view
posterior spinal fusion (PSF)
posterior spinal line
posterior spinocerebellar tract
posterior sternoclavicular ligament
posterior subluxation
posterior superior humeral head defect
posterior supraclavicular nerve
posterior talofibular ligament
posterior talotibial ligament
posterior third frontal gyrus
posterior thoracic nerve
posterior tibial artery
posterior tibial muscle
posterior tibial nerve entrapment
posterior tibial pulse
posterior tibial slope
posterior tibial tendon dysfunction
  (PTTD)
posterior tibial translation
posterior tibiofibular ligament
posterior tibiotalar ligament
posteroanterior (PA) view
posterolateral aspect
posterolateral corner of knee
posterolateral interbody fusion (PLIF)
posterolateral sclerosis of the spinal
  cord
posterolateral spinal artery (PLSA)
posteromedial pivot-shift test
posteromedial release (PMR)
posterosuperior
posteroventral pallidotomy
postfracture osteomyelitis
postfracture swelling
postfracture syndrome
postganglionic gray fibers
posthemiparesis syndrome

postherpetic facial pain
postherpetic neuralgia (PHN)
posthypoxic myoclonic seizures
posthypoxic myoclonus
postictal alpha slowing
postictal bisynchronous slow wave
postictal cerebral blood flow scan
postictal confusion
postictal depression
postictal drowsiness
postictally
postictal mutism
postictal paralysis
postictal period
postictal slowing
postictal state
postinfectious cerebellitis
postinfectious encephalitis
postinfectious encephalopathy
postinfectious leukoencephalopathy
postinjection reflex sympathetic
  dystrophy
postischemic cerebral hypoperfusion
postischemic flap necrosis
postlaminectomy instability
post-LP (lumbar puncture) headache
postmenopausal
postmetrizamide CT scan
postneuritic atrophy
postneurosurgical evaluation
postoperative flexor tendon traction
  brace
postoperative neovascularization
postoperative wound care
postpartum pituitary apoplexy
postpolio fatigue
postpoliomyelitic muscle contracture
postpoliomyelitis muscular atrophy
  (PPMA)
postpolio syndrome
postreduction ischemic necrosis
postreduction x-ray
postrema of medulla
postrolandic parietal cortex
POSTs (positive occipital sharp
  transients)
postsphenoidal bone

postsphenoid bone
poststress ankle/arm Doppler index
postsynaptic cortical neuronal potential
postsynaptic dopamine receptors
postsynaptic neuronal membrane patch
postsynaptic potential (PSP)
postsynaptic receptor
post-tetanic potentiation
Post total shoulder arthroplasty
post-traumatic amnesia (PTA)
post-traumatic angulation
post-traumatic apoplexy of Bollinger
post-traumatic arthritis
post-traumatic arthropathy
post-traumatic arthrosis
post-traumatic cavus
post-traumatic cerebral syndrome
post-traumatic chronic disability
post-traumatic chronic osteomyelitis
post-traumatic cortical dysfunction
post-traumatic encephalopathy
post-traumatic epilepsy
post-traumatic fibrosis
post-traumatic headache
post-traumatic neck pain
post-traumatic neuroma
post-traumatic osteoarthritis
post-traumatic osteoporosis
post-traumatic spondylitis
post-traumatic stress disorder
post-traumatic vertigo
post-treatment evaluation
post-treatment neuropsychologic
   evaluation
postulnar bone
postural awareness
postural fixation
postural instability
postural seizure
postural tone
postural tremor
posture, posturing
   batrachian
   benediction
   benedictory
   decerebrate
   decorticate and decerebrate

posture *(continued)*
   dystonic
   extensor
   flexor dystonic
   forward-head
   good
   limb
   opisthotonic
   poor
   round-back
   stooped
   tonic
Posture Curve lumbar cushion
Posture Pulley neck exerciser
Posture Pump spine trainer
posture-related overdrainage of shunt
Posture-Rite lap desk
Posture S'port
Posture Training Support (PTS)
Posturite paper holder
Posturite writing board device
posturography
postvaccinial leukoencephalitis
potential
   acoustic evoked
   action
   attack-specific
   auditory evoked
   bias
   biphasic
   brain stem auditory evoked (BAEP)
   brain stem evoked
   bursts of muscle
   cerebral
   compound muscle action (CMAP)
   compound nerve action (CNAP)
   cortical evoked
   cortical somatosensory evoked
     (CSSEP)
   denervation
   difference between
   EEG
   electrical
   EMG
   evoked
   excitatory postsynaptic (EPSP)
   extracerebral

potential *(continued)*
    far-field
    fasciculation
    fibrillation
    glossokinetic
    high frequency
    inhibitory postsynaptic (IPSP)
    localized evoked
    long duration
    median mixed nerve action
    membrane
    microvolts of sensory
    millivolts of motor response
    miniature endplate (MEPP)
    motor evoked (MEP)
    motor nerve evoked
    motor unit action (MUAP)
    near-field
    nerve action (NAP)
    neurogenic motor evoked
    NMEP (neurogenic motor evoked)
    normal motor (on EMG)
    P100
    piezoelectric
    polyphasic
    polyphasic motor unit
    posterior tibial nerve-evoked
    postsynaptic (PSP)
    postsynaptic cortical neuronal
    propagated volley
    recruitment of motor unit
    resting
    satellite
    scalp
    sensory evoked (SEP)
    sensory nerve action (SNAP)
    serrated
    short-duration motor unit
    skin
    somatosensory
    somatosensory evoked (SEP, SSEP)
    spinal dorsal horn
    spinal evoked (SEP)
    spinal sensory evoked
    visual evoked (VEP)
    voluntary motor unit
potential cumulative trauma disorders

potential P300 latency
potentiation, post-tetanic
Potenza arthrodesis
Pott (18th century British surgeon)
Pott abscess
Pott disease
Potter arthrodesis
Pott fracture of fibula
Pott paralysis
Pott paraplegia
Pott puffy tumor
Potts (20th century pediatric surgeon)
Potts eversion osteotomy
Potts rib shears
Potts scissors
Potts-Smith dressing forceps
Potts-Smith scissors
Potts splint
Potts tenotomy scissors
Potts tibial osteotomy
Potts-Yasargil scissors
pouce flottant (floating thumb)
pouch
    dural root
    Rathke (in the brain)
    suprapatellar
pound, foot
pounds of traction
Poupart inguinal ligament
Pourcelot resistance index
Pourfour du Petit syndrome
pout sign
poverty of movement
powder
    bone
    cranioplastic
    thrombin
    zinc peroxide
power
    motor
    muscle
PowerCut drill blade
power-driven saw
Powered Metaphyseal Stapler
powered shaver
power feedback
Powerflex CPM exerciser

power grip of hand
Power-Grip pliers
Power Node AcuVibe massager
Power Pillow cervical massager
PowerTrack Commander strength
    tester
power-train
Power Web Jr. upper extremity
    exerciser
Pozzi muscle
PPIVMs (passive physiological inter-
    vertebral movements)
PPMA (postpoliomyelitis muscular
    atrophy)
PPPMA (progressive postpolio muscle
    atrophy)
PPRF (paramedian pontine reticular
    formation)
PPRF (pontine parareticular
    formation)
PPT/Rx Firm Molded Insole
pQCT (peripheral quantitative
    computed tomography)
PRA (proximal reference axis)
Prader-Willi syndrome
pragmatic
pramipexole (Mirapex)
Pratt technique
Pravachol (pravastatin sodium)
pravastatin sodium (Pravachol)
praxis
    constructional
    ideational
    ideomotor
praxis testing
PRC (proximal row carpectomy)
preauricular point
preaxial polydactyly
precentral glioma
precentral gyrus
precentral seizure
precentral sulcus
precession
precessional frequency
Prechtl method
precipitate a migraine
precision grip

Precision Osteolock femoral prosthesis
precision radiotherapy for skeletal
    tumors
Precision Tack transvaginal anchor
    system
Precision Twist transvaginal anchor
    system
precoated femoral stem prosthesis
precoated layer
precommunicating segment of anterior
    cerebral artery
precuneate
precuneus
precursor
    neuronal
    serotonin
precursor sign to rupture of aneurysm
predental space
Predictive Salvage Index (PSI)
predisposition to migraine
predominance
    anterior
    posterior
    temporal
predormital sleep paralysis
predormition
predrilling
preexisting
preferential use of right/left hand
prefrontal bone of von Bardeleben
prefrontal function
pregabalin
prehensile hand movements
prehension
preinterparietal bone
Preiser disease
premature suture synostosis
premaxillary bone
premedullary arteriovenous fistula
premonition of seizure
premonitory sign
premonitory symptoms
premorbid level of functioning
premorbid traits
premotor area
preneurosurgical evaluation
prenylation

Prenyl jacket
preoccipital notch
preoperative autologous blood
    donation
prepared and draped (also prepped and
    draped)
Prep-Assist leg positioner
prepatellar bursa
prepatellar bursitis
prepontine cistern
prereduction x-ray
prerubral field nucleus
presacral nerve
PREs (progressive resistive exercises)
presacral mass
presacral neurectomy
presbyophrenia
Presbyterian Hospital staphylorrhaphy
    elevator
prescapula
presenile dementia
presenile onset of dementia
preservation of insight
preservation of nerve
Preservex
pre-slip changes
presphenoid bone
PRESS-CSI sequence
Press-Fit component
Press-Fit Condylar Total Knee
press-fit mode
Press-Fit stem
pressoreceptor nerve
pressor nerve
pressor reflex
pressure
    ankle systolic
    bone marrow (BMP)
    central venous (CVP)
    cerebral perfusion (CPP)
    cerebrospinal fluid
    closing p. on lumbar puncture
    colloid oncotic
    compartmental
    continuous positive airway (CPAP)
    cranial perfusion (CPP)
    Doppler ankle systolic

pressure *(continued)*
    Doppler calf systolic
    Doppler thigh systolic
    elevated intracranial
    epidural
    forefoot peak
    increased interstitial
    increased intracranial
    interstitial fluid hydrostatic
    intracranial (ICP)
    intracranial epidural (ICEDP)
    intradiskal
    intraneural
    intraspinal epidural (ISEDP)
    manual
    opening p. on lumbar puncture
    perfusion
    photoelectric skin
    regional cerebral perfusion (rCPP)
    spinal cord perfusion
    spinal tap opening
    TMA
    toe systolic
    tourniquet
pressure-controlled roller pump
pressure fracture
pressure monitor, subdural
pressure necrosis
pressure needles (teishein)
pressure-relieving orthosis
pressure sella
pressure sensor
pressure sore
pressure wave
presternal notch
Preston ligamentum flavum forceps
Preston pinch gauge
Preston Traveler CPM exerciser
prestyloid recess
presynaptic neurons
presynaptic terminal
presyncope
pretectal area
pretectal lesion
pretectal nucleus
pretectal region
pretendinous bands

pretendinous cord
pretensioning of graft
pretibial edema
pretibial region
pretreatment evaluation
pretreatment neuropsychologic
  evaluation
PRE 2 suture
Prevent Recurrence of Osteoporotic
  Fractures (PROOF) group
prevertebral fascia
prevertebral soft tissue
prevertebral space
Prévost sign
PreVue *B. burgdorferi* antibody
  detection assay
pre-walking treatment of pronated feet
  in infancy
PRG (phleborheography)
PRGR (percutaneous retrogasserian
  glycerol rhizolysis)
Pribham suction tubes
Price muscle biopsy clamp
prickling
primary aminoaciduria
primary auditory cortex
primary brain tumor
primary, cancer of unknown (CUP)
Primary Care Evaluation of Mental
  Disorders (PRIME)
primary central nervous system
  lymphoma
primary closure
primary craniosynostosis
primary degenerative dementia
primary fibromyalgia syndrome (PFS)
primary gain
primary gout
primary intention, healing by
primary metallic fixation
primary myopathies
primary optic atrophy
primary rigid fixation
primary sarcoma
primary suture of ruptured tendons
primary visual cortex

PRIME (Primary Care Evaluation of
  Mental Disorders)
PRIME-MD (computerized version of
  Primary Care Evaluation of Mental
  Disorders)
prime movers (agonist muscle groups)
primidone (Mysoline)
primitive dislocation
primitive neuroectodermal tumor
  (PNET)
primitive reflexes
primitive stem cell migration
principle
  axial compression
  Enneking
prion (slow virus) disease
prism, Fresnel
Pritchard Mark II pin
Pritchard score
Pritchard-Walker total elbow prosthesis
Private Practice vibration reminder
  disk
proband genotype
probe
  Acufex
  angled
  arthroscopic
  Arthrocare Wand
  bipolar cautery (BICAP)
  Bunnell
  Bunnell dissecting
  Bunnell forwarding
  Dandy
  dissecting
  electromagnetic focusing field (EFF)
  Endotrac
  forwarding
  Frigitronics
  hemispherical contact
  high frequency
  intraosseous
  Jacobson
  Jacobson micro
  Jannetta
  laser Doppler
  Laserflo Doppler

probe *(continued)*
    LDF (laser-Doppler flowmetry)
    malleable
    McCain TMJ
    micro
    Mitek Vapor
    Neurotrend
    Nucleotome aspiration
    Nucleotome Flex II cutting
    OCT surgical imaging
    Oratec electrocautery
    pedicle
    polarographic P(ti)O$_2$ catheter
    radiofrequency
    skin temperature monitoring
    Steffee
    Surgical Dynamics aspiration
    telomere-specific
    thermal
    tulip
    ultrasonic
probenecid (Benemid)
probe-to-bone test
procaine-phenol motor point injection
Procare orthopedic accessories
procedure (see also *operations*)
    ablative
    activating
    arthroscopic
    balloon-assisted
    chiropractice adjustment
    computerized dynamic
        posturography
    crossfire radiation therapy
    debulking
    Dockery
    electrocorticography
    endoscopic
    gasless
    isotopic cisternography
    laparoscopic
    laser Doppler fluxmetry
    magnetic resonance imaging
    magnetic resonance neurography
        (MRN)
    magnetic source imaging

procedure *(continued)*
    manipulative (chiropractic)
        adjustment
    organ harvesting
    porte manteau
    posturography
    salvage
    takedown
procedural memory
procedure time
procerus muscle
process (pl. processes)
    accessory
    acromial
    alar
    angular orbital
    articular
    ascending
    basilar
    bony
    calcaneal
    caudate
    clinoid
    concrete thought
    condyloid
    coracoid
    coronoid
    costal
    cytoplasmic
    diffuse encephalopathic
    ethmoidal
    falciform
    fibroplastic
    frontal
    frontonasal
    frontosphenoidal
    glenoid
    inflammatory
    interspinous
    lumbar transverse
    monarthric
    neoplastic
    odontoid (dens)
    olecranon
    osseous destructive
    pathomechanical

process *(continued)*
  pterygoid
  radiostyloid
  sacral
  SinterLock CSTi bonding
  spinous
  Steida bony
  styloid
  Ti-Nidium surface hardening
  transverse vertebral
  trochlear
  Tutoplast tissue preservation
  uncinate
  vertebral
  vertebrospinous
  xiphoid
  zygomatic
processing, higher integrative language
ProCol bovine bioprosthesis tendon
procollagen I aminoterminal propeptide (PINP)
procollagen I carboxyterminal propeptide (PICP)
procurvature deformity
Prodigy densitometer
prodromal symptom
prodrome
  affective
  epileptic
  irritability
  migraine headache
  visual
product
  fibrin degradation
  mammalian cell
  nonglycosylated bacterial cell
Pro-8 ankle brace
Profex arthroscopic leg positioner
Profex arthroscopic tourniquet
profile, Profile
  Functional Limitation (FLP)
  Maryland Foot Score
  Nottingham Health (NHP)
  PULSES
  rotational
  Sickness Impact (SIP)
  Staheli rotational

Profile hip prosthesis
Profile stapler
profilometer, laser stylus
Profix mobile-bearing knee implant
profound
progenitor skin cells
prognosticator
program
  exercise
  home exercise
  treatment
  weight-training
  Williams exercise
programmed cell death
progression to full weightbearing
progressive cerebral poliodystrophy
progressive dementing illness
progressive diaphyseal dysplasia
progressive external ophthalmoplegia
progressive hydrocephalus
Progressive Matrices Test
progressive multifocal leukoencephalopathy (PML) viral encephalitis
progressive myoclonic epilepsy
progressive osseous heteroplasia
progressive osteolysis
progressive resistance
progressive resistive exercises (PREs)
progressive rostral-caudal brain stem
  dysfunction
progressive supranuclear palsy
progressive weights
Prohance contrast medium
proinflammatory cytokines tumor
  necrosis factor
Project, Human Genome
projection system, diffuse thalamic
prolactinoma
prolactin-secreting adenoma
Prolene suture
proliferation
  angiofibroblastic
  myointimal
  osteophytic
  Schwann cell
  synovial
  villous

Proline Stomatex shoulder brace
prolotherapy
ProMem (metrifonate)
PROM (passive range of motion)
  exercise
prominence
  bony (spur)
  tibial tubercle
prominence of forehead
prominent xiphoid process
promontory, sacral
Promycin (porfiromycin)
pronated foot
pronated grip x-ray
pronated straight flatfoot
pronation and supination
pronation
  hallucal
  rearfoot
  subtalar joint
pronation-external rotation (P-ER)
  injury
pronation sign
pronator drift
pronator muscle
pronator quadratus
pronator reflex test
pronator sign
pronator teres syndrome
prone lateral view
prone position
prone scapular retraction exercises
prone view
Pronex pneumatic cervical traction
prong, modified tonsil
pronosupination
PROOF (Prevent Recurrence of
  Osteoporotic Fractures) group
Pro Osteon 500 bone graft substitute
propagation, seizure
Propel cannulated interference screw
propeller, orthopedic
propentofylline
proper palmar digital nerve
prophylactic antibiotic therapy
prophylactic anticoagulation
Proplast prosthesis

propofol
proportionality, cephalofacial
propranolol (Inderal)
proprioception
  afferent
  foot
  joint
proprioceptive defect
proprioceptive end organs
proprioceptive neuromuscular
  facilitation (PNF)
proprioceptive rehabilitation
proprioceptive sense of muscles and
  ligaments
proprioceptive vertigo
proprius, nucleus
propulsion of gait
propulsive foot
propulsive forces
propulsive phase of gait
prosencephalon
prosody
ProSom (estazolam)
prosopagnosia
Prosorba
prostacyclin
prostaglandin endoperoxide
prostaglandin E_1
PROSTALAC (prosthesis of
  antibiotic-loaded acrylic cement)
prosthesis (pl. prostheses)
  above-elbow
  above-knee
  acetabular
  ACG knee replacement
  advanced mobile-bearing knee
  Advance PS total knee
  Advantim total knee system
  Aesculap-PM noncemented femoral
  AFI total hip replacement
  AGC (anatomically graduated
    component)
  AGC femoral
  AGC knee
  AGC tibial
  AHP (American Hand Prosthesis)
  AHP digital

prosthesis *(continued)*

AHSC (Arizona Health Science
Center-Volz) elbow
Airprene hinged knee
Aliplast insoles
Alivium implant metal
alumina-alumina total hip
replacement
AMC total wrist
American Hand Prosthesis (AHP)
AML (anatomic medullary locking)
hip
AML Tang femoral
Amstutz cemented hip (TR-28)
Anametric total knee
anatomic surface
Anderson acetabular
Angelchik antireflux
ankle
aortic valve
Apollo knee and hip systems
APR (anatomic porous replacement)
APR acetabular
APR femoral
APR II
APRL hand
Arafiles elbow
Arizona Health Science Center-
Volz (AHSC) elbow
Arthopor acetabular cup
Arthopor cup (I, II, III)
Atkinson endoprosthesis
Attenborough knee
Aufranc cobra hip
Aufranc-Turner
Aufranc-Turner cemented hip
Austin Moore hip
Autophor ceramic total hip
Autophor femoral
Averett hip
ball-and-socket ankle
Bankart shoulder
Bateman UPF
Bateman UPF II bipolar hip
Bateman UPF II shoulder
BDH (biologically designed hip)
bead-blasted

prosthesis *(continued)*

Bechtol hip
Bechtol shoulder
Becker hand
Beck-Steffee total ankle
below-elbow
below-knee
Bi-Angular shoulder
Bias hip
Biaxial Weave composite
bicentric
bicompartmental knee implant
bicondylar ankle
bicondylar knee
Bi-Metric hip
Bio-Chromatic hand
biodegradable implant
biodegradable self-reinforced
polyglycolide rod
Biofit press-fit acetabular
Bio-Groove Macrobond HA
femoral
Biomet
Biomet AGC
Biomet hip
Biometric
Biophase implant metal
Biotex implant metal
bipolar femoral head
bipolar hip replacement
Blazina
Bock knee
Bombelli-Mathys-Morscher hip
bovine collagen material
Brigham
Bryan total knee implant
Buchholz ankle
Buchholz hip
Buechel-Pappas ankle
CAD (computer-assisted design)
femoral
CAD femoral stem
Caffinière
Calandruccio cemented hip
calcar replacement femoral
Callender hip
Calnan-Nicolle metatarsophalangeal

prosthesis *(continued)*
    Calnan-Nicolle synthetic joint
    capitellocondylar unconstrained
      elbow
    carpal lunate implant
    carpal scaphoid implant
    Cathcart Orthocentric hip
    cementless
    Centralign Precoat Hip
    ceramic femoral head
    Ceramion
    Charnley cemented
    Charnley low friction hip
    Charnley-Hastings
    Charnley-Mueller hip
    Chatzidakis hinged Vitallium
      implant
    Chopart partial foot
    Christiansen hip
    Cintor knee
    CKS (Continuum knee system)
    Cloutier unconstrained knee
    Coballoy implant metal
    CoCr alloy (cobalt-chromium)
    Co-Cr-Mo alloy (cobalt-chromium-
      tungsten-nickel)
    Co-Cr-W-Ni alloy (cobalt-
      chromium-tungsten-nickel)
    Cofield shoulder
    cold-mold
    cold-weld
    collar-calcar support femoral
    Compartmental II
    compression-molded
    Conaxial total ankle
    constrained hinged
    Continuum knee system (CKS)
    Continuum P/S total knee
    Contour internal
    Coonrad hinge
    Coonrad semiconstrained elbow
    CSF (contoured femoral stem) hip
    C-2 OsteoCap hip
    custom-threaded
    Cutter-Smeloff cardiac valve
    DANA (designed after natural
      anatomy) shoulder

prosthesis *(continued)*
    D'Aubigné femoral
    Deane unconstrained knee
    debonded femoral stem
    Dee totally constrained elbow
    De La Caffinière trapezio-
      metacarpal
    Deon hip
    DePalma
    DePuy AML Porocoat stem
    DF80 (Wilson-Burstein) hip
    digital
    Dimension hip
    Dimension/C femoral stem
    doffing (taking it off)
    donning (putting it on)
    Dorrance hand
    double pearl-face hip joint
    Dow Corning implant
    Dow Corning Wright finger joint
    DRUJ (distal radioulnar joint)
    dual-lock hip
    Dupaco knee
    Duracon
    Dynaplex knee
    Eaton
    Eaton finger joint replacement
    Eicher femoral
    elbow
    ELP femoral
    Endo-Model rotating knee joint
    endoprosthesis
    Engelhardt femoral
    Eriksson knee
    Evolution hip
    Ewald unconstrained elbow
    Exeter cemented hip
    femoral
    Fett
    finger
    finger-joint implant
    Finn hinged knee replacement
    FIRST knee
    fixed femoral head
    Flatt finger joint
    Flatt finger/thumb
    Flexfoot foot

prosthesis *(continued)*

FLEX H/A total ossicular
fluid
forearm lift-assist
forged cobalt-chromium alloy
four-bar linkage on knee
Freehand system
Freeman modular total hip
Freeman-Samuelson
Freeman-Swanson knee
F.R. Thompson femoral
fully constrained tricompartmental
    knee
Gaffney ankle
Gemini hip system
Gemini MKII mobile-bearing knee
Genesis knee
Geomedic total knee
geometric total knee
Gerard
Gianturco
Giliberty femoral
Giliberty hip
Gillette joint
Gore-Tex knee
great toe implant
Gripper acetabular cup
grit-blasted
Gritti-Stokes knee
GSB (Gschwind-Scheier-Bahler)
    elbow
Guepar hinged knee
Gunston-Hult knee
Gunston knee
Gustilo hip
Gustilo knee
Hamas
hand
hand-glove
Harris (HD-2) cemented hip
Harris-CDH hip
Harris Design 1 (or 2) femoral
Harris-Galante hip
HA 65101 implant metal
Hastings hip
Haynes-Stellite (HS) implant metal
Hedley-Hungerford hip

prosthesis *(continued)*

Henschke-Mauch SNS knee
Herbert knee
Hexcel knee
HG Multilock hip
hinged implant
hinged knee
hip replacement
Hittenberger
Howmedica Kinematic II knee
HPS II hip
HSS knee
Hunter tendon
Hydra-Cadence knee
Hydroxial hip
ICLH (Imperial College London
    Hospital)
ICLH ankle
ICLH knee
Impact total hip
Implex hip or knee
Indiana conservative
Indong Oh
Insall/Burstein II modular total
    knee
Insall-Burstein semiconstrained
    tricompartmental knee
Integrity acetabular cup
Interax Integrated Secure Assym-
    metric (ISA) mobile-bearing
    knee implant
Intermedics Natural-Knee
Inter-Op acetabular
Iowa
Ishizuki unconstrained elbow
Jaffe-Capello-Averill hip
J-FX bipolar head
Joplin toe
Judet press-fit hip
Kessler
Kinematic fully constrained
    tricompartmental knee
Kinematic II rotating hinge total
    knee
Kinemax Plus knee
Kirschner Medical Dimension
KMC femoral stem

prosthesis *(continued)*
KMP femoral stem
KMW/PC femoral
knee
Koenig MPJ
Kudo unconstrained elbow
Küntscher humeral
Lacey fully constrained tricompart
mental knee
LaPorte total toe
LCS New Jersey knee
LCS Total Knee Systems
Leeds-Keio ligament
Leinbach femoral
Lewis expandable adjustable
(LEAP)
Lewis Trapezio
Ling cemented hip
Link cementless reconstruction hip
Link Endo-Model rotational knee
Lippman hip
Lisfranc below-knee
Liverpool elbow
Liverpool knee
Lo Bak spinal support
locking
London unconstrained elbow
Lo-Por vascular graft
Lord Press-Fit hip
Lord total hip
Lowe-Miller unconstrained elbow
low-neck femoral
low profile femoral
Lubinus knee
lunate acrylic cement wrist
Lunceford-Pilliar-Engh hip
MacIntosh knee
MacNab-English shoulder
Macrofit hip
madreporic hip
Mallory-Head total hip
manual locking knee
MAPF femoral stem
Marmor modular knee
Matchett-Brown cemented hip
Mathys
Matrol femoral head

prosthesis *(continued)*
Mayo ankle
Mayo semiconstrained elbow
Mazas totally constrained elbow
MBK mobile-bearing knee implant
McBride femoral
McCutcheon SLT hip
McGehee elbow
McKee-Farrar total hip
McKeever Vitallium cap
McKeever Vitallium knee
Mecring acetabular
Mediloy implant metal
medium profile femoral
metal
metal femoral head
Metasul hip
MG II knee
Michael Reese articulated
Microknit vascular graft
Microloc knee
migration of
Miller-Galante hip or knee
Milliknit vascular graft
Minneapolis
Mittlemeir ceramic hip
Mittlemeir noncemented femoral
modular total hip
modular unicompartmental knee
Monk hip
monoblock femoral stem
monolithic A1203 cup
Moore femoral
Moore hip
MP35N implant metal
MST-6A1-4V
Mueli wrist
Mueller (Müller) Duo-Lock hip
Mueller total hip replacement
Muhlberger orbital implant
multiaxis
MultiLock hip
myoelectric control for upper arm
Naden-Rieth hip
Natural-Knee
NEB (New England Baptist) hip
Neer I and II shoulder replacement

prosthesis *(continued)*
    Neer umbrella
    Neer Vitallium humeral
    NeuFlex metacarpophalangeal joint
      implant
    NeuroCybernetic Prosthesis (NCP)
    Neville tracheal and tracheo-
      bronchial
    New Jersey LCS knee
    Newton ankle
    Nexus hip
    Niebauer
    Noiles fully constrained
    Noiles posterior stabilized knee
    Noiles rotating-hinge total knee
    nonhinged knee
    nonhinged linked
    Normalize press-fit hip
    nudge control on
    Odland ankle
    Oh cemented hip
    Oh press-fit hip
    Oklahoma ankle
    Omnifit HA hip stem
    Omnifit knee
    Optifix femoral
    Oregon Poly II ankle
    Orthochrome implant metal
    Orthofix
    Ortholoc implant metal
    orthopedic
    osseointegrated
    OsteoCap hip
    Osteolock femoral
    Osteonics hip
    Otto Bock modular PTB
    Overdyke hip
    Panje voice button
    partial ossicular replacement
    patellar
    PCA E-Series femoral
    PCA knee (porous-coated anatomic)
    PCA unconstrained tricompartmental
    PCA unicompartmental knee
    pegged tibial
    Perfecta hip
    Performance knee

prosthesis *(continued)*
    Phoenix hip
    Pillet hand
    Plastiport TORP
    PMI-6A1-4V implant metal
    polycentric knee
    Poly-Dial acetabular cup
    polyethylene patellar implant
    Porocoated AML noncemented
    Porometal noncemented femoral
    porous-coated anatomic (PCA) knee
    porous-coated hip
    porous-surfaced
    PORP (partial ossicular replacement)
    Precision Osteolock femoral
    Precision Osteolock hip
    precoated femoral stem
    precoat hip
    Press-Fit condylar total knee
    Press-Fit implant
    Pritchard-Walker semiconstrained
      elbow
    ProCol bovine bioprosthesis
    Profile hip
    Profix mobile-bearing knee implant
    PROSTALAC (prosthesis of anti-
      biotic-loaded acrylic cement)
    Protasul-10 noncemented femoral
    Protasul-64 WF Zweymuller
    provisional
    proximally coated femoral stem
    PTB (patellar tendon-bearing)
      strap of
    PTB supracondylar (SC)
    PTB suprapatellar (SP)
    PTS soft wedge
    radial head implant
    RAM knee
    Ranawat-Burstein hip
    Re-Flex VSP
    Richards hip
    Richards hydroxyapatite PORP
    Richards hydroxyapatite TORP
    Richards Spectron metal-backed
    Richards Zirconia femoral head
    Ring total hip
    RM isoelastic hip

prosthesis *(continued)*
Robert Brigham total knee
Rosenfeld hip
Rotaglide knee
rotating femoral head
rotating hinge
Rothman Institute femoral
Sabolich socket system
SACH (solid-ankle, cushioned heel) foot
SAF (self-articulating femoral)
SAL (Self-Aligning) mobile-bearing knee implant
Sarmiento (STH-2) hip
Sauerbach
Savastano Hemi-Knee
Sbarbaro hip
Sbarbaro tibial plateau
Schlein elbow
Schlein semiconstrained elbow
Scorpio total knee system
seated
seating of the
Seattle foot
Select ankle
Select shoulder
Self-Aligning (SAL) mobile-bearing knee implant
self-bearing ceramic hip
semiconstrained tricompartmental
Sense-of-Feel
Sharrard-Trentani
Sheehan knee
Sheehy incus replacement
Sherfee
Shier total knee
shoulder disarticulation
Silastic
Silastic ball spacer
Silastic HP-100 finger joint
Silastic radial head
Silflex intramedullary
silicone elastomer rubber ball
silicone trapezium
single-axis ankle
single pearl-face hip joint
single smooth-face hip joint

prosthesis *(continued)*
sintered implant
SinterLock implant metal
Sivash hip
SKI knee
SMA
Smith ankle
Smith-Petersen
Sorbie-Questor total elbow system
Souter unconstrained elbow
Spectron hip
Speed
spherocentric fully constrained
spherocentric knee
S-ROM femoral stem
stainless steel implant metal
Stanmore elbow
Stanmore totally constrained
Starr-Edwards Silastic ball valve
STD hip
Steeper powered Gripper
stemmed
stemmed tibial
Stevens-Street elbow
St. George-Buchholz ankle
St. George total elbow
STH-2 (Sarmiento) hip
St. Jude Medical valve
Street-Stevens humeral
SuperCup acetabular cup
Surgitek
Sutter double-stem silicone implant
Sutter MCP joint
Sutter silicone metacarpophalangeal joint
Sutter-Smeloff heart valve
Swanson great toe
Swanson metacarpal
Swanson metatarsal
Swanson T-shaped great toe
Swanson wrist
Syme amputation
Syme foot
Synatomic knee
synthetic
TACK (Translating and Congruent [Mobile-Bearing] Knee) implant

prosthesis *(continued)*
    talar part of ankle
    Taperloc femoral
    TARA (total articular replacement arthroplasty) hip
    Tavernetti-Tennant
    TCCK unconstrained knee
    Thackray hip
    Tharies hip replacement
    thermomechanical implant metal
    Thompson femoral neck
    Thompson hip
    threaded titanium acetabular (TTAP)
    Thurst plate femoral
    Ti-BAC II hip
    tibial part of ankle
    tibial plateau
    Ti-Con
    Tilastin hip
    Tillman
    Titan cemented hip
    titanium hip
    titanium implant
    TMJ fossa-eminence
    TORP (total ossicular replacement)
    Total Condylar Knee
    Total Condylar semiconstrained tricompartmental
    total hip replacement
    total joint replacement
    total knee replacement
    Total Rotating Knee (TRK) mobile-bearing
    Townley TARA
    TPR ankle
    Trac II knee
    trapezium implant
    Trapezoidal-28 hip
    Triad hip
    trial
    Tri-Axial
    triaxial semiconstrained elbow
    tricompartmental knee
    Tricon-M patellar
    Tri-Lock
    TR-28 hip
    TTAP-ST acetabular

prosthesis *(continued)*
    two-prong stem finger
    UCI ankle
    UHMWPE (ultrahigh molecular weight polyethylene)
    ulnar head implant
    unconstrained tricompartmental knee
    unicompartmental knee
    Universal hip
    UPF (universal proximal femur)
    Valls hip
    Vanghetti
    Varikopf
    Vinertia implant metal
    Vitallium-W implant metal
    Vocare neuroprosthetic bladder system
    Volz wrist
    Wada valve
    Wadsworth unconstrained elbow
    Wagner
    Wall stent biliary endoprosthesis
    Walldius knee
    Waugh total ankle replacement
    Wayfarer modifiable foot
    Weaveknit vascular
    Wehrs incus
    Weil-type Swanson-design hammertoe implant
    well-seated
    Whiteside knee
    Whiteside Ortholoc II condylar femoral
    William Harris hip
    Wilson-Burstein (DF80) hip
    Wright titanium
    wrist joint implant
    wrought cobalt-chromium alloy
    Xenophor femoral
    YIS knee
    Young hinged knee
    Young-Vitallium hinged
    Zimalite implant metal
    Zimaloy implant metal
    Zimmer
    Ziramic femoral head

prosthesis *(continued)*
  Zirconia femoral head
  Zirconia orthopedic
  zirconium oxide ceramic
  Z stent
  ZTT I and ZTT II acetabular cups
  Zweymuller cementless hip
prosthesis cup
prosthesis dehiscence
prosthesis of antibiotic-loaded acrylic
  cement (PROSTALAC)
prosthetic articulation
Prosthetic Disc Nucleus (PDN)
prosthetic femorodistal graft
prosthetic fixation
prosthetic hook
Prosthetic Problem Inventory Scale
prosthetics and orthotics (P&O)
prosthetic sheath/liner, Silipos Distal
  Dip
prosthetic support
prosthetist
Protasul implant metal
ProtectaCap
protection, radiologic
  adequate collimation
  filtration
  gonadal shielding
protective knee guard (PKG)
protective limitation of range of
  motion
protective spasm
protective weightbearing
protector
  Adson drill guide and dura
  Adson dural
  Alvarado collateral ligament
  Ankle Ligament (ALP)
  collateral ligament
  dural
  grooved
  heel
  Heelbo decubitus heel/elbow
  M-F Athletic heel
  Ortho-Foam
  PRN

protector *(continued)*
  self-retaining
  tissue
Pro-Tec support
Protector meniscus suturing system
Protecto splint
Protect Point needle
protein
  amyloid precursor
  antiglial fibrillary acidic
  APP (platelet amyloid precursor
    protein)
  Bence Jones
  bone morphogenetic
  COMP (cartilage oligomeric
    matrix protein)
  C-reactive (CRP)
  EMBP (estramustine binding
    protein)
  Endostatin
  enhanced green fluorescent
  ENP (extractable nucleoprotein)
  GFAP (glial fibrillary acidic
    protein)
  heat-shock
  natural antiangiogenic protein
  neuron-specific
  oncoprotein
  p-glycoprotein
  S-100
  sialoprotein
  viral envelope
  voltage-gated calcium channel
    (VGCC)
proteinase-K extraction method
protein C (functional)
protein kinase C
protein marker for Alzheimer
  A68
  ALZ-50
protein monomers of fibrillin (FBN1)
protein S deficiency
protein truncation test (PTT)
proteoglycan, disk matrix
proteoglycan gel of nucleus pulposus
proteolysis

proteolytic enzymes
Proteus syndrome
prothrombic state
protocol
  Bruce
  IDE
  Madden dynamic splint
  Marx osteoradionecrosis
  telomere repeat amplification
  Walsh
proton
Protoplast cement
Protouch synthetic orthopedic padding
Pro-Trac cruciate reconstruction system
Pro-Trac measurement device
Pro-Trac system for knee surgery
protrusion
  disk
  hip
  navicular   *protrusio*
  spicular   *acetabuli*
protrusio shill
protuberance, occipital
protuberans, enchondroma
proud flesh
proud graft
proverb interpretation testing
  abstract responses
  concrete responses
  semi-abstract responses
Provigil (modafinil)
provocative diskography
provocative maneuvers
provocative test for epilepsy
prow effect
proximal anterior tibial artery
proximal articular set angle (PASA)
proximal bow position
proximal carpal row
proximal denervation
proximal-end tibia fracture
proximal femoral focal deficiency
proximal first metatarsal osteotomy
proximal focal femoral deficiency
  (PFFD)
proximal interphalangeal (PIP) joint
proximally

proximal phalangeal osteotomy
proximal phalanx, duplicated
proximal phocomelia
proximal popliteal artery
proximal radioulnar articulation
proximal radioulnar joint
proximal row carpectomy (PRC)
proximal tibiofibular joint
proximal weakness
Prozac (fluoxetine hydrochloride)
PRS (Photon Radiosurgery System)
Pruitt-Inahara shunt
psammoma body
psammomatous meningiomas
PSA (power spectral analysis) thermoplastic orthosis
PSE (portal-systemic encephalopathy)
pseudarthrosis
  ball-and-socket giant
  congenital
  Girdlestone
  interspinous
pseudoachondroplasia
pseudoaddiction
pseudoaneurysm
pseudo-Argyll Robertson pupil
pseudoarthrosis (see *pseudarthrosis*)
pseudoathetosis
pseudo-Babinski sign in poliomyelitis
pseudobulbar affect
pseudobulbar palsy
pseudobulbar paralysis
pseudobulbar signs
pseudocapsule
pseudocapsulectomy
pseudocholinesterase syndrome
pseudoclaudication
pseudocoma
pseudocortex
pseudodementia, hysterical
pseudodislocation
pseudodura
pseudodynamic imaging
pseudoepileptogenic pattern
pseudoepiphysis
pseudofacilitation
pseudo-Foster-Kennedy sign

pseudo-Foster-Kennedy syndrome
pseudofracture artifact
pseudoglenoid
pseudogout
pseudo-Hurler deformity
pseudohypertrophic dystrophy
pseudohypertrophic musculature
pseudohypertrophy of calves
pseudohypoparathyroidism
pseudo-internuclear ophthalmoplegia
pseudojoints
pseudoluxation
pseudomalignant, non-neoplastic
    osseous soft tissue tumors
pseudomeningocele
pseudomigraine
Pseudomonas aeruginosa osteomyelitis
pseudomotor (cf. *sudomotor*)
pseudomyasthenic symptom
pseudomyotonia, Debré-Sémélaigne
pseudomyotonic reflex
pseudonephritis, athlete's
pseudoneurasthenic syndrome
pseudoneuroma
pseudo-orbital tumor
pseudopapilledema
pseudophlebitis syndrome
pseudopollicization
pseudosclerosis, spastic
pseudoseizure
pseudosheath
pseudosubluxation
pseudotabes, diabetic
pseudothrombophlebitis
pseudotumor cerebri (PTC)
pseudotumor, orbital
pseudoxanthoma elasticum
PSF (posterior spinal fusion)
PSH-25GT transcranial imaging trans-
    ducer
PSI (Predictive Salvage Index)
psittacosis encephalitis
psittacosis viral encephalitis
P6 acupressure point
psoriatic arthritis
psoriatic onychopachydermoperiostitis
psoas abscess

psoas muscle
PSP (postsynaptic potential)
PSP (progressive supranuclear palsy)
psyche, tumor
psychiatry, rehabilitation (RP)
psychic disturbance
psychic equivalent
psychic seizure
psychogenic amnesia
psychogenic hyperventilation
psychogenic rheumatism
psychogenic seizure
psychogenic tremor
psychogenic unresponsiveness
psychogenic vertigo
psychometric testing
psychomotor activity
psychomotor attacks
psychomotor epilepsy
psychomotor fit
psychomotor phenomena
psychomotor retardation
psychomotor seizure
psychomotor slowing
psychomotor symptom
psychomotor variant of epilepsy
psycho-optical reflex controls
psychosensory aphasia
psychosensory stimuli
psychosensory symptom
psychosis
    Korsakoff
    levodopa-induced
PT (physical therapy)
PT (prothrombin time)
PTA (post-traumatic amnesia)
PTB (patellar tendon-bearing) ankle-
    foot orthosis
PTB brace
PTB-SC-SP prosthesis
PTB supracondylar (SC) prosthesis
PTB suprapatellar (SP) prosthesis
PTC (pseudotumor cerebri)
PtcO$_2$ (transcutaneous oxygen)
pterion
pterional approach
pterional craniotomy

pterygoid bone
pterygoid canal
pterygoid muscle
pterygoid nerve
pterygoid notch
pterygomandibular ligament
pterygopalatine neuralgia
pterygopalatine nerves
pterygospinal ligament
PTFE (polytetrafluoroethylene) graft
PTF (posterior talofibular) ligament
P-3 suture
P-31 magnetic resonance spectroscopy
P300 latency, potential
P300 test for dementia
ptosis
    bilateral
    ipsilateral
    myasthenic
    unilateral
    upside-down
ptosis of eyelid
ptosis of third nerve paresis
    complete
    partial
PTS (patellar tendon stabilization)
PTS (Posture Training Support)
PTS soft wedge prosthesis
PTT (partial thromboplastin time)
PTT (patellar tendon transfer)
PTT (protein truncation test)
PTTD (posterior tibial tendon
    dysfunction)
PTTT (posterior tibialis tendon
    transfer)
PTV (posterior terminal vein)
P-type (persistent) alpha rhythm
puberty, precocious
pubic bone
pubic nonunion
pubic ramus (pl. rami)
pubic symphysis
pubic tubercle
pubis
    ramus of
    symphysis
pubocapsular ligament

pubocervical ligament
pubococcygeal line
pubococcygeal muscle
pubofemoral ligament
puboischial area
puboprostatic ligament
puboprostatic muscle
puborectal muscle
pubovaginal muscle
pubovesical ligament
pubovesical muscle
Puddu tendon technique
Puddu x-ray view of knee
pudendal nerve
pudendal neurogram
Pudenz flushing chamber
Pudenz peritoneal catheter
Pudenz shunt
Pugh plate
Pugh sliding nail
Pugh traction
pudic nerve
puerperal hemiplegia
Puka chisel
puller
    CNS pin and wire
    Miltex pin
pulley
    annular
    A1-A5
    cruciate
pulley exercises
pulley of fingers
pullout technique
Pulmonair 40-bed
pulmonary embolism (PE)
pulmonary ligament
pulmonary parenchymal window
pulp
    finger
    thumb
pulpiform nucleus forceps
pulposus
    nucleus
    proteoglycan gel of nucleus
pulp-plasty
pulp space

pulsatile exophthalmos
pulsatile lavage
pulsatile tinnitus
pulsation
Pulsavac lavage
Pulsavac III wound debridement
    system
pulse (pl. pulses)
    carotid
    dorsalis pedis
    EEG calibration
    posterior tibial
    radiofrequency
pulsed electromagnetic field (PEMF)
    stimulation
pulsed-field gel electrophoresis
pulsed gradients
pulsed low-intensity ultrasound
pulsed ultrasound
pulse generator, NeuroCybernetic
    Prosthesis
pulse lavage irrigation
pulse lavage system
pulse length
pulseless disease
pulseless electrical activity (PEA)
PULSES disability profile
    P   physical condition
    U   upper extremity function
    L   lower extremity function
    S   sensory and communication
        abilities
    E   excretory control
    S   social support
pulse sequences
pulse volume waveforms
pulse width
pulsing current (electrostimulation) for
    nonunion of fracture
Pulver-Taft fish-mouth stitch
Pulver-Taft weave
pulvinar region
pumice stone
pump
    ankle
    antithrombotic
    arthroscopic

pump *(continued)*
    calf muscle (anatomical)
    cement
    IES PowerPump
    Infusaid continuous flow drug
    intermittent compression
        (mechanical)
    intrathecal infusion
    intrathecal morphine
    Jobst antithrombotic
    knee
    Medtronic programmable drug
    pneumatic foot (mechanical)
    pressure-controlled roller
    programmable drug
    Secor drug (I or II)
    Servo
    Synchromed programmable drug
    Therex programmable drug
    Vacu-Mix cement
    venous
pump bump (retrocalcaneal exostosis)
pump standby
punch
    Acufex rotary
    bone
    bone graft
    boxer's (fracture of the fifth
        metacarpal)
    Caspari suture
    cervical laminectomy
    Charnley femoral prosthesis neck
    Cone skull
    disk
    dural
    DyoVac suction
    Hajek-Koffler
    Hajek laminectomy
    Hardy sellar
    Hirsch hypophyseal
    intervertebral disk
    Kerrison
    laminectomy
    Raney laminectomy
    Rhoton sellar
    rotary basket
    Rowe glenoid

punch *(continued)*
   Sauerbruch-Frey bone
   Schlesinger
   sellar
   skull
   suture
   tibial
   tubular
   Yankauer
punch-drunk syndrome of boxers
punch forceps
puncta dolorosa of Valleix (trigeminal
   neuralgia)
puncture
   bloody lumbar
   cisternal
   dry lumbar
   dural
   intraventricular
   lumbar (LP) (spinal tap)
   opening pressure on lumbar
   stereotactic
   traumatic lumbar
puncture fracture
puncture wound (types I-IV)
puncture-wound osteochondritis
pupil (pl. pupils)
   Adie
   Adie-Holmes
   Adie tonic
   Argyll-Robertson
   bilaterally dilated
   bilaterally fixed and dilated
   blown
   briskly reactive
   consensual response
   corn-picker's
   curtsying
   dilated
   dilated and fixed
   fixed
   Holmes-Adie
   Hutchinson
   inequality of
   inverse Argyll Robertson
   isocoric
   light reaction of opposite

pupil *(continued)*
   Marcus Gunn
   midposition
   moderately dilated
   myotonic
   pinpoint
   poorly reactive
   pseudo-Argyll Robertson
   reactive
   reactivity of
   sluggishly reactive
   tonic
   tonically dilated
   tonohaptic reaction of
   unequal
   unilaterally fixed and dilated
pupil check
pupillary areflexia
pupillary change
pupillary constriction
pupillary dilatation
pupillary escape
pupillary light reaction
pupillary light response
pupillary near-reflex
pupillary reaction
pupillary reflex
pupillary response
pupillary sign
pupillary-skin or ciliary reflex
pupillometric signs of brain activation
pupillomotor fibers
pupils nonreactive to light
pupils nonresponsive to light
pupils responsive to light
pupils unreactive to light
pupils unresponsive to light
purchase, bicortical
Purdue Pegboard Test
pure athetoid palsy
pure autonomic failure
pure hemisensory stroke
pure limb apraxia
pure motor hemiplegia
pure sensory stroke
pure spastic palsy
pure-tone threshold

pure word deafness
purine-free diet
Purkinje cells of cerebellum
purse-string closure (or pursestring)
pursuit movements, visual
purulent drainage
purulent material
purulent meningitis
pus, puric
pusher
    Charnley femoral prosthesis
    femoral
    femoral component
    femoral prosthesis
    Jacobson suture
    knot
    suture
    trochanter position
    trochanteric
push-off by great toe
push-off during walking
push-off of the foot in gait
push-off phase of gait
push-off strength
push-off velocity
push-pull tip coagulator
putamen
    medial
    posterior
putaminal hemorrhage, nondominant
putative effect
putative factors
Putnam-Dana syndrome
Putti arthrodesis
Putti bone plast
Putti bone rasp
Putti-Platt arthroplasty
Putti-Platt shoulder procedure
putty, BeOK hand exercise
PVA (polyvinyl alcohol) splinting
    material
PVA strip
PVB (pigmented villonodular bursitis)
PVG (periventricular gray) matter

PVS (persistent vegetative state)
PVS (pigmented villonodular synovitis)
PWB (Puno-Winter-Byrd)
PWB awl
PWB fixation system
PWB rod
PWB screw
pyarthrosis
pyencephalus
pygalgia
pyknodysostosis
pyknoepilepsy
pyknolepsy
pyknomorphous
pyknophrasia
pylon attachment plate
pylon, metal
pyloric sphincter muscle
pyocephalus
pyoderma gangrenosum
pyogenic arthritis
pyogenic granuloma
pyogenic meningitis
pyogenic spondylitis
pyoventricle
PYR (person years at risk)
pyramid, petrous
pyramidal auricular muscle
pyramidal bone
pyramidal cell
pyramidal fracture
pyramidal layer of cerebral cortex
pyramidal lobe
pyramidal neurons
pyramidal sign
pyramidal tract
pyramis
pyranocarboxylic acid class
pyridinoline test
pyridoxine dependency
pyriform (see *piriform*)
Pyrilinks-D assay
Pyrost bone graft material
pyruvate dehydrogenase stimulator

Q, q

Q angle test
QALYs (Quality Adjusted Life Years)
QCT (quantitative computed tomography) test for bone loss
QDR-1500 or QDR-2000 bone densitometer
QEEG (quantitative electroencephalogram)
qi (Chi) (Chinese medicine term)
Qiaex gel extraction kit
qi deficiency (Chinese medicine term)
qi gong therapy (Chinese medicine term)
qi stagnation (Chinese medicine term)
QL Index
QTR (quadriceps tendon rupture)
quad cane
quad (quadriceps) sets
Quadramet (samarium Sm 153 lexidronam)
quadrangle cartilage
quadrangular positioning plate
quadrangular space
quadrant of death (anterosuperior quadrant of hip)
quadrant on EEG
quadrant-position test
Quadrant shoulder brace

quadrantanopia
quadrantanopsia
    contralateral homonymous inferior
    contralateral homonymous superior
    homonymous
quadrantic hemianopia
quadrapod cane
quadrate gyrus
quadrate ligament of Denuce
quadrate muscle
quadrature detector
quadratus femoris muscle
quadratus fascia
quadratus, pronator
quadriceps apron
quadriceps De Lorme boot
quadriceps graft
quadriceps mechanism
quadriceps muscle
quadricepsplasty
    Thompson
    V-Y
quadriceps retinaculum
quadriceps, short arc
quadriceps stretch reflex
quadriceps tendon rupture (QTR)
quadriceps torque
quadriceps wasting

quadrigeminal plate
quadrilateral brim
quadrilateral space of Marie
quadriparesis, spastic
quadriparetic
quadriphasic wave
quadriplegia
  high level
  spastic
  traumatic
Quality Adjusted Life Years (QALYs)
quality factor
quality of gait
quality of life assessment
Quality of Well-Being Scale
QUANTAP computerized questionnaire
quantitative computed tomography
  (QCT)
quantitative electroencephalogram
  (QEEG)
Quantum foot
quarter (part of shoe)
quartet, digital flexor tendon
Quartet sleep apnea system
quasipurposive movement
quaver, nystagmoid
Quebec Back Pain Disability Scale
Queckenstedt sign
Queckenstedt test
quenching
Quengel cast
Quengel hinge
Quenu nail-plate removal technique
Quervain disease (see *de Quervain*)
Quervain fracture (see *de Quervain*)
questionnaire, Questionnaire (see also
   assessment, index, scale, score)
  AAOS/HKOD
  AAOS POI (American Academy
    of Orthopedic Surgeons Pedi-
    atrics Outcomes Instrument)
  AIMS II
  Beck
  Behavioral Risk Factor Surveillance
    System (BRFSS)

questionnaire *(continued)*
  Campbell
  CFQ (Child Health Questionnaire)
  Chesworth Functional Index
  Child Health Questionnaire PF-50
  cognitive failures (CFQ)
  CSQ (Coping Strategies Question-
    naire)
  Disabilities of Arm, Shoulder and
    Hand
  Dutch Vocational Handicap
  Euroqol
  everyday memory
  FAB (Fear Avoidance Behavior)
  FIQ (Fibromyalgia Impact
    Questionnaire)
  Foot Function Index
  Foot Health Status
  Fracture Intervention Trial (FIT)
  Frank Noyes function
  Functional Status (FSQ)
  General Health (GHQ)
  Health and Labor
  Health Assessment (HAQ)
  Health Assessment Questionnaire
    for Spondyloarthropathies
    (HAQ-S)
  IKDC (International Knee Docu-
    mentation Committee)
  International Knee Ligament
    Standard Evaluation
  ISOA
  Johns Hopkins National Low Back
    Pain Study
  Kenny Self-Care
  Lambeth Disability Screening
  Levine
  LISREL
  MACTAR
  McGill Pain (MPQ)
  McMaster Health Index
  mental status
  Michigan Hand Outcomes
  Modified Health Assessment
    (MHAQ)
  MSTS/ISOLS

questionnaire *(continued)*
   Musculoskeletal Outcomes Data
      Evaluation and Management
      System (MODEMS) spine
      outcomes
   Noyes function
   OKQ (Osteoporosis Knowledge
      Questionnaire)
   quality of life
   QUANTAP computerized
   Oswestry Low Back Pain Disability
   Radiographs Outcomes Data
      Collection
   Rosenstiel Coping
   SF-36 (Short-Form 36 Health
      Survey)
   Short Form-12 general health
      survey
   Sleep Habits (SHQ)
   Speech

questionnaire *(continued)*
   Toronto Functional Capacity (TFCQ)
   Tremor Disability
   Varni Pediatric Pain
   Ways of Coping Checklist
   WOMAC (Western Ontario and
      McMaster)
   WOSI (Western Ontario Instability
      Index)
Questus Leading Edge instruments/
   devices
quetiapine fumarate (Seroquel)
quiescence
quiescent
Quiet interference screw
Quigley traction
Quincke lumbar puncture needle
quiritarian epilepsy
QUS-2 calcaneal ultrasonometer

R, r

RA (rheumatoid arthritis) factor
RAB (remote afterloading brachy-
    therapy)
rabies (hydrophobia)
rabies viral encephalitis
Rabiner neurological hammer
Rabot disease
raccoon eyes sign (periorbital
    ecchymosis)
rachialgia
rachicentesis
rachiocampsis
rachiochysis
rachiodynia
rachiokyphosis
rachiomyelitis
rachioparalysis
rachiopathy
rachioplegia
rachioscoliosis
rachiotomy
rachisagra
rachischisis
rachitic rosary sign
rachitic scoliosis
rachitomy
    Capener
    decompression

rack, bow boring
racquetball
RADAR (Rapid Assessment of Dis-
    ease Activity in Rheumatology)
radial bone
radial bursa
radial club hand
radial collateral ligament
radial deviation
radial drift
radial epiphyseal displacement
radial extensors
radial facing of metacarpal heads
radial flexor muscle
radial forearm flap
radial head dislocation
radial head fracture
radial head subluxation (RHS)
radialis sign
radialized
radial metacarpal ligament
radial nerve palsy
radial nerve paresis
radial notch
Radial Osteo Compression (ROC)
    soft tissue anchor
radial polydactyly
radial ray defect

radial recession osteotomy
radial styloid process fracture
radial synovial recess
radial trio
radial tuberosity
radial tunnel syndrome
radian
radiata, corona
radiate sternocostal ligament
radiating "burner" down an extremity
  (paresthesia)
radiation
  adjuvant
  auditory
  myelopathy
  neutron capture
  optic
  whole-brain
  visual
radiation edema
radiation of pain
radiation osteonecrosis
radical extirpation
radical nail-bed ablation
radicals, free
radicotomy
radicular compression
radicular neural deficits
radicular neuropathy, familial sensory
radicular pain
radicular symptom
radicular syndrome
radicular vessel
radiculectomy
radiculitis
  cervical
  manual traction test for cervical
radiculomedullary artery
radiculoneuritis
radiculopathy
  compressive cervical
  lumbar
  lumbosacral
  radiation-induced
  S1
  spondylitic caudal
  spondylotic

radiculospinal artery
radioactive sequencing
radioactive xenon clearance
radiocapitellar joint
radiocapitellar line
radiocarpal angle
radiocarpal articulation
radiocarpal dislocation
radiocarpal joint
radiocarpal ligament
radiocarpal portal
radioccipital
radiofrequency (RF)
radiofrequency arthroscopic tool
radiofrequency coil
radiofrequency pulse
radiogram, radiograph
  oblique
  plain film
  soft tissue
  stress
  tilted lateral
  weightbearing
radiographically firm synostosis
Radiographs Outcomes Data
  Collection Questionnaire
radiography
  high resolution, low speed
  upright skeletal
  Yochum chiropractic
radiohumeral articulation
radioimmunoassay (RIA)
radioimmunoassay of cerebrospinal
  fluid
radioiodinated serum albumin (RISA)
radioisotope cisternography
radioisotope clearance assay
radioisotope (static) scanning
radioisotope uptake
radiolabeled fibrinogen technique
Radiological Society of North America
  (RSNA)
radiologic protection
  adequate collimation
  filtration
  gonadal shielding
radiology, interventional

radiolucency
radiolucent area
radiolucent hand table
radiolucent spine frame
RadioLucent wrist fixation system
radiolunate joint
radiolunotriquetral ligament
radiomuscular
radionecrosis, cerebral
Radionics CRW stereotactic head
  frame
Radionics fiducial localizer
Radionics radiofrequency electrode
Radionics stereotactic frame
radionuclide blood flow (dynamic)
  studies
radionuclide cisternography, Katzman
  infusion of
radionuclide flow scan
radionuclide, HMPAO (hexamethyl
  propylene amine oxime)
radiopaque
radioresistant
radioscaphocapitate ligament
radioscaphoid joint
radioscaphoid ligament
radioscapholunate ligament
radioscintigraphy
radiosensitive
radiosensitivity
radiostyloid process
radiosurgery
  Bragg peak
  charged particle
  dynamic stereotactic
  Gamma Knife
  heavy charged particle Bragg peak
  helium-ion particle beam
  interstitial
  LINAC (linear accelerator)
  linear accelerator
  multiarc LINAC
  stereotactic or stereotaxic
radiosurgical corpus callostomy
radiosurgically
radiosynovectomy
radiotelemetry EEG

radiotherapy
  fractionated
  fractionated external beam
  hyperfractionated
  neuroaxis
  palliative
radioulnar articulation
radioulnar joint
radioulnar subluxation
radioulnar surface
radioulnar synostosis
radiowave tracking system
radius
radius inclination
radius length
radius tilt
radius width
Radley-Liebig-Brown resection
Radolf nail-pulling forceps
Raeder paratrigeminal syndrome
RA (rheumatoid arthritis) factor
ragged red fibers (RRFs)
Ragnell handheld retractor
RAI (Ritchie Articular Index)
RAI (Rivermead ADL Index)
rail, Lumex Tub-Guard safety
railroading of tendon
railroad track pattern
railway (physiological) nystagmus
Raimiste sign
Raimondi infant scalp hemostatic
  forceps
Raimondi spring peritoneal catheter
Raimondi ventricular catheter
Rainbow cast sandal
Rainin clip-bending spatula
raised and padded toilet seat
raised intracranial pressure
raising
  crossed straight leg
  straight leg (SLR)
rake, Israel
rales and rhonchi
Ralk hand drill
Ralks mallet
Ralston-Thompson pseudarthrosis
  technique

RAM (rapid-alternating movements)
  knee prosthesis
rami of lateral sulcus
ramp
  folded step
  half-pipe snow
  Mini-Ramp
  Porta-Deck
Ramsay Hunt cerebellar myoclonic
  dyssynergia
Ramsay Hunt progressive cerebellar
  tremor
Ramsay Hunt syndrome
Ramsay Hunt type of inherited
  dentatorubral degeneration
ramus (pl. rami)
  dorsal
  dorsal primary
  inferior
  inferior pubic
  ischiopubic
  pubic
  superior
  ventral
  ventral primary
Ranawat-Burstein hip prosthesis
Ranawat-DeFiore-Straub technique
Rancho cube
Rancho fixation system
Rancho mounting technique for
  Ilizarov apparatus
Rancho pin-gripper cube
Rancho swivel hinge
Rancho system modification of
  Ilizarov external fixation
Rancho trocar-drill sleeve
Rancho-type anklet foot control device
Rand Functional Limitations Battery
Rand microballoon
Rand Physical Capacities Battery
Rand Social Health Battery
randomized clinical trial (RCT)
random letter test
Raney clip-applying forceps
Raney coagulating forceps
Raney cranial drill
Raney-Crutchfield drill point

Raney-Crutchfield skull tongs
Raney forceps
Raney hemostatic clip
Raney laminectomy punch
Raney laminectomy rongeur
Raney perforator drills
Raney rongeur forceps
Raney saw guide
Raney scalp clip-applying forceps
Raney stirrup-loop curet
range
  alpha frequency
  delta frequency
  frequency
  theta frequency
range of excursion
range of flexion and extension
range of motion (ROM)
  active (AROM)
  active and passive
  active-assisted
  passive
  restricted
range of motion therapy
Ranke angle
Ranke complex
Rankin Scale
Ransford loop
Ranvier groove
Ranvier node
Ranvier segment
raphe nucleus of midbrain
raphe
  tendinous
  ventral median
rapid-alternating movements (RAM)
Rapid Assessment of Disease Activity
  in Rheumatology (RADAR)
Rapide suture
rapid eye movement (REM) sleep
rapid onset dystonia-parkinsonism
rapid saccades
RapiScan roadside saliva drug test
Rappaport Disability Rating Scale
raptus of attention
rarefaction, fluffy
rarefaction of cortex

RAS (reticular activating system)
Rascal scooter
Rasch analysis
rash
    dermatomal
    discoid
    heliotrope
    macular
Rasmussen encephalitis
Rasmussen syndrome
rasp, raspatory
    Acufex
    Acufex convex
    Alexander
    Alexander-Farabeuf
    angled
    Aufricht glabellar
    Austin Moore
    Bacon
    Bardeleben
    Black
    Bristow
    Brown
    carbon-tungsten
    Charnley
    convex
    Coryllos
    costal
    Cottle-MacKenty
    DePuy
    diamond
    Doyen costal
    Doyen rib
    Endotrac
    Epstein bone
    Farabeuf
    Farabeuf bone
    Farabeuf-Collin
    Farabeau-Lambotte
    Filtzer interbody
    Fisher
    Fomon
    Gallaher
    glabellar
    Good
    Herczel
    Herczel rib

rasp *(continued)*
    Hylin
    interbody
    intramedullary
    Israel
    Jansen
    Key
    Kirmission periosteal
    Kleinert-Kutz
    Koenig
    Lambotte
    Langenbeck
    Lewis
    Lewis periosteal
    Mallory-Head
    Maltz
    Mathieu
    McCabe-Farrior
    McKenty
    micro
    Miller
    Nicoll
    Nicola
    Olivecrona
    Phemister
    Plenk-Matson
    power
    Putti bone
    rib
    Rubin
    Schneider
    Schneider-Sauerbruch
    Seawell
    Semb rib
    Thompson
    Yasargil micro
    Zoellner
RAT (right anterior temporal) EEG
    lead
ratchet, bone graft T-handle
ratchet knot
ratchet spanner
ratchet syndrome
rate
    alternating motion (AMR)
    click stimulus
    sed (sedimentation)

rate and rhythm of breathing
Rathke cleft cyst
Rathke pouch
rating
  SANE (Single Assessment Numeric
    Evaluation)
  Single Assessment Numeric
    Evaluation (SANE)
  UCLA (University of California at
    Los Angeles) activity
rating scale
rating system, Iowa hip status
ratio
  ankle-brachial pressure
  arch height
  brain-to-background
  C/N (contrast-to-noise)
  carpal interval
  CBV/CBF
  cerebral blood volume/cerebral
    blood flow
  choline/creatine (Cho/Cr)
  contrast-to-noise (C/N)
  dome-to-neck
  FL/AC (femur length to abdominal
    circumference)
  glutamine/glutamate/creatine
  gray/white matter activity
  gyromagnetic
  hamstring/quadriceps torque
  HC/AC (head circumference to
    abdominal circumference)
  Holdaway
  Insall patella alta
  Insall-Salvati
  international normalized (INR)
  lesion-to-muscle
  lesion-to-nonlesion count
  maximum diameter to minimum
    diameter
  metatarsal length
  MMP-1/TIMP-1 (matrix metallo-
    proteinase-1 to tissue inhibitor
    of metalloproteinase-1 (TIMP-1)
  myoinositol/creatine (Myo/Cr)

ratio *(continued)*
  P:A (peroneal to anterior compart-
    ment)
  patellar ligament-patellar
  Poisson
  recruitment
  serum glucose:CSF glucose
  signal-to-noise
  TME (trapezium-metacarpal
    eburnation)
  tumor-to-normal brain
ratio scales in rehabilitation testing
Ratliff classification of avascular
  necrosis
Rau, apophysis of
Rauchfuss sling
ray (pl. rays)
  central
  digital
  hypermobile first
  long axis
  pollicized
ray amputation
Ray brain spatula spoon
Rayleigh scattering law
Raymond-Céstan syndrome
Raymond shoulder immobilizer
Raynaud disease
Raynaud phenomenon
  bilateral
  unilateral
Raynaud syndrome
Ray-Parsons-Sunday staphylorrhaphy
  elevator
Ray pituitary curet
Rayport dural dissector and knife
Rayport muscle biopsy clamp
ray resection
Ray-Tec sponge
Ray TFC (threaded fusion cage)
Ray ventricular cannula
RBC protein band 4.1
rBPI-21 (Neuprex)
RC (rehabilitation counseling)
RCA (retained cortical activity)

RCA (*Ricinus communis* agglutinin 1) antibody
RCA lectins
RCB (Rotator Cuff Buttress)
rCBF (regional cerebral blood flow) PET scan
rCBV (regional cerebral blood volume) PET scan
RCC (Rathke cleft cyst)
RCI titanium soft tissue interference screw
RC Mini-Open lighted retractor
rCMRO$_2$ (regional cerebral metabolic rate for oxygen)
rCPP (regional cerebral perfusion pressure)
RCT (randomized clinical trial)
RCT (retinocortical time)
rCVR (regional cerebral vasoreactivity)
RDF (registered deafness specialist)
RE (rehabilitation engineering)
reabsorption, bony
Reach Easy massager
re-arthroscoped
ReAct neuromuscular stimulator
reaction
  acute exogenous
  catastrophic
  cell-mediated
  doll's eye
  equilibrium
  groping
  hypersensitivity
  hysterical conversion
  id
  immune-mediated systemic
  Jarisch-Herxheimer
  lamellar
  light
  magnetic
  migrainous
  migrainoid
  PCR (polymerase chain reaction)
  periosteal
  pupillary
  pupillary light

reaction *(continued)*
  synovial inflammatory
  tonohaptic
  tyramine
  Weil-Felix
reactive disease of smooth muscle
reactive pupils
reactivity of pupils
Read gouge
reading comprehension impairment
reading epilepsy
reading impairment
readout delay
realign
realignment
  joint surface
  patellofemoral
real strabismus
ream
reamed and rasped
reamed, sequentially
reamer
  acetabular
  Anspach
  Arthrex coring
  Aufranc
  Austin Moore
  ball
  barrel
  blunt tapered T-handled
  bone
  brace-type
  calcar
  Campbell
  cannulated Henderson
  chamfer
  Charnley
  Charnley deepening
  Charnley expanding
  Charnley taper
  Charnley trochanter
  Christmas tree
  congruous cup-shaped
  conical
  corrugated
  cup
  deepening

reamer *(continued)*
 DePuy
 expanding
 female
 femoral shaft
 fenestrated
 flexible medullary
 grater
 Gray
 grooving
 Hall Versipower
 handle-type
 Harris center-cutting acetabular
 hemispherical
 hollow mill
 Indiana
 Intracone intramedullary
 intramedullary
 Küntscher intramedullary
 male
 Marin
 medullary canal
 Micro-Aire
 Mira
 Moore bone
 multisized
 Norton ball
 Perthes
 power
 power-driven
 progressively larger
 Richards
 rigid
 Rotalink flexible-shaft
 Rush awl
 self-centering
 Smith-Petersen
 spherical
 spiral cortical
 spiral trochanteric
 square
 starting
 step-cut
 straight
 Swanson
 T-handled
 tapered

reamer *(continued)*
 tapered hand
 triangular bone
 trochanter
 trochanteric
 Wagner acetabular
reaming awl
reanastomosis
reapproximation
rearfoot eversion
rearfoot pronation
rearfoot striker
rearfoot varus
Rebel knee orthosis
Rebif (recombinant interferon beta-1a)
rebleeding of aneurysm
recalcitrance of syndromes
recalcitrant pain
recall of events
recall of information
recanalization, angiographic
receiver coil
recent memory
recentralization, tendon
receptive aphasia
receptive aphasic disorder or impairment
receptive language
receptor
 acetylcholine (ACh)
 dopaminergic
 ETA
 ETB
 ETB1
 ETB2
 Krause sensory
 Meissner corpuscle sensory
 Merkel disc sensory
 pacinian corpuscle sensory
 postsynaptic dopamine
 Ruffini corpuscle sensory
receptor site
recess
 accessory
 acetabular
 attic
 central

recess *(continued)*
    cerebellopontine
    costodiaphragmatic
    costomediastinal
    dorsal proximal synovial
    infraglenoid
    lateral
    popliteal
    prestyloid
    radial synovial
    sacciform
    subscapularis
    triangular
    ulnar synovial
    volar synovial
recessive dystrophic epidermolysis
    bullosa
recheck
recipient team
reciprocal agonist-antagonist relaxation
Reciprocal Coordination Test
reciprocal loading pattern
reciprocally innervated
reciprocating gait orthosis (RGO)
reciprocating saw
Reci-Vacette
Recklinghausen disease of bone
recombinant hirudin
recombinant human bone morpho-
    genetic protein (rhBMP)
recombinant human bone morpho-
    genetic protein-2 (rhBMP-2)
recombinant human interferon-a2a
    (rhIFN-a2a)
recombinant interferon beta-1a (Rebif)
recombinant prourokinase
recombinant tissue plasminogen
    activator (alteplase)
recombinant tissue-type plasminogen
    activator (rt-PA)
reconstruction (see *operations*)
reconstructive surgery
record, recording
    all-night sleep
    ambulatory EEG
    artifact-free
    bipolar EEG

record *(continued)*
    cassette EEG
    clinical EEG
    ear reference EEG
    electroencephalographic (EEG)
    electromyographic (EMG)
    epidural pressure
    evoked potential
    flat (isoelectric) EEG
    intraoperative microelectrode
    microelectrode
    multichannel EEG
    neonatal EEG
    referential EEG
    scalp EEG
    serial EEG
    single-unit microelectrode
    waking baseline
recording channel
recovery, functional
Recovery Locus of Control
recrudescence
recruiting response
recruitment of motor unit potential
recruitment pattern
recruitment ratio
recruitment spasm in tetanus
rectal diazepam
rectangle
    Hartshill
    Luque
rectilinear bone scan
rectococcygeus muscle
rectourethral muscle
rectouterine muscle
rectovesical muscle
rectus abdominis muscle
rectus abdominis musculocutaneous
    free flap
rectus femoris muscle
rectus muscle flap
rectus position
recumbency
recumbent position
recumbent view
recur, recurred
recurrence, local

recurrent artery of Heubner
recurrent dislocation
recurrent laryngeal nerve
recurrent meningeal nerve
recurrent ophthalmic nerve
recurrent torsion spasms
recurvatum deformity
recurvatum during gait
Red Cross freeze-dried allograft
Reddick-Saye screw
Reddick-Saye suture
red erythrocyte-fibrin thrombus
Redi-Around finger splint
Redi-Drape
Redigrip knee pad
Redigrip pressure bandage
Redi head halter
redistribution image
Redi-Trac traction device
Redi-Vac cast cutter
Redi-Vacette
red light neon laser
red migraine
red muscle
red nucleus syndrome
reduced subluxation
reduction (see also *operations*)
   anatomic
   closed
   concentric
   congruent
   fracture
   Kocher
   manual
   manual fracture
   open
   stable
   Stimson
   surgical
   trial
REE (resting energy expenditure)
Reebok shoes
Reed cast belt
re-education, neuromuscular
reefing, capsular
reefing of medial retinaculum of knee
reefing procedure

Reese dermatome
Reese osteotomy guide
Reese stimulator
reevaluate
reexploration
reference
   Goldmann-Offner
   Stephenson-Gibbs
   sternospinal
reference electrode
reference line
reference, sternospinal
referential alternating montage
referential block montage
referential montage
referred neuritic pain
referred pain
refill, capillary
refixation of chondral fragments
refixation saccade
refixation reflexes
refixational shift of gaze
ReFix stereotactic head holder
reflect, reflected
reflected inguinal ligament
reflecting edge of ligament
reflective marker
reflex (pl. reflexes)
   abdominal
   absent
   accommodation
   Achilles tendon
   adductor
   anal wink
   ankle jerk
   asymmetric tonic neck
   automatic bladder
   Babinski
   Bekhterev-Mendel
   biceps stretch
   blink r. to corneal stimulation
   brachioradialis
   brain stem
   brisk
   bulbar
   bulbocavernous
   cervico-ocular

reflex *(continued)*
    Chaddock
    chewing
    ciliary or pupillary-skin
    ciliospinal or pupillary-skin
    consensual light
    contralateral grasp
    corneal
    cough
    cremasteric
    crossed
    cubital tendon
    deep tendon (DTRs)
    delayed
    deltoid
    depressed
    diminished
    diving
    doll's eye
    dorsal
    elbow
    equivocal plantar
    exaggerated deep tendon
    extensor plantar
    facial
    fencing posture
    fixation
    flexion
    flexor
    frontal lobe
    gag
    gastrocnemius
    glabella
    glabellar
    Golgi
    Gordon
    grasp
    H reflex (Hoffmann monosynaptic)
    hamstring
    Hirschberg
    hung-up (slowed)
    hyperactive deep tendon
    hypoactive deep tendon
    intramuscular recording
    jaw jerk
    Kimura blink
    knee jerk

reflex *(continued)*
    Landau
    laryngeal-tracheal
    lengthening
    ligamentomuscular protective
    masseter-temporalis stretch
    Mayer
    Mendel-Bekhterev
    monosynaptic
    Moro
    motor
    muscle stretch
    myotatic
    near
    neck righting
    neonatal
    nociceptive
    nuchocephalic
    oculocephalic
    oculovestibular (OVR)
    Oppenheim
    optokinetic
    orbicularis pupillary
    palmomental
    parachute
    patellar
    patelloadductor
    pathologic
    pathological
    pectoral
    pectoralis
    pendular
    periosteal
    plantar
    polykinetic
    pressor
    primitive
    pseudomyotonic
    psycho-optical
    pupillary light
    pyramidal tract
    quadriceps stretch
    radial
    refixation
    Remak
    righting
    rooting

reflex *(continued)*
 rotular
 scapular
 scapulohumeral
 silent
 snout
 somatovisceral
 spinal
 spindle system
 stepping
 sternutatory
 Stookey
 stretch
 suck
 sucking
 superficial abdominal
 suprapatellar
 swallow
 tendon
 toe
 tonic neck
 triceps
 triceps surae
 ulnar
 vasovagal
 ventral suspension
 vestibulo-ocular (VOR)
 viscerosomatic
 von Bekhterev
 Wartenberg
 withdrawal
 mass limb
reflex arc, monosynaptic
reflex controls
 psycho-optical
 static
 statokinetic
reflex epilepsy
Reflex exercise and rehab equipment
reflex eye movement
reflexic
reflex inguinal ligament
reflex inhibition
reflex iridoplegia
reflex neurologic activity
reflexology, full-spectrum
reflex paralysis

ReflexPro linear percussion device
reflex rebound component of whiplash
reflex relaxation delay
reflex sympathetic dystrophy (RSD)
reflex sympathetic dystrophy
 syndrome (RSDS)
Re-Flex VSP prosthesis
refluxing spastic neurogenic bladder
reflux, venous
refractory
refracture
refrigerant, skin
Refsum disease
Refsum syndrome
regenerating peripheral fibers
regeneration
 axon
 imperfect
 neural
Regen flexion exercises
regimen
 Duran
 force
 Strickland
region
 anesthesic
 anterior head
 Broca
 central head
 centroparietal head
 cervical
 cervicothoracic
 clival
 craniofacial
 frontal
 frontocentral head
 frontotemporal
 frontozygomatic
 geniculocalcarine
 hippocampal
 insular
 interseptal
 lumbar
 lumbosacral
 mesiotemporal
 midbrain subthalamic
 midfrontal

region *(continued)*
    occipital
    orbitofrontal
    paracervical
    parasagittal head
    parasellar
    paraspinal
    paravermian
    paravertebral
    patellofemoral
    periaqueductal
    petroclival
    petrous
    pineal
    pontomedullary
    prestyloid
    pretectal
    pretibial
    retrosellar
    retrostyloid
    rolandic head
    sacral
    septal
    subfrontal
    subthalamic
    supramalleolar
    suprasellar
    task-activated brain
    temporal
    temporozygomatic
    thoracolumbar
    Wernicke
regional cerebral blood flow (rCBF)
    PET scan
regional cerebral blood volume
    (rCBV) PET scan
regional cerebral metabolic rate for
    oxygen (rCMRO$_2$)
regional cerebral oxygen saturation
regional cerebral perfusion pressure
    (rCPP)
regional cerebral vasoreactivity
    (rCVR)
regional sympathetic blockade
register, Autologous Chondrocyte
    Implantation (ACI)
registered deafness specialist (RDF)

registration
    image
    spatial
registry
    Cochrane Controlled Trials
    Pediatric Rheumatology Disease
    Registry of Interpreters for the Deaf
        (RID)
Regnauld degeneration of MTP joint
Regnauld modification of Keller
    arthroplasty
Regnauld-type degeneration of great
    toe
regress
regression analysis
regression modeling
regressive remodeling
rehabilitation (rehab)
    aquatic
    community
    Engineering and Assistive Tech-
        nology Society of North
        America (RESNA)
    free weight
    muscular
    neurological
    Office of Vocational (OVR)
    swallowing
    vestibular
    vocational (VR)
rehabilitation assessment
rehabilitation behaviors
rehabilitation care
rehabilitation counseling (RC)
rehabilitation engineering (RE)
rehabilitation evaluation
rehabilitation interventions
rehabilitation planning
rehabilitation psychiatry (RP)
Rehabilitation Services Administration
    (RSA)
rehabilitation treatment
Rehbein rib spreader
Reichenheim-King procedure
Reichert-Mundinger biopsy needle
Reichert-Mundinger-Fischer stereotactic
    frame

Reichert-Mundinger hematoma
  evacuator
Reichert-Mundinger stereotactic head
  frame
Reil, island of
Reimer migration index
reimplantation
Reiner bone rongeur
Reiner plaster knife
reinforcement ring
reinnervation after nerve injury
reinnervation, motor
Reintegration to Normal Living Index
re-irrigation
Reisseisen muscles
Reiter syndrome
Reitan trail-making test
relapsing course
relapsing-remitting multiple sclerosis
relation, phase
relationship
  force-strain
  stress-strain
relative elective mutism
relative scotomata
Relax-A-Bac posture support
relaxation rate
relaxation, reciprocal agonist-
  antagonist
relaxation techniques
relaxation time
Re-Lax-O chiropractic table
Relay packaging
release (see also *operations*)
  abductor hallucis muscle
  adductor tendon and lateral capsular
  brevis
  capsular
  carpal tunnel
  clubfoot
  Dupuytren contractor
  fascial
  flexor-pronator origin
  glenohumeral
  hamstring
  key
  lateral capsular

release *(continued)*
  lateral retinaculum
  plantar plate
  posteromedial (PMR)
  retinacular
  snapping tendon
  soft tissue
  tendon
  trigger finger
  trigger thumb
  ulnar nerve
relevant; understandable; measurable;
  behavioral; achievable (RUMBA)
reliability of rehabilitation testing
relocation test
Relton-Hall frame
remacemide
remaining lifetime fracture probability
Remak paralysis
Remeron (mirtazapine)
Remicade (infliximab)
Reminyl (galantamine)
remineralization
remission, endocrinological
remitting course
remnants, notochordal
remodeling
  bone
  craniofacial
  occipital vault
  para-articular bone
  regressive
remote afterloading brachytherapy
  (RAB)
remote lower motor neuron lesion
remote memory
removal key
removal, subtotal, of tumor
remover
  cast
  Wolfe-Boehler cast
REM (rapid eye movement) sleep
  bursts of
  periods of
REMstar Reliance CPAP system
remyelination
renal osteodystrophy

Renee creak sign (friction rub in knee)
Renografin contrast media
Renshaw cell
Reopro (abciximab)
repair (see *operations*)
repeated FID (free induction decay)
repeated microtraumas
reperfusion injury
repetitive impulse loading
repetitive microtrauma to the knee
repetitive seizures
repetitive strain (or stress) injury (RSI)
repetition time (TR)
rephasing gradient
replacement (see *operations*)
replacement bone
replantation of amputated digit or
  extremity
replantation of finger
replant splint
Repose surgical system
reprep and drape
Repro head halter
Requip (ropinirole hydrochloride)
rerotation, varus
reroute
rerouting, lateral band
rerouting of the tibialis anterior tendon
rerupture of aneurysm
resected, surgically
resecting fracture
resection (see *operations*)
  anteromedial temporal lobe
    (AMTR)
  bone wedge
  epileptogenic foci
  en bloc
  first rib
  iliopsoas tendon
  meniscus
  microsurgical
  panmetatarsal head
  ray
  subtotal
  surgical
  synostotic suture
  temporal bone

resection *(continued)*
  tumor
  volumetric stereotactic surgical
  wafer distal ulna
resection arthroplasty
resector
  Accu-Line femoral
  Accu-Line tibial
  femoral
  full radius
  orthotome
  synovial
  tibial
reservoir (also pouch)
  Accu-Flo CSF
  Braden flushing
  Cordis implantable drug
  CSF (cerebrospinal fluid)
  double-bubble flushing
  flush
  flushing
  Foltz flushing
  McKenzie
  Ommaya ventriculostomy
  Rickham intraventricular
  Salmon Rickham ventriculostomy
  Secor implantable drug
  ventricular catheter
residual artery lumen
residual cement
residual hemiparesis
residual interstitial changes
resiniferatoxin (RTX)
resin, polyacetal
resistance
  flexion against
  isodynamic
  progressive
  strength against
  tensile stretch
resistive exercise table
resistive magnet
RESNA (Rehabilitation, Engineering
    and Assistive Technology Society
    of North America)
resolution, spatial
resonance, nuclear magnetic (NMR)

resonant frequency
resorbable pin
resorbable plate
resorbable rod
resorbable screw
resorption
  bone
  osteoclastic
  osteoclast-mediated bone
respiration
  ataxic
  hissing, in uremic coma
respiratory depression
respiratory embarrassment
Respond Select neuromuscular
  stimulator
response
  adaptive
  brain stem auditory-evoked
  bulldog (chewing reflex)
  clasp knife
  corneal
  Cushing
  cyclic creep of graft
  decremental
  driving
  EEG augmenting
  EEG recruiting
  evoked (ER)
  evoked cortical (ECR)
  extensor plantar
  F wave
  focal epileptiform
  galvanic skin (GSR)
  ice water caloric
  jittery
  mass motor reflex
  M-
  obliterative
  oculocephalic
  on-and-off
  pattern reversal visual-evoked
  photic pattern-evoked
  photoconvulsive
  photomyoclonic
  photoparoxysmal
  placebo

response *(continued)*
  prominent flash-evoked
  psychogalvanic skin
  pupillary
  recruiting
  short latency somatosensory-evoked
  somatosensory-evoked (SER)
  steal
  sympathoadrenal
  triple
  visual-evoked (VER)
Response Abdominal Back/Side
  Combo
Response Cervical 8-Way Machine
Response Multi-Hip
Response rehab and fitness equipment
Response Rotary Torso
Response Seated Leg Curl & Leg
  Extension
Response Single Cable Column
responsive
responsiveness, reduced
rest
  foot
  Greenberg hand
  hand
  head
  horseshoe head
  kidney
  Mayfield horseshoe head
  Mayfield tic head
  tic head
  tumor
Restcue bed
rest, ice, compression, elevation
  (RICE)
restiform body
resting ankle/arm Doppler index
resting calcaneal stance position
resting energy expenditure (REE)
resting pan splint
resting potential
restive
restless legs syndrome (RLS)
restlessness
Reston dressing
Reston foam-padded headrest

restorator
Restore ACL guide system
Restore tools for knee surgery
restraint, Posey
restriction
  activity
  shoe
restrictor
  cement
  plastic marrow canal
rest splint
rest tremor
resurfacing, carbon fiber
resurrection bone
retained cortical activity (RCA)
retained foreign body
retardation
  mental
  profound mental
  psychomotor
  severe mental
rete (pl. retia)
rete pegs
rete ridges
reticular activating formation (RAF)
reticular activating substance
reticular activating system (RAS)
reticular formation of brain stem
reticulated bone
reticulin
reticulocortical pathway
reticulocytosis, cerebroside
reticulospinal tract
reticulum cell sarcoma
reticulum, hematopoietic
retina, angiomatosis of
retinacular disruption
retinacular ligament
retinaculum
  avulsed
  extensor
  flexor
  patellar
  superior peroneal (SPR)
retinitis pigmentosa
retinoneuropathy, toxic
retinopathy, venous stasis

retraction exercises, prone scapular
retractor
  Adson
  Adson-Anderson cerebellar
  Adson brain
  Adson cerebellar
  Adson hemilaminectomy
  Allport
  Alm wound
  amputation
  Anderson-Adson scalp
  angled
  appendiceal
  Army-Navy
  Aufranc cobra
  Badgley laminectomy
  Ballantine hemilaminectomy
  Bankart shoulder
  Beckman
  Beckman-Adson laminectomy
  Beckman-Eaton laminectomy
  Beckman-Weitlaner laminectomy
  Bennett bone
  Bennett tibial
  blade
  Blount anvil
  Blount hip
  Blount knee
  Bodnar
  bone
  brachial plexus root
  brain
  Budde-Greenberg-Sugita
  bunion
  Campbell nerve root
  carotid
  Carroll-Bennett
  Carroll hand
  centrum
  cerebellar
  cervical disk
  Chandler knee
  Charnley horizontal
  Charnley initial incision
  Charnley knee
  Charnley pin
  Charnley self-retaining

retractor *(continued)*
   Charnley vertical
   Cherry brain
   Cherry laminectomy
   Cloward blade
   Cloward brain
   Cloward cervical
   Cloward-Cushing vein
   Cloward dural
   Cloward-Hoen hemilaminectomy
   Cloward-Hoen laminectomy
   Cloward lumbar lamina
   Cloward nerve root
   Cloward skin
   Cloward small cervical
   Cloward tissue
   cobra
   Collis-Taylor
   Cone laminectomy
   Cone scalp
   Contour scalp
   Cooley rib
   Crego
   curved
   Cushing brain
   Cushing decompression
   Cushing nerve
   Cushing vein
   Davis brain
   Davis scalp
   Deaver
   decompression
   D'Errico-Adson
   D'Errico nerve root
   Doane knee
   Dohn-Carton brain
   Dott
   double-ended right-angle
   double-hook Lovejoy
   Downey hemilaminectomy
   Downing
   dural
   East-West
   Echols
   Elite Farley
   endaural
   Endotrac

retractor *(continued)*
   Enker brain
   eXpose
   Fahey
   fat pad
   finger
   Finochietto laminectomy
   Frazier laminectomy
   Frazier lighted brain
   Fujita snake
   Fujita suction
   Fukushima
   Gelpi pediatric
   Gifford mastoid
   Gilvernet
   Glaser automatic laminectomy
   Goulet
   Greenberg Universal
   hand
   Hands Free knee
   Hardy spinal
   Harrington
   Haverfield-Scoville hemilaminectomy
   Hayes
   Hays hand
   heavy-duty two-tooth
   Hedblom rib
   Heiss soft tissue
   hemilaminectomy
   Henley carotid
   Henning meniscal
   Hertzler rib
   Hibbs
   Hoen hemilaminectomy
   Hoen scalp
   Hohmann bone
   Holscher knee
   Holscher nerve root
   Holzheimer
   horizontal
   House-Fisch dura
   humeral head
   humpback Weitlaner
   Inge laminectomy
   initial incision
   Israel
   Jannetta posterior fossa

retractor *(continued)*
  Jansen mastoid
  Jansen scalp
  Jansen-Wagner
  Johnson
  Kasdan
  Kennerdell-Maroon orbital
  Kleinert-Ragdell
  Klemme laminectomy
  knee
  Knighton hemilaminectomy
  Knighton laminectomy
  Kocher
  Kuz-Medics total knee
  lamina
  laminectomy
  Lange-Hohmann bone
  Langenbeck
  lateral collateral ligament
  Leyla
  Leyla brain
  Love nerve root
  lower hand
  Lowman hand
  lumbar lamina
  Luongo hand
  Maison
  Malis brain
  Markham-Meyerding hemi-
    laminectomy
  Martin nerve root
  Mark II Chandler
  Mark II distal femur
  Mark II PCL
  Mark II S
  Mark II Z knee
  mastoid
  Mayo-Collins
  meniscus
  metacarpal
  Meyerding finger
  Meyerding laminectomy
  Meyerding self-retaining
  Miller-Senn
  mini-Hohmann podiatric
  Miskimon cerebellar
  Morris

retractor *(continued)*
  Myers knee
  narrow blade
  narrow neck mini-Hohmann
  Nelson rib
  nerve root
  North-South
  Oberhill laminectomy
  Oldberg brain
  Ollier rake
  Omni
  orbital
  Paulson knee
  PCL (posterior collateral ligament)
  Penfield
  Percy amputation
  pin
  pitchfork
  Poppen-Gelpi laminectomy
  posterior fossa
  Ragnell handheld
  rake
  RC Mini-Open lighted
  rib
  Richardson
  right-angle
  Robotrac
  Roos brachial plexus root
  Rosenberg
  Rowe capsular
  Rowe humeral head
  S-shaped brain
  Sachs vein
  Sauerbruch
  scalp
  Schink
  Schwartz laminectomy
  Scoville cervical disk
  Scoville-Haverfield hemilaminectomy
  Scoville hemilaminectomy
  Scoville nerve root
  Scoville-Richter laminectomy
  Seletz-Gelpi laminectomy
  self-retaining
  Senn double-end
  sharp
  Sheldon hemilaminectomy

retractor *(continued)*
  Sherwin knee
  Sims
  single-hook auto
  skid humeral head
  Smillie knee
  Smillie meniscus hook
  Smith nerve root suction
  snake
  Snitman endaural
  Sofield
  Spurling nerve root
  Stack hand
  staple-shaped
  stiff ribbon
  Stiwer
  straight
  Stryker illuminated
  Stuck laminectomy
  suction
  Taylor self-retaining spinal
  Taylor spinal
  Teflon-coated brain
  Temple-Fay laminectomy
  tibial
  Tiemann shoulder
  toothed
  tracheal
  trigeminal nerve
  Tuffier laminectomy
  Tuffier-Raney
  two-prong rake
  U-shaped
  U.S. Army
  universal
  upper-hand
  Valin hemilaminectomy
  vein
  Verbrugge-Hohmann bone
  Versatrac lumbar
  vertebral body
  vertical
  vessel
  Volkmann rake
  Wagner
  Weary nerve root
  Weitlaner-Beckman

retractor *(continued)*
  Wilson gonad
  Wiltse-Bankart
  Wiltse-Gelpi
  Wink
  wishbone
  Zinn
re-treating
retrieval task
retriever
  Carroll tendon
  Kleinert-Kutz tendon
retrobulbar hemorrhage
retrobulbar neuritis
retrocalcaneal bursa
retrocalcaneal bursitis, chronic
retrocalcaneal exostosis
retrocalcaneal spur
retrochiasmal lesion
retrochiasmal visual pathway
retroclavicular
retrocolic spasm
retrogeniculate pathway
retrograde amnesia
retrograde Beaver blade
retrograde femoral nailing
retrograde perfusion
retrolaminar fat
retrolisthesis
retromastoid craniectomy
retromedullary arteriovenous
  malformation
retronuchal muscle
retro-orbital space
retropatellar fat pad
retroperfusion
retropharyngeal space
retropubic space
retropulsed bony fragment
retropulsion of bone fragment into
  spinal canal
retropulsion of gait
retrosellar region
retrostyloid region
retroversion, femoral
retrovestibular neural pathway
retroviral-mediated gene therapy

Retrox Fractal active fixation lead
Retter aneurysm needle
Retter knot tier and ligature carrier
Retzius ligament
revascularization
    cerebral
    endosteal
revascularization of foot
revascularization of graft
revascularized tissue
Revelation hip system
Revel Functional Index (RFI)
Reverdin epidermal free graft
Reverdin-Green osteotomy
reversal
    instrumental phase
    letter
    phase (on EEG)
    shunt
    true phase
reverse Barton fracture
reverse Colles fracture
reverse Hill-Sachs
reversal of cervical lordosis
reversal of fore-aft shear phase of gait
reverse-last shoes
reverse Mauck knee procedure
reverse pivot-shift test
reverse transcription polymerase chain
    reaction
reverse urea syndrome
reversible inactivation of subthalamic
    nucleus neurons
reversible ischemic neurologic deficit
    (RIND)
reversible organic brain syndrome
revision of total hip
revision, stump
revision total hip surgery
Revo retrievable cancellous screw
Rey and Taylor Complex Figure Test
Rey Auditory Verbal Learning Test
Rey Osterrieth Complex Figure Test
Reye syndrome, adult
Reynolds skull traction tongs
REZ (root exit zone)
Rezinian external fixation

Rezinian interbody device
RF (radiofrequency) coil
RF (radiofrequency) pulse
RF (rheumatoid factor) test
RF (right frontal) EEG lead
rhBMP (recombinant human bone
    morphogenetic protein)
rhBMP-2 (recombinant human bone
    morphogenetic protein-2)
RFE (radiofrequency electro-
    coagulation)
RFG-3CF radiofrequency generator
RFI (Revel Functional Index)
RGO (reciprocating gait orthosis)
rhabdoid suture
rhabdomyolysis
rhabdomyoma
rhabdomyosarcoma, alveolar
rheumatic chorea
rheumatic fever (RF)
rheumatic gout
rheumatism
    palindromic
    psychogenic
rheumatoid arthritis (RA) factor
rheumatoid arthritis agglutinin test
rheumatoid factor (RF)
rheumatoid neuropathy
rheumatoid nodule
rheumatoid scoliosis
rheumatoid spondylitis
rheumatoid synovitis
rheumatoid vasculitis
rheumatologist
rhIGF-1 (Myotrophin)
Rhinelander pin
Rhinelander wire tightener
rhinencephalic mamillary body
rhinocerebral mucormycosis
rhinophyma
Rhino Triangle polypropylene hip
    abduction brace
rhizolysis
    percutaneous radiofrequency
        trigeminal
    percutaneous retrogasserian
        glycerol

rhizomelic spondylitis
rhizomelic spondylosis
rhizotomy (radicotomy)
   chemical
   dorsal root
   functional posterior
   glycerol
   intracranial glossopharyngeal
   percutaneous high frequency
   percutaneous thermal
   selective dorsal (SDR)
   surgical
   thermal
   vagal
rhombencephalon
rhomboid fossa
rhomboid ligament
rhomboid major muscle
rhonchus (pl. rhonchi)
Rhoton ball dissector
Rhoton bayonet scissors
Rhoton bipolar forceps
Rhoton cup forceps
Rhoton curet
Rhoton-Cushing forceps
Rhoton dissecting forceps
Rhoton elevator
Rhoton enucleator
Rhoton forceps
Rhoton fork
Rhoton hook
Rhoton loop curet
Rhoton-Merz suction tube
Rhoton micro curet
Rhoton microdissector
Rhoton needle holder
Rhoton osteotome
Rhoton pituitary curet
Rhoton punch
Rhoton scissors
Rhoton sellar punch
Rhoton spatula dissector
Rhoton spoon curet
Rhoton suction tip
Rhoton-Tew bipolar forceps

RHS (radial head subluxation)
rhythm
   alpha
   alpha variant
   alphoid
   arceau
   attenuation of alpha
   attenuation of background
   Berger (on EEG)
   beta
   circadian
   comb
   EEG
   fast alpha variant
   focal parietal theta
   frontal beta
   gamma
   kappa
   M-type (minimal) alpha
   midline theta
   monorhythmic occipital
   mu (μ)
   occipital
   P-type (persistent) alpha
   paradoxical alpha
   paradoxical mu (μ)
   persistent slowing of alpha
   posterior beta
   posterior theta
   postictal slowing of alpha
   projected EEG
   R-type (reactive) alpha
   regular sinus
   scapulohumeral
   sigma
   slow alpha variant
   spike and slow wave
   theta
   trains of mu (μ)
   wicket
   widespread beta
rhythmical spindle-shaped activity
rhythmicity of wave
rhythmic handgrip endurance/work
rhythmic (jerk) nystagmus

RIA (radioimmunoassay)
rib (pl. ribs)
  angle of
  bed of
  bicipital
  bifid
  cervical
  facet for head of
  false
  first
  floating
  fused
  head of
  hypoplastic horizontal
  lumbar
  minced
  neck of
  notching of
  periosteum of
  retracted
  rudimentary
  shaft of
  slipping
  sternal
  Stiller
  superior
  true
  tubercle of
  vertebral
  vertebrocostal
  vertebrosternal
rib belt orthosis
rib belt, Zim-Zap
Ribble bandage
ribbon muscles
rib contusion
rib fracture
rib guillotine
rib notching
rib penciling
rib recession
rib spaces, narrowed
rib view
RICE (rest, ice, compression, elevation)
rice bodies
Richards angle guide

Richards compression screw
Richards curet
Richards hip prosthesis
Richards-Hirschhorn plate
Richards hydroxyapatite PORP
  prosthesis
Richards hydroxyapatite TORP
  prosthesis
Richards mallet
Richards modular hip system (RMHS)
Richards reamer
Richards reconstruction nail
Richards self-tapping screw
Richards Solcotrans Plus
Richards Spectrum metal-backed
  acetabular prosthesis
Richards Zirconia femoral head
  prosthesis
Richardson retractor
Richardson rod
Riche-Cannieu anastomosis
Riches artery forceps
Richet bandage
Richet, tibioastragalocalcaneal
  canal of
Richmond subarachnoid screw
  instruments
Richter laminectomy punch forceps
Rich theory of tuberculous meningitis
Ricinus communis agglutinin 1 (RCA)
  antibody
rickets, familial hypophosphatemic
rickettsial infections of the central
  nervous system
  murine typhus
  Rocky Mountain spotted fever
  scrub typhus (tsutsugamushi)
Rickham reservoir
RID (Registry of Interpreters for the
  Deaf)
Ridaura (auranofin)
rider's bone
rider's muscles
ridge, ridging
  alveodental
  alveolar
  apical ectodermal (AER)

ridge *(continued)*
  basal
  bisagittal
  broad maxillary
  buccocervical
  bulbar
  cerebral
  cranial
  dental
  dorsal
  epicondylar
  fibrocartilaginous
  fibromuscular
  ganglion
  gluteal
  greater multangular
  humeral
  interarticular
  interosseous
  intertrochanteric
  longitudinal
  marginal
  mylohyoid
  Outerbridge
  petrous
  radial
  sagittal
  septal
  sphenoid
  supracondylar
  supraorbital
  tentorial
  transverse
  triangular
  trochlear
  ulnar
  vastus lateralis
ridge augmentation procedure
Ridley sinus
Ridlon hip reduction
Ridlon plaster knife
Riel index
Rienhoff rib spreader
rifaximin
right and left respiratory nerves
right anterior temporal (RAT)
  EEG lead

right-bearing nystagmus
right frontal (RF) EEG lead
right-hand dominant
right-handed patient
right hemiplegia
righting reflex
right lateral decubitus view
right-left disorientation
right motor (RM) EEG lead
right occipital (RO) EEG lead
right parietal (RP) EEG lead
right posterior oblique (RPO) position
right posterior temporal (RPT)
  EEG lead
right respiratory nerve (phrenic nerve)
right-side-down decubitus position
right-sided weakness
right triangular ligament
rigid bars
rigid flatfoot
rigid internal fixation
rigidity
  axial
  clasp knife
  cogwheel
  decerebrate
  decorticate
  lead pipe
  nuchal
  ratchet
  reflex
rigidity predominant Parkinson disease
rigid-lens endoscope
rigid neuroendoscope
Riley-Day syndrome
Rilutek (riluzole)
rim
  capsule
  dark signal intensity
  glenoid
  sclerotic
  signal enhancement
riMLF (rostral interstitial nucleus of
  medial longitudinal fasciculus)
RIND (reversible or resolving
  ischemic neurologic deficit)

ring (pl. rings)
 abdominal
 Ace-Colles half
 arc
 BRW (Brown-Roberts-Wells) head
 cartilaginous
 CBI stereotactic
 centering
 Charnley centering
 common tendinous
 constriction
 doughnut
 drop lock
 femoral
 fibrocartilaginous
 fibrous
 foramen magnum
 fracture
 Fischer
 half
 halo
 Ilizarov
 ischial weightbearing
 Kayser-Fleischer (K-F)
 Mose concentric
 olive
 orthosis drop lock
 pelvic
 perichondral
 periosteal bone
 proximal to distal
 reinforcement
 stereotactic or stereotaxic
 vertebral
ring apophysis
ring blush on cerebral arteriography
ring curet, Cloward-Cone
Ringer's injection, lactated
Ringer's irrigation
ring fracture
ring ligament
ring-man shoulder
Ring total hip prosthesis
Ring UPM hip (or knee) replacement
Rinne hearing conduction test
Riolan bone
Riolan muscle

Riordan classification of club hand
Riordan finger flexion
Riordan finger opponensplasty
Riordan finger pollicization
Riordan tendon transfer technique
rippling muscle disease
RISA (radioiodinated serum albumin)
Riseborough-Radin classification of
 intercondylar fracture
risedronate (Actonel)
riser, stress
Rish osteotome
risorius muscle
risperidone (Risperdal)
Risser-Ferguson scoliosis measuring
 technique
Risser localizer scoliosis cast
Risser sign
Risser table
Ritcher screwdriver
Ritchie Articular Index (RAI)
Ritchie index for rheumatoid arthritis
Ritchie nail starter
rivastigmine tartrate (Exelon)
Rivermead ADL Index (RAI)
Rivermead Behavioral Memory Test
Rivermead Mobility Index (RMI)
Rivermead Motor Assessment
Rivermead Perceptual Assessment
 Battery (RPAB)
rivet, pop
RLE (right lower extremity)
RLS (restless legs syndrome)
RM (right motor) EEG lead
RM isoelastic hip prosthesis
RM (Reichert/Mundinger) stereotaxic
 system
RMC knee replacement device
RMHS (Richards modular hip system)
RMI (Rivermead Mobility Index)
RMTD (rhythmical midtemporal
 discharge)
RO (right occipital) EEG lead
R/O (rule out)
roadmapping
 biplane
 digital

Robaxacet (methocarbamol and aceta-
   minophen)
Robert Brigham total knee prosthesis
Robert Jones dressing
Robert ligament
Roberts-Gill periosteal elevator
Robertson suture
Roberts rib shears
Roberts technique
Robin Hood phenomenon (steal
   syndrome)
Robinson anterior cervical discectomy
Robinson arthrometer
Robinson cervical spine fusion
Robinson-Chung-Farahvar clavicular
   morcellation
Robinson-Riley cervical arthrodesis
Robinson-Riley spinal fusion
Robinson-Southwick fusion
Robodoc instrument holder
robot
   Grenoble stereotactic
   Kwoh-Young stereotactic
   Lausanne stereotactic
   Long Beach stereotactic
   Mayo Clinic stereotactic
   neurosurgical stereotactic
   stereotactic
   3 Degree of Freedom
   4 Degree of Freedom
   5 Degree of Freedom
   6 Degree of Freedom
Robotrac passive retraction system
ROC (Radial Osteo Compression)
   fastener/soft tissue anchor
Rocephin (ceftriaxone)
Rochester bone trephine
Rochester-Carmalt forceps
Rochester compression system
Rochester harvest bone cutter
Rochester HKAFO (hip-knee-ankle-
   foot orthosis)
Rochester lamina dissector
Rochester lamina elevator
Rochester-Ochsner forceps
Rochester-Pean forceps
Rochester recipient bone cutter

Rochester spinal elevator
rocker, Carolina
rocker foot
rockerbottom flatfoot
rockerbottom foot
RocketSoc ankle brace
Rockwood classification of acromioclavicular injury
Rockwood-Green technique
Rocky Mountain spotted fever
   meningoencephalitis
rod
   absorbable
   acetabular cup detaching
   acetabular cup push (pushing)
   Acufex TAG
   alignment
   Alta tibial/humeral
   Amset R-F
   auto-reinforced polyglycolide
   bendable metallic
   Bickel intramedullary
   biodegradable
   C-D or CD (Cotrel-Dubousset)
   compression
   Dacron-impregnated silicone
   degradable polyglycolide
   distraction
   Edwards-Levine
   Edwards reverse ratchet
   Ender
   Fixateur Interne
   fluted medullary
   grooved titanium
   Hall
   Harrington compression
   Harrington distraction
   Harris condylocephalic
   Hartshill rectangle
   hinge
   humeral
   Hunter Silastic
   Hunter tendon
   Ilizarov telescoping
   IM (intramedullary)
   impactor
   Isola

rod *(continued)*
  Jacobs distraction
  Kaneda
  Knodt compression
  knurled
  Kostuik
  Küntscher condylocephalic
  Luque
  Moe distraction
  Moe-modified Harrington
  Moss
  Mouradian
  Olerud PSF
  partially threaded
  pedicular
  PMMA (polymethylmethacrylate)
  polyglactin
  polyglycolide, self-reinforced
  PWB (Puno-Winter-Byrd)
  rectangular
  resorbable
  Richardson
  Rogozinski spinal
  Rush
  Russell-Taylor reconstruction
  Sage
  Schanz
  Schmidt
  Schneider
  Seidel humeral
  Seidel intramedullary
  Selby I and II
  Serrato forearm
  Silastic
  silicone flexor
  Smith & Nephew Richards
  spinal
  Steffee pedicular
  Stenzel
  straight threaded
  Synthes
  telescopic
  telescoping medullary
  tendon
  threaded
  titanium alloy
  top-loading

rod *(continued)*
  True/Fit femoral intramedullary
    rod system
  TSRH (Texas Scottish Rite
    Hospital)
  U Luque vertebral
  Ultimax distal femoral intra-
    medullary rod system
  V-A alignment
  VDS (ventral derotating spinal)
    compression
  VSF (Vermont spinal fixator)
  Wiltse
  Wissinger
  Zickel
  Zielke
rod bender
roentgen knife
roentgenogram, two-plane
roentgen stereophotogrammetric
  analysis (RSA)
rofecoxib (Vioxx)
Roger Anderson compression device
Roger Anderson external fixation
  apparatus
Rogers cervical fusion technique
Rogers wire-cutting scissors
Rogozinski hook
Rogozinski screw
Rogozinski spinal fixation system
Roho cushion
Rokitansky pelvis
Roland index of low back pain
rolandic cortex
rolandic dip transient
rolandic epilepsy
rolandic epileptiform discharges
rolandic fissure
rolandic seizure
rolandic sharp transient
rolandic sharp wave
rolandic spike
rolandic sulcus
rolandic vein syndrome
Rolando angle
Rolando area
Rolando cell

Rolando fissure
Rolando fracture
Rolando line
Rolando point
Rolando tubercle
Rolando zone
rolandoparietal glioma
Rolator walker
rolfing (massage) therapy
Rolimeter
roll
  axillary
  chest
  cotton
  hand
  hip
  iliac crest
  palmar
  positioning
  radiolucent
  towel
rollback, femoral
roller
  cranioplastic
  Spence cranioplastic
Rolyan Firm D-Ring wrist support
Rolyan Gel Shell splint
Rolyan tibial fracture brace
ROM (range of motion) walker brace
Romano surgical curved drilling
  system
Romazicon (flumazenil)
Romberg sign
Romberg station
Romberg syndrome
Romberg tandem
Romberg test
Rome criteria for rheumatoid arthritis
rongeur (see also *forceps*)
  Adson cranial
  angled jaw
  angled pituitary
  angular bone
  Bacon bone
  Bacon cranial
  Baer bone
  Bane-Hartmann bone

rongeur *(continued)*
  Bane mastoid
  basket
  bayonet
  Beyer-Stille bone
  Blumenthal bone
  Boehler bone (Böhler)
  bone-nibbling
  Bruening-Citelli
  Bucy laminectomy
  Campbell
  cervical laminectomy
  Cherry-Kerrison laminectomy
  Cicherelli bone
  Cintor bone
  Cleveland bone
  Cloward intervertebral disk
  Cloward large cervical
  Cloward-English laminectomy
  Cloward-Harper laminectomy
  Cloward pituitary
  Codman-Harper laminectomy
  Codman-Kerrison laminectomy
  Codman-Leksell laminectomy
  Codman-Schlesinger cervical
    laminectomy
  Cohen
  Colclough-Scheicher laminectomy
  Corbett bone
  cranial
  curved bone
  Cushing cranial
  Cushing intervertebral disk
  Cushing pituitary
  Dahlgren cranial
  Dale first rib
  Dean bone
  Decker microsurgical
  Decker pituitary
  Defourmentel bone
  DeVilbiss cranial
  disk
  double-action
  downbiting
  duckbill
  Echlin bone
  Echlin duckbill

rongeur *(continued)*
  Echlin laminectomy
  Echlin-Luer
  Ferris Smith intervertebral disk
  Ferris Smith laminectomy
  Ferris Smith-Kerrison laminectomy
  Ferris Smith pituitary jaw
  Ferris Smith-Spurling disk
  first rib
  Fisch bone
  FlexTip intervertebral
  Friedman bone
  Frykholm bone
  Fulton laminectomy
  Geiger
  gooseneck
  Gruenwald neurosurgical
  Guleke bone
  Hajek antrum
  Hajek-Koffler laminectomy
  Hakansson bone
  Hartmann bone
  Hein
  Hoen intervertebral disk
  Hoen laminectomy
  Horsley bone
  Hudson cranial
  Husk bone
  intervertebral disk
  Jackson intervertebral disk
  Jansen
  Jarit-Kerrison laminectomy
  Jarit-Liston bone
  Jarit-Ruskin bone
  Kerrison down-biting
  Kerrison laminectomy
  Kleinert-Kutz bone
  Kleinert-Kutz synovectomy
  laminectomy
  Lebsche
  Leksell laminectomy
  Leksell-Stille thoracic
  Lempert bone
  Liston bone
  Liston-Littauer bone
  Littauer-West
  Love-Gruenwald intervertebral disk

rongeur *(continued)*
  Love-Gruenwald pituitary
  Love-Kerrison cervical
  Love-Kerrison laminectomy
  Luer bone
  Luer-Friedman bone
  Luer-Hartmann
  Markwalder bone
  Marquardt bone
  Mayfield
  McIndoe bone
  Mead bone
  micro-Kerrison
  microlaminectomy
  Miltex-Kerrison cervical
  mini-Ruskin
  Montenovesi
  Mount laminectomy
  Mueller (Müller)
  Nicola pituitary
  Oldberg intervertebral disk
  Oldberg pituitary
  Olivecrona
  osteophyte nipper
  peapod intervertebral disk
  Peiper-Beyer laminectomy
  Pilling-Liston
  pituitary
  Poppen intervertebral disk
  Raney laminectomy
  Reiner bone
  Rottgen-Ruskin bone
  Ruskin-Jansen bone
  Ruskin-Jay
  Ruskin-Liston bone
  Ruskin-Rowland bone
  Rust
  Sauerbruch-Coryllos
  Sauerbruch rib
  Sauerbruch-Stille
  Schell bone
  Schlesinger cervical
  Schlesinger intervertebral disk
  Schlesinger laminectomy
  Schlesinger pituitary
  Selverstone intervertebral disk
  Semb-Stille bone

rongeur *(continued)*
  Shearer
  single action
  Smith-Petersen laminectomy
  Spence intervertebral disk
  Spurling intervertebral disk
  Spurling-Kerrison laminectomy
  Spurling-Kerrison up-biting and
    down-biting
  Spurling pituitary
  Stellbrink synovectomy
  Stille-Horsley bone
  Stille-Leksell
  Stille-Liston bone
  Stille-Luer bone
  Stille-Luer duckbill
  Stille-Luer-Echlin
  Stille-Ruskin bone
  Stookey cranial
  straight bone
  straight pituitary
  Strully-Gigli
  Strully-Kerrison
  synovectomy
  Takahashi
  thoracic
  upbiting
  Urschel first rib
  Walton-Liston bone
  Walton-Ruskin bone
  Watson-Williams intervertebral disk
  Weil-Blakesley intervertebral disk
  Whitcomb-Kerrison laminectomy
  Wilde intervertebral disk
  Yasargil pituitary
  Zaufel-Jansen bone
rongeur forceps
roof
  acetabular
  intercondylar
roof arc measurement
roof of insula
roof of ventricle
room
  Allender vertical laminar flow
  Charnley laminar flow
Roos approach

Roos brachial plexus root retractor
Roos first rib shears
root (pl. roots)
  cervical nerve
  compression of nerve
  cranial
  extrathecal nerve
  fila of nerve
  impingement on nerve
  injury to nerve
  intradural nerve
  intrathecal
  motor
  neoplastic invasion of
  nerve
  posterior
  somatosympathetic fibers of nerve
  spinal
  ventral nerve
root compression syndrome
root entry zone
root exit zone (REZ)
root fiber
root irritation
root lesion
rootlets of nerve
root level motor impairment
Root-Siegal osteotomy
root sleeve
ropinirole hydrochloride (Requip)
rosary, rachitic
Rose foot procedure
Rose, lateral mamillary nucleus of
Rosenberg retractor
Rosen bur
Rosen elevator
Rosenfeld hip prosthesis
Rosenmüller, fossa of
Rosenstiel Coping Questionnaire
Rosenthal, basal vein of (BVR)
Rosenthal fiber formation in
  leukodystrophy
Rosenthal vein (basal vein)
rosette Beaver blade
rosette strain gauge
Rose-Waaler test
Rosomoff cordotomy

Rosser classification of illness states
Rosser crypt hook
Rossolimo contraction
rostral brain stem
rostral brain stem ischemia
rostral cervical nerve
rostral connection
rostral hypothalamus
rostrally
rostral medulla
rostral neuropore
rostral pons
rostral spinal cord
rostral terminus
rostrum of corpus callosum
Rotablator rotating bur
Rotaglide knee implant
rotary chair test
rotary gamma scalpel
rotary instability
rotary joint
rotary scoliosis
rotary subluxation
rotary thoracolumbar scoliosis
rotating frame of reference
rotation
    axis of
    eccentric axis of
    external
    functional axial
    hip lateral
    hip medial
    internal
    internal femoral
    inward
    lateral
    medial
    neutral
    outward
    passive head
    pelvic
    tibiofibular
    transverse
rotational alignment
rotational flaps
rotational force

rotational interface
rotational scarf bunionectomy
rotationplasty
rotator
    external
    internal
    Jarit
    long external
    short external
Rotator Cuff Buttress (RCB)
rotator cuff calcific tendinitis
rotator cuff impingement syndrome
rotator cuff tear
rotator cuff tendinopathy
rotator cuff tendon
rotator muscle
rotatory joint
rotatory load on spine
rotatory nystagmus
Rotes scale for joint mobility
Roth-Bernhardt disease
Rothman Institute femoral prosthesis
RotoRest bed
rotoscoliosis
Rottgen-Ruskin bone rongeur
Rouget muscle
roughened surface
roughening
rouleaux formation
round-back posture
round cell tumors
round ligament
round pronator muscle
Rousek extraction set
Rousek extractor
Roussy-Dejerine thalamic pain
    syndrome
Roussy-Lévy disease
Roussy-Lévy hereditary areflexic
    dystasia
Roussy-Lévy syndrome
Rouviere, ligament of
Roux-duToit staple capsulorrhaphy
Roux-Goldthwait procedure
roving eye movements
roving ocular movements

row
 carpal
 proximal carpal
 suture
Rowe calcaneal fracture classification
Rowe capsular retractor
Rowe disimpaction forceps
Rowe fusion
Rowe glenoid punch
Rowe glenoid-reaming forceps
Rowe-Harrison bone-holding forceps
Rowe humeral head retractor
Rowe-Lowell fracture-dislocation
 classification system
Rowe modified-Harrison forceps
Rowe score
Rowe-Zarins shoulder immobilization
 technique
Rowland-Hughes splint
Roxiam (remoxipride)
Royalite body jacket
Roy-Camille cervical plate
Roy-Camille occipitocervical plate
Roy-Camille pedicle plate
Roy-Camille screw placement
 technique
Royle-Thompson transfer technique
RP (rehabilitation psychiatry)
RP (right parietal) EEG lead
RPAB (Rivermead Perceptual
 Assessment Battery)
RPS (reverse pivot shift) test
RPT (right posterior temporal)
 EEG lead
RRFs (ragged red fibers)
RSA (Rehabilitation Services
 Administration)
RSA (roentgen stereophotogrammetric
 analysis)
RSA calibration cage
RSD (reflex sympathetic dystrophy)
RSDS (reflex sympathetic dystrophy
 syndrome)
RSI (repetitive stress injury)
RSNA (Radiological Society of North
 America)
RT (repetition time)

rt-PA (recombinant tissue-type
 plasminogen activator)
RTX (resiniferatoxin)
R-type (reactive) alpha rhythm
rubber-band technique, Kleinert
Rubbermaid adjustable bath/shower
 seat
rubber-shod (protected) clamp
rubella, congenital
rub, friction
Rubin bone planer
Rubin cartilage planer
Rubin gouge
Rubin rasp
Rubinstein-Taybi syndrome
rubor
rubral tremor
rubrospinal tract
rubrous
rucksack paralysis
rudimentary bone
rudimentary postaxial polydactyly
rudimentary rib
Rud syndrome
RUE (right upper extremity)
Ruedi-Allgower tibial plafond fracture
 classification
Ruffini corpuscle sensory receptor
Ruffini mechanoreceptor
Ruffini terminals
rugger jersey spine
Ruiz-Mora procedure
rule of squares to plot scotomas
ruler
 Berndt hip
 stainless steel
RUMBA (relevant; understandable;
 measurable; behavioral; achievable)
Rumel aluminum splint
runner (pl. runners)
 extrinsic-dominant
 heel-toe
 intrinsic-negative
 intrinsic-positive
runner's bump
runner's knee
running epilepsy

running lock suture
running-related injury
running seizures
rupture
  Achilles tendon
  arch
  attrition
  brain aneurysm
  buttonhole
  chordae tendineae
  complete Achilles tendon
  contained aneurysmal
  plantaris (tennis leg)
ruptured Achilles tendon
  complete
  partial
ruptured disk
ruptured intracranial aneurysm
Rush awl
Rush driver-bender-extractor
Rush mallet
Rush pin
Rush rod
Ruskin bone-cutting forceps
Ruskin bone-splitting forceps
Ruskin-Jansen bone rongeur

Ruskin-Liston bone-cutting forceps
Ruskin-Liston rongeur
Ruskin rongeur
Ruskin-Rowland bone-cutting forceps
Russe approach
Russe bone graft
Russell-Rubinstein classification of
  cerebrovascular malformation
Russell-Taylor interlocking nail
Russell-Taylor reconstruction rod
Russell traction for femoral fracture
Russian forceps
Russian stimulation
Rust amputation saw
Rust rongeur
Rust saw
Rust sign
Ruysch muscle
RVBF (reversed vertebral blood flow)
Rydell nail
Ryder needle holder
Ryder test
Ryerson graft
Ryerson tenotome
Ryerson triple arthrodesis

S, s

SAB (short-acting block) anesthesia
Sabel cast walker
sabeluzole
saber shin
Sabin-Feldman dye test for congenital
    toxoplasmosis
Sabolich socket system
sac
    bursal
    common dural
    cystic
    dural
    effacement of dural
    narrowing of thecal
    spinal
    thecal
    tight dural
SAC (short arm cast)
saccade (pl. saccades)
    adduction
    back-to-back
    contralateral
    corrective
    dysmetric
    hypermetric
    hypometric
    optic dysmetric
    rapid (corrective)

saccade *(continued)*
    rapid lateral
    refixation
    volitional
saccade velocity
saccadic blur
saccadic breakdown of pursuit
saccadic corrections
saccadic eye movements
saccadic oscillations
saccadic palsy
saccadic slowing
saccadic snap
saccharopinuria
sacciform recess
saccular aneurysm
saccular nerve
SACH (solid-ankle, cushioned-heel)
    foot prosthesis
SACH heels
Sachs brain suction tip
Sachs dural hook
Sachs dural separator
Sachs nerve separator-spatula
Sachs suction tube
Sachs vein retractor
sacral alae
sacral cyst

sacral dermatomes
sacralgia
sacral gutter
sacral insufficiency fracture (SIF)
sacralization of transverse process of
    vertebra
sacralization of vertebra
sacralized transverse process
sacral nerve stimulation (SNS) therapy
sacral plexus
sacral promontory
sacral sparing (in sensory loss)
sacral splanchnic nerves
sacrectomy
    complete
    hemisacrectomy
    partial
    subtotal
sacrifice, parent vessel
sacroabdominoperineal pull-through
sacrococcygeal chordoma
sacrococcygeal joint
sacrococcygeal junction
sacrococcygeal muscle
sacrococcygeal remnant tumor
sacrococcygeal teratoma
sacrococcyx
sacrodural ligament
Sacro-ease pillow
Sacro-Eze lumbar support
sacroiliac (SI)
sacroiliac articulation
sacroiliac disease
sacroiliac joint syndrome
sacroiliac resisted abduction test
sacroiliac sprain
sacroiliac stretch test
sacroiliac subluxation
sacroiliac syndrome
sacroiliitis
sacropubic diameter
sacrosciatic foramen
sacrosciatic notch
sacrospinalis muscle
sacrospinous ligament
sacrospinous ligament suspension
sacrotuberous ligament

sacrouterine
sacrovertebral angle
sacrum
    alae of
    assimilation
    cornua of
    promontory of
    scimitar
    tilted
saddle anesthesia
saddle-area anesthesia
saddle-area sensory loss
saddle block
saddle clamp
saddle coil
saddle distribution of sensory loss
saddle hypesthesia
saddle joint
saddle points
saddle, trapezial
SADIA (small angle double incidence
    angiograms)
SAD (seasonal affective disorder)
SAE (subcortical atherosclerotic
    encephalopathy)
Saethre-Chotzen syndrome
SAFE (stationary attachment flexible
    endoskeletal) foot
SAF (self-articulating femoral) hip
    replacement
SafeTap tapered spinal needle
Safe-T-Wheel pinwheel
SAFHS (sonic-accelerated fracture-
    healing system) 2000
Safil suture
safranin O stain
Sage-Clark technique
Sage radial nail
Sage-Salvatore classification of
    acromioclavicular joint injury
Sager traction splint
sagittal band reconstruction
sagittal orientation
sagittal plane faults
sagittal roll spondylolisthesis
sagittal sinus
sagittal T1-weighted image

SAH (subarachnoid hemorrhage)
Sahara clinical bone sonometer
Sahara portable bone densitometer
Saha transfer technique
SAID (specific adaptation to imposed
    demands) of disability
sailorman's (or sailor's) knot
sail sign
Saint (St.)
    St. George-Buchholz ankle
        prosthesis
    St. George total elbow prosthesis
    St. John's wort (*Hypericum
        perforatum*)
    St. John's transdermal patch
    St. Jude Medical valve prosthesis
    St. Louis encephalitis
    St. Louis encephalitis antibody
    St. Louis viral encephalitis
    St. Vitus dance
    Ulrich-St. Gallen forceps
Sakellarides classification of calcaneal
    fracture
salaam attack
salaam seizures
Salenius meniscus knife
Salibi carotid artery clamp
salicylic acid plaster for plantar warts
salicylic acid tape
salient antecedents to injury
saline
    heparinized
    sterile
saline-enhanced MR arthrography
saline flush
saline hot bath
saline-soaked Weck spears
saline torch
SAL (self-aligning) mobile-bearing
    knee implant
salmon calcitonin nasal spray
Salmonine (calcitonin salmon)
Salmon Rickham ventriculostomy
    reservoir
salmonella arthritis
salmonella osteomyelitis
salpingopharyngeal muscle

saltatory nerve conduction
saltatory spasm
salt bridges connecting EEG electrodes
Salter fracture (I-VI)
Salter-Harris classification of fracture
    (I-VI or 1-6)
Salter-Harris classification of tibial-
    fibular injury
Salter-Harris-Rang classification of
    epiphyseal fracture
Salter innominate osteotomy
Salter radiographic criteria for
    avascular necrosis
Saltiel brace
salts, gold
salt wasting, cerebral
salvage
    interventional limb
    limb
    tibiotalar
salvage reconstruction
salvo (pl. salvos)
Salzer prosthesis
Salzer resurfacing procedure
samarium Sm 153 lexidronam
    (Quadramet)
same-day microsurgical arthroscopic
    lateral-approach laser-assisted
    (SMALL) fluoroscopic diskectomy
Samilson osteotomy
Sam Jr. posture analyzer
sample, Pennsylvania bimanual work
sampling rate on EEG
Sampson medullary nail
Sam splint
Samuels forceps
sandal, Rainbow cast
sandbagging fracture of long bones
Sanders computed tomography
    classification of fracture
SANE (Single Assessment Numeric
    Evaluation) score/assessment/
    rating/method
Sanfilippo syndrome
sanguineous
SANS (Stoller afferent nerve stimula-
    tion) device

Santa Casa distractor
Santavuori-Haltia-Hagberg disease
Santorini ligament
Santorini muscle
saphenous nerve
saphenous vein extracranial-
  intracranial bypass graft
Sappey ligament
Sarbo sign
sarcoid arthritis
sarcoid, Boeck
sarcoid flexor tenosynovitis
sarcoidosis, spinal cord
sarcoma
  alveolar soft part
  botryoid
  classic Kaposi
  clear cell
  epidemic Kaposi
  epithelioid
  Ewing
  extraosseous Ewing
  fibromyxoid
  high grade surface osteogenic
  intracortical osteogenic
  juxtacortical
  Kaposi
  low grade central osteogenic
  malignant myeloid
  multicentric osteogenic
  osteogenic
  Paget-associated osteogenic
  parosteal osteogenic
  postirradiation osteogenic
  primary
  reticulum cell
  small cell osteogenic
  soft tissue
  spindle cell
  synovial
sarcomere
sarcopenia
sarcopenic
sarcotubular myopathy
sardonicus, risus
Sargent knee procedure
Sarmiento (STH-2) hip prosthesis

Sarmiento short leg patellar tendon-
  bearing cast
sartorius muscle
sartorius nerve
sartorius tendon
S.A.S. shoes
SAS software
Sassouni analysis
SAS II (shoulder arm system) brace
Sat-A-Lite cushion (by Bodyline)
Sateen knee immobilizer
satellite plantar wart
Satterlee amputating saw
Satterlee bone saw
saturation
  jugular bulb oxygen (SjO$_2$)
  jugular venous oxygen
  regional cerebral oxygen
saturation recovery
saturation transfer
Saturday night paralysis
Saturday night radial palsy
Saturn splint
saucerization of vertebra
saucerize
Sauerbruch-Britsch rib shears
Sauerbruch-Coryllos rongeur
Sauerbruch-Frey bone punch
Sauerbruch-Frey rib shears
Sauerbruch rib elevator
Sauerbruch rib forceps
Sauerbruch rib rongeur
Sauerbruch rib shears
Sauerbruch-Stille rongeur
Saunders Cervical Hometrac traction
Saunders digital inclinometer
Saunders lumbar traction device
Saunders Posture S'port
sausage finger
Sauvé-Kapandji (S-K) reconstruction
  of distal radioulnar joint
Savastano Hemi-Knee prosthesis
Saver, Haemonetics Cell
saw
  Adams
  Adson wire
  Aesculap

saw *(continued)*
   air-powered
   amputating
   Bailey-Gigli
   Bailey wire
   bayonet
   Beaver
   Bier amputation
   Bishop
   bow-type
   cast
   Charriere amputating
   Charriere bone
   circular
   Cottle
   counter rotating
   craniotomy
   crosscut
   Cushing
   Davis
   DeMartel wire
   electric cast
   end-cutting reciprocating
   Engel plaster
   fenestration
   Gigli wire
   Hall air-driven oscillating
   Hall Micro E oscillating
   Hall Micro E reciprocating
   Hall Micro E sagittal
   Hall Versipower oscillating
   Hall Versipower reciprocating
   Herbert
   Langenbeck metacarpal
   Lebsche wire
   Luck-Bishop bone
   metacarpal
   Micro-Aire oscillating
   micro-oscillating
   micro sagittal
   Midas Rex craniotomy
   Mueller (Müller)
   Olivecrona-Gigli
   Orthair oscillating
   oscillating
   Oscillo III plaster
   Percy amputating

saw *(continued)*
   plaster
   Poppen
   power oscillating
   power-driven
   Raney
   reciprocating motor
   Rust amputation
   sagittal surgical
   Satterlee amputating
   single-blade
   straight oscillating
   Strully-Gigli
   twin-blade oscillating
   Tyler-Gigli
   Weiss amputation
   Wigmore plaster
   wire
   Zimmer oscillating
SAWA shoulder brace
sawcut
saw guide
   Bailey Gigli
   Poppen Gigli
saw handles, Strully Gigli
Sayk preparation of CSF cells
Sayre periosteal elevator
Sayre splint
Sayre traction
Sbarbaro tibial plateau prosthesis
SBO (spina bifida occulta)
SBRN (sensory branch of radial
   nerve)
SCA (superior cerebellar artery)
scaffold
   bone
   endoluminal
   3D porous Chitosan
Scaglietti closed reduction technique
scale (see also *assessment, index,*
     questionnaire, score)
   Abbreviated Injury Scale (AIS)
   Abnormal Involuntary Movement
     (AIMS)
   ADAS noncognitive subscale
   AIMS2 (Arthritis Impact Measure
     ment Scales-Symptoms [Pain])

scale *(continued)*
  AIMS2 Hand Subscale
  ALS Functional Rating Scale
    (ALSFRS)
  American Musculoskeletal Tumor
    Society rating
  Arthritis Impact Measurement
    (AIMS)
  Arthritis Quality of Life
  Ashworth
  Behavioral Pathology in Alz-
    heimer's Disease Rating Scale
  Blessed Behavior Scale
  Blessed Dementia Rating (BDRS)
  Blessed-Roth Dementia Scale
    (BRDS)
  Bonney hallux valgus outcome
  Brief Cognitive Rating Scale
    (BCRS)
  Brink-Yesavage Geriatric Depres-
    sion Scale
  Canadian Neurological Scale
  CATCH (Chedoke-McMaster
    Attitudes Toward Children with
    Handicaps)
  Charnley-Merle D'Aubigné
    disability grading
  Charnley pain and function grading
  Chronic Pain Self-Efficacy Scale
  CINA (Clinical Institute Narcotic
    Assessment)
  Clinical Dementia Rating (CDR)
  Columbia neurologic rating
  Comprehensive Level of
    Consciousness (CLCS)
  Constant-Murley rating
  Cornell Scale for Depression,
    Dementia (CSDD)
  Cox multivariate regression
  Cronbach alpha
  Crosby-Insall rating
  Crowe hip
  CRP concentration
  DASH (Disabilities of the Arm,
    Shoulder, and Hand)
  Dementia Behavior Disturbance
    (DBD)

scale *(continued)*
  Dementia Mood Assessment
    (DMAS)
  Drake
  Edinburgh Rehabilitation Status
  EIS (Emotional Intimacy Scale)
  Exercise Self-Efficacy Scale
  Expanded Disability Status
  Fibromaylgia Self-Efficacy Scale
  Ficat grading
  Gait Abnormality Rating (GARS)
  Glasgow Coma (GCS)
  Glasgow Outcome
  Gross Motor Function Measure
  Guttman
  Hallux Metatarsophalangeal-
    Interphalangeal Scale
  Hamilton Rating Scale for
    Depression
  Harris hip
  hierarchical s. of ADLs
  Hoehn and Yahr Staging of
    Parkinson's Disease
  Hospital Anxiety and Depression
  HSC (Hospital for Sick Children)
    Scale
  HSS (Hospital for Special Surgery)
    ligament rating
  Hunt-Hess subarachnoid
    hemorrhage
  Injury Severity Scale (ISS)
  Insall-Crosby
  International Knee Documentation
    Committee
  interval rehabilitation testing
  Jadad
  Japanese Orthopaedic Association
    (JOA) functional
  Johnson-Boseker
  Kellgren
  LEFS (Lower Extremity Functional
    Scale)
  LIDO
  ligament sizing
  Likert
  linear analog pain
  linear analog self-assessment

scale *(continued)*
    Lovett's clinical s. of strength
    Lower Extremity Functional Scale
      (LEFS)
    Lubben
    Lysholm knee function
    Lysholm II
    MAS (Motor Assessment)
    Mattis Dementia Rating
    McGowan
    Medical Outcome
    Merle D'Aubigné pain and mobility
      rating
    Mississippi Scale for Combat-
      Related Posttraumatic Stress
      Disorder
    modified Ashworth s. for grading
      spasticity
    Montefiore Organic Brain Scale
      (MOBS)
    Motor Assessment (MAS)
    Neurobehavioral Rating
    NIH (National Institutes of Health)
      Stroke
    Nottingham Ten-Point ADL Scale
    Noyes knee rating
    Outerbridge
    Oxford
    Peabody Developmental Motor
    Perceived Therapeutic Efficacy
      Scale
    Prosthetic Problem Inventory
    Quality of Well-Being
    Quebec Back Pain Disability Scale
    Rankin
    Rankin Scale
    Rappaport Disability Rating
    Rotes
    Rowe-Zarins
    Scandinavian Stroke Scale
    Semmes-Weinstein
    Short-Form 36 Health Survey
      (SF-36)
    Social Adjustment Scale
    Sports Activity Scale
    Symptoms and Sports Participation
      Rating Scale

scale *(continued)*
    Tegner activity level
    UCLA (University of California
      at Los Angeles)
    Unified Huntington's Disease
      Rating Scale
    VASHD (Visual Analog Scale
      of Handicap)
    Visual Analog Scale of Handicap
    Wechsler Adult Intelligence Scale
    Weschler Memory Revised
    Wechsler Memory Scale or Test
    Western Ontario Instability Index
      (WOSI)
    Wilson-Krout grading
    Yesavage Geriatric Depression
      Scale
    Yesavage-Brink Geriatric Depres-
      sion Scale
    Zuckerman
    Zung Depression Scale
    Zung Self-Rating Depression
scalene block
scalene fat pad
scalene muscle
scalene musculature
scalenus anticus syndrome
scalenus anticus test
scalenus minimus
scalloping of margin of vertebral body
scalloping of vertebrae
scalp clip
    Children's Hospital
    Raney
scalp clip applicator
scalp edema
scalp EEG (SEEG)
scalpel
    LaserSonics Nd:YAG LaserBlade
    rotary gamma
scalp electrode
scalp-electrode interface
scalp hematoma
scalp inclusion cyst
scalp muscle
scalp recording
scalp slips, LeRoy

scalp vein
scan, scanning (see *scanner*)
  bone
  brain
  CAT (computerized axial
    tomographic)
  contrast material enhanced
  CT (computed tomography)
  CT (computerized tomography)
  CTAT (computerized transverse
    axial tomography)
  DEXA (dual-energy x-ray
    absorptiometry)
  duplex
  duplex carotid
  fluorodopa PET
  gallium
  gallium-67 bone
  high resolution ultrasound
  indium-111-labeled leukocyte bone
  isotope
  isotope bone
  isotope shunt
  linear
  MRI (magnetic resonance imaging)
  NeuroSector
  nuclear bone
  PET (positron emission tomography)
  positron emission transaxial
    tomography
  postmetrizamide CT
  radioisotope gallium
  radioisotope indium-labeled white
    blood cell
  radioisotope (static)
  radioisotope technetium
  radionuclide
  radionuclide brain
  rectilinear bone
  sector
  serial
  SPECT (single photon emission CT)
  stacked
  technetium
  technetium-99m diphosphonate
  technetium-99m MDP bone
  technetium-99m pyrophosphate

scan *(continued)*
  technetium-99m sulfur colloid
  three-phase bone
  total body
  triple-phase bone
  TSPP rectilinear bone
  unenhanced
  ventilation-perfusion lung
Scandinavian Stroke Scale
scanner
  ATL real-time Neurosector
  GE (General Electric) Advance
    PET
  GE CT Advantage
  GE CT 8800
  GE CT Hi-Speed Advantage
  GE CT Max
  GE CT Pace
  GE detector
  GE gamma camera
  GE HiSpeed Advantage helical CT
  GE HiSpeed CT
  GE Medical Systems
  GE MR Max
  GE MR Signa
  GE MR Vectra
  GE 9800 high resolution CT
  GE Omega 500 MHz
  GE QE 300 MHz GE PET
  GE Signa 1.5 T magnet
  GE Signa 1.5 tesla
  GE Signa 4.7 MRI
  GE Signa 5.2 with SR-230 3-axis
    EPI gradient upgrade
  GE Signa 5.4 Genesis MR imager
  GE Signa 5.5 Horizon EchoSpeed
    MR imager
  GE single axis SR-230 echo-planar
  GE single-detector SPECT-capable
    camera
  GE SPECT (single-photon emission
    computerized tomography)
  GE Spiral CT
  GE Starcam single-crystal tomo-
    graphic scintillation camera
scanning densitometry
scanning speech

Scan-O-Grams of lower extremities
scanography
scaphocapitate joint
scaphocephalic head shape
scaphocephaly
scaphoid bone
    pole of
    waist of
scaphoid cookie in shoe
scaphoid humpback deformity
scaphoid impaction syndrome
scaphoiditis
Scaphoid-Microstaple system
scaphoid shift test
scapholunate arthritic collapse (SLAC)
    wrist
scapholunate dissociation
scapholunate ganglion
scapholunate (SL) joint
scapholunate ligament (LSS)
scapholunate space
scapholunate widening
scapho-trapezium-trapezoid (STT) joint
scaphotrapezoid-trapezial (STT) joint
scapula
    body of
    inferior tip of
    margin of
    high-riding
    winged
    winging of the
scapular bone
scapular flap
scapular notch
scapular winging
scapulectomy
    Das Gupta
    Phelps
scapuloclavicular
scapulocostal stabilization
scapulocostal syndrome
scapulohumeral rhythm
scapuloperoneal muscular atrophy
scapulothoracic arthrodesis
scapulothoracic bursitis
scapulothoracic joint
scapulothoracic motion

scapulovertebral border
scar
    dural
    endovascular
    incisional
    retractile
    scarring
Scarborough total hip replacement
scar contracture
scarf osteotomy-bunionectomy
scarf rotational bunionectomy
scarified
Scarpa fascia
Scarpa ganglion
Scarpa ligament
Scarpa nerve
scarred
scarring
scattered dysrhythmic slow activity
Scerratti goniometer
SCFE (slipped capital femoral
    epiphysis)
Schaberg-Harper-Allen technique
Schaltenbrand atlas of stereotaxy for
    neurosurgery
Schanz angulation osteotomy
Schanz brace
Schanz collar
Schanz metaphyseal screws
Schanz rod
Scharff microbipolar and suction
    forceps
Schatzker fracture classification system
Schauwecker patellar wiring technique
Schede bone curet
Schede hip osteotomy
Schedule
    General Well-Being
    Glasgow Assessment
Scheffe test
Scheicker laminectomy punch forceps
Scheie syndrome
Schell bone rongeur
Scheuermann disease
Scheuermann juvenile kyphosis
Schiefferdecker disk
Schiek back support

Schiff-Sherrington phenomenon
Schilder disease
Schilder encephalitis
schindyletic joint
Schink retractor
Schirmer test
schistosomiasis, spinal
schizencephaly
  closed-lip (type I)
  open-lip (type II)
Schlatter-Osgood disease
Schlein clamp
Schlein elbow arthroplasty
Schlein prosthesis
Schlemm ligament
Schlesinger cervical punch forceps
Schlesinger cervical rongeur
Schlesinger intervertebral disk rongeur
Schlesinger laminectomy rongeur
Schlesinger pituitary rongeur
Schlesinger rongeur forceps
Schlesinger sign
Schlesinger vein
Schmeisser spica
Schmidt rod holder
Schmidt syndrome
Schmieden dural scissors
Schmieden-Taylor dissector
Schmitt disease
Schmorl disease
Schmorl node
Schmorl nodule
Schneider arthrodesis
Schneider driver-extractor
Schneider nail
Schneider rasp
Schneider rod
Schneider-Sauerbruch rasp
Schnidt forceps
Schnute wedge resection technique
Schober index
Schober test of lumbar flexion
Schoeber sign
Schoemaker-Burkart marker
Scholl's pads
Schreiber maneuver
Schrock procedure

Schrötter chorea
Schuchart rib shears
Schuhli implant system
Schuknecht wire-cutting scissors
Schuller view
Schultze bundle
Schumacher criteria for diagnosis of
  multiple sclerosis
Schumacher rib shears
Schutte basket, shovel nose
Schwab and England Activities of
  Daily Living Score
Schwalbe nucleus of cerebellum
Schwann cell body
Schwann cell of myelin sheath
Schwann cells, proliferation of
Schwann cell tube
Schwann tumor
schwannoma
  dumbbell
  facial nerve
  intraosseous
  melanotic
  orbital
  vestibular
Schwartz aneurysm clip
Schwartz clip-applying forceps
Schwartze chisel
Schwartz intracranial clamp
Schwartz-Jampel syndrome (SJS)
Schwartz laminectomy retractor
Schwartz temporary clamp-applying
  forceps
Schwartz temporary intracranial artery
  clamps
Schwarz finger extension bow
Schweitzer spring plate
SCI (spinal cord injury)
sciatica
sciatic endometriosis
sciatic foramen
sciatic nerve irritation
sciatic notch
sciatic plexus
sciatic scoliosis
sciatic stretch test
SCICU (spinal cord intensive care
  unit)

scimitar sign on x-ray
scintigraphy
  bone
  bone marrow
  brain perfusion
  cortical
  gated blood pool
  indium-111
  indium scintigraphy with [111]In
    white blood cells (^{111}In-WBC)
  pyrophosphate
  SPECT brain perfusion
  technetium ^{99m}Tc-PYP
    (pyrophosphate)
  three-phase bone (TPBS)
  white blood cell (WBCS) with
    indium-111
scintilla
scintillating scotoma (pl. scotomata)
scissor gait
scissoring of legs
scissors
  Acufex
  Adson ganglion
  Adson-Toennis
  alligator
  arthroscopic
  Babcock wire-cutting
  bandage
  Bantam wire-cutting
  bayonet-shaped
  Beebe wire-cutting
  Bellucci alligator
  Bergmann plaster
  bipolar cautery
  blunt-tipped iris
  brain
  cartilage
  circumflex
  Crafoord thoracic
  crown and collar
  curved Mayo
  Dandy neurosurgical
  Dandy trigeminal nerve
  Dean
  DeBakey endarterectomy
  Decker alligator

scissors *(continued)*
  Decker micro
  Decker microsurgical
  DeMartel neurosurgical
  dissecting
  dural
  endarterectomy
  ENT (ear, nose, and throat)
  Esmarch plaster
  face-lift
  Fiskars Softouch
  F. L. Fischer microsurgical
    neurectomy bayonet
  Frazier dural
  Giertz-Stille
  Halsey nail
  Harvey wire-cutting
  hook
  iris
  Jacobson microneurosurgical
  Jannetta-Kurze dissecting
  Kelly fistula
  Koenig nail-splitting
  Kreuscher
  Kurze dissecting
  LaserScissors 390/20
  Lister
  Luque rod
  Malis bipolar cautery
  Malis neurological
  Martin cartilage
  Mayo
  McCain TMJ
  McIndoe
  Medi plaster
  meniscectomy
  meniscus
  Metzenbaum
  micro
  microneurosurgical
  Micro-One
  microsurgery or microsurgical
  Micro-Two
  moleskin
  nail
  nail splitting
  Nelson

scissors *(continued)*
  neurological or neurosurgical
  Nicola
  Olivecrona dural
  Olivecrona trigeminal
  operating
  Oxo kitchen
  Penn wire-cutting
  pituitary
  plaster
  Potts-Smith
  Potts tenotomy
  Potts-Yasargil
  Rhoton bayonet
  Rogers wire-cutting
  Schmieden dural
  Schuknecht wire-cutting
  Seutin plaster
  Slip-N-Snip
  Smillie meniscus
  Smith wire-cutting
  spring-handled
  Stevens
  Stiwer
  strabismus
  Strully dissecting
  Strully dural
  Strully neurological
  suture
  Sweet pituitary
  Take-apart
  Taylor brain
  Taylor dural
  tenotomy
  thoracic
  Tindall
  Toennis dissecting
  trigeminal
  Walton
  Webster meniscectomy
  Weck microsuture cutting
  Weller cartilage
  Wiet otologic
  wire
  wire-cutting
  Yasargil bayonet
  Yasargil micro

scissors gait
SCIWORA (spinal cord injury without radiologic abnormality) syndrome
scleroderma
sclerosant
sclerosing nonsuppurative osteitis
sclerosing nonsuppurative osteomyelitis
sclerosis
  Ammon horn (mesial temporal)
  amyotrophic lateral (ALS) (Lou Gehrig disease)
  Baló
  congenital hippocampal
  diffuse
  disseminated
  familial amyotrophic lateral
  hippocampal
  incisural
  Krabbe diffuse
  lobar
  mesial temporal
  Mönckeberg
  multiple (MS)
  pedicle
  posterolateral
  subchondral
  tuberous
sclerotherapy, transvenous retrograde
  nidus
sclerotic area
sclerotic reactive line
sclerotic rims in gout
sclerotomal diagram of pain
sclerotomal pain
sclerotome area
SCNB (stereotactic core needle biopsy)
SCOI (Southern California Orthopedic Institute))
SCOI arthroscopic tenodesis
SCOI shoulder brace
scoliorachitis
scoliosis
  adolescent idiopathic (AIS)
  Aussies-Isseis unstable
  Brissaud

scoliosis *(continued)*
   cicatricial
   Cobb measurement of
   collapsing
   coxitic
   dextrorotary
   dextroscoliosis
   Dwyer correction of
   empyematic
   endoscopic correction of
   Fergusson method for measuring
   fixation of
   functional
   idiopathic
   inflammatory
   ischiatic
   King classification of thoracic
   King-Moe
   levorotary
   levoscoliosis
   lumbar
   lumbar component of
   Moe and Kettleson distribution of
      curves in
   myopathic
   osteopathic
   paralytic
   rachitic
   rheumatoid
   rotary
   sciatic
   S-shaped
   static
   thoracic
   thoracic component of
   thoracolumbar
   traumatic
   uncompensated rotary
   Winter-King-Moe
scoliosis correction with Dwyer cable
scoliosis curve pattern
Scoliosis Research Society
scoliotic spine
scoop
   bone
   Cushing pituitary
   intervertebral disk

scoop *(continued)*
   Scoville intervertebral disk
   Yasargil
scooter
   Lark
   Rascal
scope
   Doppler
   Harris
   Hughston knee
   Lysholm knee joint instability
scopolamine (Transderm-Scop)
score (see also *assessment, index,*
      questionnaire, scale)
   AAOS Knee Society Clinical
      Rating
   American Knee Society
   American Orthopaedic Foot and
      Ankle Society (AOFAS) ankle-
      hindfoot
   Ankle Score
   ASES (American Shoulder and
      Elbow Surgeons) shoulder
   Ashworth muscle spasticity
   Athlete Shoulder Scoring System
   Bandi patellofemoral
   Beck Cognitive
   Bray
   Broberg
   Carter-Rowe shoulder
   Champion Trauma (CTS)
   Charlson Comorbidity Score
   Child-Pugh
   Children's Coma (CCS)
   Cincinnati
   composite knee
   Constant
   Constant-Murley
   Denis
   Diabetic Quality of Life (DQOL)
   DQOL (Diabetic Quality of Life)
   D'Aubigne-Postel postoperative
      function
   ECLAM
   Ewald
   FFI (Foot Function Index)
   Foot Function Index

score *(continued)*
  Frank Noyes function
  Functional Rating Score
  Gillquist-Lysholm
  Hachinski ischemia
  Hannover Polytrauma
  Harris Hip Score
  Hawkins-Warren athlete's shoulder
  HHS (Harris Hip Score)
  HSS (Hospital for Special Surgery) knee
  Hughston knee
  IKDC
  injury-severity
  ISS
  Jäger-Wirth
  Jebson Taylor
  JOA (Japanese Orthopaedic Association) knee
  Karnofsky performance (KPS)
  Knee Society Score
  Kurtzke disability
  Larsen hip
  Lysholm knee joint instability
  Lysholm-Gillquist
  Mangled Extremity Severity (MESS)
  Mankin
  Marshall knee
  Mayo Elbow Performance Index
  Mayo wrist
  McGill-Melzack scoring system
  Merle D'Aubigne
  modified Harris Hip Score
  modified Rowe shoulder
  Mohtadi Quality of Life Assessment Score
  Molander-Olerud ankle
  Morrey
  MSTS
  Nottingham Health Profile (NHP)
  Noyes function
  OAK (Orthopädische Arbeitsgruppe Knie)
  Olerud-Molander ankle
  Oswestry Disability
  pain

score *(continued)*
  Patte
  Pritchard
  Rankin
  Rowe
  SANE (Single Assessment Numeric Evaluation)
  Schwab and England Activities of Daily Living
  SF-36 (Short-Form 36 Health Survey)
  Single Assessment Numeric Evaluation (SANE)
  skeletal injury
  T
  Tapper-Hoover
  Taylor vertebral body
  Tegner activity s. for knee reconstruction
  UCLA
  VAS (visual analog score)
  WOSI (Western Ontario Instability Index)
  Z
SCORE (Simple Calculated Osteoporosis Risk Estimation)
scoring incision
scorings on bone
Scorpio total knee system
Scotchcast 2 casting tape
Scotchcast splint
scotoma (pl. scotomata)
  absolute
  bilateral
  cecocentral
  central
  dense
  fortification
  homonymous scintillating
  march of
  mental
  negative
  paracentral
  relative
  scintillating
scotomata of action
scotometry

scotomization
Scott ankle splint
Scott cock-up wrist splint
Scott contoured cervical collar
Scott double-strap ankle support
Scott elastic ankle strap
Scott glenoplasty technique
Scott hinged knee support
Scottish Rite hip orthosis
Scott lumbosacral support
Scott-McCracken periosteal elevator
Scott serpentine cervical collar
Scott silicone ventricular catheter
Scott tennis elbow sleeve with tension
    wrap
Scott Unifoam tennis elbow splint
Scott universal cervical collar
Scott ventricular cannula
Scott wrist wrap
scout electrode
scout film
ScoutView targeting
Scoville blade
Scoville brain clip-applying forceps
Scoville brain spatula forceps
Scoville cervical disk retractor
Scoville clip-applying forceps
Scoville disk curet
Scoville dissector
Scoville-Haverfield hemilaminectomy
    retractor
Scoville intervertebral disk scoop
Scoville nerve root hook
Scoville nerve root retractor
Scoville retractor
Scoville-Richter laminectomy retractor
Scoville ruptured disk curet
Scoville skull trephine
Scoville spatula forceps
Scoville ventricular needles
Scranton-McDermott classification
scraped
scraping toe gait
scratching automatism
    blood
    drug
    Lanex

screen, screening
    Gait Arms Legs and Spine (GALS)
    genome
    mutation
Screening Examination of the
    Musculoskeletal System (SEMS)
Screening Test, Halstead-Wepman
    Aphasia
screw
    Ace
    AcroMed VSP
    Aesculap
    AMBI hip
    Amset R-F
    AO-ASIF
    AO cancellous
    AO cortical
    AO lag
    AO spongiosa
    arthrodesis
    ASIF cancellous
    ASIF cortical
    Asnis 2 guided
    Asnis cannulated
    Aten olecranon
    Barouk cannulated bone
    Barouk micro
    Basile
    Bechtol
    bicortical
    biodegradable
    Bio-Interference tibial
    Bionx absorbable cannulated
    BioScrew absorbable interference
    BioSorbFX SR self-reinforced plate
    bone mulch
    Bosworth
    breakable
    breakout of
    buttress
    Calandruccio compression
    Campbell cannulated
    cancellous bone
    cannulated
    Carrell-Girard
    Caspar cervical
    C-D (Cotrel-Dubousset)

screw *(continued)*
  chrome cobalt
  Collison
  compression hip
  compression lag
  Concept cannulated
  Concise compression hip
  cortex
  cortical bone
  cortical cancellous
  Cotrel-Dubosset vertebral
  Coventry
  cross slot
  cruciate head
  cruciform head
  Cubbins
  DDT (device for transverse
    traction)
  DeMuth
  dome
  double-fluted tip
  double-threaded Herbert
  Duo-Driv
  DuVal
  Dwyer cable and
  dynamic condylar
  dynamic hip
  ECT (European compression
    technique) bone
  Edwards
  Eggers
  EndoFix bioabsorbable
  epidural
  Fixateur Interne
  fretted
  fully threaded
  Geckler
  Gentle Threads interference
  Glasgow
  Glass-Bessen transfixion
  Guardsman femoral
  Hahn
  Hamilton
  Hedrocel titanium
  Henderson lag
  Herbert bone
  Herbert-Whipple bone

screw *(continued)*
  hex (hexagonal)
  hex head
  hexagon
  hexagonal slot cap
  hollow mill Asnis cannulated
  home run
  Howmedica ICS
  Howmedica VSF
  Ilizarov
  In-Fast bone
  interference
  interfragmentary
  Isola vertebral
  Jeter lag or position
  Johansson lag
  Jones
  Kaessmann
  KLS Centre-Drive
  Knöringer
  Kostuik
  Kristiansen eyelet lag
  Kurosaka fixation
  LA (ligament anchor)
  lag
  Lane bone
  large-headed
  Leibinger Micro Plus
  Leibinger mini-Wurzburg
  Leinbach
  Lindorf lag or position
  Lorenz cranial
  Lorenzo
  Luhr
  Lundholm
  Luque II
  Maconor
  Magerl transarticular
  Magna-Fx cannulated
  malleolar
  Marion
  Martin
  McLaughlin
  metallic
  micro self-tapping
  Mille Pattes
  mini AO

screw *(continued)*
   Morris biphase
   Morris biplane
   Moss
   Mouradian
   navicular
   Neufeld
   NoLok
   Olerud PSF
   Orthofix
   pedicle
   PerFixation interference
   Phillips
   Phillips recessed head
   pitch of threads on
   polylactide
   Propel cannulated interference
   PWB (Puno-Winter-Byrd)
   Quiet interference
   RCI titanium soft tissue inter-
      ference
   Reddick-Saye
   Revo retrievable cancellous
   resorbable
   Richards compression
   Richards self-tapping
   Rockwood
   Rogozinski
   Salzburg
   Schanz metaphyseal
   Selby I and II
   self-tapping bone
   SemiFix
   Shelton bone
   Sherman bone
   Simmons
   sliding compression hip
   small fragment
   small-headed
   SmartScrew resorbable
   Spiessel lag or position
   stainless steel
   Steffee pedicle
   Steffee plate and
   Steinhauser cranial
   Steinhauser lag or position
   Storz

screw *(continued)*
   strip-out of
   Stryker
   subarachnoid
   subdural pressure
   suprasyndesmotic
   Swiss cancellous
   syndesmosis
   syndesmotic
   Synthes compression hip
   Sysorb
   tension
   Thornton
   threaded cancellous
   thumb
   tibial head
   tip of
   titanium lag
   top-loading
   Townley
   Townsend-Gilfillan
   transarticular
   transfixing
   transfixion
   transpedicular
   transsyndesmosis
   transsyndesmotic
   triangulated
   Tronzo VLC cannulated
      compression
   TSRH (Texas Scottish Rite
      Hospital) pedicle
   TSRH vertebral
   Tunneloc bone mulch
   unicortical
   Universal fixation
   varus-valgus adjustment
   VDS (ventral derotating spinal)
   Venable-Stuck
   Vitallium
   von Bahr
   VSF (Vermont spinal fixator)
   VSP (variable screw placement)
   Wagner-Schanz
   Wiltse
   wood
   Woodruff

screw *(continued)*
   Wurzburg
   Zimmer compression hip
   Zuelzer
screw and keel fixation
screw and plate (screw-plate)
screwdriver
   automatic
   Becker
   Bosworth
   cannulated
   Cardan
   collet adapter
   Collison
   cross slot
   cruciform
   Flatt self-retaining
   Ken
   Phillips head
   Ritcher
   self-retaining
   single-slot
   torque
   VDS (ventral derotating spinal)
   Wera-Werk torque
   Williams
screw fixation
screw head
   countersink
   Phillips
screwhome mechanism
screw-in ceramic acetabular cup
screw placement, variable (VSP)
screw-plate
   Calandruccio impaction
   pedicle
   Zimmer impaction
screw pullout
screw-rod
   Edwards D-L modular
   Wiltse
screw tap
screw toggle
Scrip Muscle Master massager
scriptorius, calamus
scroll bones

scrub
   Betadine
   Hibiclens
scrum ear (in rugby players)
SCT (spinal cord tether)
SCT (star cancellation test)
Scuderi technique for repair of
   ruptured quadriceps tendon
Scully Hip S'port
scultetus bandage/binder
scurvy
SDAT (senile dementia, Alzheimer
   type)
SDEEG (stereotaxic depth electroencephalogram)
SDH (subdural hemorrhage)
SDRI (small, deep, recent infarct)
S*D*sorb meniscal stapler
SDS-PAGE test
SEA (spinal epidural abscess)
sealant
   fibrin
   Tisseel fibrin sealant
seasonal affective disorder (SAD)
seat
   Heffington lumbar surgical
   ischial-bearing
   LiteNest portable
   Rubbermaid adjustable bath/shower
   sigmoid
   ulnar
   Wayne laminectomy
seat-belt fracture
seat-belt injury
seat-belt sign
seated prosthesis
seating of prosthesis
   adaptive
   proper
seating site
seat surface
Seattle foot prosthesis
Seattle orthosis
Seawell rasp
sebaceum, adenoma (in tuberous
   sclerosis)

Sebileau muscle
Sebileau periosteal elevator
Seckel syndrome
secondary brain tumor
secondary cartilaginous joint
secondary closure
secondary contractures
secondary fracture
secondary gain
secondary gout
secondary intention, healing by
secondary metatarsalgia
secondary or acute hematogenous
  osteomyelitis
secondary suture of ruptured tendons
secondary union
second compartment
second cranial nerve
second double support of gait
second impact syndrome
second tibial muscle
Secor drug pump (I and II)
Secor implantable drug reservoir
secreting neurons
secretomotor fibers
secretomotor nerve
secretory nerve
sectioning of tight filum terminale
section, permanent
sector
  lower field visual
  Sommer sector of the hippocampus
sed (sedimentation) rate
Sedan goniometer
Sedan-Vallicioni cannula
Seddon classification of nerve injuries
Seddon coin stereognosis test
sedentary lifestyle
Sedillot periosteal elevator
seeding
  intracranial
  metastatic
  tumor
seeds, "melon"
SEEG (scalp EEG)
SEEG (stereotactic electroencephalogram)

seesaw nystagmus
Seever disease
SEG-CES (segmented cement extraction system)
segmental bone loss
segmental branch of vertebral artery
segmental distribution of
  syringomyelia
segmental ectasia
segmental epidural nerve block with
  local anesthesia
segmental fracture
segmental narrowing
segmental sign
segmental spinal instrumentation (SSI)
segmental symptoms
segmental tract of trigeminal
segment distraction
segmented orthopaedic system (SOS)
segment fixation
segment, transected
Segond fracture
segregation analysis
Seguin sign
SEH (spinal epidural hemorrhage)
Seidel humeral locking nail
Seidel intramedullary fixation
Seidel intramedullary rod
Seinsheimer classification of femoral
  fracture
Seitelberger disease
seizure (see also *epilepsy*)
  absence
  acute
  adversive motor
  akinetic
  alcohol as cause of
  alcohol-related
  alcohol withdrawal
  alimentary
  aphasic
  apneic
  astatic
  asymptomatic
  atonic absence
  atypical absence
  audiogenic

seizure *(continued)*
    auditory
    benign neonatal familial
    bilateral myoclonic
    cardiovascular
    centrencephalic
    cephalgic
    cerebellar fits
    cerebral
    cessation of
    chewing automatism during
    chewing during
    clonic
    clonic-tonic-clonic
    complex partial (CPS)
    continuing petit mal
    contraversive
    convulsive
    cryptogenic
    diencephalic
    drug-induced
    drug withdrawal
    ectopic foci of
    electrodecremental
    electrographic
    emotion as cause of
    epigastric sensation prior to
    epileptic
    epilepsia partialis continua
    extratemporal origin of
    eye movements during
    facial expression automatism during
    fatigue as cause of
    febrile
    fecal incontinence during
    foaming at the mouth during
    focal
    focal cerebral
    focal motor with march
    focal sensory
    focus of
    generalized
    generalized convulsive with focal onset
    generalized convulsive without focal onset
    generalized nonconvulsive

seizure *(continued)*
    generalized symmetrical and without focal onset
    generalized tonic-clonic (GTC)
    gestural automatism during
    grand mal (tonic-clonic)
    gustatory
    hippocampal
    history of
    hybrid
    hysterical
    iatrogenic
    ictal confusional
    idiopathic primarily generalized
    infantile spasms
    inhibitory motor
    intractable
    jackknife
    jacksonian
    Janz juvenile myoclonic
    laughing (gelastic epilepsy)
    lip-smacking automatism during
    long-lasting
    major motor
    menstrual cycle and occurrence of
    minor motor
    multifocal
    mumbling automatism during
    myoclonic
    myoclonic-astatic
    myoclonic jerks
    neonatal
    neonatal withdrawal
    new onset
    nonmotor somatosensory
    occult
    olfactory
    olfactory psychomotor
    parietal
    paroxysmal choreoathetosis
    partial complex
    partial elementary with motor symptoms
    partial sensory
    partial tonic
    patting automatism during
    petit mal

seizure *(continued)*
  petit mal variant
  phonatory
  photogenic
  piloerection prior to
  postdialysis
  postdiuresis
  posthypoxic myoclonic
  postictal depressive phase of
  post-traumatic
  postural
  precentral
  precipitation of
  premonition of
  primary
  psychic
  psychogenic
  psychomotor
  recurring
  reflex
  repetitive
  repetitive partial
  retropulsive absence
  rolandic
  running
  salaam
  scratching automatism during
  secondary generalization with
  secondary spread from focus of
  sensory-evoked
  simple partial
  single partial
  situation-related
  sleep-waking cycle and occurrence of
  somatosensory
  subclinical
  swallowing automatism during
  swimming movements during
  sylvian
  symptomatic
  temporal lobe
  tonal axial
  tongue biting during
  tonic
  tonic-clonic (grand mal)
  traumatic
  typical

seizure *(continued)*
  typical absence (petit mal)
  uncinate
  unilateral
  unilateral onset of
  urinary incontinence during
  versive
  vertiginous
  visual
  withdrawal
seizure disorder
seizure focus
seizure localization
seizure manifestations
seizure pattern
seizure phenomenon
seizure propagation
seizure threshold
Selby I (or II) fixation system
Selby I (or II) hook
Selby I (or II) rod
Selby I (or II) screw
Seldinger-technique angiography
Select ankle prosthesis
selective dorsal rhizotomy
selective excitation
selective imidazoline receptor agonist
  (SIRA)
selective irradiation
Selectively Lockable knee brace
selective lymphadenectomy
selective serotonin 1F agonist
  (SSOFRA)
selective serotonin reuptake inhibitor
  (SSRI)
selective traction/compression
Select joint orthosis
Select modular shoulder prosthesis
selegiline hydrochloride (Zelapar)
Seletz-Gelpi laminectomy retractor
Seletz nonrigid ventricular catheter
self-aligning (SAL) mobile-bearing
  knee implant
self-articulating femoral (SAF) hip
  replacement
self-bearing ceramic total hip
  replacement

self-care activity
self-centering bone-holding forceps
self-expanding metallic wall stent
self-feeder, Winsford
self-inflicted gunshot wound
self-reinforced polyglycolide
self-retaining screwdriver
self-tapping screw
Selig hip procedure
sella
  atrophy of
  ballooned
  ballooning of
  calcified
  decalcified
  empty
sella-nasion plane
sellar mass
sellar tomography
sellar tumor
sella turcica
Sell-Frank-Johnson extensor shift
  technique
Sellors rib contractor
Selspot System for optoelectronic
  analysis of human movement
Selverstone carotid artery clamp
Selverstone cordotomy hook
Selverstone intervertebral disk rongeur
Selverstone rongeur forceps
semantic (or verbal) paraphasia
Semb bone forceps
Semb bone rongeur
Semb rib forceps
Semb rib rasp
Semb rib shears
Semb-Stille rongeur
sEMG (surface electromyography)
semicircular canals, hydrops of the
semicoma
semicomatose
semiconscious
semiconsciousness
semidynamic splint
SemiFix screw
semi-Fowler position
semilunar bone

semilunar bony formation
semilunar cartilages
semilunar notch
semimembranous muscle
semipurposeful behavior in petit mal
  seizures
semirigid carbon fiber reinforced
  plastic plates
semirigid polypropylene ankle-foot
  orthosis
semisitting position
semispinal muscle
semitendinosus/gracilis autograft
semitendinosus tendon
semitendinosus tenodesis
semitendinosus transfer
semitendinous muscle
Semkin tissue forceps
Semmes spinal fusion curet
Semmes-Weinstein esthesiometer
Semmes-Weinstein monofilament hair
  test of sensory loss
Semmes-Weinstein scale
Semon law
SEMS (Screening Examination of the
  Musculoskeletal System)
SEMs (slow lateral eye movements)
Senegas approach to hips
senile ankylosing hyperostosis of spine
senile chorea
senile dementia, Alzheimer type
  (SDAT)
senile osteoporosis
senile paraplegia
senile subcapital fracture
senile tremor
Senn double-end retractor
sensation
  altered
  buzzing
  catching
  deep
  diminished
  dysesthesic
  epigastric (prior to seizure)
  facial
  fine tactile

sensation *(continued)*
  impaired
  light touch
  pain
  phantom
  pinprick
  pins and needles
  pins sticking
  popping
  return of
  superficial
  temperature
  tingling
  touch
  vibration
  vibratory
sensation of heat; warmth
sense
  joint position (JPS)
  position
  proprioceptive s. of muscles and
    ligaments
  vibration
  vibratory (pallesthesia)
Sense-of-Feel prosthesis
sense of time
sensitive plane
sensitive point
sensitive volume
sensitivity of rehabilitation testing
sensitivity, vibration
sensorial epilepsy
sensorimotor cortex
sensorimotor neuropathy
sensorimotor polyneuropathy
sensorimotor skills
sensorimotor stroke
sensorimotor syndrome
sensorimotor system
sensorineural hearing loss (SNHL)
sensorium
  altered
  changes in
  clouded
  depressed
sensor, universal force movement
sensory action potential

sensory apraxia
sensory branch of radial nerve
  (SBRN)
sensory deficit
  central
  peripheral
sensory delay
sensory-deprivation nystagmus
sensory dermatome
sensory disassociation
sensory discrimination
sensory dysphasia
sensory evoked potential (SEP)
sensory evoked seizures
sensory extinction test
sensory fibers
sensory input
sensory integration (SI)
sensory jacksonian attack
sensory level
sensory long tract
sensory loss
  cortical
  dense
  level of
  saddle area
  stocking-glove
  tactile
sensory manifestation
sensory modality
sensory nerve
sensory nerve action potential (SNAP)
sensory nerve conduction study
sensory nerve-endings
sensory nerve fiber
sensory neuropathy
Sensory Organization Test (SOT)
sensory or motor deficit
sensory paralysis
sensory paralytic bladder
sensory shocks of predormitum
sensory stimulation, double simultaneous
sensory stroke, pure
sensory symptoms
sensory transcortical aphasia
sentence closure tasks
sentence closure test

Sentence Repetition Test
sentences, Babcock
sentinel headache
SEP (sensory evoked potential)
SEP (somatosensory evoked potential)
separation
    AC (acromioclavicular)
    atlantoaxial
    atlanto-occipital
    costochondral junction
    fracture fragment
    physeal
    shoulder
    spinal
separator
    Davis nerve
    Dorsey dural
    dural
    Frazier dural
    Hoen dural
    Horsley dural
    Hunter dural
    nerve
    Sachs dural
    Sachs nerve
    toe
    Woodson dural
separator-spatula
    Sachs nerve
    Woodson dural
sepsis, pin-tract
Septacin implant to treat osteomyelitis
septal area
septal bone
septal region
septic arthritis
septum
    intermuscular
    internal intermuscular
    medial intermuscular
    posterior median
septum hematoma, nasal
septum pellucidum
sequela (pl. sequelae)
sequence
    Alu 1
    genomic

sequence memory
sequence time
sequencing
    gene
    radioactive
sequential compression device
sequentially reamed
sequential plane imaging
sequential point imaging
sequestered disk fragment
sequestra (pl. of sequestrum)
sequestrated disk
sequestration
sequestrectomy
sequestrotomy
sequestrum (pl. sequestra)
    associated
    bone
    bony
    necrotic
    primary
    secondary
    tertiary
sequestrum forceps
SER (somato-emotional release)
SER (somatosensory evoked response)
SER (supination, external rotation-
    type) fracture), I-IV
serendipity view
SergiScope robotic microscope
serial casts
serial EEG recording
serial sevens test
serial splinting
serial subtractions
serial threes test
seriation tests
Series-II humeral head
series, Valpar component work sample
Serlect (sertindole)
seropositive rheumatoid arthritis
Seroquel (quetiapine fumarate)
serosanguineous
serotonergic activity
serotonin (5-HIAA)
serous ligament
serpentine aneurysm

serpentine deformity
serpentine foot
serration
Serrato forearm pin
Serrato forearm rod
serratus muscle
Serter, C-wire
sertindole (Serlect)
sertraline hydrochloride (Zoloft)
serum osteocalcin
serum 25-hydroxyvitamin D test
serum YKL-40
Servo pump
Servox device
Serzone (nefazodone)
sesamoid bones of foot
  accessory
  bipartite
  entrapped plantar
  fibular
  great toe
  hallux
  Hardy-Clapham classification of
  quadripartite
  symptomatic bipartite
  tibial
  tripartite
sesamoid bones of hand
sesamoid complex
sesamoidectomy dissector
sesamoiditis
sesamoid ligament
sesamoid migration
sesamoidometatarsal joint
sesamophalangeal ligament
sessile
set (pl. sets)
  acetabular trial
  AO minifragment
  Hollywood bed extension hook
  Mira Mark V craniotome
  Moore nail
  nail
  quad
  Rousek extraction
  spondylophyte impaction
set angle of toes

Seton hip brace
set-shifting
  ideational
  motor
setter, bone plug
setting sun phenomenon
Seutin plaster shears
sevens test, serial
seventh cranial nerve (facial nerve)
Sever disease
severe ataxia
severe diffuse brain dysfunction
severe dysarthria
severe headache
Sever-L'Episcopo repair of shoulder
Sever modification of Fairbank
  technique
Sevrain cranial clamp
Sewall brain clip-applying forceps
SEWHO (shoulder-elbow-wrist-hand
  orthosis)
SFA (subclavian flap aortoplasty)
SFEMG (single-fiber electromyography)
S-fluoxetine (racemic fluoxetine)
SFS (small fragment system)
SF-36 Health Functional Outcomes
  Scoring System
SF-36 orthopedic outcomes questionnaire
shadowing
  acoustical
  paraspinal soft tissue
Shaeffer rigid orthosis
shaft
  bone
  distal third
  femoral
  French
  middle third
  ministem
  proximal third
shaft fracture
shaft of bone
SHAFT (sad, hostile, anxious, frustrating, tenacious) syndrome
shagreen patches in tuberous sclerosis
shakes, morning

shank bone
shank of shoe
shank, steel
Shannon 44 bur
Shanz dressing
Shanz pin
Shanz screw
shao yang disorder (Chinese medicine
   term)
shape
   brachycephalic head
   head
   mesocephalic head
   scaphocephalic head
shaper, interbody
shark mouth of myotonic dystrophy
Sharp angle
Sharpey fibers
Sharplan ultrasonic aspirator
Sharp-Purser test
sharp trocar
sharp waves, interictal paroxysmal
Sharrard transfer technique
Sharrard-Trentani prosthesis
Sharrard-type kyphectomy
shaver
   automated
   Concept
   Dyonics
   femoral
   intra-articular (IAS)
   motorized meniscus
   motorized suction
   patellar
   powered
   sucker
   synovial
   whisker
shaving
   arthroscopic
   femoral condylar
   patellar
shaving of patella
Shaw aneurysm needle
Shaw catheter
shawl muscle

shear
   anterior
   transitional
Shearer rongeur
shear examination
shear fracture
shearing forces
shearing of white matter
shearing stress
shear motion
shear rate
shear stress
shears
   Bacon thoracic
   Baer rib
   Bethune-Coryllos rib
   Bethune rib
   biarticular bone
   Brunner rib
   Bruns plaster
   Collins rib
   Cooley rib
   Coryllos rib
   Esmarch plaster
   first rib
   Giertz-Shoemaker rib
   Gluck rib
   Hercules plaster
   Horsley-Stille rib
   Lefferts rib
   Liston-Key-Horsley rib
   plaster
   Potts rib
   rib
   Roberts rib
   Roos first rib
   Sauerbruch-Britsch rib
   Sauerbruch-Frey rib
   Schuchart rib
   Schumacher rib
   Semb rib
   Seutin plaster
   Shoemaker rib
   Stille-Giertz rib
   Stille plaster
   Stille rib

sheath (pl. sheaths)
  arthroscope
  carotid
  flexor tendon
  ganglionic cyst in synovial tendon
  intratendon
  muscle
  myelin
  nerve root
  neural
  obturator
  periradicular
  plicated dural
  Schwann cell of myelin
  synovial
  tendon
  unplicated
sheath ligament
sheath of muscle
Sheehan chisel
Sheehan gouge
Sheehan knee prosthesis
Sheehan osteotome
Sheehy incus replacement prosthesis
  cranial incise
  fenestrated
  head
  laparotomy
  Silastic
  Silastic gel
  split
  sterile
  tantalum
Sheffield collimator helmet
Sheffield Gamma Knife unit
Sheffield hand elevator
Sheldon hemilaminectomy retractor
Sheldon-Spatz vertebral arteriogram
  needle
shelf
  Blumer
  lateral
  Mayeda
  medial
  patellar
shelf procedure

shell
  acetabular
  isodose
  Vitalock solid back
shelling off of cartilage
Shelton femur fracture classification
shelving edge of Poupart ligament
shen (Chinese medicine term)
Shenton line
shepherd's crook deformity
Shepherd fracture
Shepherd internal screw fixation
Sherfee prosthesis
Sherk-Probst technique
Sherlock threaded suture anchor
Sherman block test
Sherman bone plate
Sherman bone screw
Sherwin knee retractor
Shiatsu therapeutic massage
shield
  AME PinSite
  arthroscopic
  Faraday
  splash
Shields knee support
Shier total knee prosthesis
Shifrin wire twister
shift
  anterior capsular
  arthroscopic capsular
  intracranial
  laser-assisted capsular
  midline
  pivot
  plantar
  reverse pivot (RPS)
  ventricular
  weight
shift of midline structures
shift of pineal gland
shift of ventricle
shift to the left (on white count)
shift to the right (on white count)
shill, protrusio
shim coil

shim effect
shimmering, visual
shin bone
shingles (herpes zoster)
shin, saber
shin soreness
shin splints
Ship hammertoe implant
Shirley drain
shirt, EZ "T" orthopedic
shock
    neurogenic
    spinal
    sensory
shock absorbent heel pad
shock blocks
shod, rubber
shoe (pl. shoes)
    accommodative
    Acor Quikform I or II
    Ambulators
    Anti-Shox cushion for
    balmoral laced
    balmoral throat opening of
    Bebax (for forefoot deformity)
    Bevin
    blucher laced
    blucher throat opening of
    broad-toed
    Comed postoperative
    corrective
    counter of
    custom-made
    custom-made insert for
    custom-molded
    cut-out
    Darco surgical
    Depth
    depth inlay
    dress
    extended-counter
    extra depth
    half-shoe
    heel-lift with
    high heel
    high-heeled
    ill-fitting

shoe *(continued)*
    infant clown cast
    low-heeled
    Markell Mobility
    Markell open-toe
    Markell tarso medius straight
    Markell tarso pronator outflare
    metatarsal bar for
    Moon Boot
    narrow toebox
    normal last
    open-toe
    orthopedic
    orthopedic oxford
    oversize tennis
    oxford
    Pelite liner for
    plaster sole of
    Plastizote/PTT insert for
    pointed-toe
    postoperative
    PRN
    Reece postoperative
    reverse last
    ribbed-sole
    rocker
    rockerbottom sole of
    S.A.S.
    shank of
    soft sole or soft-soled
    soft vamp
    space
    Spenco insert for
    standard shell orthopedic
    stiff-soled
    straight last
    tarsal pronator
    therapeutic
    throat of
    toe box of
    torque-heel
    vamp of
    Vibram rockerbottom
    Viking postoperative
    Viva
    WACH (wedge adjustable
        cushioned heel)

shoe *(continued)*
 wedged
 wide toebox
 wooden
 wooden-soled
 Zimmer postoperative
shoe build-up
shoe cookie
shoe extension, Legg-Perthes
shoe filler
shoe floor interface
shoe heel height
shoe insert
 cushioned
 UCB
shoelace fasciotomy technique
Shoemaker rib shears
shoemaker's swan
shoe modification
shoe restriction
shoe sandal
shoe size
shoe wear, abnormal
shoe width
short adductor muscle
short arc progressive resistive
 exercises
short arc quadriceps
short arm cast
short arm splint
short bone
short ciliary nerve
shortening
 Achilles tendon
 Hoffa tendon
 leg
 phalangeal
 radial
 skeleton
 suboccipital
 tendon
 vertebral
short extensor muscle
short fibular muscle
short flexor muscle
Short Form 12 (SF-12) general health
 survey

Short Form 36 (SF-36) Health Survey
short head of biceps
short increments sensitivity index
 (SISI) measurement
short leg brace
short leg cast (SLC)
short leg polypropylene splint
short leg walking cast
short limb dwarfism
short orientation-memory-concentration
 (OMC) test
short palmar muscle
short peroneal muscle
short radial extensor muscle of wrist
short rib polydactyly syndrome
short-rod/two-claw technique
short saphenous nerve
short-term memory
short vessel graft bypass
short wave diathermy
"shot, hot" (cervical or brachial
 plexus injury)
shot, tetanus booster
shoulder
 apprehension
 baseball
 drop
 flail
 frozen
 knocked-down
 Little Leaguer
 loose
 Neviaser classification of frozen
 ring man (in gymnasts)
 sprained
 swimmer's
 tennis
shoulder arthroplasty, UCLA anatomic
shoulder capsular shrinkage procedure
shoulder compression test
shoulder depression test
shoulder disarticulation prosthesis
shoulder-hand-finger syndrome
shoulder immobilizer
shoulder joint
shoulder pointer
shoulder prosthesis

shoulder repair
shoulder rock test
shoulder separation
shoulder shrugs, repetitive
shoulder spica cast
Shoulder Therapy Kit
shoulder-upper extremity-thoracic
  outlet syndrome
Shriner pin
shrinkage, collagen
shrinkage of ganglion cells
shrinker, stump
Shriver-Johnson interphalangeal
  arthrodesis
shroud cast
shrugging sign
shucking
shuck test
Shuffors internal screw fixation
shunt
  barium sulfate impregnated
  CSF (cerebrospinal fluid)
  cysto-atrial
  cystoperitoneal
  Denver hydrocephalus
  DVP flush
  endarterectomy
  endolymphatic
  Hakim-Cortis ventriculoperitoneal
  hermetic external
  Heyer-Schulte neurosurgical
  high pressure
  infant
  Javid
  low pressure
  lumbar arachnoid peritoneal
  lumbar thecoperitoneal
  lumboperitoneal (LP)
  medium pressure
  migration of
  Ommaya ventriculoperitoneal
  one-piece
  posterior fossa-atrial
  Pruitt-Inahara
  Pudenz
  silicone elastomer
  Spetzler lumboperitoneal

shunt *(continued)*
  subdural-to-peritoneal
  Sundt loop
  T-tube
  thecoperitoneal
  UNI-SHUNT hydrocephalus
  ventriculoatrial (VA)
  ventriculojugular (VJ)
  ventriculoperitoneal (VP)
  ventriculosubarachnoid (VS)
  ventriculovenous
shunt failure, intermittent
shunt function, cerebrospinal fluid
shunting of cerebrospinal fluid
shunting procedure
shunt malfunction
shunt-related metastasis
shunt reservoir
shunt reversal
shunt revision
shunt syndrome, lumbar thecoperitoneal
shunt tap
shunt valve
Shutrack carbon paper
Shutt Mantis retrograde forceps
Shy-Drager atrophy
Shy-Drager neuropathy
Shy-Drager syndrome
SI (sacroiliac) joint
SI joint-to-sacrum ratio
SI-LOC sacroiliac belt
SI (sensory integration)
SIADH (syndrome of inappropriate
  antidiuretic hormone) excretion
sialidosis
sialoadhesin (Sn)
sialoprotein, bone
sialorrhea
SIB-1508Y
sibrafiban
SIBS (surgical isolation bubble system)
Sibson fascia
Sibson muscle
Sicard test
sick headache (migraine)
sickle cell anemia

sickle-shape Beaver blade
"sickling in" (peroneal tendinitis)
sickness
   decompression
   sleeping
Sickness Impact Profile (SIP)
side cuff
side-cutting Swanson bur
siderosis
sideswipe elbow fracture
sidewall
Siebenmann syndrome
Siemens LINAC (linear accelerator)
sieve bone
SIF (sacral insufficiency fracture)
Siffert-Forster-Nachamie arthrodesis
Siffert-Storen intraepiphyseal
sigma rhythm on EEG
sigmoid cavity of radius
sigmoid cavity of ulna
sigmoid notch and seat
sigmoid sinus
sign (see also *syndrome*; *test*)
   Achilles bulge
   Adson
   alien hand
   Allen
   Allis
   Amoss
   Anghelescu
   antecedent
   anterior drawer
   anterior foot drawer
   anterior tibial
   anvil
   Apley
   apprehension
   Ashhurst
   Babinski
   ball-bearing eye
   Bancroft
   barber's chair
   Barlow
   Battle
   bayonet
   Beevor
   bilateral Babinksi

sign *(continued)*
   bilateral pyramidal
   Bloomberg
   bow-tie
   bowstring
   Bragard
   brain stem
   brim
   Brudzinski
   Bryant
   Burton
   buttock
   camelback
   Cantelli
   cerebellar eye
   cerebral
   Chaddock
   choppy sea
   Chvostek-Weiss
   Cleeman
   cloverleaf
   Codman
   Cogan lid twitch
   cogwheel
   Collier
   commemorative
   Comolli
   contralateral
   Coopernail
   cord
   corticospinal tract
   cranial nerve
   crescent
   cross-chest impingement
   crossed-sciatica
   David Letterman
   Dawbarn
   Dejerine
   delta
   Demianoff
   dense sigmoid-sinus
   dense vein
   Desault
   Deyerle
   dimple
   doll's eyes
   doorbell

sign *(continued)*
  dorsal column
  double anterior horn
  double camelback
  double-lumen
  drawer (ankle or knee)
  drop Lasègue
  Duchenne
  Dupuytren
  echo
  Egawa
  empty delta
  Erb
  Erichsen
  extrapyramidal tract
  fabere (flexion, abduction, external rotation, extension)
  fadir (flexion, adduction, internal rotation)
  Fajersztajn crossed sciatic
  false localizing
  fan
  fat-fluid level
  fat pad
  Finkelstein
  Fleck
  flipped meniscus
  focal
  focal motor
  focal neurologic
  Forestier bowstring
  fragment-in-notch
  Fränkel (Fraenkel)
  Friedreich
  Froment paper
  Froment ulnar nerve function
  frontal lobe
  frontal release
  Gaenslen
  Gage
  Galant
  Galeazzi hip dislocation
  Goldthwait
  Gordon
  Gowers'
  Green-Joynt
  Griesinger

sign *(continued)*
  Guilland
  H
  Hamman
  harlequin eye
  Hart
  Hawkins impingement
  head-at-risk
  Helbing
  Hirschberg
  Hoffmann
  Homans'
  Honda
  Hoover
  hot cross bun skull
  Hueter fracture
  Huntington
  internal rotation lag
  J
  Jeanne
  Jenet
  jump
  Kanavel
  Kaplan
  Keen
  Kehr
  Kellgren
  Kernig
  Kerr
  knee jerk
  Kocher-Cushing
  Lachman
  lag
  Langoria
  Lasègue
  lateralizing
  Laugier
  Lazarus
  Leichtenstern
  Leri
  Lhermitte
  light bulb
  Linder
  LMN (lower motor neuron)
  localizing
  localizing neurological
  long tract

sign *(continued)*
- Lorenz
- Lowenberg
- lower motor neuron
- Ludloff
- Macewen
- Maisonneuve
- Marie
- Marie-Foix
- McMurray
- Mendel-Bekhterev
- meningeal
- meningeal irritation
- meningoencephalitic
- Mennell
- Minor
- Morquio
- Morton-Horwitz nerve crossover
- motor
- movie
- Mulder
- mute toe
- Myerson
- Naffziger
- Neer impingement
- negative delta (on CT)
- Negro
- Nelson
- Neri bowing
- neurologic soft
- obturator
- oculomotor
- Oppenheim
- orbicularis
- organic (of brain damage)
- Ortolani
- parietal
- parietal lobe
- Parrot
- pathognomonic
- pathologic lid retraction
- Patrick fabere
- Payr
- pearl and string
- percussion
- peroneal
- perpendicular

sign *(continued)*
- Phalen
- phonatory
- piano key
- Piotrowski
- piston
- pivot-shift
- plane
- Plummer
- positive bottle
- postural motor
- pout
- precursor
- premonitory
- Prévost
- pronation
- pronator
- pseudobulbar
- pseudo-Babinski
- pseudo-Foster-Kennedy
- pseudo-Romberg
- pupillary
- pupillometric
- pyramidal
- Queckenstedt
- raccoon eyes
- rachitic rosary
- radialis
- Raimiste
- release
- Renee creak
- ring
- Rinne
- Riordan
- Risser
- Romberg
- Rust
- sail
- Sarbo
- Schlesinger
- Schoeber
- scimitar
- seat-belt
- segmental
- Seguin
- setting sun
- shrugging

sign *(continued)*
  soft neurologic
  somatic
  Soto-Hall
  Spalding
  Speed
  spine
  spread suture
  Spurling
  stairs
  Steinberg thumb
  Steinmann
  Sterling-Okuniewski
  Stewart-Holmes
  Strunsky
  Strümpell (Struempell)
  tandem Romberg
  Terry fingernail
  Terry Thomas
  theater
  Thomas
  thorn
  Thurston-Holland
  tibialis (of Strümpell)
  Tinel percussion
  toe
  toe spread
  trefoil
  tripod
  tripoding
  Trömner (Troemner)
  Trousseau
  Turyn
  Uhthoff
  UMN (upper motor neuron)
  unilateral Babinski
  upper motor neuron
  vacant glenoid cavity
  VAD (voluntary anterior drawer)
  Valleix
  Vanzetti
  Vaughn-Jackson
  versive motor
  voluntary posterior drawer (VPD)
  Voshell
  VPD (voluntary posterior drawer)

sign *(continued)*
  Waddell
  Walter-Murdoch wrist
  Wartenberg
  Weber
  Weiss
  wet leather
  white matter
  Wilson
  windshield wiper
  winking-owl spinal
  Yergason
signal
  antiphase EEG
  differential
  disk water
  out-of-phase EEG
  random
  T2 SPIR signal
  water
signal characteristics of lesion
signaling, TNFa/NFkB
signal intensity curve
signal propagation
signal transduction
Signa Special Procedures (SP) MRI
  system
signal-to-noise ratio (SNR or S/N
  ratio) on MRI
Sigvaris compression stockings
Silastic ball spacer prosthesis
Silastic ball therapy
Silastic button
Silastic drip drain
Silastic finger joint
Silastic gel sheeting
Silastic HP-100 finger joint prosthesis
Silastic radial head prosthesis
Silastic rod
Silastic sheeting
Silastic sleeve
silence, electrocerebral (ECS)
silent areas of brain
"silent epidemic" of Alzheimer disease
silent reflex
Silesian bandage prosthetic support

Silflex intramedullary prosthesis
Silfverskiöld Achilles tendon
   reconstruction
silhouette capsulectomy
Silhouette therapeutic massage system
silicone elastomer cerebrospinal fluid
   shunt
silicone elastomer rubber ball implant
silicone flexor rod
silicone gel
silicone gel pocket insert
silicone-related syndrome
silicone synovitis
silicone trapezium prosthesis
Silipos Distal Dip prosthetic
   sheath/liner
Silkam suture
silk suture
Silopad friction pad
Silver bunionectomy
silver fork deformity
silver fork fracture
Silverman placement of electrodes
Silver osteotome
silver ring splint
Silverstein facial nerve monitor and
   probe
Silver syndrome
Simal cervical stabilization system
simian griffe (ape hand)
similarities mental status testing
Simmonds-Menelaus metatarsal
   osteotomy
Simmonds test
Simmons fixation system
Simmons keystone technique
Simmons plate
Simmons screw
Simmons Vari-Hite orthopedic bed
Simms-Weinstein monofilament hair
   test of sensory loss
Simonart ligament
Simon curet
Simons subtalar clubfoot release
Simple Calculated Osteoporosis Risk
   Estimation (SCORE)
simple dislocation

simple fracture, complex
simple joint
simple knee test
simple shoulder test
simple skull fracture
Simplex adhesive
Simplex cement
Simplex P bone cement
Simpson catheter
Simpson sugar tong splint
Simpulse S/I pulsing lavage system
Simpulse suction irrigator
Simpulse system
Sims retractor
simulation of minimally invasive
   neurosurgery
simulator
   BTE Work (Baltimore Therapeutic
     Equipment)
   Work Seat driving
simultagnosia
simultanagnosia
simultaneous volume imaging
simvastatin (Zocor)
Sinding-Larsen-Johansson disease
   (SLJD)
Sinequan (doxepin)
Singh index of osteoporosis
Single Assessment Numeric Evaluation
   (SANE) score/assessment/rating/
   method
single axis foot
single axis on knee prosthesis
single base pair insertion mutation
single bundle PCL reconstruction
   technique
single channel stimulator
single contrast arthrography
Single-Day Baxter infuser in forefoot
   operations
single fiber electromyography
single hook auto retractor
single leg horizontal hop
single level decompressive laminectomy
single limb stance of gait
single limb support time
single nerve trunk

single panel knee immobilizer
single pearl-face hip joint
single pedicle subtraction osteotomy
single plantar verruca
single plantar wart
single smooth-face hip joint
single strand conformation polymorphism (SSCP) analysis
single unit microelectrode recording
sinogenic meningitis
sinogram
sintering
Sinterlock CSTi bonding process
Sinterlock implant metal
sinus
  atlas articular
  basilar
  Breschet
  cavernous
  cerebral
  cerebral venous
  cervical
  circular
  coccygeal
  convexity
  costomediastinal
  cranial
  dominant
  dura mater venous
  dural venous
  inferior sagittal (ISS)
  lateral
  lumbosacral dermal
  marginal
  osteomyelitic
  paranasal
  petrosal
  pilonidal
  piriform
  precoronal sagittal
  pyriform
  Ridley
  sagittal
  sigmoid
  sphenoparietal
  sphenopetrosal
  superior petrosal

sinus *(continued)*
  superior sagittal (SSS)
  tentorial
  transverse
  venous
  vertebral articular
sinus histiocytosis with massive
  lymphadenopathy
sinus lesion, cavernous
sinus nerve of Hering
sinus tarsi syndrome
sinus thrombosis
  cavernous
  intracranial
sinus tract
sinuvertebral nerve of Luschka
SIP (Sickness Impact Profile)
siphon, carotid
SIRA (selective imidazoline receptor
  agonist)
Siri formula for percentage of body fat
SISI (short increments sensitivity
  index) measurement
Sisson fracture-reducing elevator
site
  donor
  fracture
  nociceptor
  nonunion of fracture
  operative
  pin
  previous surgical
  recipient
  seating
  surgical
  nociceptor
SITEtrac spinal surgery system
sitting balance
  reclined
  supported
sitting SLR test (straight leg raising)
Sivash hip prosthesis
Sivash stem
Sivash total hip prosthesis
6 Degree-of-Freedom robotic
  manipulator arm
6-MNA

six-strand suture
sixth compartment
sixth cranial nerve (abducens nerve)
sixth intercostal space
sixth nerve palsy
size
   increased head circumference
   ventricular
size and reactivity of pupils
sizer, graft
SJO_2 (jugular bulb venous oxygen
   saturation)
Sjögren-Larsson syndrome
Sjögren syndrome
SJS (Schwartz-Jampel syndrome)
skateboarding accident
skeletal amyloidosis
skeletal bed
skeletal defects
skeletal deformity
skeletal disruption
skeletal emphysema
skeletal growth factor
skeletal hyperostosis
skeletal hypoplasia
skeletally immature
skeletally mature
skeletal lymphangiomatosis
skeletal metastases
skeletal muscles
skeletal radiology
skeletal survey, isotopic
skeletal traction
skeleton
   appendicular
   articulated
   axial
   bony
   cardiac
   fibrous
   gill arch
   spidering
   spiky
   sulcal
   visceral
skeletonize

skeletonizing
skeleton shortening
Skelid (tiludronate disodium)
skew deviation of eyes
skewer
skewering
skew foot
skew, ocular
skid
   bone
   hip
   Meyerding bone
   Murphy-Lane bone
skier's fracture
skier's injury
skier's tear
skier's thumb
SKI knee prostheses
skill (pl. skills)
   articulatory
   ambulation
   ball
   bed mobility
   motor
   physical daily living (PDLs)
   sensorimotor
   transfer
   word-finding
skilled nursing facility (SNF)
Skillern fracture
Skil Saw
skin blade knife
skin blood flow determination
skin bridge
skin depth
skin, dysesthetic
skinfold thickness monitoring
skinned
skin refrigerant
skin-rolling scapular tenderness
skive (shave), skived
Sklar surgical instruments
Skoog release of Dupuytren
   contracture
S-K (Sauvé-Kapandji) reconstruction
   of distal radioulnar joint

SKT (Simple Knee Test)
skull
    asymmetry of the
    base of
    beaten-silver appearance of
    cloverleaf
    foramen magnum of
    hammer-marked
    hot cross bun
    kleeblattschädel
    molded
    sonolucent
skull asymmetry
skull base reconstruction
skullcap
skull clamp pin
skull defect, postoperative
skull films
skull fracture
    basilar
    compound
    depressed
    linear
    simple
    stellate
    undepressed
skull hyperostosis
skull plate
    stainless steel preformed
    tantalum preformed
skull plate anvil
skull tongs
    Gardner-Wells
    Raney-Crutchfield
skull trephine
    D'Errico
    Scoville
skyline view of patella
Skytron bed
Skytron operating room table
slab, plaster
SL (scapholunate) joint
SLAC (scapholunate arthritic collapse)
    wrist
slap-foot gait
SLAP lesion (superior labrum anterior
    posterior)

Slatis pelvic fracture frame
Slattery-McGrouther dynamic flexion
    splint
SLC (short leg cast)
SLE (systemic lupus erythematosus)
    nephritis
sleep
    active
    arousal from
    arousing from
    benign epileptiform transients of
        (BETS)
    deep
    depth of
    descending into
    descent through non-REM to REM
    disorder of initiating and maintaining
        (DIMS)
    disturbed
    dreamless
    indeterminate
    non-REM (non-rapid eye
        movements)
    NREM (non-rapid eye movement)
    onset of
    paradoxical (REM sleep)
    quiet
    rapid eye movement (REM)
    REM (rapid eye movement)
    REM onset
    slow wave
    stage I (drowsiness)
    stage I of non-REM (drowsiness)
    stage II of non-REM (light sleep)
    stage III of non-REM (deep sleep)
    stage IV of non-REM (very deep)
    stage of REM
    stage W (wakefulness)
    transiting through
    transitional
    very deep
    very light
sleep apnea
sleep arousal disorder
sleep attacks (epilepsy)
sleep cycle
sleep deprivation

sleep disorder
sleep disturbance
sleep fragmentation
sleep, fragmented
sleep habit
Sleep Habits Questionnaire (SHQ)
sleep onset episode
sleep onset REM period (SOREMP)
sleep paralysis
    postdormital
    predormital
sleep pattern
Sleepscan Traveler ambulatory
    polysomnography system
sleep spindle
sleep state
sleep study, polysomnographic
sleep-wake cycle
sleep-wakefulness cycle
sleep-waking cycle
Sleeper II sleep support
sleepiness, daytime
sleeping sickness
sleeplessness
sleeptalking
sleepwalking
sleeve
    alignment
    circumferential ligamentous
    distal
    drill
    dural root
    Edwards-Levine
    guide
    Kendall pneumatic compression
    metaphyseal
    nerve root
    obturator
    periosteal
    polyethylene
    Rancho trocar-drill
    root
    Silastic
    taper
    2T
sleeve fracture
sleeve of drillbit

slice fracture
slide, vastus
sling
    arm elevator
    Barton
    buckle
    collar-and-cuff
    cradle arm
    Envelope arm
    extra-articular lateral
    fascial
    felt
    foam
    foot
    Glisson
    Haacker
    immobilizer
    Kenny Howard shoulder
    knee
    Kodel knee
    Legg-Perthes
    muslin
    Pavlik
    pelvic
    Rauchfuss
    rubber
    shoulder
    sleeve
    Slingers arm
    stockinette
    strap
    Teare
    tendon
    thigh
    Thomas
    Thomas buckle
    tibialis anterior tendon
    triangle
    triangular
    UltraSling
    Velpeau
    Velpeau shoulder
    Vogue arm
    volar
    volar ulnar
    Weil pelvic
    Westfield envelope

sling-and-swathe bandage
Slingers arm sling
Slingshot shoulder immobilizer
slip angle
slip knot
Slip-N-Snip scissors
slip of tendon
slip-on finger splint
slipped capital femoral epiphysis
   (SCFE)
slipped disk
slipped tendon
slipped upper femoral epiphysis
   (SUFE)
slipped vertebral apophysis
slippers, Bunnell tendon
slipper-type cast
   kite
   plaster-of-Paris
slipping-rib syndrome
slit-catheter system for compartment
   syndrome of foot
sliver of bone
SLJD (Sinding-Larsen-Johansson
   disease)
Slocum knee procedure
Slocum lateral pivot-shift test
Slocum meniscal clamp
slope, tibial
Slot distraction device
slotted cannula
slotted mallet
slough, skin
slowing
   bilateral theta
   delta
   diffuse delta
   generalized background
   monorhythmic frontal
   postictal
   psychomotor
   saccadic
   scattered
slow muscle
slow spike-and-wave pattern
slow virus infection of nervous system
slow wave activity

slow wave, phase reversing
SLR (straight leg raising) test
SLRT (straight leg raising test)
Sluder neuralgia
Sluder sphenopalatine syndrome
Sluder syndrome
sluggish
slump test
slurred speech
Sluyter-Mehta thermocouple electrode
SLWC (short leg walking cast)
SMA (spinal muscular atrophy)
SMA (supplementary motor area)
   prosthesis
small deep petrosal nerve
SMALL (same-day microsurgical
   arthroscopic lateral-approach laser-
   assisted) fluoroscopic diskectomy
small patella syndrome
small sciatic nerve
small vessel disease of the diabetic
   foot
small vessel stroke
SmartBrace
SmartScope digital imaging micro-
   scope
SmartScrew resorbable screw
SmartSpot high resolution digital
   imaging system
SmartTack fixation device
SmartWrap elbow brace
SMAS (superficial musculoaponeurotic
   system)
SMAS (superior mesenteric artery
   syndrome)
smear for parasites and fungi
Smedberg hand drill
Smedberg twist drill
SMI 3000 bed
SMI 5000 bed
Smiley-Williams arteriogram needle
Smillie-Beaver blade
Smillie cartilage knife
Smillie knee retractor
Smillie meniscotomy chisel
Smillie meniscus hook retractor
Smillie meniscus knife

Smillie nail
Smillie retractor
Smith air craniotome
Smith & Nephew bracing and support
systems
Smith & Nephew Richards rod
Smith ankle fracture
Smith ankle prosthesis
Smith automatic perforator drills
Smith bone clamp
Smith cartilage knife
Smith classification of sesamoid
position
Smith cranial drill
Smith-Davis Converta-Hite orthopedic
bed
Smith fracture
Smith-Lemli-Opitz syndrome
Smith nerve root suction retractor
Smith-Petersen chisel
Smith-Petersen femoral neck nail
Smith-Petersen gooseneck gouge
Smith-Petersen gouge
Smith-Petersen impactor
Smith-Petersen intertrochanteric plate
Smith-Petersen laminectomy rongeur
Smith-Petersen nail with Lloyd adapter
Smith-Petersen osteotome
Smith-Petersen rongeur
Smith-Petersen surgical approach
Smith-Petersen test
Smith physical capacities evaluation
(PCE)
Smith-Robinson diskectomy
Smith-Robinson interbody fusion
Smithwick button hook
Smithwick clip-applying forceps
Smithwick dissector
Smithwick nerve hook
Smithwick sympathectomy hook
Smith wire-cutting scissors
SMo (stainless steel and molybdenum)
SMO (supramalleolar orthosis)
SMON (subacute myelo-optico–
neuropathy)
smoother, Gore
smooth muscle

smooth pursuit eye movements
SNA cephalometric measurement
SNAP (sensory nerve action potential)
amplitude
snapping hip syndrome
snapping of tendon
snapping scapula syndrome
snapping tendon release
snapping thumb flexor
snap, saccadic
SNB cephalometric measurement
SNCV (sensory nerve conduction
velocity)
Sneppen fracture of talus
SNF (skilled nursing facility)
SNHL (sensorineural hearing loss)
Snitman endaural retractor
SN-MPA cephalometric measurement
Sno-Traks wheelchair chains
snout reflex
snowboarder's ankle
snowboarder's fracture
snowboarding injury
SNR (signal-to-noise ratio)
SNSF (second neuroma, same foot)
snuffbox, anatomical
snuff taker's pituitary disease
Snugs wrap
SNX-111 (ziconotide)
Snyder classification of SLAP lesions
Snyder labral-biceps detachment
soap, Betadine
soap bubble appearance
Social Adjustment Scale in brain-
injured patients
socialization skills
Social Security Disability Insurance
(SSDI)
society (see also *academy, association*)
ACSM (American College of
Sports Medicine)
American Autonomic Society
American Knee Society
AOFAS (American Orthopaedic
Foot and Ankle Society)
ASES (American Shoulder and
Elbow Surgeons)

society *(continued)*
   ASSH (American Society for
     Surgery of the Hand)
   Musculoskeletal Tumor Society
   National Ankylosing Spondylitis
     Society
   National Multiple Sclerosis Society
     (NMSS)
   Scoliosis Research Society
sock
   cast
   Orlon with Lycra stump
   Spandex Lycra three-ply stump
   stump
Sock-Assist device
socket
   check
   Poly-Dial
   modular
   quadrilateral
   Sabolich
   threaded
   total contact
socket joint
socket wrenches
SOD (superoxide dismutase)
sodium hyaluronate (Hyalgan)
sodium urate crystals
Soemmerring ligament
Soemmerring muscle
Sofamor Danek instruments
Sofamor spinal instrumentation
Sof-Gel palm shield
Sofield osteotomy
Sofield retractor
Sofrature ointment gauze
Sof-Rol cast padding
Sof-Rol dressing
Sofsilk nonabsorbable silk suture
Sofsponge material
Softcat suture material
soft clavus
soft corn
Soft Delivery System
soft disk herniation
softening of brain

soft neurologic sign
soft opposition of thumb muscle
soft tissue abnormality
soft tissue ankle injuries
soft tissue attachment, Hedrocel
soft tissue contracture
soft tissue contusion
soft tissue defect
soft tissue entrapment
soft tissue infection
soft tissue interposition
soft tissue mass
soft tissue mobilization
soft tissue necrosis
soft tissue osteochondroma
soft tissue plication
soft tissue radiograph
soft tissue realignment
soft tissue reconstruction
soft tissue sarcoma
soft tissue shortening
soft tissue swelling
soft tissue window
software
   AtlasPlan neurosurgery
   ImageFusion
   LabView
   SAS
   XPlan radiation treatment planning
Solcotrans closed vacuum drainage
   system
Solcotrans drainage/reinfusion system
Solcotrans Plus autotransfusion system
sole
   shock absorbent
   shoe
soleal line
solenoid coil
sole of foot
soleus muscle
solid ankle, cushioned heel (SACH)
solid bone
solidifier, ArthroSorb
solitary circumscribed neuroma
solitary neurofibroma
solitary plasmatoma

Solu-Medrol (methylprednisolone)
solution
  antibiotic
  Betadine Helafoam
  dilute heparin
  Hank buffered saline
  hypo-osmolar glucose
  perfusate
Somanetics INVOS cerebral oximeter
SomaSensor
somatagnosia (corporal agnosia)
somatectomy
somatesthetic fiber
somatic alpha fiber
somatic denervation
somatic dysfunction
somatic muscle
somatic nerve
somatic nerve fiber
somatic sensory seizures
somatic sign
somatic therapy
somatization disorder
somatoemotional release (SER)
somatoform disorder
SomatoKine (IGF-BP3 complex)
somatomedin-C
somatosensory cortex
somatosensory evoked potential
  (SEP or SSEP)
somatosensory evoked response (SER)
somatosensory parietal cortex
somatosensory seizure
somatosensory symptoms
somatosympathetic fibers of nerve root
somatotopic arrangement of GPi
somatotopic organization
somatovisceral reflexes
Somerville procedure
SOMI orthosis (sternal occipital
  mandibular immobilization)
Sommer sector of hippocampus
somnambulism
somniloquy
somnolence, excessive
somnolent
S-100 protein

S1-S5 (five sacral vertebrae)
Songer spinal cable system
sonic accelerated fracture-healing
  system (SAFHS) 2000
sonic massager reflexology device
sonicated tendon
Sonicator muscle stimulation
  ultrasound
Sonocut ultrasonic aspirator
sonography
  color-coded duplex
  transcranial color-coded
  transcranial Doppler
sonometer (see *imaging*)
Sony digital still image capture system
Sophy programmable pressure valve
Sorbie calcaneal fracture
Sorbothane heel cushions
Sorbothane II heel cup
SOREMP (sleep onset REM period)
soreness, delayed-onset muscle
  (DOMS)
sore, pressure
Sorrel-type snowboard boot
SOS (Segmented Orthopaedic System)
  total hip and knee systems
SOT (Sensory Organization Test)
Soto-Hall bone graft
Soto-Hall sign
sound
  cracked-pot
  tearing
SoundScan Compact bone sonometer
SoundScan 2000 bone sonometer
Souter hip procedure
Souter unconstrained elbow prosthesis
southern access to hip joint in surgery
Southern California Orthopedic
  Institute (SCOI)
Southwick biplane osteotomy
Southwick-Robinson anterior cervical
  approach
SPA (speech pathology/audiology)
space
  antecubital
  axillary
  bregmatic

space *(continued)*
  capsular
  cartilage
  Colles
  dead
  disk
  dorsal subaponeurotic
  dorsal subcutaneous
  echo-free
  epicerebral
  epidural
  epispinal
  extradural
  fifth intercostal
  first intercostal
  first web
  foraminal
  fourth intercostal
  hyperintense marrow
  iliocostal
  increased lateral joint
  intercondylar (ICS) joint
  intercostal
  intermetatarsal
  interosseous
  interpeduncular
  intervertebral disk
  intrathecal
  joint
  Larrey
  lateral joint
  left intercostal (LICS)
  marrow
  medial joint
  midpalmar
  Mohrenheim
  narrowing of joint
  palmar
  Parona
  patellofemoral joint
  periaxial
  pharyngomaxillary
  popliteal
  predental
  presacral
  prevertebral
  pulp

space *(continued)*
  quadrangular
  retro-orbital
  retroparotid
  retropharyngeal
  retropubic
  retrosphenoidal
  scapholunate
  subarachnoid
  subdural
  subepicranial
  submandibular
  submaxillary
  submental
  subtendinous
  syndesmotic clear
  thenar
  tibiocalcaneal
  ventricular
  Virchow-Robin
  web
space deficits
space nerve
space-occupying lesion
space of Marie
space of Poirier
spacer
  acetabular
  anchovy
  Barouk
  cement
  GAIT (great toe arthroplasty
    implant technique)
  joint
  PMMA
  tibial
  titanium interbody (TIS)
spacer between toes
spacer tensor jig IV
space shoes
Spalding sign
Spalteholtz technique
span
  attention
  ventricular
Spandex Lycra three-ply stump sock
spanner, socket

sparing, sacral (in sensory loss)
Spartaject (busulfan)
spasm
    carpopedal
    cerebrovascular
    convergence
    dystonic
    facial
    flexion
    habit
    hamstring
    hemifacial
    infantile massive
    intercostal
    intrinsic muscle
    involuntary flexor
    lightning-like flexion
    medial facial (of Meige)
    mobile
    muscle
    nodding
    paraspinal muscle
    paravertebral muscle
    peripheral facial
    protective
    recruitment (in tetanus)
    recurrent torsion
    saltatory
    torsion
spasmodic flexion
spasmodic torticollis
spastic ataxia, familial
spastic diparesis
spastic diplegia
spastic equinovarus deformity
spastic gait
spastic hand
spastic hemiparesis
spastic hemiplegia, Wernicke-Mann
spastic hindfoot valgus deformity
spasticity
    limb
    nocturnal leg muscle
    spinal
spasticity of extremities
spastic neurogenic bladder, refluxing

spastic palsy
spastic paralysis
spastic paraparesis
spastic paraplegia and distal muscle
    wasting
spastic paraplegia, familial
spastic paresis
spastic pseudosclerosis
spastic state
spatial accuracy
spatial disorganization
spatial disorientation
spatial distortion
spatial neglect
spatial orientation
spatial registration
spatial resolution
spatula
    brain
    cement
    Children's Hospital brain
    clip-bending
    Cushing brain
    D'Errico brain
    Davis brain
    Davis nerve
    dura
    endarterectomy
    House-Fisch dura
    Jacobson endarterectomy
    malleable
    Mayfield brain
    nerve
    nerve separator
    Olivecrona brain
    Peyton brain
    Rainin clip-bending
    Ray brain
    Rhoton
    S-shaped brain
    Sachs nerve
    Scoville brain
    Weary brain
spatula spoon
    Cushing brain
    Ray brain

Speare dural hook
Spearman rank correlation coefficient
   analysis
spears, saline-soaked Weck
special leads
Special Olympics, National
specialist, registered deafness (RDF)
specific thalamic nuclei
specimen
   biopsy
   grossly resected
specious finding
SPECT (single photon emission
   computed tomography)
spectacular shrinking deficit syndrome
SPECT brain perfusion scintigraphy
SPECT determination of cerebral
   blood flow
spectra (see *spectrum*)
spectral analysis
spectral array, compressed
spectral averaging
spectral peak frequency of activity
spectral plot
spectrometer
Spectron hip prosthesis
spectroscopy (see *imaging*)
   near-infrared
   phosphorus magnetic resonance
   (P-MRS)
spectrum (pl. spectra)
   fortification
   magnetic resonance
   migraine
Spectrum tissue repair system
speculum
   bivalve
   Cushing-Landolt transsphenoidal
   forceps
   Halle nasal
   Hardy
   Killian septum
   Landolt pituitary
   transsphenoidal
speech
   agrammatic
   arrest of

speech *(continued)*
   articulate
   articulation of
   ataxic
   cerebellar scanning quality of
   cerebellar scanning type of
   circumlocution of
   circumstantial
   confabulation of
   dysarthric
   dysrhythmic
   emotive
   executive
   festinant quality
   flaccid
   fluent aphasic
   fluent paraphasic
   halting
   hyperkinetic
   hypokinetic
   impaired
   incoherent
   incomprehensible
   internal
   irrelevant
   labored
   monosyllabic
   nonelaborative
   nonfluent aphasic
   nonsensical
   paraphasic
   rambling
   rhythm of
   scanning
   slurred
   spontaneous
   staccato
   tangential
   telegraphic
   unintelligible
   unvoiced
speech detection threshold
speech mannerisms
speech pathologist
speech pathology/audiology (SPA)
Speech Questionnaire
Speed-Boyd radial-ulnar technique

Speed hand splint
speed of gait
Speed's test
Speed V-Y muscle-plasty
spell (pl. spells)
  akinetic
  breathholding
  fainting
  myoclonic
  staring
Spence cranioplastic roller
Spence intervertebral disk rongeur
Spence rongeur forceps
Spencer tendon-lengthening operation
Spenco liners
Spenco shoe insert
Spetzler lumboperitoneal shunt
Spetzler-Martin classification of
  arteriovenous malformation
SpF Spinal Fusion Stimulator
sphenoethmoidal encephalocele
sphenoethmoidal suture
sphenoidal electrode
sphenoidal fissure syndrome
sphenoidal fossae EEG leads
sphenoidal wing
sphenoid bone
sphenoid ridge tumors
sphenoid sinus obliteration
sphenomandibular ligament
spheno-occipital joint
spheno-occipital suture
spheno-occipital synchondrosis
spheno-orbital encephalocele
spheno-orbital suture
sphenopalatine ganglion
sphenopalatine neuralgia
sphenopalatine notch
sphenoparietal suture
sphenopetrosal sinus
sphenopetrosal suture
sphenopharyngeal meningo-
  encephalocele
sphenosquamous suture
sphenotemporal suture
sphenoturbinal bone
sphenovomerine suture

spheres, oriented in all
spherical reamer
Spherocentric fully constrained tricompartmental knee prosthesis
spheroid articulation
spheroid joint
sphincter control, loss of
sphincter disturbance
sphincter incompetence
sphincter muscle
sphingolipids
sphingomyelin lipidosis
sphingomyelinase
spica bandage
spica cast
spica splint
spicular density on x-ray
spicule of bone
spicules of periosteal new bone
spicules on EEG
spidering skeleton
Spider Pad support
spiderweb circulation on angiography
  of glioblastomas
Spiegelberg epidural balloon
Spiegelberg intracranial pressure
  monitor
Spiegelberg pneumatic transducer
Spiegleman acromioclavicular splint
Spielberger State Anxiety Inventory
Spielmeyer-Vogt-Sjögren disease
Spier elbow arthrodesis
Spiessel screws and instrumentation
spike
  benign small sharp (BSSS)
  blind person's occipital
  bone
  centromidtemporal
  centrotemporal
  cortical
  epileptiform EEG
  focal interictal
  frontal
  generalized
  Gissane
  high amplitude
  infantile pattern of

spike *(continued)*
   interictal continuous
   interictal temporal lobe
   intermittent focal
   juvenile pattern of
   lateral rectus
   low amplitude
   multifocal independent
   negative vertex
   occipital
   polyphasic
   positive
   repetitive
   rolandic
   small sharp (SSS)
   slow waves interrupted by
   stereotyped
   temporal
   temperature
   unilateral
   wicket
spike and dome complex
spike and slow wave bursts
spike and wave complex
spike and wave discharge
spike and wave forms
spike averaging
spike discharges
spiked washer
spike of bone
spike on EEG
spike osteotomy
spike waves, interictal paroxysmal
spiky skeletons
Spiller-Frazier neurotomy
spina bifida
spina bifida anterior
spina bifida aperta
spina bifida cystica
spina bifida manifesta
spina bifida occulta (SBO)
spina bifida posterior
spinal abscess, epidural
spinal accessory nerve
spinal angiogram
spinal angiolipoma
spinal arthritis

spinal axial loading
spinal axis
spinal block by cord compression
spinal canal
spinal canal endoscopy
spinal canal narrowing
spinal column
spinal cord
   caliber of
   compression of
   decompression of
   hemisection of
   infarction of
   laceration of
   multiple focal lesions of
   myelopathy of
   posterolateral sclerosis of
   tethered
   transection of
spinal cord atrophy
spinal cord compression by lymphoma
spinal cord diameter
spinal cord ependymoma
spinal cord injured patient
spinal cord injury (SCI)
spinal cord intensive care unit
   (SCICU)
spinal cord ischemia
spinal cord lesion
Spinal Cord Motor Injury and Sensory
   Indices
spinal cord neoplasm
spinal cord parenchyma
spinal cord perfusion pressure
spinal cord stimulation
spinal cord stroke
spinal cord tumor
   intradural but extramedullary
   intramedullary
spinal degeneration
spinal dural arteriovenous fistula
spinal dysfunction
spinal dysraphism, occult
spinal elements, neoplastic destruction of
spinal ependymoma
spinal epidural abscess
spinal epidural hematoma

spinal fixation
spinal fluid cytology
spinal fluid, xanthochromic
spinal form of amyotrophic lateral
    sclerosis
spinal fusion
spinal hemiplegia
spinal hydatid cyst
spinal instability
spinal integrity
spinal lordosis
spinal manipulative therapy
spinal mobilization
spinal muscle
spinal muscular atrophy
spinal needle
spinal nerve level motor impairment
spinal neural deficits
spinal neuraxis
SpinaLogic-1000 bone growth
    stimulator
spinal osteomyelitis, *Staphylococcus
    aureus*
spinal osteotomy
spinal paraplegia
spinal retractor
spinal roots
    C1-7 (cervical)
    Co. 1 (coccygeal)
    L1-5 (lumbar)
    S1-5 (sacral)
    T1-12 (thoracic)
spinal separator
spinal shock
Spinal Stim bone growth stimulator
spinal subarachnoid hemorrhage
spinal subdural hematoma
spinal sympathetic fibers
spinal tap, traumatic
spinal tract of trigeminal
spinal tuberculosis
spinal vascular malformation
spinal videofluoroscopy
spin coupling
spin density

spindle
    asynchronous sleep
    muscle
    sinusoidal-appearing sleep
    sleep
    unilateral sleep
spindle burst
spindle cell carcinoma
spindle coma pattern
spindle-shaped muscle
spindle system reflexes
spindling of transverse process
spine
    alar
    angulation of
    anterior column of
    anterior maxillary
    anterior superior iliac
    anteroposterior iliac
    cervical (C)
    Charcot
    coccygeal
    dendritic
    dorsal (D)
    functional units of
    iliac
    ischial
    kinetic cervical
    kissing
    lateral bending views of
    lumbar (L)
    lumbarized
    lumbosacral (LS)
    mandibular
    maxillary
    nasal
    poker
    posterior column of
    posterior inferior
    rotatory loads on
    rugger jersey
    sacral (S)
    static cervical
    thoracic (T)
    thoracolumbar
    trochanteric

spine board
SpineCATH intradiscal catheter
spin echo
spin-echo imaging
spin-echo technique
SpineScope percutaneous endoscope
spine strain, lumbosacral
spin-lattice relaxation time
spinocerebellar ataxia
spinocerebellar degeneration
spinocerebellar disease
spinocerebellar tract
spinocerebellopathy
spinoglenoid ligament
spinoglenoid notch
spinographic angle
spinographic lines
spinography, digitized
spinolaminar line
spino-olivary tract
spinoreticular tract
spinotectal tract
spinothalamic tract
   anterior
   lateral
spinous process
spin-spin relaxation time
spin-warp imaging
spiral band of Gosset
spiral fracture
spiral ligament
spiral oblique fracture
Spira procedure
spirochete
Spittler procedure
splanchnic nerve
splashing bruit
splash shield
SPLATT (split anterior tibial tendon
   transfer)
splayed
splayfoot deformity
splaying of forefoot
splaying of frontal horns
splaying of pedicles
splaying of toes

spleen dampness (Chinese medicine
   term)
spleen phlegm (Chinese medicine
   term)
spleen qi deficiency (Chinese medicine
   term)
spleen yang deficiency (Chinese medicine term)
splenium of corpus callosum
splenius muscle
splenocolic ligament
splenorenal ligament
spline
   Blount
   Bosworth
   flat
   Rowland-Hughes
splint, splinting
   Abbott
   abduction
   abduction humeral
   abutment
   acrylic template
   Adam and Eve
   Adams
   adjustable
   aeroplane (also airplane)
   Agnew
   air
   AirFlex carpal tunnel
   airfoam
   airplane (also aeroplane)
   air pressure
   Alumafoam
   aluminum bridge
   aluminum fence
   aluminum foam
   anchor
   Anderson
   Angle
   anterior shin
   any angle
   Aquaplast
   armchair
   Asch
   Ashhurst

splint *(continued)*
    balanced
    Balkan
    ball peen
    banjo
    Barlow cruciform infant
    baseball
    baseball finger
    basswood
    Bavarian
    Baylor
    Bennett basic hand
    birdcage
    Bloom
    Boehler (Böhler)
    Böhler-Braun
    Bond
    Boston thoracic
    boutonnière
    Bowlby
    bowstring
    boxing glove
    bracketed
    Brady leg
    Brant aluminum
    Buck
    buddy finger
    Budin hammertoe
    bunion
    Bunnell active hand and finger
    Bunnell finger extension
    Bunnell knuckle-bender
    Bunnell outrigger
    Bunnell reverse knuckle-bender
    Bunnell safety pin
    Bunny Boot
    Burnham thumb and finger
    Cabot posterior
    Campbell
    cap
    Capner
    Carpal Lock cock-up
    Carl P. Jones traction
    Carter
    Chandler felt collar
    Chatfield-Girdlestone
    clavicle

splint *(continued)*
    clavicular cross
    Clayton greenstick
    clubfoot
    coaptation
    cock-up
    cock-up hand
    Colles
    Comforfoam
    composite spring
    conforming
    constant tension
    cool IROM
    cool TROM
    Core ambidextrous cock-up wrist
    Cosmolon closure for
    countertraction
    Craig
    Cramer wire
    Culley
    Curry
    Darco foot
    Darco medical-surgical shoe and
        toe alignment
    Darco toe alignment
    Davis
    Delbet
    Denis Browne clubfoot
    Denis Browne talipes hobble
    DePuy open spindle
    dermal interposition
    derotator
    Digit-Aid fifth toe
    DonJoy knee
    DonJoy wrist
    dorsal wrist
    Doyle Combo nasal airway
    Doyle Shark nasal
    dropfoot
    dropout
    Dupuytren
    Duran-Houser wrist
    Dyna knee
    Dyna leg
    dynamic extensor
    dynamic flexor
    Eaton

splint *(continued)*
- Eggers
- elastic
- Elastomull
- elbow
- elephant-ear clavicle
- Engelmann
- Engen palmar wrist
- Erich
- extension block(ing)
- extension lock (ELS)
- extrinsically powered
- felt collar
- fence
- Ferciot tiptoe
- fiberglass
- figure of 8
- Fillauer night
- finger
- finger cot
- finger extension
- finger knuckle-bender
- Firm D-Ring wrist support
- flexor hinge
- foot
- footdrop
- forearm
- Forrester
- Foster
- 4-point IROM
- Fox
- Frac-Sur
- fracture
- Framer
- Frejka pillow
- Friedman
- frog
- Fruehevald
- full ring leg
- functional
- Funsten
- Futura cock-up
- Futura wrist
- Gagnon
- gait lock
- gauntlet
- Gibson

splint *(continued)*
- Gilmer
- Gooch
- Gordon
- Granberry
- Gunning
- gutter
- half ring leg
- half shell
- hallux valgus night
- hammertoe
- Hammond
- hand
- Hanna night
- Hare traction
- Harrington outrigger
- Hart
- Haynes-Griffin
- hinged cylinder
- HIPciser abduction
- Hirschtick
- Hodgen
- HVO (hallux valgus orthosis)
  - in a bag
- Ilfield
- Ilfield-Gustafson
- inflatable
- IROM bilateral
- IROM Regal
- isoprene plastic
- Jacoby bunion
- Jelanko
- Joint-Jack finger
- Jonell
- Jones
- Joseph
- Kanavel cock-up
- Karfoil
- Kazanjian
- Keller-Blake half ring
- Kerr
- Keystone
- kinetic
- Kingsley
- Kleinert
- knee
- knuckle-bender

splint *(continued)*
Lambrinudi
lead hand
leg
Levis
Lewin baseball finger
Lewin finger
Lewin-Stern thumb
Liberty One
Link Stack Split
Liston
live
long arm
long leg
long opponens
loop-lock cock-up
Love
Lytle
Magnuson
malleable metal finger
Malmö hip
Mason-Allen universal
Mayer
McGee
McIntire
McLeod
metacarpal
Middeldorpf
MindSet toe
modified Oppenheimer
modified safety pin
Mohr
moldable
molded posterior plaster
munster
Murray-Jones
Murray-Thomas
Neubeiser
New Mind Set toe
night
O'Donoghue
OCL (Orthopedic Casting Lab)
OEC
Omega splinting material
Oppenheimer spring wire
Oppenheimer with knuckle-bender

splint *(continued)*
Oppenheimer with reverse knuckle-
   bender
opponens
Orfit
Ortho-Glass
Ortho-last
Orthoplast
orthoplastic
outrigger with
padded
padded tongue blade
palmar
Pavlik
Peabody
Pearson attachment to Thomas
pelvic
PF Night
Phelps
pillow
Plastalume finger
plaster
plaster slab
platform
Plexiglas
Polysar
Polysplint A
polyvinylalcohol
Pond adjustable
Ponseti
posterior
posterior shin
Potts
protective
Protecto
Putti
quick
Redi-Around finger
replant
rest
resting pan
reverse finger knuckle-bender
Roger Anderson
Rolyan Gel Shell
Rowland-Hughes
Rumel aluminum

splint *(continued)*
   safety pin
   Sager traction
   Sam
   Saturn
   Sayre
   Scotchcast
   Scott ankle
   Scott cock-up wrist
   Scott Unifoam tennis elbow
   semidynamic
   serial
   shin
   short opponens
   short arm
   short leg polypropylene
   shoulder spica
   silver ring
   Simpson sugar tong
   Slattery-McGrouther dynamic
     flexion
   slip-on finger
   Slocum
   Sof-Gel palm shield
   Speed hand
   spica
   Spiegleman acromioclavicular
   spreading hand
   spring cock-up
   spring wire safety pin
   Stack
   Stader
   static
   Stax finger
   stirrup plaster
   Strampelli
   Stromeyer
   Stuart Gordon
   Stubbs acromioclavicular
   sugar tong plaster
   suspension
   Swanson hand
   synergistic wrist motion
   Synergy
   talipes hobble
   Tauranga
   Taylor

splint *(continued)*
   thermoplastic
   Thomas half ring
   Thomas hinged
   Thomas leg
   Thomas suspension
   Thompson
   thumb
   thumb abduction
   thumb web
   ThumZ'Up
   Tobruk
   toe
   Toronto
   traction
   triangular pillow
   TROM
   turnbuckle functional position
   universal gutter
   vacuum
   Valentine
   Velcro
   VersaWrist wrist
   Vesely-Street
   volar cock-up
   volar plaster
   Volkmann
   von Rosen cruciform
   Weil
   well leg
   Wertheim
   Wilson
   wire grip finger
   wire grip toe
   wraparound
   wrist cock-up
   wrist extension
   wrist rest
   wrist-driven
   yucca wood
   Zimfoam
   Zimmer
   Zucker
splint attachment, Pearson
splint bone
splinted in position of function
splinter

splinter hemorrhage
splint in a bag
splinting material
splinting therapy
splint-like pain
splint with outriggers
splint with wrist support
split biceps tendon tenodesis
split brain perspective
split brain studies
split compression fracture
split foot
split hand deformity
split posterior tibial tendon transfer
split Russell skeletal traction
split spinal cord malformation (SSCM)
split stirrup
split, sublimus
splitter, nail
split thickness skin excision (STSE)
split thickness skin graft
spoke bone
Sponastrine dysplasia
spondylalgia
spondylarthritis
spondylarthrocace
spondylectomy
spondylexarthrosis
spondylitic change
spondylitis
  ankylosing
  Bekhterev
  hypertrophic
  Kümmell
  Marie-Strümpell
  muscular
  posttraumatic
  pyogenic
  rheumatoid
  rhizomelic
  traumatic
  tuberculous
spondylitis deformans
spondylizema
spondyloarthropathy
spondylodesis

spondylodiskitis
spondylodynia
spondyloepiphyseal dysplasia
spondylolisthesis
  congenital
  degenerative
  dysplastic
  isthmic
  Meyerding
  pathologic
  sagittal roll
  slip angle
  traumatic (grades 1-4)
spondylolisthetic crisis
spondylolisthetic habitus
spondylolisthetic pelvis
spondylolysis
spondylomalacia
spondylopathy
spondylophyte impaction set
spondyloptosis
spondyloptotic kyphosis
spondylopyosis
spondyloschisis
spondylosis
  cervical
  degenerative
  diffuse
  lumbar
  Nurick
  rhizomelic
spondylosyndesis
spondylotic bar
spondylotic myelopathy
spondylotic radiculopathy
spondylotomy
  Adaptic
  cellulose
  collagen
  gauze
  lap (laparotomy)
  Mikulicz
  Ray-Tec
  Taka microneurosurgical
  Telfa
  Vistec

sponge
  EZ Bend
  Helistat collagen
  Ivalon
  NeuroCo neurosurgical
  polyvinyl alcohol
  twisted
sponge and needle count
sponge test
spongiform encephalopathy
  amyotrophic type
  classic type (Jakob-Creutzfeldt type)
  optic type (Heidenhain type)
  subacute type (Nevin-Jones type)
spongioblast
spongioblastoma multiforme
spongioblastoma, unipolar
spongiocyte
spongiocytoma
spongy appearance
spongy bone
spongy degeneration leukodystrophy
Sponsel oblique osteotomy
spontaneity
  loss of
  reduction in
spontaneous autosympathectomization
spontaneous epidural pneumocephalus
spontaneous extracranial dissection
spontaneous fracture
spontaneous intracranial pneumocephalus
spontaneous post-fracture epiphysiodesis of the radius
spontaneous rupture of Achilles tendon
spontaneous speech
spontaneous wrist clunk
Spontastrine dysplasia
spoon
  Cushing brain spatula
  Cushing pituitary
  Hardy pituitary
  pituitary
  Ray brain spatula
  spatula
sponge and needle count
sporadic ataxia

sporadic meningioma
sporadic parkinsonism
Spork utensil
S'port Max magnetic lumbosacral
  support
sports
  lateral motion racket
  pivoting
Sports Activity Scale
Sports Brace, by Bodyline
Sports-Caster I and II knee braces
sports chiropractic
SportsFit thumb orthosis
spot
  capitate soft
  café au lait
  Cloward
SPR (superior peroneal retinaculum)
sprain
  acute
  ankle
  chronic
  chronic ankle
  eversion
  inversion
  lateral ligamentous
  major
  minor
  muscle
  sacroiliac
  syndesmosis sprain of ankle
sprain fracture
sprain strain
Spratt bone curet
Spratt mastoid curet
spray, salmon calcitonin nasal
spray stretch technique
sprays, vasocoolant
spreader
  Badgley rib
  Bailey rib
  Beeson cast
  Beeson plaster
  Blount lamina
  Bobechko
  Burford-Finochietto rib
  cast

spreader *(continued)*
  cervical lamina
  cervical vertebrae
  Cloward cervical vertebra
  Cloward lamina
  Davis rib
  DeBakey rib
  Favoloro-Morse sternal
  Finochietto rib
  Gerbode-Burford rib
  Haglund-Stille plaster
  Haight-Finochietto rib
  Haight rib
  Harken rib
  Harrington
  Henning cast
  Henning meniscal retractor
  Henning plaster
  Hoffer-Daimler cast
  Inge cervical lamina
  Inge laminectomy
  intervertebral
  lamina
  Landolt
  Lemmon sternal
  Lilienthal rib
  Miltex rib
  Morse sternal
  Nelson rib
  plaster
  Rehbein rib
  rib
  Rienhoff-Finochietto rib
  Rienhoff rib
  spinous process
  sternal
  Tuffier rib
  vertebrae
  Weinberg rib
  Wilson rib
  Wiltberger spinous process
spreader bar of Denis Browne splint
spreading, epitope
spread of tumor
Sprengel deformity
Springer fracture
spring fixation

spring-loaded lock on orthosis
spring swivel thumb
spring, Weiss
sprinter's fracture
Spri Xercise board
sprouting
  axonal
  collateral
sprouting with axonal neuropathy
spur, spurring
  acromial
  anterior
  bone
  bony
  calcaneal
  calcific
  degenerative
  heel
  hypertrophic marginal
  impingement
  inferior
  marginal
  Morand
  osteoarthritic
  plantar
  plantar calcaneal
  posterior
  prominent
  retrocalcaneal
  traction
  uncovertebral
spurious ankylosis
Spurling intervertebral disk rongeur
Spurling-Kerrison cervical rongeur
Spurling-Kerrison laminectomy
  rongeur
Spurling-Kerrison up-biting and down-
  biting rongeurs
Spurling neck compression test
Spurling nerve root retractor
Spurling pituitary rongeur
Spurling rongeur forceps
Spurling sign
Spurling test for nerve root
  compression
spurring
spurt, growth

squamosomastoid suture
squamosoparietal suture
squamososphenoid suture
square pronator
square-shaped wrist test
square wave jerks (SWJ)
squat, half
squatting ability
squeak phenomenon
squeeze test in syndesmosis ankle
  sprain
SREDA (subclinical rhythmic dis-
  charges of adults)
S-ROM cup
S-ROM femoral stem prosthesis
S-ROM hip prosthesis
SRS (stereotactic radiosurgery)
SRS (Suicide Risk Scale)
SRS injectable cement
SSCM (split spinal cord malformation)
SSCP (single strand conformation
  polymorphism)
SSDI (Social Security Disability
  Insurance)
SSEP (somatosensory evoked
  potential)
SSEP waveforms
SSFP (steady state free precession)
SSH (spinal subdural hemorrhage)
S-shaped scoliosis
SSI (segmental spinal instrumentation)
  in scoliosis treatment
SSI (Supplemental Security Income)
SSOFRA (selective serotonin 1F
  agonist)
SSP (subclavian steal phenomenon)
SSPE (subacute sclerosing pan-
  encephalitis)
SSPE viral encephalitis
SSRI (selective serotonin reuptake
  inhibitor)
SSS (small sharp spike)
SSS (subclavian steal syndrome)
SSS (superior sagittal sinus)
SSZ (sulfasalazine)
St. (see *Saint*)

stability
  lateral
  ligamentous
  subtalar joint
  varus-valgus
  viscoelastic
Stability total hip system
stabilization
  atlantoaxial
  bony
  scapulocostal
  subtalar
  surgical
stabilize, stabilized, stabilization
stabilizer
  first ray (muscles)
  forearm
  patellar
  Simal cervical
stable fracture
stable hinge joint
Stableloc external wrist fixation system
stable to motion
stab wound
stab wound arthroscopy entry portal
Stack hand retractor
Stack shoulder procedure
Stack splint
Stader pin
Stader splint
Stadol NS (butorphanol tartrate)
stage, staging (see also *grading*)
  American Joint Commision on
    Cancer (AJCC) soft tissue
    sarcoma
  Berndt-Harty talar lesion
  distraction flexion (DFS)
  Enneking soft tissue sarcoma
  FAST (Functional Assessment
    Staging) for Alzheimer's disease
  Ficat avascular necrosis
  Greulich and Pyle skeletal
    maturation
  Kadish esthesioneuroblastoma
  neuroblastoma
  Outerbridge degenerative arthritis

stage *(continued)*
   pre-slip
   trispiral tomographic
   W (wakefulness) of sleep
Stage-1 single stage dental implant
   system
Stagnara wake-up test
Staheli rotational profile
Staheli shelf procedure
Stahl index
stain, staining
   EthBr (ethidium bromide)
   Gomori
   Grimelius
   hamstring
   hematoxylin and eosin (H&E)
   Masson-Fontana
   Masson-Goldner trichrome
   Masson trichrome
   periodic acid-Schiff
   safranin O
   Syto 13
   toluidine blue
   tumor
stainless steel preformed skull plates
stainless steel staples
StairClimber assist device
stair rise/descent test
stairs, ascending and descending
stairs sign
stairstep artifact
stairstep fracture
stairstep-type fracture
stalk
   body
   infundibular
   pituitary
   tumor
stalk of meningoencephalocele
stalk of tumor
"stalk section effect"
STA-MCA (superficial temporal artery
   to middle cerebral artery) anastomosis
stammering of the bladder
Stamm intra-articular hip fusion
stamps, Gelfoam

stance (of gait)
   single limb
   terminal
stance phase of gait cycle
stance phase of walking
stance phase periods of gait
   initial contact
   loading response
   midstance
   preswing
   terminal
Stand, IMP-Turnstile Casting
standard shell orthopedic shoe
standardized growth curves
standby assist
standing balance test
standing frame orthosis
Stanley cervical ligament
Stanmore elbow prosthesis
Stanmore knee replacement
Stanmore shoulder arthroplasty
Stanmore total hip replacement
stannous pyrophosphate
Staodyn TENS electrotherapy
STA-PCA (superficial temporal artery-
   posterior cerebral artery) bypass
stapedius muscle
Sta-Peg subtalar implant
stapes
staphylococcus arthritis
Staphylococcus aureus spinal osteomyelitis
staphylorrhaphy elevator
staple
   automatic
   barb
   barbed
   Blount
   bone
   Coventry
   Day
   Downing
   duToit
   epiphyseal
   Hernandez-Ros bone
   Howmedica Vitallium
   Johannesberg

staple *(continued)*
  metallic
  Mitek
  O'Brien
  osteoclast tension
  Owestry
  power-drive
  scalp marker
  skin
  stabilizing
  Stone four-point
  tabletop Stone
  titanium
  Vitallium
  Wilberg bone
  Zimaloy
staple arthroereisis
staple fixation
staple gun
staple migration
stapler
  Auto Suture
  Biologically Quiet
  Closer
  EEA (end-to-end anastomosis)
  Endo Stitch suturing
  GIA
  Instrument Makar
  Multifire VersaTack
  Origin Tacker
  Powered Metaphyseal
  Profile
  S*D*sorb meniscal
  TA-55 Auto Suture
  VersaTack
staples
  stainless steel
  3-M
Staples-Black-Brostrom ligament repair
Staples elbow arthrodesis
stapling
  Blount
  epiphyseal
star cancellation test (SCT)
starch bandage
Stardox ankle brace

stare
  empty
  glassy
  glassy-eyed
  post basic
  posterior fossa
Stark-Moore-Ashworth-Boyes
  technique
star, macular
stars, seeing
starter, Ritchie nail
start hesitation
startle myoclonus
startle reflex
startling noise on EEG
Statak device
Statak suture
state (pl. states)
  acute confusional
  alpha
  amnestic
  apallic
  central excitatory
  confusional
  crepuscular (twilight)
  delirium-like
  disequilibrium
  dissociative
  dreamy
  epileptic fugue
  fugue
  hyperdopaminergic
  hypnagogic
  hysterical fugue
  hysteric coma-like
  lacunar
  locked-in
  marble
  moribund
  nonresponsive
  parasomniac conscious
  persistent vegetative (PVS)
  postictal
  prothrombic
  sleep
  spastic

state *(continued)*
  toxic confusional
  trance
  transient state of depersonalization
    in migraine
  twilight
  unresponsive
  vegetative
  wakeful
state of alertness
state of consciousness
state of heightened attention
state of heightened awareness
static cervical spine
static deformity of foot
static fixation
static foot deformity
static foot pain
static friction
static locking nail
static positioning
static reflex controls
static scoliosis
static splint
static standing balance
static torticollis
static traction
static two-point discrimination
static wryneck
station
  gait and
  gait, station, and base
  Romberg
  unsteadiness of gait and
station and gait
station test
statoacoustic nerve
statokinetic reflex controls
status
  absence
  altered mental
  ambulatory
  deterioration of
  intact neurovascular
  mental
  neurocirculatory
  neurologic

status *(continued)*
  off work
  permanent and stationary
  petit mal
status aura
status dysgraphicus
status dysmyelinatus
status epilepticus
  convulsive
  nonconvulsive
  subclinical
status marmoratus
status post
status spongiosus
Stax finger splint
Stayoden 9000F TENS
STD hip prosthesis
steady state free precession (SSFP)
stealing of cerebral blood by subclavian artery
steal phenomenon in diabetic microvasculature of lower extremities
steal response
steal syndrome, subclavian
Stealth knee brace
StealthStation neuronavigation system
StealthStation optical digitizer
Stecher arachnoid knife
Steele-Richardson-Olszewski disease
Steele-Richardson-Olszewski syndrome
Steelex suture
steel shank
Steel shelf procedure
steel sole plate
Steel triple innominate osteotomy
Steeper powered Gripper prosthetic
  device
steep left anterior oblique (LAO) view
steerable introducer
steering, paresthesia
Steffee pedicle plate
Steffee pedicular rod
Steffee plates and screws for lumbar
  fusion
Steida fracture
Steida bony process
Steinbach mallet

Steinberg test
Steinberg thumb sign
Steinbrocker classification of rheuma-
   toid arthritis
Steindler flexorplasty
Steindler stripping operation
Steinert classification of epiphyseal
   fracture
Steinhauser screws and instrumentation
Steinmann extension nail
Steinmann pin with Crowe pilot point
Steinmann sign
Steinmann smooth pin
Steinmann tendon forceps
Steinmann threaded pin
Stelazine (trifluoperazine hydro-
   chloride)
StelKast instruments/devices
stellate chemicals
stellate fracture
stellate ligament
stellate skull fracture
stellate sympathetic ganglion block
stellate undepressed fracture
Stellbrink synovectomy rongeur
stem
   Aufranc-Turner
   brain
   CoCrMo (cobalt-chromium-
      molybdenum)
   Continuum hip
   Exeter
   fenestrated
   fin of prosthetic
   Harris-Galante
   Implex ProxiLock
   infundibular
   Kirschner
   Linear hip
   Mallory-Head femoral
   matte
   Meridian
   metaphyseal loading
   Moore
   nonfenestrated
   Omnifit HA hip
   polished

stem *(continued)*
   Press-Fit
   regular
   reticular formation of brain
   roundback
   Sivash
   straight
   trial
   Zimmer bone
stem base plate
stem cell migration
stem cell transplantation
stem envelope
stem extender
stemmed tibial prosthesis
Stener-Gunterberg hip procedure
Stener lesion
stenosing tendovaginitis
stenosing tenosynovitis (tendosynovitis)
stenosis
   aqueductal
   bilateral carotid
   carotid artery
   central canal
   central spinal
   cerebral artery
   cervical
   congenital aqueductal
   congenital spinal
   hemodynamically significant
   spinal
   subclavian artery
   unilateral carotid
   vertebral artery
stent
   autologous vein-covered
   coronary
   endovascular
   flexible
   Gianturco-Roubin
   INR neurological
   intravascular
   neurovascular
   Palmaz
   Palmaz-Schatz
   pliable
   self-expanding metallic wall

stent-assisted angioplasty
stent dressing
Stenver view
Stenzel rod
step count
step-cut osteotomy
step-cut transection
step-down deformity of shoulder
step-down osteotomy
Stephenson-Gibbs reference electrode
step-off between bone fracture
    fragments
step-off deformity
step-off fracture
step-off in facial fracture diagnosis
step-off, orbital rim
step-osteotomy
steppage gait due to footdrop
stepped flash photic stimulation
step-up in spinous processes in
    spondylolisthesis
stepwise increasestep-second test
stereoanesthesia
stereognosis
StereoGuide stereotactic needle core
    biopsy
stereophotogrammetry
StereoPlan stereotactic surgery plan-
    ning software
stereoscopic head-mounted display
stereotactic *or* stereotaxic
stereotactic ablation
stereotactically defined intracranial
    target volume
stereotactically guided
stereotactic aspiration biopsy
stereotactic atlas
stereotactic bag
stereotactic carrier
stereotactic coordinates
stereotactic core needle biopsy
    (SCNB)
stereotactic craniotomy
stereotactic depth electroencephalogram
stereotactic endoscopy
stereotactic frame
stereotactic head frame

stereotactic implantation of ventriculo-
    peritoneal shunt
stereotactic irradiation (STI)
stereotactic method for intracranial
    navigation
stereotactic neurosurgery
stereotactic operating microscope
stereotactic pallidotomy
stereotactic percutaneous lumbar
    diskectomy
stereotactic placement of depth
    electrodes
stereotactic puncture
stereotactic radiosurgery (SRS)
stereotactic ring
stereotactic robot
stereotactic surgery
stereotactic system, CRW
stereotactic target
stereotactic thalamectomy
stereotactic thalamotomy
stereotactic tractotomy
stereotactic ventral pallidotomy
stereotaxic (or stereotactic)
stereotaxis, computer-assisted
    volumetric
stereotaxy, frameless
stereotypic behavior
Steri-Strips
sterile 4 x 4's
sterile saline solution
sternal angle of Louis
sternal border and apex
sternal cartilage
sternal edge
sternal joint
sternal lift
sternal marrow
sternal muscle
sternal notch
sternal occipital mandibular
    immobilization (SOMI)
sternal pleural reflection
sternal splitting
sternal view
sternobrachial reflex
sternochondroscapular muscle

sternoclavicular angle
sternoclavicular joint
sternoclavicular ligament
sternoclavicular muscle
sternocleidomastoid, clavicular head of
sternocleidomastoid muscle weakness
sternocostal articulation
sternocostal joint
sternohyoid muscle
sternomastoid muscle
sternopericardial ligament
sternospinal reference electrode
sternothyroid muscle
sternum, anterior bowing of
steroid block, epidural
steroid-induced bone disease
steroid injection
steroid myopathy
steroid pulse therapy
steroids
    tapering dose
    tapering regimen of
steroid therapy
STERRAD 50 Sterilization System
stertorous hyperventilation
Stevenson alligator forceps
Stevenson grasping forceps
Stevens scissors
Stevens-Street elbow prosthesis
Steward-Milford fracture classification
Stewart arm procedure
Stewart-Harley ankle arthrodesis
Stewart-Holmes sign
Stewart-Morel syndrome
STH-2 (Sarmiento) hip prosthesis
STI (stereotactic irradiation)
Stickler syndrome
stick, switching
stiffening
stiff-man syndrome
stiffness
    joint
    neck
    passive elastic
    torsional
stiffness coefficient
stiff person syndrome

stigmata of neurofibromatosis
Stiles-Bunnell transfer technique
Still-Chauffard polyarthritis syndrome
Still disease
Stille bone biter
Stille bone chisel
Stille bone drill
Stille bone gouge
Stille-Broback retractor
Stille bur
Stille chisel
Stille cranial drill
Stille drill points, burs, and trephine
Stille-Giertz rib shears
Stille gouge
Stille hand drill
Stille-Horsley bone forceps
Stille-Horsley rongeur
Stille-Lauer bone rongeur
Stille-Leksell rongeur
Stille-Liston bone-cutting forceps
Stille-Liston bone rongeur
Stille-Luer bone rongeur
Stille-Luer duckbill rongeur
Stille-Luer-Echlin rongeur
Stille-Luer rongeur forceps
Stille osteotome
Stille plaster shears
Stille probe
Stille rib shears
Stille rongeur forceps
Stiller rib
Stille-Ruskin bone rongeur
Stille-Sherman bone drill
Stille tourniquet
Stille trephine
Stim Plus stimulator
Stimson dressing
Stimson maneuver
Stimson reduction of shoulder
    dislocation
stimulated whole salivary flow rate
    test
stimulation, stimulator
    ACUTENS transcutaneous nerve
    AME bone growth
    Amrex muscle

stimulation *(continued)*
auditory
Axostim nerve
battery pack
Biolectron bone growth
Bionicare 1000
blink reflex to corneal
brain stem
capacitor plate for electrical
Coherent light point
constant direct current
CTDx electrostimulation system
deep brain
diffuse photic
digital
dorsal column (DCS)
double channel
double simultaneous
double simultaneous sensory
EBI SpF-2 implantable bone
EBI SpF-T bone
EBI spinal fusion
electrical
electrical surface
electrogalvanic
epidural spinal cord (ESCS)
epileptogenic
facial nerve
faradic current
flash
flashes of light
flashes per second of photic
galvanic
glissando photic
globus pallidus
high voltage pulsed galvanic
high volt biphasic
high volt inferential
Hilger facial nerve
interferential
intermittent flashes of light
intraoperative nerve
Intrel II spinal cord
JACE-STIM electrotherapy
Jako
magnetic
marrow

stimulation *(continued)*
Medtronic neuromuscular
Medtronic spinal cord
Micro-Z neuromusculator
multipulse
MuscleMax electrical muscle
MuscleSense electrical muscle
nerve
Neuromed
neuromuscular
neuromuscular electrical (NMES)
Ortho Dx knee rehabilitation
OrthoGen/OsteoGen
OrthoLogic 1000 bone growth
OrthoPak bone growth
OrthoPak II bone
OsteoGen bone growth
Osteo Stim bone
Osteo Stim implantable bone
growth
patterned light
patterned photic
PENS (percutaneous electrical
nerve stimulation)
photic (during EEG recording with
a stroboscopic light)
Physio-Stim Lite bone growth
piezo electrical
Pisces spinal cord
pulsed electromagnetic field
(PEMF)
ReAct neuromuscular
Reese
repetitive clicking
repetitive flashes of light
repetitive nerve
repetitive photic
Respond Select neuromuscular
Russian
SANS (Stoller afferent nerve
stimulation) device
sensory
single channel
somatosensory
SpF Spinal Fusion Stimulator
spinal cord
SpinaLogic-1000 bone growth

stimulation *(continued)*
  Spinal Stim bone growth
  startling noise
  stepped flash photic
  stepwise photic
  Stim Plus
  Stoller afferent nerve
  stroboscopic
  stroboscopic light
  subthalamic nucleus
  tactile
  TENS (transcutaneous electrical
    nerve)
  thalamic
  ThermaStim muscle
  TNMES (transcutaneous neuro-
    muscular electrical stimulation)
  touch and tickle
  transcranial magnetic (MAG)
  transcutaneous electrical nerve
    (TENS)
  TS-930 electric-powered foot reflex
  UniPuls electrostimulation
    instrument
  vagus nerve (VNS)
  VIM (ventral intermedius nucleus)
  visual
  WR nerve
stimulus (pl. stimuli)
  alerting
  auditory
  checkerboard pattern reversal
  click
  double simultaneous
  environmental
  epileptogenic
  external
  extinction of
  flickering
  full field monocular
  insensitivity to painful
  matching
  monophasic anodal
  monophasic cathodal
  musical
  noxious

stimulus *(continued)*
  outside
  painful
  psychosensory
  responded purposefully to
  sensory
  startling
  stimuli
  supramaximal
  tactile
  thermal
  threshold of
  train of repetitive
  triggering
  visual
stimulus artifact
stimulus bound
stimulus-evoked electromyography
stimulus polarity
stimulus rate, click
stinger (nerve pain from cervical or
  brachial plexus injury)
stinging
stippled epiphysis
stippling
stirrup (pl. stirrups)
  Aircast pneumatic air
  Allen
  ankle air
  Bicro-Lite ankle
  high
  split
  traction
  walking
stirrup taping
stitch (see *suture*)
  baseball
  Frost
Stiwer forceps
Stiwer retractor
Stiwer scissors
stock, poor bone
stockinette
  basket
  bias
  bias-cut

stockinette *(continued)*
  Buck traction
  sling and swathe
  tubular
stockinette cut on the bias
stockings (also called *hose*)
  antiembolic
  antiembolism
  antithrombotic
  compression
  graduated compression
  Jobst
  long leg
  Orthawear antiembolism
  Sigvaris compression
  TED (thromboembolic disease)
  thigh-high antiembolic
  Vairox high compression vascular
  Zipzoc compression dressing
    and wrap
stocking distribution
stocking-glove distribution
stocking-glove sensory loss
Stoke index
Stokes-Adams attack
Stoller afferent nerve stimulation
  (SANS) device
stomach qi deficiency (Chinese medicine term)
Stone and Neale Daily Coping
  Assessment
Stone arthrodesis
Stone bunionectomy
Stone four-point staple
stone, Whitfield ointment and pumice
Stookey cranial rongeur
stop action brace
stopcock
storiform pattern
stork's legs in Charcot-Marie-Tooth
  disease
Stork S'port maternity lumbosacral
  support
Storz arthroscope
Storz meniscotome
Storz Microsystems cranial fixation
  plate

Storz Microsystems drill bit
Storz Microsystems microplate
Storz Microsystems miniplate
Storz Microsystems plate cutters
Storz Microsystems plate-holding
  forceps
Storz Microsystems pliers
Storz screw
Storz telescope
stoved
Strümpell-Leichtenstern encephalitis
Strümpell sign
strabismus
  illusory
  kinetic
  real
straddle fracture
straddle injury
straight last shoes
straight leg raising test
straight stem femoral components
strain
  Brunhilde (type I poliomyelitis
    virus)
  foot (acute, chronic)
  hamstring
  Lansing (type II poliomyelitis
    virus)
  Leon (type III poliomyelitis virus)
  ligamentous
  lumbosacral spine
  muscle
strain energy
strain fracture
strain gauge evaluation
strain gauge extensometer
strain sprain injury
Strampelli splint
strap (see also *brace, splint, support*)
  capsular
  Cho-Pat (**cho**ndromalacia **pat**ellae)
    knee
  Chopart patellar
  clavicular
  crotch
  Gel-Bank patellar
  Meek clavicle

strap *(continued)*
  Pro-Tec patellar tendon
  PTB (patellar tendon-bearing)
  Scott elastic ankle
  suspension
  touch fastener
  Velcro
strap muscles
Strata hip system
stratigraphy
Stratis II MRI system
Strayer tendon technique
streak, meningeal
stream of thought
Streeter dysplasia
Street medullary pin
Street-Stevens humeral prosthesis
strength
  BUE
  extrinsic muscle
  fatigue
  5/5 (five over five)
  foot intrinsic muscle
  grip
  hand grasp
  hand grip
  intrinsic muscle
  isokinetic
  isometric muscle
  Lovett clinical scale of
  motor
  pinch
  tensile
  yield
strength against resistance
strength tester
  GripTrack Commander
  PinchTrack Commander
  PowerTrack Commander
Streptococcus agalactiae meningitis
Streptococcus pneumoniae meningitis
Streptococcus viridans
streptogramin
stress
  adduction
  biomechanical
  fluid shear

stress *(continued)*
  hyperextension
  laminar shear
  maximal effort key pinch
  mediolateral
  shear
  torque
  valgus
  varus
  von Mises
stress films
stress fracture
stress radiograph
stress riser
stress strain relationships
stress tolerant position
stretch
  intermittent passive muscle
  muscle
stretcher, field
stretches (see *exercises*)
stretching, tendo Achillis
stretch reflex
stretch reflex pathways
stretch test, sciatic
stria
  habenular
  longitudinal
  medullary
  meningitic
striae of Baillarger
striae of floor of ventricle
striatal activity
striatal denervation
striatal dopaminergic innervation
striatal lesion
striatal neuron
striatal nigral degeneration
striatal toe
striate cortex
striated muscle
striate hemorrhages in intracranial
  hypertension
striatocerebellar tremor
striatonigral degeneration
striatum, corpus
Strickland regimen

Strickland suture technique
Strickland tendon repair
stride characteristics
stride length of gait
strike phase of gait
striker
 forefoot
 rearfoot
string of pearls nuclear arrangement
strionigral
strip (pl. strips)
 AdTech electrode
 epidural electrode
 Fas-Trac
 4-contact electrode sentinel
 moleskin
 motor
 PVA
 subdural electrode
stripe
 paraspinal pleural
 vertebral
stripe of Baillarger
stripe of Gennari
stripe of Vicq d'Azyr
stripper
 Brand palmaris tendon
 Bunnell tendon
 cartilage
 endarterectomy
 fascia
 Fischer tendon
 Furlong tendon
 Grierson tendon
 IM tendon
 malleable
 New Orleans endarterectomy
 palmaris tendon
 plantaris
 rib
 tendon
stripping, periosteal
stroboscope
stroboscopic flashes of light in EEG
stroboscopic lamp
stroboscopic stimulation

stroke (cerebrovascular accident, CVA)
 acute
 anterior circulation
 brain stem
 cardioembolic
 cerebrovascular
 completed
 cryptogenic
 embolic
 evolving
 hemispheric
 hemorrhagic
 hyperacute
 hypertensive
 incomplete
 ischemic
 lacunar
 midbrain
 middle cerebral artery territory
 migrainous
 nonhemorrhagic
 posterior circulation
 progressing
 pure hemisensory
 pure motor
 pure sensory
 sensorimotor
 sensory
 small vessel
 spinal
 spinal cord
 subacute
 thalamocapsular
 thromboembolic (TE)
 thrombotic
 unheralded
stroke in evolution
strokes, multiple small (état lacunaire)
stroke syndrome
stroma
stromal cells
Stromeyer splint
Stromgren ankle brace
Stroop color word interference test
structural allograft
structural anterior column allograft

structural cellular biomaterial
structural epileptogenic lesion
   arteriovenous malformations
   cysts
   neoplasms
structural epilepsy
structure (pl. structures)
   bony
   cordlike
   extrapyramidal
   lateral supporting
   load-bearing
   shift of midline
   subcortical
Strully dissecting scissors
Strully dural hook
Strully dural scissors
Strully-Gigli rongeur
Strully-Gigli saw handles
Strully-Kerrison rongeur
Strully neurological scissors
Strümpell-Lorrain disease
Strümpell-Marie disease
Strümpell, tibialis sign of
Strunsky sign
strut
   autologous bone
   corticocancellous
strut bone graft
Struthers
   arcade of
   ligament of
strut-type pin
Stryker bed
Stryker cartilage knife
Stryker CPM exerciser
Stryker fracture frame
Stryker Howmedica Osteonics devices
   system
Stryker knee joint laxity machine
Stryker knee laxity arthrometer
Stryker leg exerciser
Stryker microsurgery drill
Stryker notch x-ray view
Stryker Quick Pressure Monitor Set
Stryker Surgilav machine

Stryker table
Stryker wedge suture anchor
STSE (split thickness skin excision)
STSG (split thickness skin graft)
STT (scaphotrapeziotrapezoid)
   arthrodesis
Stuart Gordon splint
Stubbs acromioclavicular splint
Stubbs elastic wrist support
Stubbs 4-way clavicle brace
Stubbs Sacro Belt
Stuck laminectomy retractor
stud, fixation
study (pl. studies)
   AAASPS (African-American Anti-
      platelet Stroke Prevention
      Study)
   air contrast
   antidromic (sensory) conduction
   biomechanical
   bone age
   brachial plexus motor
   cadaveric biomechanical
   CAPRIE (clopidogrel versus
      aspirin in patients at risk of
      ischemic events)
   continuous wave Doppler
   Cornwall hip fracture
   Doppler
   electrodiagnostic
   electromyographic
   electrophysiologic nerve
   Johns Hopkins National Low Back
      Pain Study
   kinematic
   Michigan Bone Health Study
   mixed nerve conduction
   motor nerve conduction
   musculocutaneous nerve sensory
   nerve conduction
   orthodromic sensory
   radial nerve motor/sensory
   sensory nerve conduction
   split brain
   tenographic
   tension-to-failure

study *(continued)*
   ulnar nerve motor/sensory
   Washington Heights-Inwood
     Genetic Study of Essential
     Tremor (WHIGET)
Stulberg hip classification
Stulberg hip positioner
Stulberg Mark II leg positioner
Stulberg method
stump
   bulbous
   distal
   edematous
   hypersensitive
   midfoot
   tendon
stump of bone
stump shrinker, elastic
stump sock
stupor
   alcoholic
   catatonic
stuporous patient
Sturge-Weber syndrome
Sturge-Weber telangiectasia
stuttering gait in parkinsonism
ST walker brace
STx lumbar traction device
styloauricular muscle
styloglossus muscle
stylohyoid ligament
stylohyoid muscle
styloid
   radial
   ulnar
styloidectomy, Stewart
styloid diaphragm
styloid process
stylomandibular ligament
stylomastoid foramen
stylomaxillary ligament
stylopharyngeal muscle
stylus, marking
Styrofoam filler block
sub-falcine (subfalcial) herniation
subacromial bursa
subacromial bursal adhesion

subacromial bursitis
subacromial decompression procedure
subacute combined degeneration of the
   cord
subacute granulomatous meningitis
subacute necrotizing myelitis
   (Foix-Alajouanine)
subacute sclerosing panencephalitis
   (SSPE) viral encephalitis
subacute spongiform encephalopathy
subacute stroke
subacute type (Nevin-Jones type)
   spongiform encephalopathy
subanconeus muscle
subarachnoid block
subarachnoid cavity
subarachnoid hemorrhage (SAH)
subarachnoid hemorrhage from rupture
   of mycotic aneurysm
subarachnoid instillation of contrast
   material
subarachnoid metastatic disease
subarachnoid phenol block (SAPB)
   with fluoroscopy
subarachnoid screw instruments
subarachnoid space
subarticular cyst
subastragalar dislocation
subaxial cervical pedicle
subcallosal gyrus
subcapital fracture
subchondral bone cyst
subchondral bone plate
subchondral drilling
subchondral microfractures
subchondral plate
subchondral sclerosis
subchorionic hemorrhage
subchoroidal approach to third
   ventricle
subclavian artery occlusion
subclavian artery steal of cerebral
   blood
subclavian artery stenosis
subclavian bruit
subclavian flap aortoplasty (SFA)
subclavian muscle

subclavian nerve
subclavian steal phenomenon (SSP)
subclavian steal syndrome (SSS)
subclinical EEG discharges
subclinical neuropathy
subclinical seizure activity
subclinical status epilepticus
subcollateral gyrus
subcoracoid shoulder dislocation
subcortical aphasia
subcortical atherosclerotic encephalopathy (SAE)
subcortical atrophy
subcortical cerebral infarction
subcortical dementia
subcortical infarct
subcortical intracerebral hemorrhage
subcortical intracranial lesion
subcortical ischemic vascular dementia
subcortical lesion
subcortical neuronal dysfunction
subcortical pacemaker
subcortical pathway
subcortical structures
subcostal muscle
subcostal nerve
subcrural muscle
subcutaneous fibroma
subcutaneous fracture
subcutaneous palmar fasciotomy
subcutaneous tissue gas
subcuticular closure
subdeltoid bursal adhesion
subdeltoid bursitis
subdural abscess
subdural blood
subdural cavity
subdural clot
subdural effusion
subdural electrode
subdural empyema
subdural hematoma
subdural hemorrhage
subdural hygroma
subdural pressure monitor
subdural space
subdural tap

subdural window
subependymal vein
subependymoma
subepicranial space
subfalcine (subfalcial) herniation
subfascial transposition
subforniceal approach to third
   ventricle
subfrontal meningioma
subfrontal meningioma tumor
subgaleal abscess
subgaleal CSF (cerebrospinal fluid)
subgaleal hematoma
subgaleal plane
subglenoid shoulder dislocation
subharmonic rhythm
subhyaloid retinal hemorrhage
subiculum
subjective cosmesis
subjective impairment
subjective limited movement
subjective symptoms of impairment
subjective vertigo
sublabral recess
sublamina wiring
subligamentous disk herniation
subliminal injury
sublimus split
sublingual nerve
sublux
subluxation
   atlantoaxial
   element
   forward
   occult
   patellar
   posterior
   radial head (RHS)
   reduced
   rotary
   tendon
   traumatic
   Volkmann
subluxation complex
subluxation correction
subluxing patella
subluxing tendon

submandibular ganglion
submandibular space
submandibular triangle
submaxillary space
submental space
submental vertex view
suboccipital craniectomy
suboccipital cranioplasty
suboccipital decompression
suboccipital headache
suboccipital muscles
suboccipital nerve
suboccipital shortening
suboccipital transmeatal craniotomy
subperiosteal corticotomy
subperiosteal fracture
subperiosteally
subperiosteal new bone formation
subpial plane
subpial resection
subquadricipital muscle
subsartorial tunnel
subscapularis muscle flap
subscapularis tear
subscapular muscle
subscapular nerve
subscapular recess
subscapular tendon
subspinous dislocation
substance
    anterior perforated
    posterior perforated
substance abuse
Substance P in cerebrospinal fluid
substitution bone
substitution, G to A
substrate, neurologic
subsurface white band (on degenerated
    implant)
subtalar arthralgia
subtalar arthrodesis
subtalar arthrotomy
subtalar articulation
subtalar axis
subtalar distraction bone-block fusion
subtalar instability
subtalar joint as torque converter

subtalar joint pronation
subtalar joint space
subtalar joint stability
subtalar posterior displacement
    osteotomy of the calcaneus
subtalar stabilization
subtemporal approach
subtendinous space
subtentorial lesions
subthalamic nucleus implantation
subthalamic nucleus of Luys
subthalamic region of midbrain
subtotal meniscectomy
subtotal removal of tumor
subtotal sacrectomy
subtractions, serial
subtrochanteric fracture
subtype, HLA
subungual abscess
subungual amelanotic melanoma
subungual hematoma
subungual tumor (glomus tumor)
subvertebral muscles
subxiphoid view
Sucker, KAM Super
sucker shaver
sucker tip
sucking reflex (primitive)
suck reflex
suction-irrigation system
suction-irrigator
    House
    Kurze
suction tip
    Frazier
    neurosurgical
suction tube
    Adson
    New York Glass
    Pribham
    wall
suction via trap bottle system
sudanophilic leukodystrophies
Sudeck atrophy
Sudeck disease
sudomotor (cf. *pseudo-motor*)
sudomotor autonomic hyperactivity

sudomotor nerve
SUFE (slipped upper femoral
  epiphysis)
sugar tong cast
sugar tong plaster splint
Sugioka transtrochanteric osteotomy
Sugita aneurysm clip
Sugita head frame
Sugita table
Suicide Risk Scale (SRS)
suit, isolation
Sukhtian-Hughes fixation devices
sulcal atrophy
sulcal obliteration
sulcal skeleton
sulcus (pl. sulci)
  calcarine
  callosal
  central
  cingulate
  collateral
  dilatation of the
  effacement of
  frontal
  hypothalmic
  lateral
  lateral occipital
  lips of lateral
  occipitotemporal
  olfactory
  parieto-occipital
  pontomedullary
  postcentral
  precentral
  rami of lateral
  rolandic
  superior frontal
  superior temporal
  supracallosal
  temporal
  trochlear
  ulnar
  widened, on scan
sulcus angle
sulcus calcaneus
sulcus lunatus
sulcus nail

sulcus of metatarsus
sulcus talus
sulcus test
sulfasalazine (SSZ)
sulfatide
sulfinpyrazone
sulfite oxidase deficiency
sulfur bath, hot
Sully shoulder stabilizer
Sulzer Orthopedics instruments
summation wire
sump effect of arteriovenous shunting
sunburst pattern on x-ray
Sundaresan approach
Sunday staphylorrhaphy elevator
Sunderland classification of nerve
  injury
Sunderland five-degree system
sundowning
Sundt classification of carotid
  ulceration
Sundt encircling clip
Sundt-Kees aneurysm window clips
Sundt loop endarterectomy shunt
Sundt shunt
sunrise view of patella
sunset eyes
sunset view
Supazote foam
SuperAnchor suture anchor
superantigen
Superblade
superciliary arch
superclot
superconducting magnet
SuperCup acetabular cup prosthesis
superficial back muscles
superficial cervical nerve
superficial dorsal sacrococcygeal
  ligament
superficial fasciotomy
superficial fibular nerve
superficial flexor muscle
superficial lingual muscle
superficial musculoaponeurotic system
  (SMAS)
superficial palmar arterial arch

superficial peroneal nerve
superficial posterior sacrococcygeal
ligament
superficial reflexes
superficial sensation
superficial transverse metacarpal
ligament
superficial transverse metartarsal
ligament
superficial transverse perineal muscle
Superfoam II material
Superglue (cyanoacrylate) adhesive
superimposed on EEG
superincumbent spinal curves
superior alveolar nerves
superior auricular muscle
superior cervical cardiac nerve
superior cluneal nerves
superior colliculus
superior constrictor muscle of pharynx
superior costotransverse ligament
superior dental nerves
superior facet
superior frontal gyrus
superior frontal sulcus
superior gemellus muscle
superior gluteal nerve
superior laryngeal nerve
superior-lateral brachial cutaneous
nerve
superior ligament
superior limb girdle
superior maxillary nerve
superior oblique muscle of head
superior olive in brain
superior parietal lobule gyrus
superior peroneal retinaculum
superior petrosal sinus
superior posterior serratus muscle
superior pubic ligament
superior pubic ramus
superior quadriceps retinaculum
superior radioulnar joint
superior rectus muscle
Superior Sleeprite Hi-Lo orthopedic
bed
superior tarsal muscle

superior temporal gyrus
superior temporal sulcus
superior tibial articulation
superior tibiofibular joint
superior transverse scapular ligament
supernumerary sesamoid bones
superolaterally
superomedial portal
superoxide dismutase (SOD)
SuperQuad assistive device
supersaturation, muscle glycogen
superselective catheterization
superselective embolization
superselectively introduced
Super Stimm interferential
supervised neglect
supination adduction fracture
supination deformity
supination eversion fracture
supination, external rotation-type IV
(SER-IV) fracture
supinator, assistant
supinator canal syndrome
supinator jerks
supinator muscle
supine cervical traction
supine film
Suppan foot procedure
Supplemental Security Income (SSI)
support (see also *brace; immobilizer;
orthosis; prosthesis; splint;
strap*)
Accommodator arch
Achillotrain
Act
Active Ankle
Act Knee
Aircast
AliMed wrist/thumb
Air-Stirrup ankle
alternating single leg (running gait)
ankle
arch
Arizona leg
ASO (Ankle Stabilizing Orthosis)
back
Band-It magnetic

support *(continued)*

Bauerfeind
bed cradle
billet prosthetic
Bio Skin
Body Gard neoprene
Body Glove
boomerang wrist
Breg
Cam Walker ankle or leg brace
canvas
carpal lock wrist
cervical
Cho-Pat knitted compression
CMO
cock-up hand (or wrist)
Comfy Cradle maternity lumbar
Comprifix
Compro
Compro Plus
condylar cuff prosthetic
Core elastic ankle
Core lumbosacral
Core Reflex wrist
Core universal
CorFit lumbosacral
Cryo Cuff compression
Cybertech 1000
cutout knee
DonJoy thigh
donut
Dyno-Cinch lumbosacral
elbow
Epipoint elbow
Epitrain Fiscoped
Epitrain knitted elbow
Fiscoped S
FiscoSpot
Fits-All
foam
fork-strap prosthetic
Freedom arthritis
Friedman elbow
Fromison elbow
Genutrain
hand
hinged knee

support *(continued)*

Houston halo cervical
initial double (of gait)
Innovation Sports bracing
Kerr-Lagen abdominal
knee
Kneed-It magnetic knee
ligamentous
Lo Bak spinal
lumbosacral
Lumbotrain lumbosacral
Malleoloc ankle
Malleotrain ankle
Manutrain active wrist
Markwort ankle
medial arch
metatarsal
MKG knee
Neck-Huggar cervical
neoprene
Night Splint
ObusForme back
OEC wrist/forearm
Omotrain active shoulder
open patella knee
Orthomedics cervical
OSI Well Leg
Otto Bock
Palumbo knee
Performance Wrap knee
Philadelphia collar cervical
Playmaker
Pro-Tec
Relax-A-Bac posture
rib
Sacro-Eze lumbar
Saunders Posture S'port
SCOI shoulder brace
Scott
second double (of gait)
Sheffield hand
Shields knee
shoe
Silesian bandage prosthetic
Sleeper II sleep, Bodyline
Slingshot shoulder immobilizer
Spider Pad

support *(continued)*
    standard U patellar
    Stork S'port maternity lumbosacral
    Stubbs elastic wrist
    Stubbs Sacro Belt lumbosacral
    S'port Max
    tennis elbow
    Thera-Back back
    Thermoskin
    Tulis
    TwinFlex back
    UltraSling
    Valeo CTS
    Viscoheel K
    Viscoheel N
    ViscoSpot
    waist-belt prosthetic
    walk with
    walk without
    WorkMod back
    wrist
    WrisTimer CTS
supporter, Malis vessel
supporting foot
suppressant, vestibular
suppression, burst
suppuration
suppurative periostitis
suppurative tenosynovitis
supracallosal epidermoid cyst
supracallosal gyrus
supracallosal sulcus
supraclavicular muscle
supraclavicular region
supraclavicular triangle
supracollicular spike of cortical bone
supracondylar femoral derotational
    osteotomy
supracondylar femoral fracture
supracondylar humerus fracture
supracondylar varus osteotomy
supraepicondylar
supraglenoid cyst
suprahyoid muscle
suprainterparietal bone
supraligamentous disk herniation
supramalleolar orthosis (SMO)

supramalleolar osteotomy
supramalleolar region
supramarginal gyrus
Supramid suture
supranuclear (bilateral upper motor
    neuron)
supranuclear disorders of ocular
    movement
supranuclear dysfunction
supranuclear lesion
supranuclear ophthalmoplegias
supranuclear palsy, progressive
supranuclear paralysis
supranuclear weakness
supraoccipital bone
supraorbital bar
supraorbital fissure
supraorbital nerve
supraorbital notch
supraorbital ridges
suprapatellar bursa
suprapatellar plica
suprapatellar pouch
suprapharyngeal bone
suprapubic area
suprascapular ligament
suprascapular nerve entrapment
suprascapular neuropathy
suprasellar adenoma
suprasellar aneurysm
suprasellar cistern
suprasellar extension of tumor
suprasellar lesion
suprasellar mass
suprasellar meningioma
suprasellar Rathke cleft cyst (RCC)
suprasellar region
suprasellar tumor
supraspinalis muscle
supraspinatus nerve
supraspinatus tendon
supraspinous ligament
supraspinous muscle
suprasternal bone
suprasternal window
suprasyndesmotic fixation
supratentorial approach

supratentorial arteriovenous
  malformation
supratentorial astrocytoma
supratentorial brain tumor
supratentorial cerebral blood flow
supratentorial epidermoid cyst
supratentorial primitive neuroectodermal tumor (PNET)
supratentorial glioma
supratentorial lesion
supratentorial mass
supratentorial symptoms (euphemism
  for hypochondriasis)
supratentorial tumor
supratip nasal tip deformity
supratrochlear nerve
supratubercular wedge osteotomy
sural nerve
Surbaugh leg holder
surcingle, Von Lackum
Sure Step ankle brace
Suretac suture
SureTrans autotransfusion system for
  orthopedics
Suretac bioabsorbable shoulder
  fixation device
surface
  acetabular weightbearing
  apposing articular
  articular
  bleeding bone
  bone
  bosselated
  cartilaginous joint
  contiguous articular
  endosteal
  grooving of articular
  joint articular
  parallelism of articular
  radioulnar
  roughened articular
  wear-resistant
  weightbearing
surface coil MR
surface electromyography (sEMG)
surface method of Hodes
surface shoe interaction

surfer's knot
Surfit adhesive
Surgairtome
Surg-Assist leg positioner
Surgenomic endoscope in carpal
  tunnel release
surgeon's tarsal joint
surgery (see *operations*)
  ablative
  aesthetic
  bur
  high torque burr
  image-guided
  neuroablative
  neurofunctional
  neuro-otologic
  outpatient ambulatory
  reconstructive
  salvage
  stereotactic
  thoracoscopic spine
surgibone
  Boplant
  Unilab
surgical ablation
surgical approach
surgical decompression
surgical escharotomy
surgical isolation bubble system (SIBS)
surgical neck fracture
Surgical No Bounce Mallet
surgical rhizotomy
Surgical Simplex P radiopaque bone
  cement
surgical site
surgical stabilization
Surgical Dynamics aspiration probe
surgically inaccessible region of brain
surgically resected
Surgical Simplex P radiopaque bone
  cement
Surgidac braided polyester suture
Surgilase CO$_2$ laser
Surgilav machine
Surgilene suture
Surgilift transportation system
Surgilon suture

Surgitek prosthesis
Surgitome device
Surgi-Tron instruments
Surgivac drain
survey
    bone
    four-view wrist
    joint
    metastatic bone
    osseous
    Short Form 12 Health Survey
        (SF-12)
    Short Form 36 Health Survey
        (SF-36)
survey view images
survival, hyaline cartilage
survival roles of ICIDH (International
    Classification of Impairments,
    Disabilities, Handicaps)
suspended animation
suspension
    adjustable Thomas splint
    balanced
    finger-trap
    half ring Thomas splint
    overhead
    sling
    Thomas splint
suspensory ligament
suspensory muscle of duodenum
sustentaculum, talar
sustentation (postural) tremor
Sutherland-Greenfield double
    innominate osteotomy
Sutherland hip procedure
Sutherland tendon transfer
Sutter-CPM knee device
Sutter double-stem silicone implant
Sutter MCP joint prosthesis
Sutter silicone metacarpophalangeal
    joint arthroplasty
sutural bone
sutural diastasis
sutural ligament
suture (also called *stitch*)
    absorbable
    Acufex bioabsorbable Suretac

suture *(continued)*
    apical
    baseball
    basilar
    Becker
    Bell
    bioabsorbable
    BioSorb
    Biosyn synthetic monofilament
    biparietal
    Bondek absorbable
    braided
    bregmatomastoid
    bridging
    bridle
    bundle
    Bunnell crisscross
    Bunnell wire pullout
    buried
    buried interrupted
    buried-knot
    catgut
    cerclage
    chromic catgut
    chromic interrupted
    circular wire
    Closer
    clove-hitch
    coapting
    coated Vicryl Rapide
    compression stay
    continuous
    continuous running
    coronal
    cotton
    cranial
    crisscross
    cruciate four-strand
    Czerny
    Dacron
    Dafilon
    Dagrofil
    delayed closure of
    dentate
    Dermalon
    Dexon
    diastasis of

suture *(continued)*
  Donati
  double-armed (DAS)
  dural tack-up
  dural traction
  end-to-end
  Ethibond
  Ethiflex
  Ethilon
  ethmoidolacrimal
  ethmoidomaxillary
  Excel polyester
  figure of 8
  fish-mouth
  flat
  four-strand
  four-strand Savage
  frontal
  frontoethmoidal
  frontolacrimal
  frontomaxillary
  frontonasal
  frontoparietal
  frontosphenoid
  frontozygomatic
  funicular
  Gillies
  grasping loop
  Gruber
  guy
  Hawkeye
  heavy silk
  horizontal mattress
  interparietal
  interrupted
  intracuticular
  intradermal
  intraluminal occluding
  inverted
  jugal
  Kelly plication
  Kessler
  knotless anchor
  Krackow
  Krause
  lambdoid
  lambdoidal cranial

suture *(continued)*
  lashing
  Le Dentu
  leg of
  Lembert
  Linatrix
  locking loop
  longitudinal
  loop mattress
  magnetic controlled suturing
    (MCS)
  mamillary
  mattress
  Maxon
  McLaughlin modification of
    Bunnell pullout
  Mersilene
  metopic cranial
  Miralene
  Mitek
  Mitek Mini GII
  modified Kessler
  Monocryl
  monofilament
  monofilament nylon
  multiple-strand
  muscle-to-bone
  myodesis
  near-far
  nerve
  nonabsorbable
  nonfusion of cranial
  Nurolon
  nylon
  occipital
  occipitomastoid
  occipitoparietal
  occipitosphenoid
  overlapping
  Owen silk
  parietal
  parietomastoid
  parietooccipital
  PDS
  Perma-Hand braided silk
  petrobasilar
  petrosphenobasilar

suture *(continued)*
  petrospheno-occipital
  petrosquamous
  PGA synthetic absorbable
  plain catgut
  plain gut
  plastic
  plication
  Polydek
  polyester
  polyglacine
  polyglactin 910
  polyglyconate
  polypropylene
  Polysorb
  PRE 2
  prematurely closed
  primary
  Prolene
  Protector meniscus
  P-3
  pullout
  pullout wire
  Pulver-Taft fish-mouth
  pursestring
  radiopaque
  Rapide
  Reddick-Saye
  rhabdoid
  Robertson
  running
  running lock
  Safil
  sagittal cranial
  Savage
  secondary
  serrated
  silk
  Silkam
  simple
  six-strand
  skin
  Sofsilk nonabsorbable silk
  Softcat chromic
  Softcat plain
  sphenoethmoidal

suture *(continued)*
  spheno-occipital
  spheno-orbital
  sphenoparietal
  sphenopetrosal
  sphenosquamous
  sphenotemporal
  sphenovomerine
  splayed cranial
  spread
  squamosomastoid
  squamosoparietal
  squamososphenoid
  squamous
  stainless steel
  Statak
  Steelex
  Strickland
  subcutaneous
  subcuticular
  Supramid
  Suretac
  Surgidac braided polyester
  Surgilon
  swaged-on
  Synthofil
  tack
  temporal
  Tevdek
  three-strand
  Ticron
  traction
  transfixion
  transosseous
  transverse
  twisted
  two-strand
  Tycron
  undyed
  Vascufil
  Vicryl Rapide
  vertical mattress
  Vicryl
  wire
  wire pullout
suture abscess

suture anchor (see also *anchor*)
  Mitek
  Mitek GII
  Mitek Superanchor
  Panalok
  TAG
suture bridge fixation
suture button
suturectomy
suture device, Zimmer Statak
suture hook
suture isometry
suture joint
sutureless closure
suture line
suture passer
suture punch
Suture-Self dressing
SV-40 virus
Sven-Johansson driver
Sven-Johansson extractor
Sven-Johansson femoral neck nail
Sven-Johansson finisher
swaged-on needle with suture
swaged-on suture
swallow reflex
swallowing automatism
swallowing, chin tuck
swallowing dysfunction
swallowing mechanism, video
  fluoroscopy of
swallowing rehabilitation
swan neck
swan-neck deformity
Swann-Morton surgical blade
Swanson awl
Swanson classification
Swanson Convex condylar arthroplasty
Swanson elevator
Swanson finger joint
Swanson great toe prosthesis
Swanson interpositional wrist
  arthroplasty
Swanson intramedullary broach
Swanson lunate awl
Swanson mallet
Swanson metacarpal prosthesis

Swanson metacarpophalangeal implant
Swanson metatarsal prosthesis
Swanson metatarsophalangeal joint
  arthroplasty
Swanson osteotome
Swanson osteotomy
Swanson PIP joint arthroplasty
Swanson prosthesis
Swanson reamer
Swanson scaphoid awl
Swanson Silastic prosthesis
Swanson T-shaped great toe Silastic
  prosthesis
Swanson wrist implant
Swanson wrist prosthesis
swathe *or* swath
swathe, sling and (bandage)
SWD (short wave diathermy)
sweat test for thoracic outlet syndrome
sweating of face, thermoregulatory
Swede-O Ankle Lok brace
Swede-O brace
Swede-O-Universal braces
Swedish knee cage orthosis
sweeny (shoulder slip)
Sweet pituitary scissors
Sweet sternal punch
Sweet two-point discriminator
swelling
  blennorrhagic
  boggy
  brain
  fusiform
  joint
  postfracture
  posttraumatic
  soft tissue
SwimEx aquatic therapy
swimmer's ear
swimmer's shoulder
swimmer's view on x-ray examination
SwingAlong walker caddie
swing phase control
swing phase periods of gait
  initial swing
  midswing
  terminal swing

swinging flashlight test
swings, mood
swing-through of extremity
Swiss ball therapy
Swiss cancellous screw
Swiss cheese appearance
Swiss pattern osteotome
switch stick
swivel dislocation
Swivel-Strap brace
SWJ (square wave jerks)
swollen, markedly
SXA (single energy x-ray)
    absorptiometer
SXCT (spiral x-ray computed
    tomography)
Sydenham chorea
Sygen (GM-1 ganglioside)
sylvian aqueduct syndrome
sylvian arachnoid cyst
sylvian candelabra
sylvian fissure
sylvian operculum
sylvian/rolandic junction
sylvian system
Sylvius
    aqueduct of
    cistern of fossa of
    fossa of
symbrachydactyly
Syme amputation, Wagner modification
Syme ankle disarticulation amputation
symmetrical diffuse neuropathy
symmetry of limb movements in
    infants
Symonds headache
sympathectomy
    cervical
    chemical
sympathetic chain
sympathetic denervation
sympathetic ganglia
sympathetic innervation
sympathetic nerve
sympathetic nervous system
sympatheticoblastoma
sympathetic overactivity

sympathetic reflex dystrophy
sympathetic vascular instability
sympathoadrenal response
sympathoadrenal system
symphalangia
symphalangism, multiple
symphysis, pubic
symphysis pubis
symptom (pl. symptoms)
    affective (of seizures)
    auditory
    brain stem
    Buerger
    chronic joint
    conversion
    extrapyramidal
    functionally debilitating
    gustatory
    insidious onset of
    Kanavel four cardinal
    localizing neurologic
    migrainous
    motor
    myasthenic
    neurologic
    olfactory
    parkinsonian
    premonitory
    prodromal
    pseudomyasthenic
    psychomotor
    psychosensory
    radicular
    segmental
    sensory
    supratentorial
    theater
    upper motor neuron
    visual
symptomatic bipartite sesamoids
symptomatic epilepsy
symptomatic metastatic spinal cord
    compression
symptomatology
symptom complex
Symptoms and Sports Participation
    Rating Scale

synapse
  abnormal axodendritic
  axodendritic
  excitatory
synaptic cleft
synaptic dopamine concentration
synaptic pathways
synaptogenesis
synarthrodial joint
synarthrosis
synathresis
Synatomic knee prosthesis
synchondrodial joint
synchondrosis petro-occipitalis
synchondrotomy
Synchromed programmable drug
  pump
synchronous lesions
synchronous nerve impulse
synchronous wave
synchrony
  bilateral EEG
  interhemispheric
  secondary bilateral
syncopal episode
syncope
  cough
  defecation
  hyperventilation
  micturition
  migrainous
  neck extension precipitating
  orthostatic
  sneeze
  tussive
  vasodepressor
  vasovagal
syndactylization of digits
syndactyly
  complex complete
  cutaneous
  soft tissue
syndesmectomy
syndesmodial joint
syndesmopexy
syndesmophytes, bridging
syndesmoplasty

syndesmorrhaphy
syndesmosis
  disrupted
  tibiofibular
syndesmosis sprain of ankle
syndesmotic clear space
syndesmotic diastasis
syndesmotic disruption
syndesmotic injury
syndesmotic ligament complex
syndesmotic screw
syndesmotomy
syndrome (see also *disease*)
  acrocallosal
  acute cerebellar
  acute organic brain
  Adie
  adrenogenital
  adult Reye
  AECS (acute exertional compart-
    ment)
  antiphospholipid antibody (APS)
  Aicardi
  akinetic rigid
  Albright-McCune-Sternberg
  alcohol withdrawal
  Alpers
  ALS-like (amyotrophic lateral
    sclerosis)
  amnesic
  amnestic confabulatory
  amotivational
  amyostatic
  angular gyrus
  anterior cerebellar artery
  anterior cervical cord
  anterior compartment
  anterior cord
  anterior impingement
  anterior spinal artery
  anterior tibial
  anterior tibial compartment
  Anton
  apallic
  Apert
  Arnold-Chiari
  Avellis

syndrome *(continued)*
    axonopathic neurogenic thoracic
      outlet
    Baastrupi
    Babinski-Fröhlich
    Babinski-Nageotte
    Balint
    Baltic myoclonus
    Barré-Lieou
    basilar
    Bassen-Kornzweig
    Basser
    beat-knee
    Behr
    Benedikt
    benign hypermobile joint
    benign pain
    Bernard-Horner
    bicipital
    Bing-Horton
    black heel
    Block-Sulzberger
    Bloom
    blue toe
    body cast
    brain death
    brain stem
    Brissaud
    broad thumb big toe
    Broca
    Brown-Séquard
    burning-feet
    carpal tunnel (CTS)
    carpal tunnel wrist
    Carpenter
    cast
    cauda equina (CES)
    cauda equina compression
    caudal regression
    cavernous sinus
    CECS (chronic exertional compart-
      ment)
    central cervical cord
    central cord
    central diencephalic herniation
    central pain (CPS)
    cerebellar cognitive affective

syndrome *(continued)*
    cerebellar hemorrhage
    cerebral steal
    cerebrohepatorenal
    cervical acceleration/deceleration
      (whiplash)
    cervical dorsal outlet
    Céstan-Chenais
    Charcot-Marie-Tooth
    Charles Bonnet
    Chauffard-Still (polyarthritis)
    Chédiak-Higashi
    cherry red spot myoclonus
    Chiari-Foix-Nicolesco
    choreic
    chronic brain (CBS)
    chronic fatigue
    chronic musculoskeletal pain
      (CMPS)
    chronic pain
    Claude
    clenched fist
    clumsy hand
    Cobb
    Cockayne
    Coffin-Lowry syndrome
    Cogan
    Collet-Sicard
    compartment
    complex regional pain (CRPS)
    compression
    constriction band
    conus medullaris
    cord traction
    Cornelia de Lange
    Costen
    costoclavicular
    Cotton-Berg syndrome
    cramp
    cranial nerve vascular compression
    craniofacial
    Creutzfeldt-Jakob
    Crouzon
    crush
    crying face
    cubital tunnel
    Cushing

syndrome *(continued)*

cyclops
dancing eyes, dancing feet
Dandy-Walker
dead-arm
de-efferented
dehiscence disinsertion
Dejerine anterior bulbar
Dejerine-Roussy
Dejerine-Sottas
de Lange
Denny-Brown (Denis-Brown)
depigmentation of iris with neonatal
   Horner
dialysis
dialysis encephalopathy
diffuse idiopathic skeletal
   hyperostosis (DISH)
DiGeorge
disconnection
disinhibitions of frontal lobe
dorsal midbrain
double-crush
Down
droopy shoulder (thoracic outlet)
drug withdrawal
Duane retraction
Dudley Morton
Dyke-Davidoff-Masson
dysarthria clumsy hand
dysequilibrium
dyssynergia cerebellaris myoclonia
Eaton-Lambert
Edwards
Ehlers-Danlos
Ekbom restless leg
empty sella
entrapment
eosinophilia myalgia (EMS)
epileptic
exertional compartment
extensor indicis proprius
extrapyramidal
facet
facio-auriculo-vertebral (FAV)
failed back (FBS)
failed back surgery (FBSS)

syndrome *(continued)*

familial articular hypermobility
Fanconi
Farber
fat embolism
fat toe
Fazio-Londe
Felty
femur-fibula-ulna
fetal alcohol (FAS)
fibromyalgia
filum terminale
Fisher
flat back
flexor hallucis longus entrapment
flexor origin
floppy baby
floppy infant
Foix
foramen
foraminal
forearm compartment
Foster-Kennedy
Foville
fragile
Froin
frontal lobe
frozen shoulder
Funston
Funston congenital cervical rib
GALOP (gait disorder, autoanti-
   body, late-age, onset, polyneu-
   ropathy)
Ganser approximate answers
Garcin
Gastaut HEE (hemiconvulsion,
   hemiplegia, and epilepsy)
Gerstmann-Straussler
Gilles de la Tourette
Gillespie
Goldenhar
gourmand
Gradenigo
Greig cephalopolysyndactyly
Grisel
Guillain-Barré (GBS)
Guillain-Barré-Strohl

syndrome *(continued)*
- Guillain-Garcin
- Gulf War Veteran
- Haglund
- half base
- Hallermann-Streiff-François
- hammer digit
- hand-foot
- hand-foot-uterus
- headache
- heel pain
- heel spur
- Heerfort
- hemibasal
- hemichorea hemiballism
- hemicord
- hemisensory
- hemispheric
- hereditary sensory neuropathy
- HHE (hemiconvulsions, hemiplegia, and epilepsy)
- Hoffmann
- Holt-Oram
- Horner
- Hunter
- Hurler
- hyperactive
- hyperactive dysfunction
- hypermobile joint
- iatrogenic Cushing
- ilioinguinal
- iliotibial band friction
- impingement
- infantile polymyoclonus
- infectious polyneuritis
- infrapatellar contracture (IPSC)
- inguinal ligament
- INO (internuclear ophthalmoplegia)
- insular opercular
- interosseous nerve
- inverse Marcus Gunn
- Isaacs
- ischemic
- isolation
- Ito hypomelanosis
- Jackson
- Jaccoud (arthritis)

syndrome *(continued)*
- Jackson-Weiss
- Jacod (neuralgia) *(not* Jacob)
- Jansky-Bielschowsky
- Jarcho-Levin
- joint hypermobility
- jugular foramen
- Kearns-Sayre (KSS)
- Kernohan notch
- Kiloh-Nevin
- Kinsbourne
- Kleffner-Landau
- Kleine-Levin
- Klinefelter
- Klippel-Feil
- Klippel-Trenaunay-Weber
- Klüver-Bucy ablation
- Kocher-Debré-Sémélaigne
- Koerber-Salus-Elschnig
- Korsakoff
- Kretschmer
- Kugelberg-Welander
- lacunar
- Lambert-Eaton myasthenic (LEMS)
- Lance-Adams
- Landau-Kleffner
- Landry-Guillain-Barré-Strohl
- Langer-Giedion
- Larson
- lateral medullary
- lateral pontomedullary
- Laurence-Moon-Biedl
- leg-foot-toe
- Leigh
- Lennox
- Lennox-Gastaut
- leprechaun
- Leriche
- Lesch-Nyhan
- Li-Fraumeni (LFS)
- limited joint motion
- locked-in
- Louis-Bar (ataxia-telangiectasia)
- Lowe
- lower basilar branch
- lumbar facet arthrosis
- Maffucci

syndrome *(continued)*
 malalignment
 malignant neuroleptic
 Marchand-Waterhouse
 Marchiafava-Bignami
 Marfan
 Marinesco-Sjögren
 Maroteaux-Lamy
 May-White
 McArdle
 McCune-Albright
 medial longitudinal fasciculus
 medial plantar digital proper nerve
 medial tibial stress (MTSS)
 median nerve entrapment
 medicamentosus Cushing
 medulla oblongata
 Meige
 Melkersson-Rosenthal
 Menkes kinky hair
 metatarsal overload
 Ménière
 midbrain displacement
 middle cerebral artery
 migrainous
 Milch fracture classification
 milk-alkali
 Milkman
 Millard-Gubler
 Miller-Fisher variant of Guillain-
  Barré
 MLF (medial longitudinal
  fasciculus)
 Möbius (Moebius)
 Morel
 Morquio
 Morton
 Morvan
 Mouchet
 myasthenic
 myofascial pain (MPS)
 myotonic
 Naffziger
 nail patella
 narcolepsy cataplexy
 naviculocapitate fracture

syndrome *(continued)*
 neglect
 Nelson
 neonatal neurological
 nerve compression
 nerve entrapment
 nerve root
 neurobehavioral
 neurocutaneous
 neuroleptic malignant
 neurologic paraneoplastic
 neuropsychiatric
 Niemann-Pick
 Nievergelt
 Nothnagel
 oculocerebrorenal
 oculosubcutaneous (of Yuge)
 one-and-a-half
 opsoclonus-myoclonus
 orbitofrontal
 organic brain
 organic brain, with psychosis
 organic delusional
 organic mental
 os trigonum
 otopalatodigital
 overuse
 pain
 pain amplification
 painful heel
 painful arc
 Palister-Hall
 pallidal
 Pancoast
 paraneoplastic
 paratrigeminal, of Raeder
 parenchymal brain stem
 parietal lobe
 Parinaud
 Parsonage-Turner
 patellar malalignment
 patellofemoral pain
 pectoralis minor
 periodic movements of the legs
  (PMS)
 peroneal palsy footdrop

syndrome *(continued)*
Pfeiffer
PICA (posterior inferior cerebellar artery)
pickwickian
Pillay
PION (posterior interosseous nerve)
piriformis
PLED (periodic lateralized epileptiform discharge)
Poland
pontotegmental
postcasting
postconcussion
posterior cord
posterior fossa brain stem compression
posterior inferior cerebellar artery (PICA)
posterior interosseous nerve
posterior joint
posterior midbrain compression
posterior spinal artery
postfracture
posthemiparesis
postlaminectomy
postpolio
post-traumatic cerebral
post-traumatic pain
Pourfour du Petit
Prader-Willi
primary fibromyalgia (PFS)
pronator teres
Proteus
pseudocholinesterase
pseudo-Foster-Kennedy
pseudoneurasthenic
pseudophlebitis
punch-drunk (of boxers)
Putnam-Dana
rabbit
radial tunnel
radicular
Raeder paratrigeminal
Ramsay Hunt
Rasmussen

syndrome *(continued)*
ratchet
Raymond
Raymond-Céstan
recalcitrance of
red nucleus
reflex sympathetic dystrophy (RSDS)
Refsum
Reiter
restless legs (RLS)
reverse urea
reversible organic brain
Reye
Riley-Day
rolandic vein
Romberg
root compression
rotator cuff impingement
Roussy-Dejerine thalamic pain
Roussy-Lévy
Rubinstein-Taybi
Rud
sacroiliac
sacroiliac joint
Saethre-Chotzen
Sanfilippo
scalenus anterior
scalenus anticus
scaphoid impaction
scapulocostal
Scheie
Schmidt
Schwartz-Jampel (SJS)
SCIWORA (spinal cord injury without radiologic abnormality)
Seckel
second impact
sensorimotor
SHAFT (sad, hostile, anxious, frustrating, tenacious)
shaken baby
shoulder-hand
shoulder-hand-finger
shoulder-upper extremity-thoracic outlet
Shy-Drager
Siebenmann

syndrome *(continued)*
  silicone-related
  Silver
  Sinding-Larsen-Johansson
  sinus tarsi
  Sjögren-Larsson
  sleep apnea
  Sluder sphenopalatine
  small patella
  Smith-Lemli-Opitz
  snapping scapula
  spasmus nutans
  spectacular shrinking deficit
  sphenoidal fissure
  sphenopalatine, of Sluder
  spinal cord injury without
    radiologic abnormality
    (SCIWORA)
  spinal stenosis
  squat jump
  steal (Robin Hood phenomenon)
  Steele-Richardson
  Steele-Richardson-Olszewski
  Stewart-Morel
  Stickler
  stiff man
  stiff person
  Still-Chauffard (polyarthritis)
  stroke
  Sturge-Weber
  subclavian steal (SSS)
  superior mesenteric artery
  supinator canal
  sweat test for thoracic outlet
  sylvian aqueduct
  syringomyelic
  Takatsuki
  talar compression
  Tapia
  TAR (thrombocytopenia-absent
    radius)
  tardive Tourette
  tarsal tunnel (TTS)
  temporomandibular pain and
    dysfunction (TMPDS)
  tensor fasciae latae
  Terson

syndrome *(continued)*
  tethered cord (TCS)
  tethered spinal cord
  T4
  thalamic pain
  thenar hammer
  thoracic inlet (Pancoast)
  thoracic outlet
  Tietze
  tired neck
  Tolosa-Hunt
  top of the basilar
  total cortical blindness
  Tourette
  transient bone marrow edema
  Treacher Collins
  triquetrohamate impaction
  Troyer
  Turcot
  Turner
  Uhthoff
  ulnar abutment
  ulnar impaction
  ulnar nerve entrapment
  ulnar styloid impaction
  ulnar tunnel
  ulnocarpal impaction
  unbalanced wrist
  uncal herniation
  Unverricht
  Unverricht-Lundborg
  useless hand
  uveomeningoencephalic
  VBA (vertebrobasilar artery)
  Vernet
  vertebral steal
  Villaret-Mackenzie
  Vogt-Koyanagi-Harada
  von Hippel-Lindau (VHL)
  von Recklinghausen
  Wallenberg lateral medullary
  Weber
  Werdnig-Hoffmann
  Wernicke-Korsakoff
  West
  Weyers
  whiplash

syndrome *(continued)*
    windblown hand
    withdrawal
    Wolfart-Kugelberg-Welander
    Wolf-Hirschhorn
    XXX
    XXY
    XYY
    Zellweger
syndrome of approximate answers
syndrome of Harada
syndrome of inappropriate antidiuretic
    hormone (SIADH) excretion
syndrome of sensory dissociation
syndrome of the great radicular artery
    of Adamkiewicz
syndrome of the jugular foramen
syndromic craniosynostosis
Synercid (quinupristin/dalfopristin)
synergic muscles
synergistic contraction
synergistic muscles
synergistic wrist motion splint
Synergy flexible splinting material
Synergy joint rehabilitation
Synergy posterior titanium spinal
    system
Synergy spine rehabilitation system
Synergy ultrasound system
synesthesia
synkinesis (pl. synkineses)
synkinetic arm swing
SynMesh titanium mesh
synostosis
    cervical
    congenital radioulnar
    coronal
    lambdoid
    multiple suture
    nonsyndromic bicoronal
    nonsyndromic unicoronal
    premature suture
    radiographically firm
    radioulnar
    sagittal
    single suture

synostosis *(continued)*
    terminal
    tibiofibular
Synovator curved arthroscopic blade
synovectomy
    Albright
    arthroscopic
    chemical
    open knee
    partial
    total
    wide
synovectomy blade
synovia (see *synovium*)
synovial cavity
synovial chondromatosis
synovial crystals
synovial fluid
synovial fringe
synovial frond
synovial frost
synovial hyaluronidase
synovial inflammatory reaction
synovial joint
synovial ligament
synovial lining cells
synovial plica
synovial proliferation
synovial sarcoma
synovial surface
synovial thickening
synoviochondromatosis
synoviocyte
synoviogram
synovioma
synovitis
    boggy
    carpometacarpal
    disseminated-type pigmented
       villonodular
    florid
    gonorrheal
    hypertrophic
    intra-articular pigmented villonodular
       (IPVS)
    parapatellar

synovitis *(continued)*
  pigmented villonodular (PVS)
  proliferative
  rheumatoid arthritis
  silicone
  toxic
  villonodular
  villous
synovium (pl. synovia)
  boggy
  exuberant
  hyperplastic
  opaque
syntactical disorder
Synthes cervical plate
Synthes compression hip screw
Synthes dorsal distal radius plate
Synthes drill
Synthes fixation system
Synthes Microsystem cranial fixation
  plate
Synthes Microsystem drill bit
Synthes Microsystem microplate
Synthes Microsystem plate cutters
Synthes Microsystem plate-holding
  forceps
Synthes Microsystem pliers
Synthes minifragment countersink
Synthes mini L-plate
Synthes modular spine instruments
Synthes I plate
Synthes rod
Synthes Schuhli implant system
Synthes screw
Synthes wire guide
synthetic corticotropin-releasing factor
  (Xerecept)
synthetic graft bypass to ankle
synthetic polymer, biodegradable
synthetic prosthesis
Synthofil suture
Synvisc injection
syphilis
  cerebrospinal
  meningovascular
  parenchymatous
  tertiary

syphilitic amyotrophy
syphilitic meningoencephalitis
syphilitis endarteritis, Heubner
Syracuse I plate
syringe
  bulb
  cement
syringe Avitene
syringe irrigation with deionized
  sterile water
syringobulbia
syringocele *or* syringocoele
syringoencephalia
syringoencephalomyelia
syringomeningocele
syringomyelia
  acquired (post-traumatic)
  congenital
  post-traumatic
  segmental distribution of
  traumatic
syringomyelic cavity
syringomyelic syndrome
syringomyelocele
syringomyelus
syringopontia
syrinx cavity
syrinx, traumatic
Sysorb screw
system (see also *device*)
  AccuLength arthroplasty measuring
  AccuSway balance measurement
  AcroMed VSP fixation
  Acryl-X orthopedic cement
    removal
  Activa tremor control therapy
  Acustar surgical navigation
  AddOn-Bucky digital imaging
  Advantage electromyography
  AERx pain management
  Aesculap ABC cervical plating
  Airis II open MRI
  Albert Grass Heritage digital EEG
  AlgoMed infusion
  Alice 4 diagnostic sleep
  Alphatec mini lag-screw (MLS)

system *(continued)*
    American shoulder and elbow
        (ASES)
    AMK (Anatomic Modular Knee)
        total knee
    Amset R-F fixation
    Anametric knee
    Andersson hip status
    anterior dynamized (ADS)
    anterior locking plate (ALPS)
    AOFAS hindfoot scoring
    Apollo DXA bone densitometry
    Apollo knee and hip prosthesis
    APR total hip
    APR II hip
    Ariel computerized exercise
    ArthroCare arthroscopic
    Arthro-Flo arthroscopic irrigation
    Arthro-Lok
    ArthroProbe laser
    ascending activating
    ascending reticular activating
    Ashhurst fracture classification
    ASIF
    Astro-Med Albert Grass Heritage
        digital EEG
    AuRA cemented total hip
    autonomic nervous
    AutoSuture vascular clip-applier
    autotransfusion
    axial spinal
    BacFix
    Bad Wildungen Metz (BWM) spine
    BAK/C (cervical) interbody fusion
    BAK interbody fusion
    BAK/T (thoracic) interbody fusion
    Barouk-Microscrew
    Bassett electrical stimulation
    Betaseron needle-free delivery
    Biad SPECT imaging
    Biofix
    Bionicare 1000
    BioSorbFX SR self-reinforced plate
        and screw
    BIOWARE software for Biodex
        isokinetic exercise
    Boston Classification

system *(continued)*
    Boston Children's Hospital grading
    Bowden cable suspension
    Brackmann II EMG
    Braille TeleCaption
    Bridge hip
    Brighton electrical stimulation
    Browlift Bone Bridge
    Budde halo retractor
    BWM (Bad Wildungen Metz) spine
    Cable-Ready cable grip
    cable suspension
    cannulated guided hip screw
    Cannulated Plus screw
    CarboJet lavage
    Caspari suture punch
    C-D (Cotrel-Dubousset) fixation
    Ceegraph 128 EEG
    Cemex
    central nervous (CNS)
    Charnley Howorth Exflow
    Charnley total hip
    Chattanooga Balance
    Cincinnati rating
    Closer suture-based
    Command joint replacement
        instrument
    Compass stereotactic frame
    Compumedics sleep
    Concise compression hip screw
    Cordis MPAP
    Corin hip arthroplasty
    Cotrel-Dubousset (C-D) spinal
        instrumentation
    Cotrel-Dubousset (C-D) universal
        instrumentation
    Counter Rotation (CRS)
    CPT hip
    craniosacral
    cruciate condylar knee
    CRW stereotactic
    CTDx electrostimulation
    CT-MRI-compatible stereotactic
        headframe
    Cybex I (or II+) exercise
    Cybex 340 isokinetic rehabilitation
        and testing

system *(continued)*
  Dallas grading
  Dall-Miles cable grip
  D'Aubigné hip status
  Deknatel orthopedic autotransfusion
  DePuy total hip, with porous
    coating
  diffuse thalamic projection
  dopaminergic
  double inflow cannula
  Dualer Plus
  dual-lock total hip replacement
  Duo-Lock
  DUPEL iontophoretic drug delivery
  DuPont Rare Earth Imaging
  Duracon total knee
  Dwyer-Wickham electrical
    stimulation
  Dyna-Lok spinal instrumentation
  dynamic locking (partial locking)
    nail
  Dynasplint shoulder
  Dyonics shaving
  EBI bone-healing
  EchoEye 3-D ultrasound imaging
  ECT internal fracture fixation
  Ectra endoscopic release
  Edwards fixation
  Electri-Cool cold therapy
  Emed-F foot-force measurement
  Endotrac carpal tunnel release
  Enview camera
  Equinox EEG neuromonitoring
  estimated 10-20
  Evans fracture classification
  Evolution total hip
  Ewald elbow arthroplasty rating
  Exact-Fit ATH hip replacement
  EX-FI-RE external fixation
  Extend total hip
  external jugular
  extracranial carotid
  extrapyramidal
  E-Z Flap neurosurgery mini-plate
  FASTak suture anchor
  F.A.S.T. 1 intraosseous infusion
  Fenlin total shoulder

system *(continued)*
  Ficat-Marcus grading
  Fitnet joint testing
  Fixateur Interne fixation
  fixation
  FluoroScan mini C-arm imaging
  Forte distal radius plate
  Foundation total hip and knee
  Fowler knee
  frameless stereotaxic
  Freehand prosthesis
  Freehand surgically implanted
    neuroprosthetic
  Freeman-Swanson knee
  Fuji FCR9000 computed radiology
    (CR)
  Fukushima retraction
  gamma efferent
  gamma loop nervous
  Gem total knee
  Genesis total knee
  Genucom ACL laxity analysis
  Geomedic
  Global total shoulder arthroplasty
  Golgi
  GoodKnight 318 sleep monitoring
  gray matter of central nervous
  GTS great toe two-piece implant
  Haid UBP (universal bone plate)
  Halifax interlaminar clamp
  Harris hip status
  haversian
  Hemi-Knee
  Herbert bone screw
  Herbert-Fisher fracture classification
  Hexcel total condylar knee
  Hoek-Bowen cement removal
  host immune
  Hot/Ice System III
  Howmedica knee
  Howmedica VSF fixation
  Hunt-Hess aneurysm grading
  HydroFlex arthroscopy irrigating
  Ilizarov
  image analysis
  In-Fast bone screw
  Infinity hip replacement

system *(continued)*
  Infuse-A-Port drug delivery
  Inglis-Pellicci elbow arthroplasty
  Insall-Burstein
  Insall/Burstein II modular total
    knee replacement
  InstaTrak 3000
  In-Tac bone-anchoring
  Interax total knee
  internal carotid
  International 10-20 electrode
    placement
  Intrel II spinal cord stimulation
  iontophoretic drug delivery
  Iowa hip status
  Isocam SPECT imaging
  Isola fixation
  Isola spinal instrumentation
  Judet hip status
  kallikrein-kinin (KK)
  Kambin and Gellman lumbar
    diskectomy instrumentation
  Kaneda Anterior Scoliosis System
    (KASS)
  Kaneda anterior spine stabilizing
  Kelly-Goerss Compass stereotactic
  Kendall A-V Impulse
  Kin-Com isokinetic exercise
  Kirschner Medical Dimension hip
    replacement
  Knee Signature (KSS)
  Kyle fracture classification
  Laitinen CT guidance
  laminar air flow
  Larson hip status
  LCR (ligamentous and capsular
    repair)
  Leibinger miniplate
  Leibinger Profyle
  Leksell microstereotactic
  Leksell stereotaxic
  Lido Active Multijoint
  Lidoback isokinetic dynamometry
  Lido Passive Multijoint
  Life-Port drug delivery
  ligamentous and capsular repair
    (LCR)

system *(continued)*
  limbic
  Linear total hip and hip stem
  Link Lubinus SP II hip replace-
    ment
  Luque II fixation
  Magna-Fx cannulated screw
    fixation
  Magnes 2500WH
  Malcolm-Lynn radiolucent spinal
    retraction
  MARS (Modular Acetabular
    Revision System)
  Mason fracture classification
  Masterstim chiropractic therapy
  Masterstim Micro therapy
  Max FiberScan laser
  Maxilift Combi patient-lifting
  Mayfield/ACCISS stereotactic
    workstation
  Mazur ankle evaluation or rating
  Mazur arthrodesis grading
  MCAT (modular coded aperture
    technology) collimator
  MED (microendoscopic diskec-
    tomy)
  Mednext bone-dissecting
  Medtronic Activa tremor control
    therapy implant
  Meniscus Mender II
  MG II total hip and knee
  Micro-Aire pulse lavage
  Miller Galante I condylar total
    knee
  Mini-Acutrak small bone fixation
  Miniport drug delivery
  Mitek anchor
  MKM AutoPilot stereotactic
  modified 10-20
  Modulock posterior spinal instru-
    mentation
  Monticelli-Spinelli
  Morrey arthritis grading
  Morrey elbow arthroplasty rating
  MosaicPlasty
  Moss fixation

system *(continued)*

Moss Miami load-sharing spinal
    implant
motion capture
MPAP (multipurpose access port)
Multi Podus boot
Multitak suture
Natural-Hip
Natural-Knee
Natural-Knee II
Navigator virtual endoscopic
    visualization
NC-stat nerve conduction
Neck-Trac passive motion
NECKSYS home neck care
Neer fracture classification
NeuroCybernetic Prosthesis (NCP)
NeuroLink II EEG data acquisition
NeuroMap
neuronavigational
NeuroPlan
NeuroPro rigid fixation
NeuroSector ultrasound
Neurotrend
N fiducial localization stereotactic
NightOwl pocket polygraph
nigrostriatal
NK hand evaluation
nociceptive afferent
Nomos pin-free attachment
    stereotactic
Norian SRS (skeletal repair system)
Novus LC threaded interbody
    fusion cage
Nucleotome
OATS (Osteochondral Autograft
    Transfer System)
Olerud PSF fixation
Omega compression hip screw
Omnifit Plus hip
Operating Arm
Opmilas 144 Plus laser
Optical Tracking System neuro-
    surgery
Option hip
optoelectronic
Orth-evac autotransfusion

system *(continued)*

Orthodoc presurgical planning
Ortho Dx electrotherapy
Ortholoc Advantim knee revision
OrthoPAT perioperative autotrans-
    fusion
OSCAR ultrasonic bone cement
    removal
osteochondral autograft transfer
    (OATS)
Osteo-Clage cable
Osteonics Scorpio posterior
    cruciate-retaining total knee
OsteoView 2000 digital imaging
Paramax
parasympathetic nervous
Paris ultrasound
Patil stereotaxic
PCA primary total knee
PCA universal total knee
    instrument
PCReflex infrared tracking
PEAK anterior compression plate
PEAK channeled plate
Pelorus stereotactic
PercScope percutaneous diskectomy
PFC total hip
Phoresor II iontophoretic drug
    delivery
Picket Fence fiducial localization
    stereotactic
picture archive and communication
    (PACs)
Pinn.ACL guide
Pisces spinal cord stimulation
Polarus Plus humeral fixation
Polycentric and Wide-Track knee
Polysit drug delivery
POSICAM PET
Postel hip status
posterior cruciate condylar knee
Protector meniscus suturing
Pro-Trac cruciate reconstruction
Pro-Trac knee surgery
Pulsavac III wound debridement
Pulse lavage
PWB fixation

system *(continued)*
- Quartet sleep apnea
- RadioLucent wrist fixation
- radiowave tracking
- Rancho fixation
- Repose surgical
- Restore ACL guide
- reticular activating (RAS)
- Revelation hip system
- Richards modular hip (RMHS)
- RM (Reichert/Mundinger) stereotaxic
- Robotrac passive retraction
- Rochester compression
- Rogozinski spinal fixation
- Romano surgical curved drilling
- Rowe-Lowell fracture-dislocation classification
- Russell-Taylor interlocking medullary nail
- Sabolich socket
- SAFHS (sonic accelerated fracture healing system) 2000
- Savastano Hemi-Knee
- Scaphoid-Microstaple
- Schatzker fracture classification
- Schuhli implant
- Scorpio total knee
- SEG-CES (segmented cement extraction system)
- segmented orthopaedic (SOS)
- Selby I or II fixation
- sensorimotor
- SergiScope
- SFS (small fragment system)
- shaving
- SIBS (surgical isolation bubble system)
- Signa Special Procedures (SP)
- Silhouette therapeutic massage
- Simal cervical stabilization
- Simmons fixation
- Simpulse lavage
- SITEtrac spinal surgery
- Sleepscan Traveler ambulatory polysomnography

system *(continued)*
- slit-catheter
- skeletal repair bone paste
- Smith & Nephew
- Solcotrans closed vacuum drainage
- Solcotrans Plus autotransfusion
- Songer cable
- sonic accelerated fracture-healing (SAFHS) 2000
- Sony digital still-image capture
- SOS (segmented orthopaedic system)
- Spectrum tissue repair
- Spherocentric knee
- spindle
- S-ROM total hip modular
- Stability total hip
- Stableloc external wrist fixation
- Stableloc II external fixator
- Stage-1 single stage dental implant
- static locking (complete locking) nail
- StealthStation neuronavigation
- STERRAD 50 Sterilization
- Steward-Milford fracture classification
- Strata hip
- Stratis II MRI
- suction via trap bottle
- suction-irrigation
- Sunderland five-degree
- SureTrans autotransfusion orthopedic
- surgical isolation bubble (SIBS)
- sylvian
- sympathetic nervous
- Synergy posterior titanium spinal
- Synthes fixation
- Synthes Schuhli implant
- Tarlov neurologic function grading
- TCPM pneumatic tourniquet
- 10-20
- Tetrax interactive balance
- Texas Scottish Rite Hospital (TSRH) instrumentation
- Thera-Band Resistive Therapy

system *(continued)*
 Thera-Ciser Light Exercise
 THORP (titanium hollow screw
  osseointegrating reconstruction
  plate)
 Ti-Fit modular hip
 titanium mesh bone plate and screw
 top-loading screw and rod
 Torus external fixation
 Total Condylar Knee
 Total Gym rehabilitation
 Townley anatomic knee
 TransFix ACL
 Trans Q 1 iontophoretic drug
  delivery
 transverse tripolar
 Trilogy acetabular
 Trio arthroscope
 True/Fit femoral intramedullary
  rod
 True/Flex intramedullary rod
 True/Lok external fixator
 Trunkey fracture classification
 TSRH fixation
 TSRH universal instrumentation
 Tylok high tension cerclage cabling
 UBP (universal bone plate)
 Ulson fixator
 Ultimax distal femoral intra-
  medullary rod
 Ultra-Drive bone cement removal
 Ultra-X external fixation
 unicompartmental knee
 Unicondylar Geomedic
 Unidose drug delivery
 Unilink
 Vapr
 variable axis knee
 Varigrip spine fixation

system *(continued)*
 ventricular
 Versa-Fx femoral hip fixation
 Versalok low back fixation
 Versatrac lumbar retractor
 Vertetrac ambulatory traction
 VICON three-dimensional gait
  analysis
 Viewing Wand imaging
 Vocare neuroprosthetic bladder
 VSF fixation
 VSP fixation
 WalkAide
 WarmTouch patient warming
 Washerloc
 Wiltse fixation
 Wisconsin compression
 Wisconsin spinal fracture
 Wurzburg plating
 Xact ACL graft fixation
 XPlan radiation treatment planning
 Zest Anchor Advanced Generation
  (ZAAG) bone anchoring
 Zeus microsurgery computer and
  voice-controlled robotic
 Zickel fracture classification
 Zimmer anatomic hip
 Zimmer CPT (collarless polished
  taper) hip
 ZMS intramedullary fixation
 Zone Specific II meniscal repair
 ZPLATE-ATL anterior spinal
  fixation
systemic lupus erythematosus (SLE)
systemic mastocytosis
systemic onset
System•S soft skeletal implant
systolic pressure wave
Syto 13 stain

T, t

T (temporal)
T (tesla)
T (thoracic)
TAANOS (The American Academy
  of Neurological and Orthopaedic
  Surgeons)
tabes, burned-out
tabetic arthropathy
tabetic crisis
tabetic neurosyphilis
table
  activator
  Adapta physical therapy
  adjusting
  Allen arm/hand surgery
  AlphaStar
  AM-MI orthopedic
  Andrews SST-3000 spinal surgery
  Back Specialist chiropractic
  Chick CLT operating
  Chick fracture
  Chiro-Manis chiropractic
  DC-101 chiropractic
  EZ-Up inversion
  flexion-distraction chiropractic
  fracture
  Gemini chiropractic
  hand surgery

table *(continued)*
  inner skull
  inner iliac crest
  intersegmental traction chiropractic
  Leander chiropractic
  Leander motorized flexion
  Leander 790 Series distraction
  Lloyd chiropractic
  long-axis traction chiropractic
  Mayfield-Larsen
  N-K 330 BRQ exercise
  OrthoVision orthopedic
  passive traction
  pediatric spica
  physical therapy
  radiolucent hand
  Re-Lax-O chiropractic
  resistive exercise
  Skytron operating room
  Stryker
  Sugita
  tilt
  Zenith chiropractic
table saw injury
taboparesis
Tab-Strap knee immobilizer
Tachdhian orthosis
Tacit threaded anchor

tack, Bankart
TACK (Translating and Congruent [Mobile-Bearing] Knee) implant
tackler's arm
tackler's exostosis
tacrolimus
tactile agnosia
tactile alexia
tactilegnosis
tactile information
tactile sensory loss
tactile threshold
taenia fornicis of the choroidal fissure
Taenia solium meningoencephalitis
TA-55 Auto Suture
TA-55 stapler
tag of cartilage
tag, skin
TAG suture anchor
Tai Chi Chuan exercise
tai chi martial arts
tail bone
tailor's bunion
tailor's bunionette
tailor's muscle
Tait flaps
Tait graft
Tajima stitch
Takahashi forceps
Takahashi rongeur
Takakura index
Taka sponge
Takatsuki syndrome
Takayasu arteritis
Takayasu pulseless disease
Takayasu vasculitis
Take-apart instruments
takedown procedure
TAL (tendo Achillis lengthening)
Talairach stereotactic conditions
Talairach stereotactic frame
talar compression syndrome
talar dome
talar impingement
talar neck osteotomy
talar osteochondral fractures
talar osteochondritis dissecans

talar osteotomy
talar tilt angle
talar tilt test
talectomy
talipes equinovarus, congenital
talipes hobble splint
talocalcaneal angle
talocalcaneal articulation
talocalcaneal index
talocalcaneal joint
talocalcaneal ligament
talocalcaneal osteotomy, subluxation
talocalcaneonavicular joint
talocrural angle
talocrural articulation
talocrural fusion
talocrural joint
talofibular joint
talofibular ligament
talometatarsal angle
talonavicular angle
talonavicular beaking
talonavicular capsule
talonavicular capsulotomy
talonavicular coalition
talonavicular joint
talonavicular ligament
talus
    congenital vertical
    flat-top
    neck of
    Sneppen fracture of
    sulcus
    vertical (rockerbottom flatfoot)
tamp
    Kiene bone
    wire
tandem-walking test
tangential layer of hand
tangential remarks
tangential speech
tangential view
Tangier disease
tangles, intraneuronal neurofibrillary
tank, Hubbard
Tanner-Whitehouse bone-age reference values

tantalum gauze
tantalum preformed skull plates
tantalum sheets
tantalum skull plate
tap
  bloody
  bloody lumbar
  dry lumbar
  glabellar
  reservoir
  screw
  shunt
  spinal
  subdural
  traumatic (lumbar puncture)
  ventricular
tape
  benzoin adherent
  DynaSport athletic
  Endobutton
  graded Gore-Tex
  moistened umbilical
  Morse
  nerve
  OKN (optokinetic nystagmus)
  salicylic acid
  Scotchcast 2 casting
  umbilical
tapering regimen of steroids
Taperloc femoral prosthesis
taper sleeve
Tapia syndrome
taping
  antipronation
  basket-weave ankle
  buddy
  McConnell
  stirrup
tapir's mouth (bouche de tapir) in
  muscular dystrophy
tapper
  bone
  cervical
  rectangular
  round
Tapper-Hoover changes and score

tapping, glabellar
tapping tests of arm disability
TARA (total articular replacement
  arthroplasty) prosthesis
tardive dyskinesia (oral-buccal-lingual)
tardive dystonia
tardive ulnar nerve palsy
tardy palsy
target-activated partial thromboplastin
target coordinates
  CT-derived
  MRI-derived
target disorder
Targeted Jobs Tax Credit (TJTC)
targeting, angiographic
target localization
target sign
Tarlov neurologic function grading
  system
tarsal arch
tarsal bars
tarsal bone
tarsal canal
tarsal coalition
tarsal joint
tarsal-metatarsal joint space
tarsal ligament
tarsal navicular
tarsal tunnel syndrome
tarsectomy
tarsometatarsal ligament
task (see also *test*)
  added purpose
  complex multistep
  encoding
  repetitive
  retrieval
  sentence closure
  three-step
  walking
  word retrieval
task-activated brain regions
Tasmar (tolcapone)
TAT (Thematic Apperception Test)
Taylor blade
Taylor brain scissors

Taylor dural scissors
Taylor percussion hammer
Taylor pinwheel
Taylor self-retaining spinal retractor
Taylor spinal retractor blade
Taylor vertebral body score
Tay-Sachs disease
T-bar
T-Bar trigger-point massager
TBI (traumatic brain injury)
TB montage (transverse bipolar)
TBNAA (total body neutron activation
    analysis)
TCA (transcondylar axis)
TC angle
TCBF (total cerebral blood flow)
TCCK unconstrained knee prostheses
TCD (transcranial Doppler) ultra-
    sonography
T-cell antigen receptor (TCR)
T-cell surface marker
tcMEP (transcranial motor-evoked
    potential)
TCNB (Tru-Cut needle biopsy)
T condylar fracture
TCP/IP (transmission control protocol/
    Internet protocol)
TCPM pneumatic tourniquet system
TCR (T-cell antigen receptor)
TCR (tethered cord release)
TCR (thalamocortical relay) neuron
TCR, rebound excitation of
TCS (tethered cord syndrome)
TCS knee immobilizer
TDD (telecommunication device for
    the deaf)
TDE (thiamine deficiency
    encephalopathy)
TE (echo time)
tear
    attritional
    bowstring
    bucket-handle
    cleavage
    dural
    fishtail
    flap

tear *(continued)*
    full-thickness
    L-shaped rotator cuff
    lunotriquetal
    micro
    radial meniscus
    rotator cuff
    micro
    parrot-beak meniscus
    skier's
    subscapularis
    tendon (types I-IV)
    tibiofibular ligament
    V-shaped rotator cuff
teardrop-shaped flexion-compression
    fracture
tea-tree oil (*Melaleuca alternifolia*)
Techmedica implant
technetium-99m bicisate (Neurolite)
technetium-99m (Ceretec)
technetium-99 exametazime SPECT
technetium-99 hexametazime SPECT
technetium-99 MDP bone scan
technique (see *operations*; *procedure*)
    activating, with EEG
    Amspacher-Messenbaugh
    AO/ASIF compression
    AO tension band
    Arana-Iniquez intracranial cyst
        removal
    arthroscopic inferior capsular split
    autogenous peroneus longus free
        graft
    bone-marrow stimulating
    Bunnell technique of pulley
        reconstruction
    Caspar anterior cervical plating
    Caspari transglenoid multiple-suture
    Chow modified
    Coltart fracture
    computer-assisted frameless
        navigation
    Cone-Grant
    cuboid squeeze
    cuboid whip
    Deyerle
    double-bundle PCL reconstruction

technique *(continued)*
  dowel graft
  dynamic tendon-gripping (DTG)
  free-floating forehead
  Garrett
  hamstring ACL reconstruction
    fixation
  Harmon transfer
  horizontal loop suture
  Ilizarov
  indirect reduction
  injection
  Kapandji pinning
  Karev pulley reconstruction
  Klagsbrun harvesting
  Kleinert rubber-band
  Lister pulley reconstruction
  Maquet
  Mankin scoring (cutting)
  marrow stimulation
  Meyer sublaminar wiring
  minimal incision
  modified Chow
  needle manometer
  Northern hybridization
  open-bowl cement
  partial saturation
  radiolabeled fibrinogen
  SCOI (for arthroscopic tenodesis)
  single-bundle PCL reconstruction
  Spalteholtz
  spin-echo
  spray-stretch
  standard pressurized cement
  tendon-for-ligament
  3D ultrasound reconstruction
    imaging
  two-bundle anterior cruciate
    ligament reconstruction
  two-sleeve
  two-strut tibial graft
  vacuum cement mix
  vertical loop suture
  xenon washout
  Watson matched resection
  Whitesides
  wick

technology
  electrothermal
  work evaluation systems (WEST)
tectal lesion
tectoral ligament
tectospinal tract
tectum
TED hose or stockings (thromboembolic disease)
TEE (transesophageal echocardiography)
teeth grinding, repetitive
Teflon-coated driver
Teflon felt
Teflon implant
Tegaderm dressing
tegmental tract
tegmentum
  medullary
  midbrain
  pontine
tegmentum of midbrain
tegmentum of pons and midbrain
Tegner activity level scale
Tegner knee scoring system
Tegretol (carbamazepine)
Tegtmeier hand board
teichopsia
teishein pressure needles
Tekscan in-shoe monitoring device
Tekscan pressure-sensitive insole
  sensor
telangiectasia
  ataxia (Louis-Bar syndrome)
  Sturge-Weber
telangiectatic osteosarcoma
TeleBrailler
TeleCaption TV decoders for the deaf
telecommunication device for the deaf
  (TDD)
T electrode (temporal) (T_7-T_{10})
telegraphic speech
telomerase activity
telomere repeat amplification protocol
telomere-specific probe
telemetry, EEG

teleopsia
telephone electroencephalogram
teleroentgenogram
Tele-Sensor, Cosman ICP
telescope
  Hopkins
  Lumina
  Storz
telescoped words
television-induced epilepsy
Telfa bolster
Telfa dressing
Telfa sponge
teloleukoencephalopathy, perinatal
telos radiographic stress device
Telos SE ankle stress device
TEM (terminal extensor mechanism)
Temodal (temozolomide)
temozolomide (Temodal)
temperature discrimination
temperature-gradient gel electrophoresis (TGGE)
Temperlite saw blade
template
  broach cutting
  Charnley
  fixator
  handheld
  hyperthermia
Temple-Fay laminectomy retractor
temporal area
temporal arteritis
temporal artery biopsy
temporal bone
temporal EEG lead
  left anterior (LAT)
  left posterior (LPT)
  right anterior (RAT)
  right posterior (RPT)
temporal electrode (T_7-T_{10})
temporal encephalocele
temporal gyrus
temporal horn atrophy
temporal horn neoplasm
temporal lobe contusion
temporal lobe epilepsy
temporal lobe herniation

temporal lobe lesion
temporal lobe seizure
temporal lobe status epilepticus
temporal lobe tumor
temporally
temporal muscle
temporal negative sharp transient
temporal-occipital craniotomy
temporal-occipital junction
temporal pole
temporal positive sharp transient
temporal region
temporal summation of pain
temporolimbic epilepsy
temporomandibular articulation
temporomandibular joint arthralgia
temporomandibular ligament
temporomandibular nerve
temporomandibular pain and
  dysfunction syndrome (TMPDS)
temporoparietal aphasia
temporoparietal muscle
temporoparietal region
temporopontine tract
temporozygomatic region
Temtamy-McKusick classification
tenaculum
tender, markedly
tenderness
  bony
  joint
  point
  skin-rolling scapular
tender-point criterion of fibromyalgia
  syndrome
tendinitis
  bicipital
  calcific
  chronic Achilles
  cuff
  de Quervain
  impingement
  insertional
  noninsertional
  rotator cuff calcific
  tricipital
tendinopathy, insertion

tendinoplasty
tendinosis, patellar
tendinosuture
tendinous insertion
tendo (pl. tendines)
tendo Achillis lengthening (TAL)
tendo Achillis stretching
tendo calcaneus
tendolysis
tendon
 abductor hallucis
 Achilles
 adductor
 ADQ (abductor digiti quinti)
 APB (abductor pollicis brevis)
 APL (abductor pollicis longus)
 aponeurosis of
 attenuated
 bowed
 bowing in arthritis
 brachioradialis
 bulbous
 calcaneal
 central
 central perineal
 collagen fibrils within
 common
 conjoined
 coronary
 cricoesophageal
 deep flexor
 discontinuity of
 disinsertion of
 ECRB (extensor carpi radialis brevis)
 ECRL (extensor carpi radialis
  longus)
 ECU (extensor carpi ulnaris)
 EDC (extensor digitorum communis)
 EHL (extensor hallucis longus)
 EIP (extensor indicis proprius)
 elongation of
 EPB (extensor pollicis brevis)
 EPL (extensor pollicis longus)
 EQP (extensor quinti proprius)
 extensor digitorum brevis manus
  (EDBM)
 FCR (flexor carpi radialis)

tendon *(continued)*
 FCU (flexor carpi ulnaris)
 FDC (flexor digitorum communis)
 FDI (first digital interosseous)
 FDL (flexor digitorum longus)
 FDP (flexor digitorum profundus)
 FDQ (flexor digiti quinti)
 FDS (flexor digitorum sublimis)
 FDS (flexor digitorum superficialis)
 FHB (flexor hallucis brevis)
 FHL (flexor hallucis longus)
 flexor
 flexor carpi ulnaris (FCU)
 FPB (flexor pollicis brevis)
 FPL (flexor pollicis longus)
 fraying of
 hamstring
 heel
 insertion of
 interosseous
 intra-articular subscapularis (IASS)
 membranaceous
 ODQ (opponens digiti quinti)
 open tendon repair
 palmaris longus
 patellar
 peroneal
 ProCol bovine bioprosthesis
 pulled
 quadriceps
 retraction of
 rider's
 rotator cuff
 rupture of
 ruptured Achilles (partial or
  complete)
 slipped
 snapping tendon release
 sonicated
 spontaneous rupture of Achilles
 subluxing
 subscapular
 subscapularis
 tenotomized
 tibial
 Todaro
 watershed area of Achilles

tendon *(continued)*
    Zinn
    Z-lengthening of
tendon-balancing procedure
tendon-bone attachment
tendon dislocation, peroneal
tendon-for-ligament technique
tendon gap
tendon insufficiency
tendon interposition anchovy
tendonitis (see *tendinitis*)
tendon lengthening
tendon of Hector
tendon of Zinn
tendon passer
tendonplasty
tendon railroading
tendon recentralization
tendon reflexes, deep (DTRs)
tendon rupture
tendon sheath
tendon-sheath space infection
tendon sling
tendon stretching exercises
tendon tear (types I-IV)
tendon transfer
tendoplasty
tendosynovitis (tenosynovitis)
tendovaginal
tendovaginitis, stenosing
tenectomy
tenets of treatment
Tenex (guanfacine)
teniola
Tennessee slider knot
tennis elbow
tennis elbow arm band
tennis leg
tennis shoulder
tennis toe
tenodesis (see *operation*)
tenographic study
tenography
"tenoids" (see *ctenoids*)
tenolysis
tenon

tenonitis
tenontodynia
tenorrhaphy
tenosynovial injection
tenosynovitis (also tendosynovitis)
    de Quervain stenosing
    flexor
    hypertrophic infiltrating
    sarcoid flexor
    stenosing
    suppurative
tenotome, Ryerson
tenotomized tendon
tenotomy
    adductor
    extensor
    flexor
    percutaneous
    percutaneous adductor
TENS (transcutaneous electrical nerve
    stimulation) unit, microcurrent
tense fontanelle
tensile load deformation
tensile strength
tensile stretch resistance
tensile test
Tensilon test for myasthenia gravis
tensing of muscle
tensiometer, intraoperative calibrated
tension band wiring
tensioned cross-pin
tensioner
    cable
    dynamometric wire
    graft
    wire
tension headache
tensioning device
tension migraine headache
tension myositis syndrome (TMS)
tension, neural
tension pneumocephalus
tensor fasciae latae anchovy
tensor fasciae latae flap
tensor muscle
tenth cranial nerve (vagus nerve)

tentorial edge
tentorial herniation
tentorial incisura
tentorial meningioma
tentorial nerve
tentorial notch herniation
tentorial sinus
tentorium
 cerebellar
 cerebelli
 incisura of
tentorium of cerebellum
Tenzel elevator
Tepper Wedge
teratocarcinoma, cerebral
teratologic dislocation of hip
teratoma
 congenital immature
 congenital intracranial
 cystic
 intramedullary spinal
 pineal
 sacrococcygeal
 solid
 suprasellar atypical
terbinafine
teres major muscle
teres minor muscle
teres test
terminal
 axon
 axonal
 nerve
 presynaptic
 Ruffini
terminal axonal ovoids
terminal nerves
terminal reservoir syndrome
terminal stance of gait
terminal tremor
terminus, rostral
termite forceps
"terrible triad" of shoulder
territory of artery
territory, vascular
terror, night (pavor nocturnus)
Terry fingernail sign

Terry nails
Terry Thomas sign
Terson syndrome
tertiary neuroborreliosis
tertiary syphilis
tertius, peroneus
tesla (T)
Tesla imaging system
test, testing
 abduction stress
 Abnormal Involuntary Movement
  Scale
 acetazolamide challenge
 Achilles squeeze
 Action Research Arm (ARA)
 actual leg length
 Adams forward-bending scoliosis
 Adams position
 adduction stress
 adductor sweep
 Adson
 Ad7C cerebrospinal fluid test
 AFP (alpha-fetoprotein)
 Alberts Famous Faces
 Allen
 alpha-fetoprotein
 amobarbital sodium
 Amsler grid visual
 amytal provocation
 anterior apprehension
 anterior drawer (ADT)
 anterior innominate
 antibody to VZ (varicella-zoster)
 antigen to *H. influenzae* in CSF
 antigen to meningococci in CSF
 antigen to pneumococci in CSF
 antithrombin III
 anvil
 APACHE II
 aphasia screening
 Apley grinding
 Apley scratch
 apparent leg length
 apprehension
 arm abduction
 arm roll
 Ashworth Scale

test *(continued)*

axial manual traction
Ayres tactile discrimination
stereognosis
B-cell surface marker of neoplasm
BAER (brain stem auditory-evoked
response)
ballistic dynamometer
Barlow hip instability
Barthel ADL Index
Battery of Memory Efficiency
Bayer Immuno 1 Dpd assay
Behavioral Inattention (BIT)
Behavioral Pathology in Alzheimer
Disease Rating Scale
Bekhterev sitting
belly-press
belt
bentonite flocculation (BFT)
Benton Visual Retention
bicipital groove tenderness
Bielschowsky head tilt
big toe
biomechanical extensometer
BIT (Behavioral Inattention)
Blessed Dementia Rating Scales
Blessed Information Memory
Concentration (IMC)
block design
blood level of anticonvulsant drugs
blood level of illicit drugs
blood screen for drugs
Booth
boron assay
Boston Classification system
Boston Diagnostic Aphasia
Examination
Boston Naming
bounce home
box and block tendon of arm
disability
bracelet
brain proteins 130 and 131
Brief Attention
Brunnstrom-Fugl-Meyer (BFM)
arm assessment
Bunnell-Littler

test *(continued)*

Burns bench
calculations
calf squeeze
California Verbal Learning
Callaway
caloric response
caloric stimulation
caloric vestibular function
Cambridge battery
Caregiver Strain Index
carotid Amytal procedure (CAP)
carotid balloon occlusion
carpal stretch
Carroll
CFQ-for-others
chest expansion
Childress duck waddle
chi-square
city and state
Clarke patellar compression
Clifton Assessment Procedures
for the Elderly
clonality assay
coagulate assay
cognitive failures questionnaire
cold provocation
cold water calorics
colloidal gold tendon of CSF
comb your hair
complement fixation (CF)
complex thematic pictures
compression
concealed straight leg raising
Conceptual Series Completion
mental status
confrontation naming
confrontational visual
construct validity of rehabilitation
content validity of rehabilitation
continuous performance
Controlled Oral Word Association
copy geometric designs
copy intersecting pentagons
cortical
Cotton ankle instability
cough-sneeze

test *(continued)*
    count backwards from 100
    counterimmune electrophoresis
        of CSF
    cover-uncover
    Cowdry-type intranuclear inclusion
        bodies
    COWS (cold to the opposite,
        warm to the same)
    Cozen
    Cram
    cranial nerve I (olfactory)
    cranial nerve II (optic)
    cranial nerve III (oculomotor)
    cranial nerve IV (trochlear)
    cranial nerve V (trigeminal)
    cranial nerve VI (abducens)
    cranial nerve VII (facial)
    cranial nerve VIII (vestibulo-
        cochlear)
    cranial nerve IX (glossopharyngeal)
    cranial nerve X (vagus)
    cranial nerve XI (accessory)
    cranial nerve XII (hypoglossal)
    crank
    Crawford small parts dexterity
    creep
    criterion-related validity of
        rehabilitation
    cross-chest adduction
    cross leg/straight leg raising
    crossed leg raising
    crossed straight leg raising
    CSF cryptococcal antigen titer
    CSF-serum HSV antibody ratio
    CUWD (cold up, warm down)
    Cybex isokinetic
    cytotoxic leukocyte
    D'Ambrosia
    day of month
    dexamethasone suppression (DST)
    Dexter hand evaluation
    Deyerle sciatic tension
    differential latency
    digit repetition
    digit reversal
    digit span

test *(continued)*
    digit symbol
    distraction
    DNA flow cytometry
    doll's eyes
    dorsal drawer
    double leg raise
    double Maddox rod
    double simultaneous stimulation
    Downey object recognition
        stereognosis
    Downey texture discrimination
    draw a clockface
    Draw a House
    draw a picture from memory
    Dreyer
    drop-arm
    drug screening
    duck waddle
    Dugas
    Dunnet two-sided T
    Durkan CTS (carpal tunnel
        syndrome) gauge
    dynamic visual acuity
    Eden
    Edinburgh Rehabilitation Status
        Scale
    Edinburgh-2 Coma Scale
    edrophonium chloride (Tensilon)
    elbow flexion
    electroencephalogram (EEG)
    electromyogram (EMG)
    electrophysiologic
    Elihorn Maze
    ELISA (enzyme-linked immuno-
        sorbent assay)
    Ely heel-to-buttock
    EMSA (electrophoretic mobility
        shift assay)
    ENA (extractable nuclear antigen)
    end point of
    ESR (erythrocyte sedimentation
        rate)
    everyday memory questionnaire
    Examining for Aphasia
    extensometry
    external rotation-recurvation

test *(continued)*
    face-hand
    face validity of rehabilitation
    facial recognition
    factor V Leiden
    Farr
    Fastex proprioceptive and agility
    femoral nerve stretch
    femoral nerve traction
    fibular squeeze
    50-hole peg
    finger count
    finger-to-finger
    finger-to-nose (F to N)
    Finkelstein
    Fisher exact
    Fist-Palm-Side
    Fist-Ring
    fluorescent treponemal antibody
      (FTA)
    forced duction
    forearm ischemic exercise
    forefoot adduction correction
    formal caloric
    formal visual field
    forward digit span recall
    Fournier ataxic gait
    free beta
    Frenchay Activities Index
    Frenchay Aphasia Screening
      (FAST)
    Frenchay Arm (FAT)
    Froment ulnar nerve function
    FTA (fluorescent treponemal
      antibody)
    Functional Ambulation Categories
    Functional Independence Measure
    Functional Limitation Profile
    Functional Status Questionnaire
    fund of information
    fungal culture of CSF
    Gaenslen
    Gait Abnormality Rating Scale
    Galveston Orientation and
      Awareness (GOAT)
    GBST (galvanic body sway test)
    Gilchrest

test *(continued)*
    Gillis
    Glasgow Coma Scale
    glucose level of CSF
    gluteal punch
    gluteus maximus tensing
    Godfrey
    Gram stain of CSF
    grimace
    grip pinch
    grip strength
    Guthrie bacterial inhibition
    Hachinski ischemia score
    Halstead-Reitan Battery
    Halstead-Wepman Aphasia
      Screening
    Hamilton
    Hamilton ruler
    Hauser ambulation index
    Hawiva
    head-rotation
    head-shaking nystagmus
    head-thrust
    Health Care Questionnaire
    heel walk
    heel-to-knee
    heel-to-shin
    Helfet
    hemagglutination inhibition (HI)
    hemispheric Wada
    herpes simplex antibody titer
      in CSF
    hesitation
    Hibbs
    hip abduction stress
    HIV viral antigen
    Hodkinson Mental (HMT)
    Hoffa
    hook
    Hooper Visual Organization
    Hoover
    Hopkins Verbal Learning
    HPLC
    Hughston
    Hughston knee
    Hyams esthesioneuroblastoma
    hyperemia

test *(continued)*
- hyperextension
- ice and warm water
- ice water calorics
- IFA (immunofluorescent antibody)
- IgM affinity purification
- iliac compression
- iliopsoas
- immediate memory
- Immuno 1 Dpd assay
- immunoprecipitation assay
- in a chair
- India ink examination of CSF
- Ingram-Withers-Speltz motor
- interpretation of proverbs
- intracarotid amobarbital speech
- intracarotid sodium amytal
  perfusion
- intracranial amobarbital procedure
  (IAP)
- ischemic forearm exercise
- isokinetic strength
- isolated cold stress (ICST)
- isometric muscle strength
- isotope cisternography
- isotope transfer
- Jackson compression
- Jacob shift
- Jamar grip
- Jebsen hand function
- Jebsen-Taylor hand function
- jerk
- Jobe relocation
- Johnson-Zuck-Wingate motor
- Judgment of Line Orientation
- jugular venous oxygen saturation
- Katz ADL Index
- Kaufman Adolescent and Adult
  Intelligence
- Kemp
- Kenny ADL Index
- Kenny Self-Care Evaluation
- kinase assay
- Kleiger
- knee drop
- knee flexion stress
- kneeling bench

test *(continued)*
- Knee Society Score
- Kohs block
- Kruskal-Wallis
- Kveim
- Lachman
- lactate level of CSF
- lactic dehydrogenase level of CSF
- Lambeth Disability Screening
  Questionnaire
- laser Doppler fluxmetry
- lateral pinch
- lateral pivot-shift
- latex particle agglutination
- Laugier
- LDH level of CSF
- LE prep (lupus erythematosus
  preparation)
- letter cancellation
- Lewin-Gaenslen
- Lewin punch
- Lewin reverse Lasègue
- Lewin snuff
- Lewin standing
- Lewin supine
- lick your lips
- lidocaine provocation
- Life Satisfaction Index
- lift-off
- light touch
- line bisection
- Lippman
- load-and-shift
- locking-position
- logical memory (paragraph recall)
- LOS (Lincoln-Ogeretzky Scale)
- Ludington
- lumbar puncture
- Lyme antibody
- lymphocytes in CSF
- Lysholm knee
- Maddox rod
- Magnuson
- Mann-Whitney U
- manometric
- Mantel-Haenszel Chi-square
- Mantoux

test *(continued)*
  manual muscle (MMT)
  manual percussion
  Marval
  maximum cervical compression
  maximum grip strength
  McDowell Impairment Index
  McIntosh
  McMurray
  McNemar symmetry
  Memory for Designs
  memory for digits
  Memory Impairment Screen (MIS)
  mental status examination
  metatarsal
  midtarsal movement
  Milgram
  Miller-Fisher
  Mills
  Mini-Mental State Examination
    (MMSE)
  Minnesota Multiphasic Personality
    Inventory (MMPI)
  Minnesota Rate of Manipulation
  Minnesota Test for Differential
    Diagnosis of Aphasia
  Minnesota Test of Aphasia
  misplaced objects
  Mississippi Scale for Combat-
    Related Post-traumatic Stress
    Disorder
  MMPI (Minnesota Multiphasic
    Personality Inventory)
  Moberg pick-up stereognosis
  MOBS (Montefiore Organic Brain
    Scale)
  modified anterior drawer
  modified Ashworth Scale
    for spasticity
  Moire topographic scoliosis
    screening assessment
  month of year
  Motor Assessment Scale
  Motor Club Assessment
  Motor Control Test (MCT)
  Motoricity Index
  motor performance

test *(continued)*
  Multilingual Aphasia Examination-
    Controlled Oral Word Associ-
    ation
  multiple sleep latency (MSLT)
  Murphy punch
  myelin basic protein
  Myers-Briggs Personality Inventory
  Myers-Briggs Temperament Indi-
    cator (MBTI)
  MyoForce
  Naffziger
  name the date
  naming common objects
  near card vision
  neck compression
  nerve conduction study (NCS)
  Neurobehavioral Cognitive Status
    Examination
  neuro-ophthalmological
  neuropsychologic battery of
  neuropsychological
  neuropsychometric
  neutralization antibodies to
    St. Louis encephalitis
  Nine Hole Peg (NHPT)
  Northwick Park Index of
    Independence in ADL
  Nottingham Extended ADL Index
  Nottingham Health Profile
  Nottingham Ten-Point ADL Scale
  N-telopeptide
  number 3 traced on patient's palm
  Nylen-Bárány maneuver
  Nymox urinary
  O'Brien cross-arm
  O'Brien needle
  O'Connor finger dexterity
  Ober
  obturator
  ocular tilt reaction (OTR)
  oculovestibular
  OKN (optokinetic nystagmus)
  OMC (orientation-memory-
    concentration)
  one-legged hop
  optokinetic drum

test *(continued)*
   oral potassium-loading
   Oregon Digit Recognition
   orientation-memory-concentration
     (OMC)
   Ortolani
   OsteoGram bone density
   Osteomark (NTx Assay)
   Osteomark bone-loss urine
   Osteosal
   Ottawa Ankle Rules (OARs)
   Oxford Scale
   Paced Auditory Serial Addition
     (PASAT)
   Pandy
   paragraph recall (logical memory
     after head injury)
   Parquetry Block
   passive head rotation
   patellar apprehension
   patellar inhibition
   patellar retraction
   patellar tap
   Patrick
   pattern reversal visual-evoked
     response
   peg arm disability
   pelvic-rock
   pencil Morton neuroma
   percussion
   perimetry
   Perkins
   peroneal tunnel compression
   Perthes
   PET with 3D SSP
   photometrazol
   pinch strength
   pinprick
   pinwheel
   pivot-shift
   polymorphonuclear leukocytes
     in CSF
   popliteal press
   Porch Index of Communicative
     Ability (PICA)
   Porteus Maze
   positive relocation

test *(continued)*
   posterior drawer
   posteromedial pivot-shift
   Pratt
   praxis
   preoperative balloon occlusion
   preoperative Wada
   PreVue *B. burgdorferi* antibody
     detection assay
   probe-to-bone
   Progressive Matrices
   pronator reflex
   protein C (functional)
   protein in CSF
   protein S (free antigen)
   protein truncation
   proverb interpretation
   proverbs
   provocative epilepsy
   PRP capsule of *H. influenzae*
     in CSF
   psychometric
   P300
   punch
   pupillary light
   Purdue Pegboard
   pyridinoline
   Pyrilinks-D assay
   Q angle
   quadrant-position
   Queckenstedt
   radioimmunoassay
   Rand Functional Limitations
     Battery
   Rand Physical Capacities Battery
   Rand Social Health Battery
   random letter
   Rankin Score
   RapiScan roadside saliva drug
   read a sentence
   recall 5 items after 5 minutes
   recall of information
   recent memory
   Reciprocal Coordination
   Reitan trail-making
   relocation
   remote memory

test *(continued)*

reverse digit span recall
reverse pivot-shift
reversed straight leg raising
Rey and Taylor Complex Figure
Rey Auditory Verbal Learning
Rey Osterrieth Complex Figure
RF (rheumatoid factor)
rheumatoid arthritis agglutinin
RIA (radioimmunoassay)
Rinne hearing conduction
Rivermead ADL
Rivermead Behavioral Memory
Rivermead Mobility Index
Rivermead Motor Assessment
Rivermead Perceptual Assessment
  Battery
Romberg
Rose-Waaler
rotary chair
rotatory instability
RPS (reverse pivot-shift)
RSA (roentgen stereophotogram-
  metric analysis)
Ryder
Sabin-Feldman dye test for
  congenital toxoplasmosis
sacroiliac resisted abduction
sacroiliac stretch
scalenus anticus
scaphoid shift
Scheffe
sciatic stress
sciatic stretch
SDS-PAGE
Seddon coin stereognosis
Selective Reminding
Semmes-Weinstein monofilament
  hair sensory loss
sensory extinction
Sensory Organization Test (SOT)
sentence closure
Sentence Repetition
serial sevens
serial threes
seriation
serum osteocalcin

test *(continued)*

serum 25-hydroxyvitamin D
sharp versus dull sensory
Sharp-Purser
short orientation-memory-
  concentration (OMC)
shoulder compression
shoulder depression
shoulder rock
shuck
Sicard
Sickness Impact Profile
similarities
similarities mental status
Simmonds
simple knee
simple shoulder
sit-and-reach flexibility
sitting SLR
Slocum
SLR (straight leg raising)
slump
Smith-Petersen
Speech Questionnaire
Speed
spell a word backwards
spell backwards
Spielberger State Anxiety Inventory
sponge
Spurling nerve root compression
square-shaped wrist
squat
squeeze syndesmosis ankle sprain
stair rise/descent
standing balance
star-cancellation (SCT)
static two-point discrimination
Steinberg
Steinmann
step-second
stimulated whole salivary flow rate
straight leg raising (SLR)
Stroop color-word interference
sulcus
supported Adams
supraselective Amytal
supraspinatus press

test *(continued)*
    swinging flashlight
    swinging light
    systolic toe/brachial index
    talar-tilt
    tandem Romberg
    tandem walking
    tapping
    TAT (Thematic Apperception Test)
    tensile
    thematic picture
    thenar weakness
    Thomas
    Thomas flexion
    Thompson calf squeeze
    thoracic outlet provocation
    three-point pinch
    three-stage command
    thumb-finding
    thumb-finger-approximator
    timed walking
    tiptoe
    Tobey-Ayer
    toe index
    Token aphasia
    tomodensitometric abdominal
    tourniquet
    Trail Making
    Trendelenburg
    tripod
    trunk control
    Tufts Quantitative Neuromuscular
        Exam
    Tukey
    turn
    two-part Apley
    two-point discrimination
    two-quarter
    ulnar grind
    ULTT (upper limb tension)
    understanding of similarities
    urine drug screen
    urodynamic
    valgus extension
    valgus stress
    varus stress
    varus-valgus stress

test *(continued)*
    vertebral artery
    vertical stress
    vestibular caloric
    Vironostika blood screening
    visual choice reaction time
    visual evoked response
    visual field
    Visual Neglect
    Visual Pattern Completion
    Visual Reproduction
    visual threat
    VrE (varus extension)
    VZ (varicella-zoster) antibody titer
    Wada (intracarotid amobarbital
        speech)
    WAIS-R Block Design
    wall chart vision
    Watson
    waving-hand threat
    Weber two-point discrimination
    Wechsler Adult Intelligence Scale
    Wechsler Memory Scale
    Weschler Memory Scale, Revised
    well leg straight leg raising
    Western blot
    Wide Range Achievement
    wiggle this finger
    Wilcoxon
    Wisconsin Card Sorting
    Wolf motor function
    word retrieval
    write a sentence
    xenon skin clearance
    Yergason
    YKL-40
    Zung Depression Scale
tester
    Disk-Criminator sensory
    Fitnet joint
Testut ligament
tetanus booster shot
tetanus immunization
tetanus immunoglobulin
tetanus-prone wound
tetany
tethered cord syndrome

tethered spinal cord
tethering of nerves
tether, spinal cord
tetraparesis, dense
tetraplegia
tetraspasticity
Tetrax interactive balance system
Teutleben ligament
Texas Scottish Rite Hospital (TSRH)
    instrumentation system
TFA (thigh-foot angle)
TFA (tibiofemoral angle)
TFC (theaded fusion cage)
TFCC (triangular fibrocartilaginous
    complex)
TFCQ (Toronto Functional Capacity
    Questionnaire)
T-Fix absorbable meniscal repair
    device
T4 syndrome
T fracture
TGA (transient global amnesia)
TGF-B (transforming growth factor-
    beta)
TGGE (temperature-gradient gel
    electrophoresis)
THA (total hip arthroplasty)
THA (transient hemisphere attack)
Thackray hip prosthesis
Thackray low-friction arthroplasty
thalamectomy, stereotactic
thalamic components of limbic system
thalamic deficit
thalamic dementia
thalamic disorder
thalamic fracture of calcaneal
thalamic hemorrhage
thalamic hyperpathia
thalamic infarct
thalamic inhibitory interneuron
thalamic ischemia
thalamic lesion
thalamic neural deficits
thalamic nucleus
    associational
    nonspecific
    specific

thalamic pacemaker cell
thalamic pain syndrome
thalamic projection system, diffuse
thalamic stimulation
thalamic syndrome
thalamic ulnar nerve
thalamocaudate artery
thalamocortical pathway
thalamocortical relay (TCR) neuron
thalamofrontal fibers
thalamogeniculate
thalamoperforate artery
thalamostriate vein
thalamotegmental involvement
thalamotomy
    parafascicular (PFT)
    stereotactic
    stereotaxic
    ventrolateral
thalamus
    dorsal medial nucleus of the
    intralaminar
    lateral
    nonspecific activating nuclei of
    parafascicularis of the
    thalamic
thalidomide (Thalomid)
thallium polyneuropathy
thallium SPECT (thallium 201 single-
    photon emission computed tomo-
    graphic) imaging
T-handled awl
THARIES (total hip articular replace-
    ment by internal eccentric shells)
The American Academy of Neuro-
    logical and Orthopaedic Surgeons
    (TAANOS)
theater symptom
thecal injection
thecal sac
theca, spinal
thecoperitoneal shunt
Theile muscle
Thematic Apperception Test (TAT)
thematic picture test
thenar eminence
thenar groups

thenar hammer syndrome
thenar muscle
thenar space abscess
thenar weakness test
theory
   corticoreticular
   facultative pacemaker
Thera-Back back support
Thera-Band hand exercisers
Thera-Band progressive weights
Thera-Band Resistive Therapy System
Thera-Bite wafer
Thera-Bite jaw exerciser
Thera-Bite Jaw Motion Rehabilitation
   System
Thera-Boot compression dressing or
   wrap
Thera-Cane trigger-point massager
Thera-Ciser Light Exercise System
Thera-Ciser Therapeutic Exercise
   System
TheraCool cold therapy
Therafectin (amiprilose hydrochloride)
Thera-P Bar
therapeutic aspiration
therapeutic recreation (TR)
therapeutic shoe
therapeutic ultrasound for tendon
   healing
therapist
   certified hand
   language
   occupational
   physical
   speech
TheraPulse bed
Thera-Putty CTS exerciser
therapy
   Activa tremor control
   adjuvant radiation
   antioxidant
   antithrombotic
   anti-TNF
   auriculotherapy
   boron neutron capture
   Bragg-peak photon-beam
   brisement

therapy *(continued)*
   compression
   constraint-induced movement
   deliberate
   diffusion
   disease-modifying
   electric differential (EDiT)
   electrical stimulation
   electron beam
   endovascular
   fad (spurious)
   flexion-distraction
   fomentation
   fractionated radiation
   glucocorticoid
   helmet-molding
   hot fomentation
   interferential
   interferon
   intradiscal electrothermal
   IR501 immune
   magnetic field
   Medtronic Activa tremor control
   meridian
   microcurrent interferential
   neoadjuvant chemotherapy
   neuroprotective
   occupational
   osteomanipulative
   osteopathic manipulative
   outpatient physical
   PEMF (pulsed electromagnetic
     field)
   perioperative antibiotic
   physical
   pneumatic compression
   Polar Wrap cold
   pool
   precision radiotherapy
   prolotherapy
   prophylactic antibiotic
   qi gong (Chinese medicine term)
   range of motion
   retroviral mediated gene
   rolfing (Dr. Ida Rolf)
   sacral nerve stimulation (SNS)

therapy *(continued)*
  SAFHS (sonic-accelerated fracture-
    healing system)
  Shiatsu therapeutic massage
  Silhouette therapeutic massage
  somatic
  spinal manipulative
  splinting
  steroid pulse
  SwimEx aquatic
  Swiss ball
  Thera Cool cold
  thrombolytic
  trial of conservative
  ultrasound
Thera-Soft hand/wrist orthosis
Therex programmable drug pump
thermal alteration of joint capsule
thermal asymmetry
thermal capsular plication
thermal capsular shrinkage
thermal capsulorrhaphy
thermal energy in arthroscopy
thermal modification of collagen
thermal necrosis
thermal probe (see *probe*)
thermal probe temperature
thermal procedure, Bronstrom
ThermaStim muscle stimulator
ThermaWave warming device
thermistor
  nasal
  oral
thermocoagulation, bipolar
thermocoagulative zone
thermocouple-controlled radio
  frequency device
thermocouple monitoring
thermode, Peltier
thermography
  chiropractic
  infrared electronic
  liquid crystal contact (LCT)
  low-resolution
thermolytic lesion
thermometer, low-reading
Thermophore moist heat pad

thermoplastic elastomer (TPE)
thermoplastic knee-ankle-foot orthoses
thermoplastic splint
thermoregulatory sweating of the face
thermorhizotomy
Thermoskin ankle and shoulder braces
Thermosport hot/cold wrap
theta activity
theta bursts
theta frequency band
theta index
theta pattern
theta rhythm
theta slowing
theta wave bursts
theta wave
theta waveform
thick bones
thickening
  mucoperiosteal
  neointimal
thienopyridine-derivative platelet anti-
  aggregant
thigh bone
thigh-foot angle
thigh-high antiembolic stockings
thigh joint
thinking
  abstract
  concrete
  disorganized
  forced
thin-plate spline
thin-section CT
thiopental
T1 (spin-lattice or longitudinal
  relaxation time)
T1-weighted image (short TR/TE)
T2 (spin-spin or transverse relaxation
  time)
T2-weighted image (long TR/TE)
toward the cord
third compartment
third cranial nerve (oculomotor nerve)
third intercondylar tubercle of Parsons
  (TITP)
third nerve mononeuropathy, diabetic

third nerve palsy
third occipital nerve
third peroneal muscle
third ventricle tumors
third ventriculostomy
31-P magnetic resonance spectroscopy
Thomas buckle sling
Thomas fixator
Thomas flexion test
Thomas frame
Thomas half-ring splint
Thomas heel, reverse
Thomas leg splint
Thomas rigid collar
Thomas sign
Thomas sling
Thomas suspension splint
Thomas test
Thomas traction
Thompson calf squeeze test
Thompson carotid clamp
Thompson femoral neck prosthesis
Thompson ligament
Thompson rasp
Thomsen disease
Thomsen dystrophy
thoracic bone
thoracic cardiac nerve
thoracic component of scoliosis
thoracic inlet (Pancoast) syndrome
thoracic interspinal muscle
thoracic intertransverse muscle
thoracic joint
thoracic longissimus muscle
thoracic OPLL (ossification of the
    posterior longitudinal ligament)
thoracic outlet provocation test
thoracic outlet syndrome (TOS)
thoracic rotator muscle
thoracic spinal nerve
thoracic splanchnic nerve
thoracoabdominal nerve
thoracodorsal nerve
thoracolumbar burst fracture
thoracolumbar region
thoracolumbar scoliosis
thoracolumbar spine

thoracolumbosacral orthosis (TLSO)
thoracoscopic spine surgery
thorax, muscles of
Thorazine shuffle gait
THORP (titanium hollow-screw
    osseointegrating reconstruction
    plate) system
thought processes, concrete
thought, stream of
thousand-hands Kannon universal
    headframe
THP (total hip prosthesis)
THR (total hip replacement)
thread length
three-cornered bone
3DCT (3-dimensional CT scan)
3 Degree-of-Freedom robotic
    manipulator arm
3D Fourier transformation MRI
    (3DFT MRI)
3DFT MRI (3D Fourier transforma-
    tion MRI)
3D porous Chitosan (membrane)
    scaffold
3D ultrasound reconstruction imaging
three-finger spica cast (Dehne cast)
3M modular shoulder system
3M staples
three-part fracture
three-paw bone holder
three-phase bone scan
three-phase bone scintigraphy (TPBS)
three-plane alignment
three-point pinch testing
three-point skull clamp
three-square flap
threes, serial
three-strand semitendinosus tendon
    graft
three-strand suture
threshold
    acoustic-reflex
    air-conduction
    auditory brain stem response
    bone-conduction
    cutaneous vibration
    pain

threshold *(continued)*
  perception
  pure-tone
  seizure
  speech-detection
  stimulus
  tactile
threshold intensity
thrills (murmurs)
throat clearing, repetitive
thrombectomy
thrombectomy/embolectomy
thrombi (pl. of thrombus)
thromboembolic complications
thromboembolic event
thromboembolic stroke
thromboendarterectomy
thrombolectomy
thrombolysis-associated intracerebral
  hemorrhage
thrombolytic therapy
thrombophlebitis, cerebral
thrombosis
  cavernous sinus
  central
  central retinal vein
  central venous
  cortical vein
  deep venous (DVT)
  dural sinus
  intra-aneurysmal
  intracranial sinus
  large-vessel
  sagittal sinus
  septic cavernous sinus
thrombotic microangiopathy
thrombotic stroke
thrombotic thrombocytopenic purpura
  (TTP)
thromboxane A2
thrombus (pl. thrombi)
  anterograde extension of
  intraluminal
  peroneal obliterative
  red erythrocyte-fibrin
  tibial obliterative
  white platelet-fibrin

through-and-through fracture
thrower's elbow
throwing-arm injury
thumb
  adductor sweep of
  bowler's
  cortical
  floating
  gamekeeper's
  hypoplastic
  low-set
  opposable
  skier's
  spring swivel
  trigger
  triphalangeal
  unopposable
thumb-finding test
thumb-finger-approximator test
ThumZ'Up functional thumb splint
thunderclap headache
Thurston-Holland fragment
thyrocervical trunk of subclavian
  artery
thyroid myopathy
thyroarytenoid muscle
thyroepiglottic ligament
thyroepiglottic muscle
thyrohyoid ligament
thyrohyoid muscle
thyroid notch
thyromegaly
thyrotoxicosis
T1 (inversion time)
Ti (titanium)
TIA (transient ischemic attack)
tiagabine (Gabitril)
Ti-BAC II hip prosthesis
tib-fib (tibia-fibula)
tibia coordinate system (TIBIACS)
TIBIACS (tibia coordinate system)
tibial aligner
tibial artery disease
tibial collateral ligament
tibial communicating nerve
tibial crest
tibial eminence

tibial flare
tibial hemimelia
tibialis sign of Strümpell
tibial jig
tibial muscle
tibial nerve
tibial nerve somatosensory-evoked
    potential (T-SSEP)
tibial obliterative thrombi
tibial outflow tracts, blind
tibial-peroneal trunk
tibial pilon fracture
tibial plafond fracture
tibial plateau fracture
tibial sesamoid ligament
tibial slope
tibial spacer
tibial tendon
tibial torsion
tibial tray
tibial tubercle transfer
tibial tuberosity
tibial tunnel enlargement
tibia vara, adolescent
tibioastragalocalcaneal canal of Richet
tibiocalcaneal arthrodesis
tibiocalcaneal fusion
tibiocalcaneal joint complex
tibiocalcaneal ligament
tibiocalcaneal space
tibiofemoral interaction
tibiofibular articulation
tibiofibular diastasis
tibiofibular fracture
tibiofibular ligament tear
tibiofibular overlap
tibiofibular syndesmosis
tibiofibular synostosis
tibionavicular ligament
tibioperoneal occlusive disease
tibiotalar angle
tibiotalar joint
tibiotalar ligament
    anterior
    posterior
tibiotalar salvage procedure
tibiotalocalcaneal fusion

tibiotarsal dislocation
tic
    articulatory
    chronic
    facial
    motor
    transient
    vocal
TICA (traumatic intracranial
    aneurysm)
tic douloureux, trigger zones for
tick-borne viral encephalitis
tick paralysis
ticlopidine
Ti-Cron (or Tycron) suture
tidemark, intact
Tiedemann nerve
Tiemann Meals tenolysis knife
Tiemann shoulder retractor
tier
    Adson knot
    knot
Ti-Fit modular hip system
tightener
    band
    equinus hamstring
    Kirschner
    Loute wire
    Nordt knot
    Parham band
    Rhinelander wire
    wire
tight heel cord
Tikhoff-Linberg radical arm resection
Tikhoff-Linberg shoulder resection
Tilastin hip prosthesis
Tillaux-Kleiger fracture
tilt
    bent-knee pelvic
    head
    patellar
    pelvic
    posterior pelvic
    radius
    talar
    valgus
    varus

Tilt and Turn Paragon bed
tilt board
tilted lateral radiograph
tilting angle
tiludronate disodium (Skelid)
time
    floating, in gait
    interpulse
    nerve conduction
    neuromuscular transmission
    retinocortical (RCT)
    single-limb support
    total tourniquet
timed sequential behavior
timed walking tests
time/money/number concepts
time sense
TiMesh titanium mesh bone-plate and
    screw system
Tindall scissors
tinea pedis
Tinel percussion sign
tingle, tingling
tingling in extremities
Ti-Nidium alloy
Ti-Nidium surface-hardening process
tinnitus, pulsatile
tip
    Adson brain suction
    Cloward drill
    drill
    Ferguson brain suction
    Fragmatome
    Frazier suction
    occipital
    Rhoton suction
    Sachs brain suction
    sucker
    suction
    uninsulated electrode
tip of screw
tiptoe gait
tiptoe, stand on
tiredness
TIRR foot-ankle orthosis
TIS (titanium interbody spacers)
Ti6A14V alloy for prosthesis

Tisseel fibrin sealant
Tissucol fibrin glue
tissue
    adipose
    collateral-dependent
    devitalized soft
    extrasynovial
    exuberant granulation
    fibrils of connective
    fibrocartilaginous
    fibrocollagenous connective
    granulation
    grumous
    inflammatory granulation
    intertrabecular soft
    intrasynovial
    isointense soft tissue (on MRI)
    meningeal mesenchymal
    myofascial muscular
    nociceptive
    ossification of soft
    prevertebral soft
    Tutoplast tissue preservation
        process
tissue elongation
tissue engineering
tissue expander
tissue fluorescence
tissue-type plasminogen activator
    (t-PA)
titanium (Ti)
titanium alloy rod
titanium aneurysm clip
titanium grommet
titanium interbody spacers (TIS)
titanium hip prosthesis
titanium mesh
titanium microsurgical bipolar forceps
titanium microsurgical needle holders
titanium nail
titanium plate
titanium staple
titer, Toxoplasma
TITP (third intercondylar tubercle of
    Parsons)
titubation
tizanidine

TJ (triceps jerk)
TJA (total joint arthroplasty)
TJTC (Targeted Jobs Tax Credit)
TKA (total knee arthroplasty)
TKR (total knee replacement/revision)
TLE (temporal lobe epilepsy)
TLIF (transforaminal lumbar interbody
    fusion)
TLSO (thoracolumbosacral orthosis)
TMA (transmetatarsal amputation)
TMA (transmetatarsal angle)
TMA (true metatarsus adductus)
TMA pressure
TMA-thigh angle (transmalleolar axis)
TMB (transient monocular blindness)
TME (trapezium-metacarpal eburnation)
TMJ (temporomandibular joint)
TMJ fossa-eminence prosthesis
TMJ syndrome
TMPDS (temporomandibular pain and
    dysfunction syndrome)
TMS (tension myositis syndrome)
TMS (transcranial magnetic stimula-
    tion)
TNF (tumor necrosis factor)
TNF-a (tumor necrosis factor alpha)
TNFa/NFkB signaling
TNMES (transcutaneous neuromuscu-
    lar electrical stimulation)
Tobey-Ayer test
tobramycin-impregnated PMMA
    implant
Todd motor paralysis
Todd motor weakness
Todd palsy
Todd paralysis (postepileptic)
Todd-Wells guide
Todd-Wells stereotactic frame
Tod muscle
toe (pl. toes)
    big
    clawing of
    cock-up
    congenital overlapping
    curly
    downgoing
    fanning of

toe *(continued)*
    floppy big
    hammer
    jammed
    lesser
    mallet
    marathoner's
    overlap of
    overlapping
    overriding
    searching
    splaying of
    stoved
    striatal
    tennis
    turf
    unilaterally upgoing
    upgoing
    V-Y plasty correction of varus
    Weil-type Swanson-design hammer-
        toe implant
toe box of shoe
toe cap
toe-drop
toe flexion
toe flexors
toeing-in gait
toeing-out gait
toenail
    circumferential
    ingrowing
toe-off phase of gait
toe range of motion
toe separator
toe splint, New Mind Set
toe-straight device
toe systolic pressure
toe–to–hand transfer
toe-touch ambulation
toe-touch weightbearing
toe-walking gait
toe walking, idiopathic
Toennis-Adson dissector
Toennis dissecting scissors
Toennis dura dissector
Toennis dura hook
Toennis dura knife

Toennis tumor forceps
Tofranil (imipramine)
toileting
Token Test for aphasia
tolcapone (Tasmar)
Tolosa-Hunt syndrome
toluidine blue stain
Tommy trapeze bar
tomodensitometric examination,
  abdominal
tomogram, tomography
  automated computerized axial
    (ACAT)
  computerized cranial
  electron-beam computed (EBCT)
  fludeoxyglucose F 18 positron
    emission
  positron emission
  hypocycloidal ankle
  optical coherence
  plain
  positron emission (PET)
  positron emission transaxial
  sellar
  single-photon emission computed
    (SPECT)
tomomyelography
"Tom Thumb," repeat the word
  (during EEG)
tone
  arteriolar muscle
  muscle
  postural
  symmetrically depressed
tone-reducing ankle-foot orthosis
  (TRAFO)
T1-T12 (twelve thoracic vertebrae)
tongs
  Barton skull traction
  Cherry traction
  Cone skull traction
  Crutchfield-Raney skull traction
  Crutchfield skeletal traction
  Crutchfield skull traction
  Gardner-Wells skull
  Gardner-Wells traction

tongs *(continued)*
  Mayfield
  Raney-Crutchfield skull
  Raney-Crutchfield traction
  Reynolds skull traction
  skull
  skull traction
  sugar
  traction
  Trippi-Wells
  Vinke
tongue
  beefy
  deviated to left
  deviated to right
  magenta
  muscles of
tongue-and-trough technique
tongue biting during seizure
tongue bone
tongue deviation
tongue protrusion, repetitive
tongue thrusting, repetitive
tongue-type fracture
tongue writhing, repetitive
tonic-clonic movements
tonic-clonic seizure
tonic desynchronizing input
tonic deviation of eyes
tonic neck reflex (primitive)
tonic phase-spike
tonic posturing
tonic pupils
tonic seizure
tonohaptic pupil
tonohaptic reaction of pupil
tonsil, herniated cerebellar
tonsillar herniation
tonsillar nerves
tonus
  arterial
  decreased
  increased
  muscular
Tool, Gore Smoother Crucial
Topamax (topiramate)

tophaceous deposits
tophaceous gout
tophaceous material
tophus (pl. tophi) formation
top-loading screw and rod system
topognosis
topographic mapping
topographical agnosia
topography of wave
Toradol (ketorolac tromethamine)
torch, saline
torcular Herophili
Torg classification of fracture
Torkildsen shunt procedure
tornado epilepsy
Tornwaldt bursitis
Toronto Functional Capacity
    Questionnaire (TFCQ)
Toronto Medical CPM exerciser
Toronto orthosis
Toronto parapodium
TORP (total ossicular replacement
    ˙ prosthesis)
torque
    peak
    pin extraction
torque converter, subtalar joint as
torque limit
torque measure
torque stress
torsion
    femoral
    internal tibiofibular
    lateral femoral
    malleolar
    tibial
    tibiofibular
torsional abnormalities
torsional alignment
torsional impaction force
torsional stiffness
torsional stress
torsion bar
torsion fracture
torsion spasm

torticollis
    spasmodic
    static
torula (spheroid bodies in crypto-
    coccosis)
Torula histolytica (earlier name for
    Cryptococcus neoformans)
Torus external fixation system
torus fracture
torus-type buckle fracture
TOS (thoracic outlet syndrome)
Total Anatomical Hinge knee brace
total body neutron activation analysis
    (TBNAA)
total contact cast
total cortical blindness
total fracture
Total Gym rehabilitation system
total hip arthroplasty (THA)
total hip prosthesis (THP)
total hip replacement (THR)
total joint arthroplasty (TJA)
total knee replacement/revision (TKR)
total pituitary ablation
Total Rotating Knee (TRK) mobile-
    bearing implant
total synovectomy
total tourniquet time
Toti trephine drill
touch
    dull
    light
    sharp
Tourette syndrome
tourniquet
    Accuflate
    arthroscopic
    Bodenstab
    Digikit finger
    digital
    finger
    Kidde
    Medi-Quet
    pneumatic
    pneumatic ankle

tourniquet *(continued)*
   Profex arthroscopic
   proximal thigh
   Stille
tourniquet test
tourniquet time, total
towel
   moist
   wound
towel curls (postoperative exercises)
Towne occipital view of the skull
Towne projection in skull x-rays
Towne view
Townley TARA prosthesis
Townsend knee brace
toxic amblyopia
toxic-confusional state
toxic delirium
toxic encephalopathy
toxic hypoxia
toxicity, ammonia
toxic nystagmus
toxic paraplegia
toxic retinoneuropathy
toxic synovitis
Toxoplasma gondii
Toxoplasma titer
toxoplasmosis
   acquired
   central nervous system
   cerebral
   congenital
   CSF
   glandular
Toynbee muscle
t-PA (tissue-type plasminogen
   activator)
TPBS (three-phase bone scintigraphy)
TPE (thermoplastic elastomer)
TPE ankle-foot orthosis
TPE biomechanical foot orthosis
TP electrode (temporal-posterior)
   (TP_7-TP_{10})
TPL-6 total hip replacement
TPR ankle prosthesis
TQNE (Tufts Quantitative Neuro-
   muscular Examination)

TR (repetition time)
TR (therapeutic recreation)
trabecula (pl. trabeculae)
trabecular bone
tracheal muscle
tracheloclavicular muscle
trachelomastoid muscle
tracing
   EEG (electroencephalogram)
   flattening of
Tracker 10 catheter
Tracker 18 catheter
Tracker 18 microcatheter
Tracker vascular access system
tracking of movements, visual
tracking, patellar
tract
   anterior corticospinal
   anterior spinocerebellar
   anterior spinothalamic
   ascending
   brain stem pyramidal
   central tegmental (CTT)
   cerebellar
   cerebellorubral
   cerebellorubrospinal
   cerebellospinal
   cerebellotegmental
   cerebellothalamic
   cerebral fugal
   conariohypophyseal
   corticobulbar (CBT)
   corticopontine
   corticorubral
   corticospinal (CST)
   corticotectal
   crossed pyramidal
   cuneocerebellar
   Dejerine aberrant pyramidal
   dentatothalamic
   dermal sinus
   descending
   direct pyramidal
   dorsal spinocerebellar
   dorsolateral
   extracorticospinal
   extrapyramidal

tract *(continued)*
  fastigiobulbar
  frontopontine
  frontotemporal
  Gudden
  hypothalamicohypophysial
  interstitiospinal
  lateral corticospinal
  lateral spinocerebellar
  lateral spinothalamic
  long
  long spinal white matter
  mamillothalamic
  mesencephalic
  motor
  nerve
  occipitopontine
  occipitotemporopontine
  olivocerebellar
  optic
  paraventriculohypophysial
  parietopontine
  pilonidal
  posterior spinocerebellar
  pyramidal
  reticulospinal
  reticulovestibulospinal
  rubrobulbar
  rubroreticular
  rubrospinal
  Schultze
  Schütz
  segmental tract of trigeminal
  sensory long
  spinal
  sinus
  spinocerebellar
  spinocervical
  spinocervicothalamic
  spinocuneocerebellar
  spino-olivary
  spinoreticular
  spinotectal
  spinothalamic
  tectobulbar
  tectocerebellar
  tectospinal

tract *(continued)*
  tegmental
  temporopontine
  tegmentospinal
  temporopontine
  thalamo-olivary
  trigeminal nerve
  trigeminothalamic
  tuberohypophysial
  ventral amygdalofugal
  ventral spinocerebellar
  ventral spinothalamic
  vestibulocerebellar
  vestibulospinal
traction
  Airtrac cervical/lumbar
  axial
  Back Revolution
  balanced suspension
  bidirectional
  Bremer halo crown
  Bryant
  Buck
  Buck skin
  cervical
  Chattanooga
  Cotrel
  C-TRAX
  Dunlop
  floating
  halo
  inline
  intermittent
  intersegmental
  InvertaChair
  Kuhlman cervical
  leg
  long-axis
  lumbosacral
  mechanical
  pelvic
  pin
  pounds of
  Pronex pneumatic cervical
  Quigley
  Russell
  Saunders Cervical Hometrac

traction *(continued)*
  skeletal
  skull tong
  static
  supine cervical
  Thomas
  well-leg
traction apophysitis
traction bow, Kirschner
traction/compression, selective
traction exostosis
traction suture
traction tongs, Cone skull
tractus solitarius nucleus
Trac II knee implant
trafermin (Fiblast)
TRAFO (tone-reducing ankle-foot
  orthosis) trajectory
tragicus muscle
Trail Making Test
train
  constant-frequency
  electrical stimulation
training
  concentric muscle
  eccentric muscle
  functional
  gait
  lumbar spine stabilization
  transfer
trains of flashes
trains of waves
traits, premorbid
trajectory
  foot
  lower extremity
trajectory angle
trajectory of screw
tramline calcification
trampoline
tram track pattern
trance, hysterical
trance states
transarterial embolization
transarticular screw fixation
transcallosal

transcapitate fracture
Transcend total hip system
transcervical fracture
transchondral talar fracture
transchoroidal approach
transclival approach
transcondylar axis (TCA)
transcondylar fracture
transcortical aphasia
  motor
  sensory
transcranial approach
transcranial color-coded sonography
transcranial Doppler (TCD) ultrasound
transcutaneous electrical nerve stimulation (TENS)
transcranial imaging transducer
transcranial magnetic stimulation
  (TMS)
transcranial motor-evoked potential
  (tcMEP)
transcutaneous oxygen determination
  (TCPO$_2$)
transcranial oxygen extraction
transcription-based clonality assay
transcutaneous neuromuscular electrical stimulation (TNMES)
transcutaneous oxygen (PtcO$_2$)
transcutaneous signal transmission
Transderm-Scop (scopolamine)
transducer
  Camino subdural
  digital pressure
  ergonomically-designed
  Gaeltec catheter-tip pressure
  Spiegelberg pneumatic
transduction, signal
transected segment
transection
  axon
  nerve
  spinal cord
  traumatic cord
transepiphyseal fracture
transesophageal echocardiography
  (TEE)

transethmoidal encephalocele
transfer
    autogenous osteocartilage
    Brooker-Jones tendon
    Bunnell tendon
    Chandler tendon
    flexor tendon
    foot-to-hand transfer
    free toe
    free tissue
    independent in bed
    Mustard iliopsoas
    nerve
    pivot
    split posterior tibial tendon
    Sutherland tendon
    tibial tubercle
    toe–to–hand transfer
    two-stage opposition
transfer lesion
transfer skills
transfer training
transfer ulcer
transfibular approach for arthrodesis
transfibular arthrodesis
TransFix ACL reconstruction system
transfixing screw
transfixion pin
transforaminal approach to third
    ventricle
transforaminal lumbar interbody fusion
    (TLIF)
transforming growth factor-beta
    (TGF-B)
transfusion, intraoperative autologous
    (IAT)
transglenoid
transhamate fracture
transient
    benign epileptiform
    frontal sharp
    high-amplitude
    multifocal sharp (MST)
    nonepileptiform sharp
    occipital negative sharp
    polyphasic

transient *(continued)*
    positive occipital sharp (POSTs)
    rolandic dip
    rolandic sharp
    sharp
    sleep
    spiky
    temporal negative sharp
    temporal positive sharp
    vertex sharp
transient bone marrow edema
    syndrome
transient global amnesia
transient hemisphere attack (THA)
transient ischemic attack (TIA)
transient paralysis
transient paresthesia
transient phalangeal osteolysis
transients of sleep, benign epileptiform
    (BETS)
transient states of depersonalization
transient synovitis of hip
transient tic
transient vertigo
transillumination of head
transitional shear
transitional vertebra
transition, sitting
translabyrinthine surgical approach
translation
    dorsopalmar
    posterior tibial
translation exercise
translocation, ulnar
transmalleolar axis (TMA)-thigh angle
transmetatarsal amputation (TMA)
transmissible spongiform encepha-
    lopathy (TSE)
transnasal biopsy
transosseous suture
transosseous technique
transpedal multiplanar wedge
    osteotomy/fusion
transpedicle distraction
transpedicular approach
transpedicular fixation

transphyseal neck-head femoral
　drilling
transplant
　chondrocyte
　embryonic mesencephalic
　osteoarticular
transplantation
　adrenal medulla
　allogenic
　autoadrenal
　autogenous cartilage
　autograft
　avascular chondroepiphyseal
　fetal substantia nigra
　fetal tissue
　meniscal
　osteochondral
　periosteal
　stem cell
Trans Q 1 iontophoretic drug delivery
　system
transradial styloid perilunate disloca-
　tion
transscaphoid perilunate dislocation
transsection, spinal cord
transsphenoidal approach
transsphenoidal cryohypophysectomy
transsphenoidal encephalocele
transsphenoidal hypophysectomy
transsphenoidal intraoperative color
　Doppler ultrasonography
transsyndesmotic screw fixation
transtemporal approach
transtentorial herniation
transtentorially
transthecal digital block anesthesia
transtriquetral fracture-dislocation
transvenous embolization
transvenous retrograde nidus sclero-
　therapy under controlled hypoten-
　sion (TRENSH)
transverse arch of foot
transverse arytenoid muscle
transverse atlantal ligament
transverse carpal ligament
transverse cervical artery

transverse cord lesion
transverse crural ligament
transverse diameter
transverse fracture
transverse genicular ligament
transverse humeral ligament
transverse ligament of atlas
transverse magnetization
transverse metacarpal ligament
transverse metatarsal ligament
transverse muscle
transverse myelitis
transverse nerve
transverse orientation
transverse pelvic diameter
transverse perineal ligament
transverse plane forces
transverse process
transverse rotation of the lower
　extremity
transverse section
transverse tarsal articulation
transverse tarsal joint
transverse tibiofibular ligament
transverse tripolar electrode
transverse tripolar system for spinal
　cord stimulation
transversospinal muscle
trapdoor effect
trapeze bar
trapezial saddle
trapeziectomy
trapeziolunate
trapeziometacarpal arthrosis
trapeziometacarpal joint
trapezioscaphoid joint
trapeziotrapezoid joint
trapezium bone
trapezius muscle
trapezoid bone
trapezoid body
trapezoid bone of Henle
trapezoid bone of Lyser
trapezoid ligament
trap, finger
trapping, aneurysmal

Trap Strap
Traube-Hering-Mayer waves of
  cerebrospinal fluid
Traube percussion hammer
trauma
  cerebral
  closed head
  craniocerebral
  distortion
  fracture
  head
  high-energy
  massive head
  occult head
trauma-related causalgia
traumatic avulsion
traumatic brain injury (TBI)
traumatic cord damage
traumatic dislocation
traumatic disruption
traumatic encephalopathy
traumatic injury
traumatic intracranial aneurysm
traumatic meningeal hemorrhage
traumatic neuroma
traumatic neurosis
traumatic osteoarthritis
traumatic periostitis
traumatic pseudoaneurysm
traumatic rupture
traumatic scoliosis
traumatic shearing of white matter
traumatic spondylitis
traumatic spondylolysis
traumatic subluxation
traumatic tap (lumbar puncture)
traumatic unidirectional instability
traumatologist
Trautmann chisel
traversing the fracture
tray
  DiChiara hand
  hand
  pattie
  surgical hand
  tibial
  TrayMate

trazodone (Desyrel)
Treace microdrill
Treacher Collins syndrome
treatment
  adjustive (chiropractic)
  communication/cognition
  daily
  Gamma Knife
  gate control pain
  osteopathic manipulative
  outpatient communication/cognition
  rehabilitation
  tenets of
  vasopneumatic
treatment frequency
treatment program
tree
  cedar shoe
  intracranial carotid
  lower extremity arterial
trefoil canal
trefoil sign on CT scan
Treitz ligament
Treitz muscle
Trélat-Charlin neuralgia
tremor
  action
  alcohol withdrawal
  benign essential
  cerebellar outflow
  counting-money
  dystonic
  emotional stress precipitating
  endpoint
  essential cerebellar
  familial
  flapping
  head and neck
  hepatic encephalopathy
  heredofamilial
  hysterical
  idiopathic
  intention
  kinetic
  metabolic
  no-no
  orthostatic

tremor *(continued)*
   oscillating
   parkinsonian
   perioral
   peripheral neuropathy
   physiologic
   physiological
   pill-rolling
   positional
   postural
   progressive cerebellar
   psychogenic
   rest
   resting
   rubral
   senile
   static
   striatocerebellar
   sustentation
   terminal
   to-and-fro
   tongue
   voice
   volitional
   wing-beating
   writing
   yes-yes
Tremor Disability Questionnaire
tremor-dominant Parkinson disease
tremor-related activity
tremulous movement
tremulousness
Trendelenburg gait
Trendelenburg position of weightbearing
   leg
Trendelenburg test
TRENSH (transvenous retrograde
   nidus sclerotherapy under controlled hypotension)
trephination
trephine
   biopsy
   bone biopsy
   break-screw
   D'Errico skull
   DeVilbiss skull
   Galt hand

trephine *(continued)*
   Galt skull
   iliac crest
   Michele vertebral body
   Polley-Bickel biopsy
   Rochester bone
   Scoville skull
   skull
   Stille
   Turkel bone biopsy
   winged
Trevor disease
triad
   Charcot
   O'Donohue's Unhappy (OUT)
   terrible
Triad hip prosthesis
trial, Fracture Intervention Trial (FIT)
trial prosthesis
trial reduction of prosthesis
triamcinolone (Aristospan)
triangle
   aponeurotic
   cephalic
   cervical
   clavipectoral
   Codman
   deltoideopectoral
   femoral
   Guillain-Mollaret
   iliofemoral
   inguinal
   insular
   Kager
   lumbocostoabdominal
   Mollaret
   myoclonic
   pain
   paramedian
   posterior
   submandibular
   supraclavicular
   vertebrocostal
triangular ankle fusion frame
triangular bone
triangular external ankle fixation
triangular fibrocartilage complex

triangular ligament
triangular muscle
triangular recess
triangulation, optical
tricalcium phosphate ceramic
triceps flap
triceps jerk (TJ)
triceps muscle
Trichinella spiralis meningoencephalitis
trichinosis
trichopoliodystrophy
tricipital tendinitis
Tricodur compression support bandage
Tricodur Epi (elbow) compression
    bandage
Tricodur Omos (shoulder) compression bandage
Tricodur Talus (ankle) compression
    bandage
Tricon-M patellar prosthesis
Tricophyton metagrophytes fungus
Tricophyton rubrum fungus
Tri-Core cervical pillow
tricorrectional bunionectomy
tricylic antidepressants
trifacial nerve
triflanged nail
trifluoperazine hydrochloride
    (Stelazine)
trifurcation of middle cerebral artery
trigeminal cavity
trigeminal hemangioma
trigeminal nerve (fifth cranial nerve)
    mandibular division
    maxillary division
    nucleus of
    ophthalmic division
    segmental tract of
    spinal tract of
trigeminal neuralgia
trigeminal neuroma extirpation
trigeminal notch
trigeminal paralysis
trigeminus, porous
trigger a seizure
trigger finger release
triggering conditions

triggering event
triggering mechanism
triggering stimulus
trigger point injection
trigger point mobilization
trigger point neuralgia
trigger point therapy
trigger points in paravertebral muscles
trigger thumb release
trigger zones for tic douloureux
trigonal muscle
trigone
    deltoideopectoral
    vertebrocostal
trigone of lateral ventricle
trigonocephaly
trihelical collagen fibers
trihexyphenidyl (Artane)
triiodothyronine receptor immuno-
    reactivity
Trillat osteotomy
Tri-Lock Cup
Trilogy acetabular cup
trimalleolar fracture
Trimline knee immobilizer
trimlines for ankle-foot orthoses
trimmer, meniscal
Trinkle drill
Trio arthroscope system
trio, radial
triorthocresylphosphate poisoning
triphalangism
triphasic slow wave (EEG) activity
triphasic wave complex
triplane fracture
triple arthrodesis
tripled semitendinosus autologous
    cancellous bone plug
tripod test
tripoding maneuver
Trippi-Wells tongs
triquetral bone
triquetral fracture
triquetrohamate impaction syndrome
triquetrohamate joint
triquetrohamate ligament
triquetrolunate dissociation

triquetrum, bone of wrist
tri-radial resector blade
triradiate cartilage
trismus
trisomy 13
trisomy 18
trisomy 21
trispiral tomographic staging
triton tumor
TRK (Total Rotating Knee) mobile-
  bearing implant
TR-NC (percutaneous trigeminal
  tractotomy-nucleotomy)
trocar
  brain
  DeRoyal surgical
  dull
  Frazier brain
  McCain TMJ
  Paulus
  pyramidal
  sharp
trochanter
  flare of
  greater
  lesser
trochanteric osteotomy
trochanter wire
trochlear defect
trochlear groove
trochlear nerve (fourth cranial nerve)
trochlear notch
trochlear process
trochlear ridge
trochlear sulcus
trochleocapitellar groove of humerus
trochoid articulation joint
Troemner (Trömner) percussion
  hammer
Troemner sign
troika, aponeurotic
tromethamine
TROM splint
Tronzo elevator
Tronzo VLC cannulated compression
  screw
trophic fracture

trophic skin changes
trophoblastic material
trough and peak levels
trough level of drug
trough line on x-ray
trough of wave
trousers, medical (or military) antishock (MAST)
Trousseau sign
Troyer syndrome
TR-28 total hip replacement
true acetabulum
true aphasia
True/Fit braces and supports
True/Flex intramedullary nail
True/Lok external fixator system
true metatarsus adductus (TMA)
true muscles of back
true neuroma
true ratio measures in rehabilitation
  testing
true vertigo
Tru-Fit braces and supports
truncal ataxia
truncal instability
trunk
  basilar artery
  brachiocephalic
  costocervical
  lumbosacral
  nerve
  thyrocervical
trunk control test
Trunkey fracture classification system
Tru-Support EW (elastic wrap)
  bandage
Tru-Support SA (self-adhering)
  bandage
Trypanosoma gambiense
T-score
TSE (transmissible spongiform
  encephalopathy)
T-shaped fracture
T-shaped silicone shunt tube
TS-930 electric-powered foot reflex
  stimulator
T spine (thoracic spine)

TSPP (technetium stannous pyrophosphate) rectilinear bone scan
TSRH (Texas Scottish Rite Hospital)
TSRH Crosslink
TSRH hook-rod
TSRH spinal instruments
TSRH fixation system
TSRH hook
TSRH pedicle fixation device
TSRH rod and screw
TSRH screw
TSRH universal instrumentation system
TSRH vertebral screw
T-SSEP (tibial nerve somatosensory-evoked potential)
Tsuge tendon repair (silent *t*)
TTAP-ST acetabular prosthesis
TTR (tarsal tunnel release)
TTS (tarsal tunnel syndrome)
T2 SPIR signal
tub bench
tube
   Adson brain suction
   Baron suction
   blocked shunt
   brain suction
   cement
   Cone suction
   Dawson-Yuhl suction
   feeding
   Ferguson brain suction
   Ferguson-Frazier suction
   guide
   Hardy suction
   Hemo-Drain wound
   House suction irrigation
   Jergesen
   Kam Vac suction
   ligament sizing
   Mason suction
   neural
   New York Glass suction
   obstructed shunt
   pressure-sensitive valve in shunt
   Pribham suction
   Rhoton-Merz suction

tube *(continued)*
   Sachs brain suction
   Schwann cell
   shunt
   suction
   T-shaped silicone shunt
   Vidicon vacuum chamber pickup
   Yankauer suction
   Yasargil suction
tubercle
   accessory
   amygdaloid
   articular
   calcaneal
   Chaput
   Chassaignac
   costal
   cuneiform
   dental
   greater
   iliac
   intercondylar
   lesser
   Lister
   medial calcaneal
   Parsons
   pubic
   rib
   sella turcica
   third intercondylar tubercle of Parsons (TITP)
   tibial
tuberculoma
tuberculosis
   extrapulmonary
   osteoarticular
   spinal
tuberculous arthritis
tuberculous meningitis
tuberculous osteomyelitis
tuberculous spondylitis
tuberosity (pl. tuberosities)
   bicipital
   calcaneal
   coracoid
   costal

tuberosity *(continued)*
  deltoid
  femoral
  greater
  iliac
  infraglenoid
  ischial
  lesser
  navicular
  plantar
  radial
  tibial
  ulnar
tuberosity avulsion fracture
tuberosity healing
tuberous sclerosis
Tubigrip bandage
Tubigrip dressing
Tubigrip gloves
tubular bone plate
tubular harvester
tubulation
tuck, chin
Tudor-Edwards bone cutting forceps
Tuffier inferior ligament
Tuffier laminectomy retractor
Tuffier-Raney retractor
Tuffier rib spreader
tuft fracture
tuft of synovium
Tufts Quantitative Neuromuscular
  Examination (TQNE)
Tukey test
Tuli Cheetah ankle brace
Tuli heel cups
tulip probe
Tuli support
Tumarkin crisis
tumbler flaps
tumbler grafts
tumefaction
tumor
  acidophilic pituitary
  acoustic nerve
  ACTH-producing pituitary
    adenoma
  anaplastic astrocytoma

tumor *(continued)*
  anterior cingulate gyrus
  astrocytic
  astrocytoma
  astroglial
  atypical giant cell
  ball-valve
  basal
  basicranial
  basiocciput
  basophilic pituitary
  blood vessel
  bone-forming
  brain stem glioma
  brown
  calcified glial
  capillary hemangioma
  cavernous hemangioma
  cerebellopontine angle
  cerebellum
  chondromyxoid fibroma
  chordoma
  choroid plexus papilloma
  chromophobe adenoma
  chromophobe pituitary
  classic Kaposi sarcoma
  cleavable
  clivus meningioma
  CNS (central nervous system)
  Codman
  colloid cyst
  congenital primitive neuro-
    ectodermal
  corpus callosum
  craniopharyngioma
  cutaneous neural
  cystic brain
  debulking of
  decompression of
  deep-seated
  dermoid
  dumbbell neurofibroma
  eccrine angiomatous hamartoma
  eighth nerve
  embryonal
  ependymoma
  epidemic Kaposi sarcoma

tumor *(continued)*
    epidermoid
    epilepsy-causing brain
    extension of
    extirpation of
    extracompartmental
    extradural
    extramedullary hemangioma
    fatty
    finger of
    flocculonodular
    fourth ventricle
    frontal lobe
    ganglion
    gasserian ganglion
    gender-related
    germ cell (GCT)
    giant cell malignant
    glial
    glioma
    glomus
    glomus jugulare
    granular cell
    growth-producing pituitary
    hemangioblastoma
    hematogenous spread of
    high-grade astrocytoma
    hourglass tumor of cord
    hypothalamus
    incomplete
    infratentorial brain
    infratentorial Lindau
    inoperable brain
    internal capsule and basal ganglia
    intra-axial brain
    intracompartmental
    intracranial
    intradural extramedullary
    intramedullary
    intramedullary spinal cord
    intramedullary spinal teratoma
    intrapetrous retrolabyrinthine
    intrasellar
    intraspinal
    invasive malignant sheath
    juxta-articular osteoid osteoma
    juxtacortical sarcoma

tumor *(continued)*
    lipomatous neuroectodermal
    low-grade astrocytoma
    low-grade malignant histiocytoma
    malignant glioma
    malignant peripheral nerve sheath
    medullary
    meningeal
    meningeal spread of
    meningioma
    metastatic
    microglioblastoma
    midbrain
    mixed
    nerve sheath
    neurilemmoma
    neuroectodermal
    neurofibroma
    nonacoustic cerebellopontine angle
    nongerminomatous germ-cell
    nonglial
    non-neoplastic
    occipital lobe
    occipital neuroblastoma
    oligodendroglioma
    optic chiasm
    optic glioma
    optic pathway
    orbital pseudotumor
    ossifying fibromyxoid
    osteoblastic
    osteoid
    papilloma
    parasagittal
    parasellar
    parietal lobe
    parosteal osteoma
    parosteal sarcoma
    perineurial fibroblastoma
    peripheral nerve
    peripheral nerve sheath
    peripheral neuroectodermal
    pilocytic
    pineal gland
    pinealoma
    pineal region
    pituitary gland

tumor *(continued)*
   pituitary microadenoma
   plantar malignant melanoma
   plasma cell myeloma
   pleomorphic hyalinized angiectatic
   pontine glioma
   poorly differentiated
   posterior fossa epidermoid
   posterior lobe
   Pott puffy
   primary brain
   primary sarcoma
   primitive neuroectodermal (PNET)
   prolactin-secreting adenoma
   pseudomalignant, nonneoplastic
   osseous soft tissue
   radiosensitive
   round cell
   sacrococcygeal remnant
   sarcomatous
   Schwann cell
   secondary brain
   seeding of
   sellar
   skull-base
   solid
   solitary brain
   sphenoid ridge
   spinal cord
   spread of
   subfrontal meningioma
   subtotal removal of
   subungual
   subungual amelanotic melanoma
   suprasellar extension of
   supratentorial brain
   temporal lobe
   third ventricle
   triton
   vascular hamartoma
   von Hippel
   well-circumscribed
tumoral calcinosis
tumor-bearing bone
tumor bed
tumor blush on cerebral angiography
tumor boundary

tumor cleavage plane
tumor debulking
tumor exophyte
tumor extirpation
tumor margin
tumor marker
tumor mass
tumor matrix
tumor necrosis factor (TNF)
tumor necrosis factor alpha (TNF-a)
tumor of epiconus of spinal cord
tumor of infundibulum
tumor psyche
tumor resection
tumor rest
tumor staining on cerebral
   angiography
tumor suppressor NF2 (merlin/
   schwannomin)
tumor to normal brain ratio
tumor volume
tumor volumetry
tuning
tunnel
   carpal
   cubital
   fascial
   fibro-osseous
   Guyon
   tarsal
   tibial
tunneler
   Anderson tendon
   Gude
Tunneloc bone-mulch screw
tunnel posterior cruciate ligament
   reconstruction technique
tunnel view
tunnel vision
Tuohy lumbar puncture needle
Tupper arthroplasty
Tupper hand-holder and retractor
turbinate bone
turbo-whisker
turcica, sella
Türck degeneration
Turco clubfoot operation

Turco posteromedial release operation
Turco repair of talipes equinovarus
Turcot syndrome
turf-toe
Turkel bone biopsy trephine
turkey-claw instrument
turnbuckle distractor
turnbuckle functional position splint
turned-down tendon flap
Turner marginal gyrus
turnip planter's palsy
turn test
"turn-up" plasty
turricephaly
Turvy internal screw fixation
Turyn sign
Tutofix cortical pin
Tutoplast tissue preservation process
Tuwave (programmed waveform
    TENS treatment)
Tuxedo cervical collar
twelfth cranial nerve (hypoglossal
    nerve)
21-channel EEG (electroencephalo-
    gram)
twig
    arterial
    muscular
    nerve
twilight state
Twisk surgical instruments
twisted sponge
twister (pl. twisters)
    Batzdorf cervical wire
    cable
    Cooley-Baumgarten wire
    orthotic
    wire
twitch, twitching
    facial
    focal
    involuntary
    muscle
    rhythmical

twitching of extremities
two-bellied muscle
two-bundle anterior cruciate ligament
    reconstruction
two-part Apley test
two-part fracture
two-plane alignment
two-point discrimination test
two-poster cervical orthosis
two-quarter test
two-sleeve technique
two-stage opposition transfer
two-strand suture
two-strut tibial graft technique
T wrench
Tycron suture
tylectomy
Tyler-Gigli saw
Tylok high-tension cerclage cabling
    system
tylosis
tympanic bone
tympani, chorda
tympanic membrane
tympanic nerve
typhoid osteomyelitis
typhoid spondylitis
Tyndall effect
typhus, murine (meningoencephalitis)
tyramine diet
tyramine reaction (to cheese, red
    wine)
Tyrell hook
tyrosinemia, neonatal

U, u

U approach
UBC (University of British Columbia)
   brace
UBP (universal bone plate) system,
   Haid
UCB (unilateral calcaneal brace)
UCB foot orthosis
UCBL (University of California
   Berkeley Laboratory) orthosis
UCBL (University of California
   Biomechanics Lab) orthosis
UCBL foot orthosis
UCB shoe insert
UCI (University of California, Irvine)
UCI ankle prosthesis
UCL (ulnar collateral ligament)
UCLA (University of California,
   Los Angeles)
UCLA anatomic shoulder arthroplasty
UCLA rating scale
UCP compression plate
U-drape
UE (*Ulex europaeus*) antibody
UE lectins
UE (upper extremity)
Uematsu shoulder arthrodesis
UHMWPe (ultrahigh molecular weight
   polyethylene)

Uhthoff phenomenon
Uhthoff sign
Uhthoff syndrome
UJ (uncovertebral joint)
UKA (unicompartmental knee arthroplasty)
ulcer
   decubitus
   ischemic foot
   mal perforant diabetic
   stasis
   trophic
ulceration
   neuropathic
   venous
   chronic leg
   neuropathic
   periulcer venous channels in
   venous stasis
ulcer osteoma
Ulco brand devices and instruments
Ulcus, Comfeel (occlusive dressing)
Ulex europaeus (UE) antibody
Ullman line
ulna
ulnar abutment syndrome
ulnar bone
ulnar bursa

ulnar collateral ligament of elbow
ulnar crease of hand
ulnar deviation of hand
ulnar dimelia
ulnar drift
ulnar extensor muscle
ulnar flexor muscle
ulnar grind test
ulnar impaction syndrome
ulnar nerve entrapment
ulnar nerve palsy
ulnar nerve paralysis
ulnar notch
ulnar palsy
ulnar pulse
ulnar seat
ulnar sesamoid bone
ulnar styloid impaction syndrome
ulnar styloid process
ulnar synovial recess
ulnar translocation
ulnar tubercle
ulnar variance
ulnarward
ulnocarpal arthrodesis
ulnocarpal impaction syndrome
ulnocarpal ligament
ulnoligamentous articulation
ulnolunate ligament
ulnotriquetral ligament
Ulrich bone-holding clamp
Ulrich bone-holding forceps
Ulrich-St. Gallen forceps
Ulson fixator system
Ultima C femoral component
Ultimax distal femoral intramedullary
    rod system
Ultrabrace knee orthosis
Ultra-Cut instruments
Ultra-Drive bone cement removal
    system
UltraFix MicroMite suture anchor
Ultra-Flex orthopedic bed
ultrahigh molecular weight poly-
    ethylene (UHMWPe)
UltraLite flow-directed microcatheter
Ultram (tramadol HCl)

UltraSafe anti-needlestick guard
UltraSafe injection system
UltraSafe syringe
Ultra-Sling abduction device
ultrasonic aspiration
ultrasonic assessment
ultrasonication
ultrasonography
    B-mode
    cranial
    CUSALap
    duplex carotid
    pulsed
    Sonicator portable
    therapeutic
    transcranial Doppler (TCD)
ultrasound (US)
    duplex
    Intelect Legend
    low-intensity pulsed
    Mettler
    transcranial Doppler
ultrasound-guided stereotactic biopsy
ultrasound scanning, high-resolution
ultrasound therapy
ultrastructural changes in wound
    healing
Ultra ultrasonic aspirator
Ultra-X external fixation system
ULTT (upper limb tension test)
U Luque vertebral rod
umbilical ligament
UMN (upper motor neuron)
unbalanced wrist syndrome in cerebral
    palsy
uncal gyrus
uncal herniation syndrome
unciform bone
uncinate aura
uncinate gyrus
uncinate processes
uncinate region of temporal lobe
uncinate seizure
uncommitted metaphyseal lesion
unconscious
unconsciousness
unconstrained elbow devices

unconstrained knee prostheses
uncotomy
uncovertebral joint (UJ)
uncovertebral spondylosis
uncovertebral spurring
uncus, arachnoid of
uncus of hamate bone
uncus of temporal lobe
undercorrection
under direct vision
understanding of similarities test
undersurface of patella
undifferentiated oligoarthritis
undisplaced fracture
undisputed axonopathic neurogenic
    thoracic outlet syndrome
undyed suture
unequivocal diplopia
unexplained drowsiness
unfractionated heparin
unfused physis
ungual tuberosity
ungual tuft
unguicular tuberosity
Unhappy Triad of O'Donoghue
unheralded stroke
uniaxial joint
unicameral bone cyst
unicameral brain
unicompartmental knee arthroplasty
    (UKA)
unicompartmental knee prosthesis
Unicondylar Geomedic Hemi-Knee
    system
unicoronal synostosis
unicortical screw
unidirectional instability
Unidose drug delivery system
Unified Huntington's Disease Rating
    Scale
Unified Parkinson's Disease Rating
    Scale
Unifix, Ace
Uniflex intramedullary nail
uniformly progressive deterioration
Unilab Surgibone bone replacement
    material

unilateral Babinski sign
unilateral carotid artery occlusion
unilateral carotid stenosis
unilateral enophthalmos
unilateral facial weakness
unilateral focus of EEG activity
unilateral fragmentation of apophysi
unilateral hallux valgus (HV)
unilateral hyperreflexia
unilateral lesion of the cerebellum
unilaterally fixed, dilated pupil
unilaterally upgoing toe
unilateral neglect, organic
unilateral paralysis
unilateral posteroventral pallidotomy
unilateral Raynaud phenomenon
unilateral seizure
unilateral S1 radiculopathy
unilateral spastic leg
unilateral supranuclear disease
unilateral thalamic-stimulating
    electrode implantation
unilateral visual neglect
Unilink system
unilocular joint
uninhibited ankle motion
uninhibited flexion
union
    bony
    delayed
    delayed fracture
    faulty
    fibrous
    osseous
    secondary
    vicious
union of fracture fragments
unipennate muscle
UniPuls electrostimulation instrument
UNI-SHUNT hydrocephalus shunt
unit
    AME microcurrent TENS
    Autoflex continuous passive motion
        (CPM)
    Bovie coagulating
    Cadwell 5200A somatosensory
        evoked potential

unit *(continued)*
  CPM (continuous passive motion)
  Cybex Torso Rotation Testing and
    Rehabilitation
  Dial Away Pain 400 electrotherapy
  diathermy
  Eclipse TENS
  gamma
  gravity traction
  Hounsfield
  Hydra-Cadence gait-control
  intermittent compression
  Leksell gamma
  linear accelerator
  Magnatherm diathermy
  Maxima II TENS
  musculotendinous
  neurological intensive care (NICU)
  neurological critical care (NCCU)
  postanesthesia care (PACU)
  Sheffield gamma
  TENS (transcutaneous electrical
    nerve stimulation)
  Wright Care TENS
Unitek steel crown
univalve cast
univalved
Universal drill point
Universal fixation screws
universal force-movement sensor
Universal hip prosthesis
universal proximal femur (UPF)
  prosthesis
Universal sling and swathe shoulder
  immobilizer
universal tri-panel knee immobilizer
University of California Berkeley
  Laboratory (UCBL) orthosis
University of California Biomechanics
  Lab (UCBL) orthosis
University of Florida LINAC (linear
  accelerator)
unkempt appearance
unleveling, pelvic
unloader brace
unmasking of silent inputs
unmethylated allele

unmyelinated nerve
unmyelinated nerve fibers
Unna boot
Unna boot cast
Unna boot wrap
Unna paste
unopposed
unplicated sheaths
unreactive pupils
unresponsive state
unresponsive to environment
unresponsiveness, psychogenic
unroof
unroofing of nerve
unshunted hydrocephalus
unstable fracture
unsteadiness of gait and station
unstriated muscle
unstriped muscle
unsustained clonus
untether
Unverricht disease
Unverricht-Lafora disease
Unverricht-Lundborg disease
Unverricht-Lundborg myoclonus
  epilepsy
Unverricht-Lundborg syndrome
Unverricht syndrome
unvoiced speech
unwinding of collagen triple helix
U1-L1 cephalometric measurement
U1-NA cephalometric measurement
upbeat (upbeating) nystagmus, coarse
UPDRS (United Parkinson's Disease
  Rating Scale)
UPF prosthesis (universal proximal
  femur)
upgaze, conjugate
upgoing toes
Upledger CST (craniosacral therapy)
upper extremity (UE)
upper jaw bone
upper lateral cutaneous nerve of arm
upper limb tension test (ULTT)
upper limits of normal
upper median palsy
upper motor neuron (UMN) disease

upper motor neuron impairment
upper motor neuron paralysis
upper motor neuron sign
upper motor neuron symptoms
Upper 7 head halter
upper subscapular nerve
upper thoracic splanchnic nerves
UPPP (uvulopalatopharyngoplasty)
upright skeletal radiography
uptake, radioisotope
upward and backward dislocation
upward retraction
urachal ligament
urarthritis
urate crystal
uremic amaurosis
uremic aseptic meningitis
uremic encephalopathy
uric acid crystal
urinary incontinence
urinary or fecal incontinence
urodynamic testing
urogenital diaphragm, muscles of
Urschel first rib rongeur

urticaria
U.S. Army bone chisel
U.S. Army gouge
U.S. Army osteotome
U.S. Army retractor
useless hand syndrome
U-shaped incision
U-shaped retractor
Uslenghi plate
Utah artificial arm
utensil
  Good Grips
  one-handed kitchen
  Spork
utricle
utricular nerve
utriculoampullar nerve
utriculus
uveitis, juxtapapillary
uveomeningoencephalic syndrome
uveomeningoencephalitis
uvula, cerebellar
uvulopalatopharyngoplasty (UPPP)
U wrench

V, v

vacant glenoid cavity sign
vaccine
  allogeneic cytokine-secreting
    cellular
  AnervaX
  duck embryo
Vac-Lok immobilization cushion
Vac-Pac pad
Vacu-Mix cement pump
vacuo, hydrocephalus ex
vacuolation of ganglion cells
vacuum cement mix technique
vacuum cleft
vacuum disk
vacuum, facet joint
vacuum headache
vacuum joint phenomenon
VAD (voluntary anterior drawer) sign
vagal attack
vagal dysarthria
vagal nerve implant
vagal rhizotomy
vaginal ligament
vaginal nerve
vagoglossopharyngeal neuralgia
vagus nerve (tenth cranial nerve)
vagus nerve stimulation (VNS)

vagus trunk
Vainio arthroplasty
Vairox high compression vascular
  stocking
Valenti arthroplasty
Valentine splint
Valentin nerve
Valeo CTS support
valgisation
valgus
  adolescent hallux
  hallux (HV)
  hindfoot
  metatarsus
  pes
  talipes
valgus carrying angle
valgus deformity
valgus foot
valgus fracture, impacted
valgus heel
valgus hindfoot
valgus index
valgus insert
valgus instability
valgus stress
valgus stress test

valgus tilt
validity of rehabilitation testing
  construct
  content
  criterion-related
  ecological
  face
Valin hemilaminectomy retractor
Valium (diazepam)
Valleix sign
Valls hip prosthesis
Valpar component work sample series
valproate sodium injection (Depacon)
Valsalva maneuver
Valsalva muscle
valsalva'd (slang)
value
  absolute band
  absolute perfusion
  attenuation
  relative band
valve
  anti-siphon
  Codman-Medos nonprogrammable
  Codman slit
  Cordis Orbis Sigman shunt
  differential-pressure
  dual-chamber flushing
  Equi-Flow hydrocephalus
  flushing
  Heyer-Schulte bur hole
  Heyer-Schulte in-line
  Heyer-Schulte low-profile
  low-profile
  Medtronic Delta pressure
  Medtronic PS Medical Delta
    flow-control
  Mishler flush
  Orbis-Sigma pressure
  pressure-sensitive shunt tube
  Pudenz flushing
  Sophy programmable pressure
vamp of shoe
van Bogaert encephalitis
van Bogaert leukoencephalitis
Van Beck nerve approximator

Van Buren sequestrum forceps
Vandenbos and Bowers procedure
Vanderbilt Pain Management
  Inventory
V-angle, femoral torsion
Vanghetti prosthesis
Van Ness procedure
Vanzetti sign
vapocoolant
Vapr electrohemostat
Vapr T electrode
vara, tibia
variable screw placement (VSP)
variance, ulnar
VariAnchor spinal implant device
Varian LINAC (linear accelerator)
variant
  anatomic
  fast alpha
  labrum
  ossification
  petit mal
  slow alpha
variation, phenotype
varicella-zoster (VZ) virus
varicella zoster encephalomyelitis
varicosities, superficial
VariFix spinal implant device
VariGrip spinal implant device
Varikopf hip prosthesis
VariLift spinal cage
VariLink spinal implant device
Vari-weights
varix (pl. varices), cerebral
Varney acromioclavicular brace
Varney pin
Varni Pediatric Pain Questionnaire
varum, genu
varus
  metatarsus
  rearfoot
  subtalar
  talipes
  tibial
varus angle
varus deformity

varus heel
varus metatarsophalangeal (MTP)
  angle
varus tilt
varus-valgus adjustment screw
varus-valgus instability
varus/valgus loading interface
varus-valgus stability
VAS (vestibular aqueduct syndrome)
VAS (visual analog score/visual
  analogic scale) for pain
Vascufil suture
vascular accident
vascular anomaly
vascular blush of tumor
vascular cell adhesion molecule-1
  (VCAM-1)
vascular claudication
vascular cord damage
vascular hamartoma
vascular invasion
vascularity, tumor
vascular metaphyseal bone
vascular nerve
vascular occlusion
vascular supply
vascular territory
vasculitic mononeuritis multiplex
vasculitis
  giant cell
  rheumatoid
  Takayasu
  temporal
vasculopathy, cerebral
VASHD (Visual Analog Scale of
  Handicap)
VA shunt (ventriculoatrial)
vasoconstrictor nerve
vasocoolant sprays
vasodepressor syncope
vasodilator, antidromic
vasodilator nerve
vasodilatory challenge
vasomotor changes
vasomotor headache
vasomotor instability
vasomotor nerve

vasopneumatic compression
vasopneumatic treatment
vasosensory nerve
vasospasm
  cerebral
  symptomatic
vasospastic attacks
vasovagal reflex
vasovagal syncope
VASS (video-assisted spine surgery)
Vastamaki paralysis
vastus intermedius muscle
vastus lateralis muscle
vastus medialis advancement (VMA)
vastus medialis muscle
vastus medialis obliquus (VMO)
vastus-splitting approach
Vater-Pacini bodies
VATER syndrome
  V   vertebral abnormality
  A   anal imperforation
  TE   tracheoesophageal fistula
  R   radial, ray, or renal anomaly
Vaughn-Jackson sign
vault
  cranial
  occipital
  plantar
VBI (vertebrobasilar insufficiency)
V blade plate
VCAM (circulating vascular adhesion
  molecule)
VCAM-1 (vascular cell adhesion
  moledule-1)
V capsulotomy
VCS clip adapter
VD (video densitometry)
VDRL (Venereal Disease Research
  Laboratory)
VDS (ventral derotating spinal)
VDS compression rod
VDS hex nut
VDS screw
VDS screwdriver
VDS wrench
VE (vocational evaluation)
vector

vectored adjustment
VEDA (Vestibular Disorders
   Association)
vegetative patient
vegetative state
vehicle, all-terrain (ATV)
vehicular accident
vein
   aneurysmal
   anterior terminal (ATV)
   basal vein of Rosenthal (BVR)
   bridging
   bulb of internal jugular
   common facial
   diploic
   external jugular
   Galen cerebral
   great cerebral vein of Galen
   internal cerebral (ICV)
   intussusception of
   jugular
   Labbe
   medullary
   meningeal
   palmar cutaneous
   petrosal
   posterior terminal (PTV)
   Rosenthal basal
   saphenous
   Schlesinger
   septal
   subependymal
   thalamostriate
   vermian bridging
Velcro fitting
Velcro immobilizer
Velcro splint
Velcro strap
Veleanu-Rosianu-Ionescu technique
Veley neurosurgical headrest
velocimetry, laser Doppler
velocity
   free-walking
   mean flow
   motor conduction
   motor nerve conduction (MNCV)
   muzzle v. in handgun injury

velocity *(continued)*
   nerve conduction (NCV)
   orthodromic
   peak height
   push-off
   saccade
   sensory conduction
   sensory nerve conduction (SNCV)
velocity encoding
Velpeau bandage
Velpeau cast
Velpeau dressing
Velpeau plaster
Velpeau shoulder immobilizer
Velpeau shoulder sling
velum
Venable plate
Venable-Stuck nail
Venable-Stuck pin
Venable-Stuck screw
vena comitans (pl. venae comitantes)
Venezuelan equine viral encephalitis
venlafaxine hydrochloride (Effexor
   XR) extended-release capsules
Venodyne boot
venography
   epidural
   intraosseous
   vertebral
venous ligament
venous line
venous malformation hemorrhage
venous plexus
venous pump of the foot
venous reflux
venous stasis retinopathy
venous stasis ulcers
venous thromboembolic disease
   (VTED)
venous ulceration
ventilation, mechanical
ventilation-perfusion lung scan
ventral cochlear nucleus
ventralis intermedius thalamic nucleus
ventral sacrococcygeal ligament
ventral sacrococcygeal muscle
ventral sacroiliac ligament

ventral spinocerebellar tract
ventral spinothalamic tract
ventral surface
ventricle
  absent
  atrium of
  ballooned floor of
  cerebral
  compensatory enlargement of
  dilatation of the
  dilated
  effacement of
  elongation of
  enlarged
  enlargement of
  floor of
  fourth
  frontal horn of lateral
  lateral
  loculate
  outflow of
  papilloma of the fourth
  roof of
  shift of the
  single large
  sixth
  slit
  temporal horn of lateral
  third
  tiny
  trigone of lateral
  Verga
ventricles of brain
ventricular cannula, Ford Hospital
ventricular collapse
ventricular dilatation
ventricular drain
ventricular drainage
ventricular enlargement
ventricular intracerebral hemorrhage
ventricular ligament
ventricular reservoir
ventricular right-handedness
ventricular shift
ventricular size
ventricular space
ventricular span

ventricular system
ventricular tap
ventricular wall
ventriculitis
ventriculoatrial (VA) shunt
ventriculogram
ventriculography
  intraoperative
  metrizamide
ventriculomegaly
ventriculoperitoneal (VP)
ventriculoperitoneal drain
ventriculoperitoneal shunt
ventriculoscope
ventriculostomy
ventriculovenous shunt
ventrolateral thalamic sensory nuclei
ventrolateral thalamotomy
VEP (visual evoked potential)
VER (visual evoked response)
verbal (or semantic) paraphasia
verbal command
verbal fluency
verbal learning and recall
verbally-mediated functions
verbigeration
Verbrugge bone-holding forceps
Verbrugge clamp
Verbrugge forceps
Verbrugge-Hohmann bone retractor
Verbrugge needle
Verdan technique
Verebelyi-Ogston decancellation
  procedure
Veress needle
Verga ventricle
vergence, downward
Veri-Sketch device
vermian bridging veins
vermian infarction
vermian medulloblastoma
vermian veins
vermicular movements
vermiform
vermis (midline cerebellum)
  cerebellar
  dysgenesis of

vermis *(continued)*
  folium
  hypoplastic
  superior
  tuber
  uvula of
Vermont spinal fixator (VSF)
Vernet syndrome
Verneuil neuroma
Vernier calipers
Verocay body
verruca
  mosaic plantar
  single plantar
verruca plantaris
Versa-Fx femoral fixation system
Versalok low-back fixation system
VersaPulse holmium laser
VersaTack stapler
Versatrac lumbar retractor system
VersaWrist wrist splint
version, internal and external
Versi-Splint
versive seizure
vertebra (pl. vertebrae)
  arch of
  articular process of
  basilar
  caudal
  cervical (C1-C7)
  coccygeal
  codfish
  cranial
  displaced
  dorsal (D)
  facet surface of
  false
  fractured
  fused
  last normal (LNV)
  lumbar (L1-L5)
  midbody of
  olisthetic
  pear-shaped
  sacral (S1-S5)
  scalloping of
  subluxed

vertebra *(continued)*
  thoracic (T1-T12)
  transitional
  transverse process of
  true
  wedging of olisthetic
vertebral ankylosis
vertebral arterial dissection
vertebral artery dissection
vertebral artery endarterectomy
vertebral artery occlusion
vertebral artery stenosis
vertebral artery syndrome
vertebral artery system
vertebral artery testing
vertebral-basilar artery syndrome
vertebral basilar insufficiency
vertebral-basilar ischemia
vertebral body collapse
vertebral body endplate
vertebral body impactor
vertebral collapse
vertebral column
vertebral endarterectomy
vertebral endplate
vertebral nerve
vertebral notch
vertebral pleural reflection
vertebral scalloping
vertebral segmentation anomaly
vertebral steal phenomenon
vertebral steal syndrome
vertebral stripe
vertebral system of veins
vertebral vein
vertebral venous plexus
vertebral wedging
vertebra plana fracture
vertebrectomy
  Bohlman anterior cervical
  cervical
  subtotal
vertebrobasilar circulation
vertebrobasilar disease
vertebrobasilar distribution stroke
vertebrobasilar insufficiency (VBI)
vertebrobasilar ischemia

vertebrobasilar occlusion
vertebrobasilar system
vertebrobasilar territory ischemia
vertebrocostal rib
vertebropelvic ligament
vertebrophrenic angle
vertebroplasty, percutaneous
vertebrosternal rib
Vertetrac ambulatory traction system
vertex of cranium
vertical fracture
vertical laminar air flow
vertical loop suture technique for
    meniscal repair
vertical muscle of tongue
vertical nystagmus
vertical sagittal split osteotomy (VSO)
vertical shear fracture
vertical talus (rockerbottom flatfoot)
vertiginous seizure
vertiginous sensation
vertigo
    benign functional
    benign paroxysmal
    benign paroxysmal positional
    cervical
    disabling
    episodic
    labyrinthine
    motion-induced
    objective
    ocular
    paroxysmal
    positional
    post-traumatic
    postural
    proprioceptive
    psychogenic
    reversible
    rotational
    subjective
    transient
    true
    visual
vesalianum of vertebral body
Vesalius bone

Vesely-Street nail
Vesely-Street splint
vesical paralysis as response to spinal
    injury
vesicle, pinocytotic
vesicoumbilical ligament
vesicouterine ligament
vessel
    collateral
    feeding
    moyamoya
    parent
    perforator
    pial
vessel encasement
vest
    Bremer AirFlo halo
    halo
    Minerva
    OrthoTrac pneumatic
    Vitrathene
vestibular apparatus
vestibular aqueduct syndrome (VAS)
vestibular canal
vestibular compensation
Vestibular Disorders Association
    (VEDA)
vestibular division of the eighth cranial
    nerve
vestibular end-organ nystagmus
vestibular enhancement exercise
vestibular hypofunction
vestibular ligament
vestibular nerve disorder
vestibular neurectomy
vestibular neuritis
vestibular neuronitis
    inferior
    lateral (Deiter)
    medial
    principal (Schwalbe)
    spinal
    superior (Von Bechterew)
vestibular nucleus
vestibular nystagmus
vestibular oculocephalic response

vestibular rehabilitation
vestibular schwannoma
vestibular suppressant
vestibulocerebellar ataxia
vestibulocochlear nerve
vestibulocochlear nucleus
vestibulogenic epilepsy
vestibulo-ocular maneuver
vestibulo-ocular reflex (VOR)
vestibulospinal reflex
vestibulospinal tract
vestigial commissure
vest-over-pants technique
veterinary approach
VGCC (voltage-gated calcium
    channel)
VHL (von Hippel-Lindau) disease
VHTS (volumetric hyperthermia
    treatment system)
viability, flap
Vibram rockerbottom shoe
Vibramycin (doxycycline)
vibration perception
vibration sensation
vibration sense
vibration sensitivity
vibration syndrome
vibratome
vibratory sense
vibratory threshold
Vibrio fetus meningitis
Vickers needle holder
VICON three-dimensional gait analysis
    system
Vicoprofen (hydrocodone and
    ibuprofen)
Vicq d'Azyr
    band of
    stripe of
Vicryl figure-of-8 suture
Vicryl Rapide suture
Vicryl suture
Victorian brace
Vidal-Adrey modified Hoffmann
    device
video-assisted spine surgery (VASS)

video densitometry (VD)
video-EEG monitoring and split-screen
    recording
videofluoroscopy
vidian nerve neuralgia
Vidicon vacuum chamber pickup tube
Vi-Drape
Vieussens
    annulus of
    ansa of
    circle of
    isthmus of
    limbus of
    loop of
    ring of
    valve of
view (see also *position, projection*)
    abdominal
    anterior
    AP (anteroposterior)
    apical
    apical lordotic
    AP supine
    axial sesamoid
    axillary
    baseline
    Beath
    Boehler calcaneal (Böhler)
    Boehler lumbosacral
    Breuerton
    Broden x-ray
    brow-down skull
    brow-up skull
    Bucky
    carpal tunnel
    Carter-Rowe
    cine
    clenched fist
    close-up
    coalition
    cone
    coned-down
    cranial angled
    craniocaudad, craniocaudal
    cross-table
    CTLV (cross-table lateral view)

view *(continued)*
  decubitus
  dens (cervical spine)
  dorsiflexion
  dorsoplantar
  Dunlop-Shands
  dynamic stress x-ray
  erect
  FCS (full cervical spine)
  Ferguson
  flexion
  fluoroscopic stress x-ray
  frogleg lateral
  frontal
  full length
  Harris
  Harris-Beath axial hindfoot
  hemiaxial
  hepatoclavicular
  hip-to-ankle
  Hobb
  Hughston
  infrapatellar view of knees
  intraoperative
  inversion ankle stress
  Jones
  Judet radius
  Knuttsen bending
  LAO (left anterior oblique)
  lateral
  lateral anterior drawer stress
  lateral bending
  lateral decubitus
  lateral oblique
  lateral tilt stress ankle
  limited
  long axial oblique
  long axis
  long-axis parasternal
  lordotic
  mediolateral
  mediolateral oblique
  Merchant
  mortise
  multiplanar fluoroscopic stress
  navicular
  Neer lateral

view *(continued)*
  Neer transscapular
  no-angulation
  nonstanding lateral oblique
  nonweightbearing
  notch
  oblique
  occipital
  odontoid
  open-mouth odontoid
  orthogonal
  outlet
  overhead
  overhead oblique
  PA (posteroanterior)
  parasternal long-axis
  parasternal short-axis
  patellar skyline
  plain
  planar
  plantar axial
  plantarflexion
  plantarflexion stress
  portable
  postoperative
  preliminary
  preoperative
  prereduction
  prone
  prone lateral
  Puddu
  push-pull ankle stress
  push-pull hip
  RAO (right anterior oblique)
  recumbent
  right lateral decubitus
  routine magnification
  Schüller
  serendipity
  short-axis
  short-axis parasternal
  ski-jump
  skyline
  spot
  standing dorsoplantar
  standing lateral
  standing weightbearing

view *(continued)*
   steep LAO (left anterior oblique)
   Stenver
   stress
   stress Broden
   stress eversion
   stress inversion
   Stryker notch
   submental vertex
   submentovertex
   subxiphoid
   sunrise
   sunset
   supine
   supine full
   suprasternal notch
   swimmer's
   tangential
   tangential scapular
   tomographic
   true lateral
   tunnel
   two-plane
   upright
   von Rosen
   Waters
   weightbearing
   weightbearing dorsoplantar
   West Point
   White leg-length
   x-ray
Viewing Wand surgical digitizer
vigilance (concentration)
vigil, coma
Vigilon dressing
Vigorimeter, Martin
Villaret-Mackenzie syndrome
villi, arachnoidal
villonodular synovitis
villous proliferation
villous synovitis
villus formation in rheumatoid arthritis
VIM (ventral intermedius nucleus)
   stimulation
vimentin antibody
vimentin immunostain
vincristine (Oncovin)

Vinertia implant metal
Vinke skull traction tongs
Vinke tongs
Vioxx (rofecoxib)
viral encephalitis (pl. encephalitides)
viral envelope protein
viral intracerebral arteritis
viral leukoencephalitis
Virchow law of skull growth
Virchow-Robin spaces of the brain
Vironostika blood-screening test
virtual endoscopy
Virtullene brace material
virus
   coxsackievirus A16
   ECHO (enteric cytopathic human
     orphan)
   encephalitis
   Epstein-Barr (EBV)
   herpes zoster
   SV-40
   varicella-zoster (VZ)
virus infection, slow
visceral muscle
visceral nerve
visceral tendon sheath layer
viscerosomatic reflexes
viscoelastic action
viscoelastic insole
viscoelastic property of muscles
viscoelastic stability
Viscoheel K heel cushion
Viscoheel K orthosis
Viscoheel N heel cushion
Viscoheel N orthosis
Viscoheel SofSpot heel cushion
Viscoheel SofSpot orthosis
Viscolas heel pain and disability
Viscolas orthotic
Viscoped Insole
Viscoped S support
ViscoSpot support
viscosupplementation
vise
   AlloGrip bone
   bone
   mechanic's pin

VISI (volarflexed intercalated segment
    instability) deformity
vision
    blurred
    blurring of
    cortical
    darkening of
    foveal
    hemifield of
    loss of
    sudden loss of
    tubular
    tunnel
vision disorder, cinematographic
visiospatial plane/planing
Visipaque (iodixanol)
Visiting Nurse Association (VNA)
visor, Georgiade
Vistec x-ray detectable sponge
visual acuity
    dynamic
    static
visual agnosia
visual amnesia
visual analog pain scale
Visual Analog Scale of Handicap
    (VASHD)
visual analog score (VAS)
visual blurring
visual cortex
visual deafferentiation
visual disturbance
visual epilepsy
visual evoked potential (VEP)
visual evoked response (VER)
visual field constriction
visual field cut
visual field defects
visual field disturbance
visual field test
visual impairment
visual learning and recall
visual memory
Visual Neglect Test
Visual Pattern Completion Test
visual prodrome
visual radiations

Visual Reproduction subtest
visual seizure
visual-spatial distortion
visual symptoms
visualized
visuospatial disorientation
Vitalock solid-back shell
Vitallium implant metal
Vitallium Küntscher nail
vitamin B_{12} deficiency
Vitox alumina ceramic material in
    prosthesis
Vitrathene vest
Vivalan (viloxazine)
Viva shoes
VJ (ventriculojugular) shunt
VMA (vastus medialis advancement)
V medullary nail
VMO (vastus medialis obliquus)
V nail plate
VNS (vagus nerve stimulation)
vocal ligament
vocal muscle
Vocare neuroprosthetic bladder system
vocational evaluation (VE)
vocational rehabilitation (VR)
Vogt disease
Vogt-Koyanagi-Harada syndrome
Vogue arm sling
volar angulation
volar capsule
volar carpal ligament
volarflexed intercalated segment
    instability (VISI)
volar flexion crease
volar intercalary wrist instability
volar interosseous nerve
volar ligament
volarly
volar synovial recess
volarward
volar wrist
volitional movement
volitional resisted flexion and
    extension
volitional saccade
Volkmann bone curet

Volkmann bone hook
Volkmann contracture
Volkmann deformity
Volkmann hook retractor
Volkmann ischemic contracture
Volkmann rake retractor
Volkov-Oganesian external fixation
voltage (on EEG)
   calibration
   high
   low
   medium
   very low
voltage-gated calcium channel
   (VGCC) protein
voltage-gated sodium channels
volume
   cerebrospinal fluid
   intracranial vascular
volume element (voxel)
volume imaging
volumetric hyperthermia treatment
   system (VHTS)
volumetric porosity
volumetric radiologic assessment of
   neuromas
voluntary hysterical overbreathing
voluntary anterior drawer (VAD) sign
voluntary muscle
voluntary posterior drawer (VPD) sign
Volz total wrist arthroplasty
Volz-Turner reattachment technique
Volz wrist prosthesis
vomer bone
vomiting, projectile
Vom Saal pin
von Bahr screw
von Bekhterev reflex
von Ebner glands
von Economo disease
von Economo encephalitis lethargica
von Economo influenza
von Eulenberg disease
Von Frey hair test of sensory loss

von Gierke disease
von Hippel-Lindau (VHL) disease
von Hippel tumor
von Lackum surcingle
von Lackum transection shift jacket
von Langenbeck periosteal elevator
von Mises stress
Von Recklinghausen disease (neurofibromatosis type 1)
von Recklinghausen syndrome
von Rosen cruciform splint
von Rosen view
von Schwann, law of
von Willebrand factor antigen
Voorhoeve disease
VOR (vestibulo-ocular reflex)
Voshell sign
Vostal classification of radial fracture
V osteotomy, Japas
voxel (volume element)
V phenomenon
VP (ventriculoperitoneal) shunt
VPL thalamic electrode (ventro-
   posterolateral)
VR (vocational rehabilitation)
VrE (varus extension) test
VS (ventriculosubarachnoid) shunt
VSF (Vermont spinal fixator)
VSF clamp
VSF fixation system
VSF rod
VSF screw
V-shaped fracture
V-shaped incision
V-shaped rotator cuff tear
VSO (vertical sagittal split osteotomy)
VSP (variable screw placement)
VSP fixation
VSP plate
VSP screw
VTED (venous thromboembolic
   disease)
Vulpian-Bernhardt spinal muscular
   atrophy

Vulpius Achilles tendon reconstruction
Vulpius-Compere gastrocnemius
　lengthening
Vulpius equinus deformity operation
V wave

V-Y advancement flap
V-Y plasty
V-Y quadricepsplasty
VZ (varicella-zoster) virus

W, w

Wada valve prosthesis
Waddell Chronic Back Pain Disability
  Index
Waddell sign
wadding
  cotton
  cotton sheet
waddle, duck
waddling gait
Wadsworth unconstrained elbow
  prosthesis
wafer distal ulna resection
wafer, Thera-Bite
Wagner classification of diabetic foot
  ulcers
Wagner classification of forefoot
  gangrene
Wagner distraction device
Wagner external fixator
Wagner fixer
Wagner frame
Wagner line
Wagner modification of Syme
  amputation
Wagner multiple K-wire osteosynthesis
Wagner retractor
Wagner-Schanz screw apparatus
Wagoner cervical technique

wagon-wheel fracture
Wagstaffe fracture
Wainwright plate
WAIS-R Block Design Test
waist of anatomical structure
waist of phalanx
waist of scaphoid
Wakefield Self-Assessment Depression
  Inventory
wakeful
wakefulness
  epochs of
  quiet
  resting
waking attacks (epilepsy)
waking frequency on EEG, dominant
Waldemar Link GmbH instruments/
  devices
Waldenström staging or classification
walk, walking (see *gait*)
  heel
  heel and toe
  nonweightbearing crutch
  toe
WalkAide system
walker
  Aircast pneumatic
  Cam Walker

walker *(continued)*
  Castaway ankle
  Castaway leg
  Charcot restraint orthotic (CROW)
  DH pressure relief
  four-point
  Guardian Red Dot
  Hi-Top foot/ankle
  ORLAU swivel
  Rolator
  rubber wedge
  swivel
Walker, Cam (leg or ankle brace)
Walker disk curet
Walker-Murdoch wrist sign
Walker ruptured disk curet
Walker-Sonix UBA 575+ ultrasound
walking aids
walking cast
walking components
  energy conservation
  progression
  standing stability
walking cycle
walking footprints classification
walking mechanics
walking, stance phase
walking tasks
"walking up the thighs" (Gowers sign)
walking without support
walking with support
wall
  aneurysmal
  cyst
  cystic
  ventricular
Walldius knee prosthesis
Wallenberg lateral medullary
  syndrome
wallerian degeneration
Wall stent biliary endoprosthesis
Walsh, protocol of
Walther oblique ligament
Walton cartilage clamp
Walton-Liston bone rongeur
Walton maneuver
Walton meniscus clamp

Walton-Ruskin bone rongeur
Walton-Ruskin forceps
Walton scissors
Walton wire-pulling forceps
Wangensteen needle holder
Ward periosteal elevator
Ward triangle
Warm 'n Form lumbosacral corset
Warm Springs brace
warmth, joint
WarmTouch patient warming system
Warner-Farber ankle fixation
  technique
Warren-Marshall classification
Warren White Achilles tendon-lengthening operation
wart
  mosaic plantar
  mother-daughter-type plantar
  satellite plantar
  single plantar
Wartenberg neurological pinwheel
Wartenberg reflex
Wartenberg sign
washboard effect on myelography in
  cervical spondylosis
washer
  oval
  resin
  slotted
  spiked
  toothed
Washerloc system
washing out of accumulated
  metabolites
Washington Heights-Inwood Genetic
  Study of Essential Tremor
  (WHIGET)
Washington regimen following tendon
  repair
wasp-tail deformity in Duchenne
  dystrophy
Wassel classification of thumb
  duplication
  type I (bifid distal phalanx)
  type II (duplicated distal phalanx)
  type III (bifid proximal phalanx)

Wassel *(continued)*
   type IV
   type V (bifid metacarpal)
   type VI (duplicated metacarpal)
   type VII (triphalangism)
Wasserstein fixation device
wasting
   hypothenar eminence
   muscle
   thenar eminence
wasting disease
Watanabe classification of discoid
   meniscus
Watco brace
Watco 2001 knee immobilizer
water, deionized sterile
water intoxication
water jet tissue cutter
Waterman osteotomy
water on the brain
waterpick
Water-Pik
watershed area of Achilles tendon
watershed infarct
watershed infarction
watershed area paresis
watershed areas between main arterial
   territories
water signal on MRI scan
Waters x-ray view
Watkins fusion technique
Watson-Cheyne technique
Watson-Jones ankle tenodesis
Watson-Jones approach
Watson-Jones bone gouge
Watson-Jones classification of spinal
   fractures
Watson-Jones fracture repair
Watson-Jones navicular fracture
Watson-Jones tenodesis
Watson matched resection technique
Watson test
Watson-Williams intervertebral disk
   rongeur
Waugh ankle prosthesis

Waugh knee prosthesis
wave
   A
   alpha
   alpha spindles
   amplitude of
   anterior predominance of
   aperiodic
   apiculate
   arch-shaped
   arrhythmical repetitive
   asymmetric
   asynchronous
   asynchronous delta
   asynchronous slow
   B
   beta spindles
   bilateral
   bilaterally synchronous
   bilaterally synchronous slow
   biparietal hump
   biphasic
   bisynchronous
   bisynchronous delta
   bisynchronous slow
   brain
   bursts of delta
   bursts of theta
   C
   centroparietal slow
   cerebrospinal fluid
   clipping of
   complex of EEG
   cone
   configuration of
   contoured
   delta
   diphasic
   distribution of
   duration of
   EEG
   epileptiform
   F
   fast
   flattened top of EEG

wave *(continued)*
  focal sharp
  focal slow
  frequency of
  frontal sharp
  frontocentral slow
  generalized asynchronous slow
  generalized fast
  generalized slow
  harmonics of
  high-amplitude
  ictal focal slow
  in-phase
  independent
  interictal focal epileptiform
  interictal focal slow
  interictal generalized epileptiform
  interictal paroxysmal sharp
  interictal paroxysmal spike
  intermittent temporal slow
  intracranial pressure B
  irregular
  lambda
  lambdoid
  larval spike-and-slow
  local ictal slow
  local slow
  localized
  low-amplitude
  low-voltage
  M
  monomorphic
  monophasic
  monorhythmic
  monorhythmic frontal delta (MFD)
  morphology of
  O
  occipital
  out-of-phase
  paroxysmal rhythmical
  peak of
  periodic
  periodic generalized sharp
  periodic slow
  persistence of
  phase-reversing slow
  plateau

wave *(continued)*
  polarity of
  polymorphic
  polyphasic
  polyrhythmic
  positive occipital spike-like sleep
  positive sharp
  posterior predominance of
  postictal bisynchronous slow
  pulse volume
  quadriphasic
  quasiperiodic
  regularity of
  repetitive
  rhythmical
  rhythmical repetitive
  rhythmical slow
  rhythmicity of
  rolandic sharp
  saw-tooth
  saw-toothed
  shape of
  sharp
  sharply contoured
  shut eye
  simultaneous
  sine
  sinusoidal
  slow
  spike-like
  sporadic
  sporadic generalized slow
  spread of
  symmetry of
  synchronous
  synchrony of
  systolic pressure
  temporal predominance of
  theta
  topography of
  trains of
  Traube-Hering-Mayer cerebrospinal
    fluid
  triangular
  triphasic
  troughs of
  unilateral

wave *(continued)*
  V
  vertex
  very slow
wave discharge on EEG
waveform amplitude
waveform, SSEP
waveform superimposed on waveform
wavelength
waves of youth, posterior slow
wax, bone
waxy flexibility
Wayfarer modifiable foot prosthesis
Wayne laminectomy seat
Ways of Coping Checklist
WBAT (weightbearing as tolerated)
WBCS (white blood cell scintigraphy)
  with indium-111
W/C (wheelchair)
WCh (wheelchair)
WCS (Wisconsin Compression
  System)
WDE (wound dressing emulsion)
weakness
  asymmetric
  breakaway
  central origin
  facial movement
  flaccid
  focal
  hemifacial
  infranuclear
  left-sided
  motor
  myopathic
  nuclear
  central origin
  peripheral origin
  progressive
  proximal
  right-sided
  supranuclear
  Todd motor
  unilateral facial
  upper motor neuron

weakness of one side of face
  central origin
  peripheral origin
wear-and-tear
wearing-off effect of L-dopa in
  parkinsonism
wear-resistant surface
Weary brain spatula
Weary cordotomy knives
Weary nerve hook
Weary nerve root retractor
weather-ache
Weaveknit vascular prosthesis
weave, Pulver-Taft
Weaver-Dunn acromioclavicular
  technique
weaver's bottom
web
  finger
  thumb
web-area of hand
Webb-Andreesen condylar bolt
webbed toes
webbing of fingers
web-border of hand
Webb stove bolt
web creep
Weber-Brunner-Freuler-Boitzy
  technique
Weber, circle of
Weber esthesiometer
Weber fracture (A-C)
Weber paralysis
Weber sign
Weber syndrome
Weber two-point discrimination test
Weber-Vasey traction-absorption
  wiring technique
Webril bandage
Webril dressing
webspace
Webster meniscectomy scissors
Webster needle holder
Wechsler Adult Intelligence Scale
Wechsler Memory Scale (WMS)

Wechsler Memory Scale, Revised
Weck clip
Weck microsuture cutting scissors
Weck osteotome
Wedeen wire passers
wedge
  bed
  compensatory
  Duo-Cline bed
  Hapad heel
  heel
  heel to toe medial shoe
  lateral (for sole or heel of foot)
  medial heel
  shoe
  tibial
  Yancy cast
wedge allograft
wedge-and-groove joint
wedge bone
wedge compression fracture
wedged shoes
wedge excision
wedge fixation
wedge flexion-compression fracture
wedge fracture
wedge osteotomy, supratubercular
wedge-shaped vertebra
wedging deformity
wedging of olisthetic vertebra
wedging of vertebral interspace
wedging, vertebral
weekend athlete
weekend diarrhea (migraine
  equivalent)
Wegener granulomatosis-associated
  peripheral neuropathy
Wehbe arm holder
Wehrs incus prosthesis
weight acceptance (of gait)
weightbearing (also weight-bearing)
  partial
  progression to
  progressive
  protective

weightbearing *(continued)*
  spinal x-ray with
  toe-touch
  touchdown
weightbearing as tolerated (WBAT)
weightbearing crutches
weightbearing dome of acetabulum
weightbearing films
weightbearing radiograph
weightbearing rotational injury
weightbearing surface
weightbearing with crutches
weightbearing x-ray
weight-loading, axial
weight-relieving calipers
weights
  handheld (HHW)
  progressive
  Thera-Band progressive
weights and pulleys
weight shift
weight shifting
weight-training program
weight transfer
Weil-Blakesley intervertebral disk
  rongeur
Weil-Felix reaction
Weil osteotomy
Weil pelvic sling
Weil procedure with modified Ronconi
  technique
Weil-type Swanson-design hammertoe
  implant
Weinberg rib spreader
wei qi (Chinese medicine term)
Weiss amputation saw
Weiss sign
Weiss spring
Weit-Arner retractor
Weitbrecht cord
Weitbrecht ligament
Weitlaner-Beckmann retractor
Welander disease
Welander distal muscular atrophy
Well-Being, Index of (IWB)

Weller cartilage forceps
Weller cartilage scissors
well leg cast
well leg straight leg raising test
well leg traction
Wells traction
Wenger plate
Wera-Werk torque screwdriver
Werdnig-Hoffmann disease
Werdnig-Hoffmann spinal muscular
  atrophy
Werdnig-Hoffmann syndrome
Wernicke aphasia
Wernicke area
Wernicke dementia
Wernicke encephalopathy
Wernicke-Korsakoff encephalopathy
Wernicke-Korsakoff syndrome
Wernicke-Mann predilection paralysis
Wernicke-Mann spastic hemiplegia
Wernicke region
Wernicke syndrome
Wertheim splint
WEST (work evaluation systems
  technology)
West and Soto-Hall patella operation
West bone chisel
West bone gouge
Western blot test
western equine encephalitis
western equine viral encephalitis
Western Ontario Instability Index
  (WOSI)
Western Ontario Rotator Cuff Index
  (WORC)
Westfield acromioclavicular
  immobilizer
Westfield envelope sling
WEST-foot sensory nerve tester
West hand dissector
West Haven-Yale Multidimensional
  Pain Inventory
Westin tenodesis
Westin-Turco category
West Nile encephalitis
West Nile viral encephalitis
West osteotome

Westphal-Edinger nucleus
West Point x-ray view
West syndrome
wet gangrene
wet smear for parasites and fungi
Weyers syndrome
WFC (World Federation of Chiropractic)
WFL (within functional limits)
Wheaton brace
Wheaton Pavlik Harness
wheel
  Carborundum grinding
  grinding
  pin
  Wartenberg pin
wheelchair (W/C)
  Adorno Rogers
  Amigo mechanical
  confinement to
  electric
  HiRider motorized/lift
  Kusch'kin Ace
whettle bone
WHIGET (Washington Heights-
  Inwood Genetic Study of Essential
  Tremor)
whiplash
  acute
  chronic
  reflex rebound component of
whiplash injury
whiplash syndrome
Whipple disease
whipstitch
whirlpool bath
whisker shaver
Whitacre spinal needle
Whitcomb-Kerrison laminectomy
  rongeur
White and Panjabi cervical spine
  criteria
white-appearing blood pool
white band on degenerated implant
white blood cell scintigraphy (WBCS)
  with indium-111
white cerebellum sign

Whitecloud-LaRocca cervical arthrodesis
white commissure of spinal cord
white count with left shift
White epiphysiodesis
white fibers (type II muscle fibers)
White leg-length view
white light
white matter of central nervous system
white migraine
white muscle
white platelet-fibrin thrombus
Whitesides-Kelly cervical technique
Whitesides Ortholoc II condylar
    femoral prosthesis
Whitesides technique
Whitesides tissue pressure determination
Whitesides total knee prosthesis
white-white zone of bucket-handle tear
Whitfield ointment and pumice stone
whitlow
    herpetic
    melanotic
Whitman femoral neck reconstruction
WHO (World Health Organization)
WHO classification of astrocytoma
WHO Handicap Scales
    economic self-sufficiency
    mobility
    orientation
    physical independence
    social integration
WHO/LAR (World Health Organi-
    zation/International League Against
    Rheumatism) Response Criteria for
    Rheumatoid Arthritis
whole-body hyperthermia
whole-body imaging
whole-body PET scan
whole-body 1.5T Siemens Vision MRI
    scanner
whole-body 3T MRI system scanner
whole-bone transplant
whole-brain mean CBF
whorl, coccygeal
Wiberg, CE angle of
Wiberg classification of patellar types
    I-III

Wiberg periosteal elevator
Wiberg type II patellar contour
wicket rhythm on EEG
wicket spike on EEG
wick, saline-soaked cotton
wick technique
wide-based gait
wide excision of lesion
wide-necked intracranial artery
    aneurysm
widened joint space
widened mediastinum
widened sulci
widened thoracic outlet
widening
    ankle mortise
    crural cistern
    growth plate
    interpedicular distance
    interspinous
    joint
    mediastinal
    tibial tunnel
Wide Range Achievement Test
wide toebox shoe
Widowitz sign for brain stem damage
width, radius
Wiet cup forceps
Wiet graft-measuring instrument
Wiet otologic scissors
Wigmore plaster saw
Wilberg bone staple
Wilco ankle exerciser
Wilco ankle machine
Wilcoxon test
Wilde ethmoid forceps
Wilde intervertebral disk rongeur
Wilke boot
Wilkins classification of radial fracture
Willauer-Gibbon periosteal elevator
William Harris hip prosthesis
Williams exercise program
Williams flexion exercises
Williams-Haddad technique
Williams screwdriver
Williger bone curet
Williger bone mallet

Williger periosteal elevator
Willis
   antrum of
   arterial circle of
   artery of
   nerve of
Willis headache
willow fracture
Wilmington arthroscopic portal
Wilmington jacket
Wilmington scoliosis brace
Wilson-Burstein (DF80) hip prosthesis
Wilson convex frame
Wilson disease
Wilson double oblique osteotomy
Wilson frame
Wilson-Jacobs tibial fracture fixation
Wilson-Johansson-Barrington cone
   arthrodesis
Wilson-Krout grading scale
Wilson-McKeever arthroplasty
Wilson-McKeever shoulder technique
Wilson muscle
Wilson procedure for extra-articular
   fusion of elbow
Wilson rib spreader
Wilson sign
Wiltberger anterior cervical approach
Wiltberger spinous process spreader
Wiltse approach in lumbosacral fusion
Wiltse-Bankart retractor
Wiltse fixation system
Wiltse-Gelpi retractor
Wiltse osteotomy of ankle
Wiltse rod
Wiltse screw-rod
Winberger line
wince, wincing
wind (Chinese medicine term)
windblown hand syndrome
wind-cold (Chinese medicine term)
wind-heat (Chinese medicine term)
windlass mechanism
window
   bone
   brain

window *(continued)*
   cortical
   soft tissue
   subdural
windowshade pulled down on visual
   field
windup injury
wing
   iliac
   sphenoid
   sphenoidal
wing-beating tremor of Wilson
   disease
winged iliac crest trephine
winged scapula
Wingfield frame
winging of the scapula
wing of ilium
wing of sphenoid bone
wink, anal
wink reflex, anal
Wink retractor
Winograd technique for ingrown nail
Winquist-Hansen classification of
   femoral fracture
Winsford self-feeder device
Winslow ligament
Winston-Lutz for LINAC-based
   radiosurgery
Winter-King-Moe scoliosis
Winter spondylolisthesis technique
wire, wiring
   Babcock stainless steel
   band
   bayonet-point
   beaded transfixion
   bind
   bone suturing
   braided
   Brook
   Bunnell pull-out
   calibrated guide
   cerclage
   chisel-tip
   circular
   Compere fixation

wire *(continued)*
    compression
    conical-point
    crossed
    crossed Kirschner
    diamond-point
    double-strand
    double-stranded
    double-twisted
    Drummond
    encircling
    figure-of-8
    fixator
    gauge of
    Ilizarov
    interfragment
    interfragmentary
    interspinous
    Isola
    K (Kirschner)
    lead
    Luque
    Luque cerclage
    Magnuson
    monofilament
    ninety-ninety (90/90) intraosseous
    Nitinol flexible guide
    nonthreaded
    oblique
    olive
    Oppenheimer spring
    percutaneous Kirschner (K)
    pull-out
    Schauwecker patellar tension
    Selby I
    Semmes-Weinstein monofilament
    sharp-pointed
    smooth transfixion
    stainless steel
    steel
    sublamina
    summation
    suture
    tension band
    Thiersch
    threaded
    transfixion

wire *(continued)*
    transosseous
    triple
    trocar-point
    trochanter
    unthreaded
    Wisconsin interspinous
    Wisconsin spinous process
wire crimper, Caparosa
wire cutter
wire driver
    Hall Micro E
    Micro Series
    Orthairtome
wire fixation
Wirth-Jager tendon technique
Wisconsin button
Wisconsin Card Sorting Test
Wisconsin Compression System
    (WCS)
Wisconsin interspinous wire
Wisconsin-Luque instrumentation
Wisconsin spinal fracture system
Wisconsin spinous process wire
Wisconsin wire fixation
wishbone retractor
Wissinger rod
Wister wire/pin cutter
withdrawal
    alcohol
    drug
withdrawal movements
withdrawal seizures
within functional limits (WFL)
Wits cephalometric measurement
witzelsucht
Wixson hip positioner
WMS (Wechsler Memory Scale)
wobble board
Wolf arthroscope
Wolfart-Kugelberg-Welander
    syndrome
Wolfe-Boehler cast breaker (Böhler)
Wolfe-Boehler cast remover
Wolfe-Boehler mallet
Wolfe hand surgery graft
Wolfe-Kawamoto bone graft

Wolff headache
Wolff law of bone structure
Wolf-Hirschhorn syndrome
Wolf motor function test
Wolin meniscoid lesion
Wolman disease
WOMAC (Western Ontario and
    McMaster) Questionnaire
Wood alloy
wood probe reflexology device
wood screw
Woodson dissector
Woodson dural separator-spatula
Woodson elevator
Woodson separator
Woodward technique
wool, lamb's
woozy feeling
WORC (Western Ontario Rotator Cuff
    Index)
word blindness
word deafness, pure
word, difficulty finding the right
word-finding ability
word-finding difficulty
word-finding skills
word retrieval tasks
word retrieval test
words
    inappropriate (paraphrasia)
    nonsensical (neologisms)
    telescoped (festinant quality in
        parkinsonian speech)
word substitution
Workers' Compensation
work evaluation systems technology
    (WEST)
work hardening
working orthopedic surgery film
WorkMod back support
workplace
work, rhythmic handgrip
Work Seat driving simulator
workstation, Mayfield/ACCISS
    stereotactic
World Federation of Chiropractic
    (WFC)

World Federation of Neurology
World Health Organization (WHO)
wormian bone
wound
    ballistic
    clean
    closed
    contaminated
    craniocerebral penetrating
    cross-irrigation of
    depths of
    exit
    gunshot (GSW)
    high-energy gunshot
    high-velocity gunshot
    incised
    military missile head
    open
    plantar puncture
    puncture (types I through IV)
    stab (arthroscopy entry portal)
    tetanus-prone
wound dressing emulsion (WDE)
Wound-Evac drain
wound towels
woven bone
W-plasty
wrap (bandage)
    Ace
    Coban
    Dura-Kold
    Elasto-Gel shoulder therapy
    Electro-Link joint
    gauze
    joint
    Kerlix
    neck
    Nylatex nylon-latex
    Scott
    Snugs
    Thermoskin
    Thermosport hot/cold
    Unna
    Unna boot
wrap-around splint
wrap-around toe transfer

wrapping
  compressive centripetal
  stump
wrapping of aneurysm
wrench
  Allen
  box-end
  cannulated
  conical nut
  Fox
  Harrington flat
  hex
  Key-loc
  locknut
  Mueller (Müller)
  open-end
  socket
  U
  VDS (ventral derotating spinal)
wrenched knee
wrestler's ear
wrestler's elbow
Wright-Adson test
Wright Care TENS unit
Wrightlock posterior fixation system
Wright plate
Wright titanium prosthesis
wringer-type injury
wrinkler muscle of eyebrow
Wrisberg cardiac ganglion
Wrisberg, intermediate nerve of
Wrisberg ligament
Wrisberg nerve
wrist
  gymnast's
  oarsman's
  palmar

wrist *(continued)*
  SLAC (scapholunate arthritic
    collapse)
  unbalanced
  volar
  Volz
wrist arthroscopy
wrist capsule
wristdrop (sign of radial nerve
  paralysis)
wrist flexion contracture
wrist-guard-top fracture
WrisTimer carpal tunnel support
  system
WristJack (see *Agee-WristJack*)
wrist joint
wristlet, elastic
Wrist Pro wrist support device
wrist rest splint
writhing
  limb
  sinuous
  tongue
writhing of extremities
Writing-Bird device
WR nerve stimulator
wryneck (torticollis)
W-sitting position
Wu bunionectomy
Wurzburg plate
Wurzburg screw
Wurzburg titanium craniomaxillofacial
  plate and screws
Wyburn-Mason arteriovenous
  malformation
Wynne-Davies joint laxity technique

X, x

x (by)
x (times)
Xact ACL graft fixation system
xanthochromia of cerebrospinal fluid
  (CSF)
xanthochromic spinal fluid
xanthoma, malignant fibrous
xanthomatosis, cerebrotendinous
xanthomatosis of long bones with
  spontaneous fracture
Xe-CT (xenon-enhanced computed
  tomography)
Xenoderm acellular dermal allograft
xenon-enhanced computed tomography
  (Xe-CT)
xenon-133 single-photon-emission
  computed tomography
xenon skin clearance test
xenon washout technique measurement
Xenophor femoral prosthesis
Xercise Bands
Xerecept (synthetic corticotropin-
  releasing factor)
Xeroform gauze dressing
xerography
xeroradiography
xerosis
X-inactivation

XIP (x-ray in plaster)
xiphicostal ligament
xiphisternal joint
xiphoid angle
xiphoid bone
xiphoid cartilage
xiphoid ligament
xiphoid process syndrome
xiphopubic area
x-irradiation
Xiu cervical vertebral instruments
X-linked recessive adrenoleukodystrophy
XMB tibial reaming guide
Xomed NIM-2 (nerve integrity
  monitor)
XOP (x-ray out of plaster)
XPlan radiation treatment planning
  system
x-ray (see *imaging*)
  AP (anteroposterior)
  AP inversion stress
  brow-down skull
  brow-up skull
  coronal bending
  CTLV (cross-table lateral view)
  dorsiflexion stress ankle
  dorsoplanar

x-ray *(continued)*
    FCS (full cervical spine)
    full length
    Harris-Beath axial hindfoot
    hip-to-ankle
    intraoperative
    lateral
    lateral anterior drawer stress
    lateral tilt stress ankle
    mortise
    mortise view
    nonweightbearing
    patellar skyline
    plain
    plantarflexion stress ankle
    postoperative
    preoperative

x-ray *(continued)*
    prereduction
    standing
    stress
    stress Broden
    stress eversion
    stress inversion
    weightbearing
x-ray in plaster (XIP)
x-ray tray, Bucky
x-ray view (see *view*)
X-TEND-O knee flexer
Xubix (sibrafiban)
XXX syndrome
XXY syndrome
Xyrem (gamma hydroxybutyrate)
XYY syndrome

Y, y

YAG (yttrium-aluminum-garnet) laser
Yale brace
Yamanda myelotomy knife
Yancy cast wedge
yang meridian
Yankauer periosteal elevator
Yankauer punch
Yankauer suction tube
Yasargil arachnoid knife
Yasargil artery forceps
Yasargil bayonet forceps
Yasargil bayonet scissors
Yasargil carotid clamp
Yasargil clip-applying forceps
Yasargil dissector
Yasargil elevator
Yasargil hypophyseal forceps
Yasargil knotting forceps
Yasargil Leyla retractor arm
Yasargil ligature carrier
Yasargil ligature guide
Yasargil microclip
Yasargil microcuret
Yasargil microdissector
Yasargil microforceps
Yasargil microrasp
Yasargil microscissors
Yasargil microvascular knife

Yasargil needle holder
Yasargil pituitary rongeur
Yasargil rasp
Yasargil scissors
Yasargil scoop
Yasargil spring hook
Yasargil suction tube
Yasargil tissue lifter
Yasargil tumor forceps
Yasargil vessel clip
Y bone plate
Y-box mutation
Y connector, universal
Yeager test
Yee posterior shoulder approach
yellow fever encephalitis
yellow fever viral encephalitis
Yellow IRIS workstation
Yergason sign
Yergason test of shoulder subluxation
Yesavage-Brink Geriatric Depression
    Scale
Yesavage Geriatric Depression Scale
Y fracture
yield strength
Y incision
yin meridian
YIS knee prosthesis

YKL-40, serum
Y line
Yochum chiropractic radiography
yoke bone (zygomatic bone)
yoked muscles
Yoke transposition procedure
Y osteotomy
Young hinged knee prosthesis
Young modulus

Young-Vitallium hinged prosthesis
Yount procedure
Y plate
Y-shaped incision
Y-shaped ligament
Y-T fracture
yttrium-aluminum-garnet (YAG) laser
Yucca board

Z, z

Zadik foot procedure
Zadik total nail-bed ablation
Zaglas ligament
Zahn, line of
ZA (zygapophyseal) joint
Zanaflex (tizanidine hydrochloride)
Zancolli capsuloplasty
Zancolli procedure for clawhand
    deformity
Zaricznyj ligament technique
Zarins-Rowe ligament technique
Zaufel-Jansen bone rongeur
Zazepen-Gamidov technique
Z bunionectomy
Z disk
ZD neurosurgical localizing unit
zebra body myopathy
Zebutal
Zeier transfer technique
Zeiss OPMI surgical microscope
Zelapar (selegiline hydrochloride)
Zeldox (ziprasidone hydrochloride)
Zellballen
Zellweger syndrome
Zenith chiropractic table
Zenotech biomaterial for synthetic
    ligaments
Zervas hypophysectomy kit

Zest Anchor Advanced Generation
    (ZAAG) bone anchoring system
zeugmatography, Fourier
    transformation
Zeus microsurgery computer- and
    voice-controlled robotic system
Z fixation nail
Z foot
Zickel fracture classification system
Zickel intramedullary nail
Zickel nail fixation
Zickel subtrochanteric fracture fixation
ziconotide (SNX-111)
Zielke derotation level
Zielke distraction device
Zielke gouge
Zielke instrumentation for scoliosis
    spinal fusion
Zielke rod
Zielke VDS (ventral derotating spinal)
    implant
zigzag finger incision
Zimalite implant metal
Zimaloy implant metal
Zimaloy prosthesis
Zimfoam head halter
Zimfoam padding
Zimmer anatomic hip system

Zimmer CAPE (continuous anatomical
   passive exerciser)
Zimmer caudal hook
Zimmer Cebotome bone cement drill
Zimmer CPT (collarless polished
   taper) hip system
Zimmer gouge
Zimmer hip prosthesis
Zimmer knee immobilizer
Zimmer low viscosity adhesive
Zimmer low viscosity cement
Zimmer microsaw
Zimmer Osteo Stim bone growth
   stimulator
Zimmer Statak suture device
Zimmer Y plate
Zimmerman pericyte
Zim-Zap rib belt
Zinco Air Cam brace
Zinco Airprene brace
Zinco CAM Walker brace
Zinco Castaway D brace
Zinco Hi-Top brace
Zinco Minerva cervical brace
Zinco Multi-Lig brace
Zinco Pin Cam Walker brace
Zinco thumb-wrist immobilizer
zinc peroxide powder
Zinn ligament
Zinn, tendon of
ziprasidone hydrochloride (Zeldox)
Zipzoc stocking compression dressing
   and wrap
Ziramic femoral head
Zirconia orthopedic prosthetic heads
zirconium oxide ceramic prosthesis
Z lengthening of tendon
Zlotsky-Ballard classification of
   acromioclavicular injury
ZMC (zygomatic-malar complex)
   fracture (of the face)
ZMS intramedullary fixation system
Zocor (simvastatin)
Zoellner rasp
Zollinger leg holder
zolmitriptan (Zomig)

Zoloft (sertraline hydrochloride)
Zomaril (iloperidone)
Zomig (zolmitriptan)
zone
   chemoreceptor trigger
   dorsal root entry (DREZ)
   epileptogenic
   fracture
   ictal onset
   Looser
   root entry
   root exit (REZ)
   thermocoagulative
   trigger (for tic douloureux)
   white-white (of bucket-handle tear)
Zonegran (zonisamide)
zone of denervation
zone of partial preservation (ZPP) in
   spinal cord injury
zone phenomenon
Zone Specific II meniscal repair
   system
zone therapy
zonisamide (Zonegran)
zoom disorder of visual perception in
   migraine
Zoroc plaster
zoster
   geniculate herpes
   herpes
Zostrix
Z-plasty
   Cozen-Brockway
   four-flap
Z-plasty closure
Z-plasty incision
Z-plasty local flap graft
Z-plasty release
Z-plasty tenotomy
Z plate
ZPLATE-ATL anterior spinal fixation
   system
ZPP (zone of partial preservation) in
   spinal cord injury
Z-score
Z slide lengthening in hallux limitus

Z stent prosthesis
ZTT I and ZTT II acetabular cups
Zuckerkandl convolution
Zuckerman scale
Zucker splint
Zuelzer awl
Zuelzer hook plate
Zung Depression Scale
Zung Self-Rating Depression Scale
Zweymuller cementless hip prosthesis
Zydone (hydrocodone and aceta-
    minophen)
zygapophyeal (ZA) joint
zygapophysis

zygoma
zygomatic arch
zygomatic bone
zygomatic muscle
zygomatic nerve
zygomaticomalar area
zygomaticomaxillary fracture
zygomaticotemporal nerve
zygomatic process
Zyloprim (allopurinol)
ZY plane
Zyprexa (olanzapine)
Zyranox zirconia material in prosthesis

Appendix

Table of Bones

bone (region)	os (pl. ossa)
acetabulum	os acetabuli
acromial bone	os acromiale
	os acromiale secondarium
ankle bone	talus
atlas (neck)	atlas
axis (neck)	axis
basilar bone	os basilare
Bertin's bone	
blade bone	scapula
breast bone	sternum
Breschet's bone	os suprasternale
calcaneus (foot)	calcaneus; os calcis; os tarsi fibulare
capitate bone (wrist)	os capitatum; os carpale distale tertium
carpal bones (wrist)	ossa carpi; ossa carpalia
central bone (wrist)	os centrale
clavicle (shoulder)	clavicula
coccyx (lower back)	os coccygis
compact bone	substantia compacta
concha, inferior nasal (skull)	concha nasalis inferior
cortical bone	substantia corticalis
cranial bones	ossa cranii; ossa cranialia
cuboid bone (foot)	os cuboideum
cuneiform bone, intermediate (foot)	os cuneiforme intermedium
cuneiform bone, lateral (foot)	os cuneiforme laterale
cuneiform bone, medial (foot)	os cuneiforme mediale
digits, bones of	ossa digitorum
elbow bone (olecranon process of ulna)	cubitus
epipteric bone (Flower's bone)	
ethmoid bone	os ethmoidale
fabella (knee)	
facial bones	ossa facialia; ossa faciei
femur (thigh)	femur

bone (region)	os (pl. ossa)
fibula (leg)	fibula
flat bone	os planum
Flower's bone (epipteric bone)	
foot, bones of	ossa pedis
frontal bone (skull)	os frontale
digits of hand	ossa digitorum manus
digits of foot	ossa digitorum pedis
Goethe's bone (preinterparietal bone)	
greater multangular bone	trapezium
hamate bone (wrist)	os hamatum; os carpale distale quartum
hand, bones of (carpals, metacarpals, phalanges)	ossa manus
heel bone	calcaneus
hip bone (pelvis and hip)	os coxae
hollow bone (pneumatic bone)	
hooked bone (hamate bone)	
humerus (arm)	humerus
hyoid bone (neck)	os hyoideum
iliac bone; ilium (pelvis)	os ilii; os ilium
incisive bone	os incisivum
incus (ear)	incus
inferior limb, bones of (os coxae, pelvis, patella, tibia, fibula, tarsus metatarsus, digits of foot)	ossa membri inferioris
innominate bone (hip bone)	os coxae
intermaxillary bone	os incisivum
interparietal bone	os interparietale
irregular bone	os irregulare
ischial bone; ischium (pelvis)	os ischii
jaw bone (mandible)	mandibula
jugal bone (zygomatic bone)	os zygomaticum
Krause's bone (small bone)	
lacrimal bone (skull)	os lacrimale
lamellar bone	
lesser multangular bone (trapezoid)	os trapezoideum
lingual bone (hyoid bone)	
long bone (pipe bone)	os longum
lunate bone (wrist)	os lunatum
malar bone	os zygomaticum

bone (region)	os (pl. ossa)
malleus (ear)	malleus
mandible (lower jaw)	mandibula
mastoid bone of occipital bone	margo mastoideus squamae occipitalis
maxilla (skull, upper jaw)	maxilla
metacarpal bones (hand)	ossa metacarpalia
metacarpal bone, third or middle	os metacarpale tertium
metatarsal bones (foot)	ossa metatarsalia
nasal bone (nose)	os nasale
navicular bone of foot	os naviculare; os centrale tarsi
navicular bone of hand	os scaphoideum
nonlamellar bone (woven bone)	
occipital bone (skull)	os occipitale
palatine bone (skull)	os palatinum
parietal bone (skull)	os parietale
patella (knee)	patella
pelvis	os pelvicum
penis bone	os penis
perichondral bone (periosteal bone)	
periosteal bone (perichondral bone)	
peroneal bone (fibula)	
petrosal bone	
phalanges (pl. of phalanx) (fingers, toes)	ossa digitorum
phalanx, proximal	os phalanx proximalis
phalanx, middle	os phalanx media
phalanx, distal	os phalanx distalis
ping-pong bone	
pipe bone (long bone)	
Pirie's bone (dorsal talonavicular bone)	
pisiform bone (wrist)	os pisiforme
pneumatic bone	os pneumaticum
postsphenoid bone	
preinterparietal bone (Goethe's bone)	
premaxillary bone	os incisivum
presphenoid bone	
pubic bone (pelvis)	os pubis; mons pubis
pyramidal bone (triquetral bone)	os triquetrum
radius (forearm)	radius
replacement bone (endochondral bone)	
reticulated bone (woven bone)	

bone (region)	os (pl. ossa)
rib, ribs	os costae, os costale; ossa costalis
rider's bone (cavalry bone, exercise bone)	
Riolan's bone	
sacrum (lower back)	os sacrum
scaphoid bone (wrist)	os scaphoideum
scapula (shoulder)	scapula
scroll bones	
septal bone (interalveolar septum)	
sesamoid bones of hand	ossa sesamoidea manus
sesamoid bones of foot	ossa sesamoidea pedis
shank bone (cannon bone; tibia)	
shin bone (tibia)	
short bone	os breve
sieve bone	
skull, bones of	ossa cranii
sphenoid bone (base of skull)	os sphenoidale
splint bone (fibula)	
spongy bone	
stapes (ear)	stapes
sternum (chest)	sternum
superior limb, bones of (humerus, radius, ulna, carpus, metacarpus, digits of hand)	ossa membri superioris
suprainterparietal bone	
suprasternal bones	ossa suprasternalia
sutural bones	ossa suturalia; ossa fonticulorum
tail bone (coccyx)	os coccygis
talus (ankle)	talus; os tarsi tibiale
tarsal bones (ankle and foot)	ossa tarsi
temporal bone (skull)	os temporale
thigh bone (femur)	
thoracic bones	ossa thoracis
three-cornered bone (triquetral bone)	os triquetrum
tibia (leg)	tibia
tongue bone (hyoid bone)	
trabecular bone	
trapezium bone (wrist)	os trapezium; os carpale distale primum
trapezoid bone (wrist)	os trapezoideum; os carpale distale secundum

bone (region)	os (pl. ossa)
triangular bone	os trigonum
triquetral bone (wrist)	os triquetrum
turbinate bone, inferior	
(inferior nasal concha)	
tympanic bone	
ulna (forearm)	ulna
unciform bone (hamate bone)	
upper jaw bone (maxilla)	
vertebrae (back)	
vertebrae, cervical	vertebrae cervicales
vertebrae, thoracic (dorsal)	vertebrae thoracicae
vertebrae, lumbar	vertebrae lumbales
vertebrae, sacral	vertebrae sacrales
vertebrae, coccygeal	vertebrae coccygeae
Vesalius' bone; vesalian bone	os vesalianum pedis
vomer (skull)	vomer
wedge bone (intermediate cuneiform)	
woven bone (nonlamellar; reticulated)	
yoke bone (zygomatic bone)	
zygomatic bone (skull)	os zygomaticum

Table of Muscles

muscle	musculus (pl. musculi)
anterior serratus muscle	musculus serratus anterior
anterior tibial muscle	musculus tibialis anterior
antigravity muscles	
antitragus muscle	musculus antitragicus
arrector pili muscles	musculi arrectores pilorum
(erector muscles of hairs)	
articular muscle	musculus articularis
articular muscle of elbow	musculus articularis cubiti
articular muscle of knee	musculus articularis genus
articular muscle of knee	articularis genu musculus
aryepiglottic muscle	musculus aryepiglotticus
auditory ossicles, muscles of	musculi ossiculorum auditus
axillary arch muscle	pectorodorsalis musculus
back muscles	musculi dorsi
Bell's muscle (ureteric bridge)	
biceps brachii muscle	musculus biceps brachii
(biceps muscle of arm)	
biceps femoris muscle	musculus biceps femoris
(biceps muscle of thigh)	
bipennate muscle	musculus bipennatus
Bochdalek's muscle	musculus triticeoglossus
Bovero's muscle ("sucking muscle")	musculus cutaneomucosus
Bowman's muscle (ciliary muscle)	musculus ciliaris
brachial muscle (brachialis)	musculus brachialis
brachiocephalic muscle	musculus brachiocephalicus
brachioradial muscle (brachioradialis)	musculus brachioradialis
Braune's muscle	musculus puborectalis
broadest muscle of back	musculus latissimus dorsi
bronchoesophageal muscle	musculus bronchoesophageus
Brücke's muscle (Crampton's muscle)	
buccinator muscle	musculus buccinator
buccopharyngeal muscles	musculi pars buccopharyngea
(also, constrictor muscles	
of pharynx, superior)	
bulbocavernous muscle	musculus bulbospongiosus
canine muscle	musculus levator anguli oris
cardiac muscle	
Casser's perforated muscle	musculus coracobrachialis
(casserian muscle)	(ligamentum mallei anterius)

muscle	musculus (pl. musculi)
ceratocricoid muscle	musculus ceratocricoideus
cervical iliocostal muscle	musculus iliocostalis cervicis
cervical interspinal muscles	musculi interspinalis cervicis
	musculus longissimus cervicis
cervical muscles	musculi colli
cervical rotator muscles	musculi rotatores cervicis
Chassaignac's axillary muscle	
chin muscle	musculus mentalis
chondroglossus muscle	musculus chondroglossus
chondropharyngeal muscles	musculi pars chondropharyngea
(constrictor muscle of pharynx, middle)	(constrictor pharyngis medius)
ciliary muscle	muscularis ciliaris
coccygeal (coccygeus) muscle(s)	musculus coccygeus, musculi coccygei
Coiter's muscle	musculus corrugator supercilii
compressor muscle of naris	
congenerous muscles	
constrictor muscle of pharynx, inferior	musculus constrictor pharyngis inferior
constrictor muscle of pharynx, middle	musculus constrictor pharyngis medius
constrictor muscle of pharynx, superior	musculus constrictor pharyngis superior
coracobrachial muscle (coracobrachialis)	musculus coracobrachialis
corrugator muscle	corrugator supercilii musculus
corrugator cutis muscle of anus	musculus corrugator cutis ani
corrugator supercilii muscle	musculus corrugator supercilii
Crampton's muscle (Bruecke's muscle)	
cremaster muscle (Riolan's muscle)	musculus cremaster
cricoarytenoid muscle, lateral	musculus crico-arytenoideus lateralis
cricoarytenoid muscle, posterior	musculus crico-arytenoideus posterior
cricopharyngeal muscle	musculus cricopharyngeus
cricothyroid muscle	musculus cricothyroideus
cruciate muscle	musculus cruciatus
cutaneomucous muscle	musculus cutaneomucosus
(the "sucking muscle," also called Aeby's muscle, Bovero's muscle, Klein's muscle, Krause's muscle, mucocutaneous muscle)	
cutaneous muscle	musculus cutaneus
dartos muscle of scrotum	musculus tunica dartos
deep muscles of back (true back muscles)	musculi dorsi
deep flexor muscle of fingers	musculus flexor digitorum profundus

muscle	musculus (pl. musculi)
deep transverse perineal msucle	musculus transversus perinei profundus
deltoid muscle	musculus deltoideus
depressor muscle of angle of mouth	musculus depressor anguli oris
depressor muscle of epiglottis	musculus thyroepiglottic
depressor muscle of eyebrow	musculus depressor supercilii
depressor muscle of lower lip	musculus depressor labii inferioris
depressor muscle of septum of nose	musculus depressor septi
depressor superciliary muscle	musculus depressor supercilii
detrusor muscle of urinary bladder	musculus detrusor urinae
	(musculus detrusor vesicae)
diaphragm, diaphragmatic muscle	diaphragma
digastric muscle	musculus digastricus
dilator muscle	musculus dilatator
dilator muscle of ileocecal sphincter	musculus dilator pylori ilealis
dilator muscle of pupil	musculus dilator pupillae
dilator muscle of pylorus	musculus dilator pylori gastro-duodenalis
dorsal interosseous muscles of foot	musculi interossei dorsalis pedis
dorsal interosseous muscles of hand	musculi interossei dorsalis manus
dorsal muscles (muscles of back)	musculi dorsi
dorsal sacrococcygeal muscle	musculus sacrococcygeus dorsalis
Dupré's muscle	musculus articularis genu
Duverney's muscle	musculus orbicularis oculi
elevator muscle of anus	musculus levator ani
elevator muscle of prostate	musculus levator prostatae
elevator muscles of rib	musculi levatores costarum
elevator muscle of scapula	musculus levator scapulae
elevator muscle of soft palate	musculus levator veli palatini
elevator muscle of upper eyelid	musculus levator palpebrae superioris
elevator muscle of upper lip	musculus levator labii superioris
elevator muscle of upper lip and wing of nose	musculus levator labii superioris alaeque nasi
emergency muscles	
epicranial muscle	musculus epicranius
epimeric muscle	
epitrochleoanconeus muscle	musculus epitrochleoanconaeus
erector muscles of hairs (arrector pili)	musculi arrectores pilorum
erector muscle of penis	musculus ischiocavernosus
erector muscle of spine	musculus erector spinae

839

muscle	musculus (pl. musculi)
eustachian muscle	musculus tensor tympani
expression, muscles of	musculi faciales
extensor muscle of fingers	musculus extensor digitorum
extensor muscle of great toe, long	musculus extensor hallucis longus
extensor muscle of great toe, short	musculus extensor hallucis brevis
extensor muscle of hand, short	musculus extensor digitorum brevis
(Pozzi's muscle)	manus
extensor muscle of index finger	musculus extensor indicis
extensor muscle of little finger	musculus extensor digiti minimi
extensor muscle of thumb, long	musculus extensor pollicis longus
extensor muscle of thumb, short	musculus extensor pollicis brevis
extensor muscle of toes, long	musculus extensor digitorum longus
extensor muscle of toes, short	musculus extensor digitorum brevis
extensor muscle of wrist, radial, long	musculus extensor carpi radialis longus
extensor muscle of wrist, radial, short	musculus extensor carpi radialis brevis
extensor muscle of wrist, ulnar	musculus extensor carpi ulnaris
external intercostal muscles	musculi intercostales externi
external oblique muscle	musculus obliquus externus abdominis
external obturator muscle	musculus obturator externus
external pterygoid muscle	lateral pterygoid musculus
external sphincter muscle of anus	
extraocular muscles	musculi bulbi
extrinsic muscles	
eyeball muscles (extraocular muscles)	
facial and masticatory muscles	musculi faciales et masticatores
facial expression, muscles of	musculi faciales
facial muscles	musculi faciales
fast muscle (white muscle)	
fauces (the throat), muscles of	musculi palati et faucium
femoral muscle	musculus vastus intermedius
fibular muscle, long	musculus peroneus longus
fibular muscle, short	musculus peroneus brevis
fibular muscle, third	musculus peroneus tertius
fixation muscles, fixator muscles	
fixator muscle of base of stapes	musculus fixator baseos stapedis
flexor muscle of fingers, deep	musculus flexor digitorum profundus
flexor muscle of fingers, superficial	musculus flexor digitorum superficialis
flexor muscle of great toe, long	musculus flexor hallucis longus
flexor muscle of great toe, short	musculus flexor hallucis brevis

muscle	musculus (pl. musculi)
flexor muscle of little finger, short	musculus flexor digiti minimi brevis manus
flexor muscle of little toe, short	musculus flexor digiti minimi brevis pedis
flexor muscle of thumb, short	musculus flexor pollicis brevis
flexor muscle of thumb, long	musculus flexor pollicis longus
flexor muscle of toes, short	musculus flexor digitorum brevis
flexor muscle of toes, long	musculus flexor digitorum longus
flexor muscle of wrist, radial	musculus flexor carpi radialis
flexor muscle of wrist, ulnar	musculus flexor carpi ulnaris
Folius' muscle	ligamentum mallei laterale
fusiform muscle (spindle-shaped muscle)	musculus fusiformis
Gantzer's muscle	
gastrocnemius muscle	musculus gastrocnemius
Gavard's muscle	
gemellus muscle, inferior	musculus gemellus inferior
gemellus muscle, superior	musculus gemellus superior
genioglossal muscle	musculus genioglossus
geniohyoid muscle	musculus geniohyoideus
glossopalatine muscle (palatoglossus)	musculus palatoglossus
glossopharyngeal muscle	pars glossopharyngea musculi constrictoris pharyngis superioris
gluteal muscle, greatest	musculus gluteus maximus
gluteal muscle, least	musculus gluteus minimus
gluteal muscle, middle	musculus gluteus medius
gracilis muscle	musculus gracilis
great adductor muscle	musculus adductor magnus
greater pectoral muscle	musculus pectoralis major
greater posterior rectus muscle of head	musculus rectus capitis posterior major
greater psoas muscle	musculus psoas major
greater rhomboid muscle	musculus rhomboideus major
greater zygomatic muscle	musculus zygomaticus major
Guthrie's muscle	sphincter urethrae
hamstring muscles	
head, muscles of	musculi capitis
Hilton's muscle	musculus aryepiglotticus
Horner's muscle	musculus orbicularis oculi
Houston's muscle	compressor venae dorsalis penis
hyoglossal (hyoglossus) muscle	musculus hyoglossus

muscle	musculus (pl. musculi)
iliac muscle	musculus iliacus
iliacus minor muscle	musculus iliacus minor
iliococcygeal muscle	musculus iliococcygeus
iliocostal muscle	musculus iliocostalis
iliocostal muscle of neck	musculus iliocostalis cervicis
iliocostal muscle of loins	musculus iliocostalis lumborum
iliocostal muscle of thorax	musculus iliocostalis thoracis
iliopsoas muscle	musculus iliopsoas
incisive muscles of inferior lip	musculi incisivi labii inferioris
incisive muscles of lower lip	musculi incisivi labii inferioris
incisive muscles of superior lip	musculi incisivi labii superioris
incisive muscles of upper lip	musculi incisivi labii superioris
index extensor muscle	musculus extensor indicis
inferior constrictor muscle of pharynx	musculus constrictor pharyngis inferior
inferior gemellus muscle	musculus gemellus inferior
inferior longitudinal muscle of tongue	musculus longitudinalis inferior
inferior oblique muscle	musculus obliquus inferior
inferior oblique muscle of head	musculus obliquus capitis inferior
inferior posterior serratus muscle	serratus posterior inferior musculus
inferior rectus muscle	musculus rectus inferior
inferior tarsal muscle	musculus tarsalis inferior
infrahyoid muscles	musculi infrahyoidei
infraspinous muscle	musculus infraspinatus
innermost intercostal muscle	musculus intercostalis intimus
inspiratory muscles	
intercostal muscles	musculi intercostales
interfoveolar muscle	ligamentum interfoveolare
intermediate great muscle	musculus vastus intermedius
internal intercostal muscle	musculus intercostalis internus
internal oblique muscle	musculus obliquus internus abdominis
internal obturator muscle	musculus obturator internus
internal pterygoid muscle	musculus pterygoideus medialis
interosseous muscles	musculi interossei
interspinal muscles	musculi interspinales
intertransverse muscles	musculi intertransversarii
intra-auricular muscles	
intraocular muscles	
intrinsic muscles	
intrinsic muscles of foot	

muscle	musculus (pl. musculi)
involuntary muscles	
iridic muscles	
ischiocavernous muscle	musculus ischiocavernosus
Jarjavay's muscle	
Jung's pyramidal auricular muscle	
Klein's cutaneomucous muscle	
Kohlrausch's muscle	
Koyter's muscle	musculus corrugator supercilii
Krause's cutaneomucous muscle	musculus cutaneomucosus
Landstrom's muscle (umlaut o)	
Langer's axillary arch muscle	
larynx, muscles of	musculi laryngis
lateral cricoarytenoid muscle	musculus cricoarytenoideus lateralis
lateral great muscle	musculus vastus lateralis
lateral lumbar intertransversarii muscles	musculi intertransversarii laterales lumborum
lateral pterygoid muscle	musculus pterygoideus lateralis
lateral rectus muscle	musculus rectus lateralis
lateral rectus muscle of the head	musculus rectus capitis lateralis
lateral vastus muscle	musculus vastus lateralis
latissimus dorsi muscle	musculus latissimus dorsi
lesser rhomboid muscle	musculus rhomboid minor
lesser zygomatic muscle	musculus zygomaticus minor
levator ani muscle	musculus levator ani
levator muscles (see *elevator muscles*)	
lingual muscles	musculi linguae
long abductor muscle of thumb	musculus abductor pollicis longus
long adductor muscle	musculus adductor longus
long extensor muscle of great toe	musculus extensor hallucis longus
long extensor muscle of thumb	musculus extensor pollicis longus
long extensor muscle of toes	musculus extensor digitorum longus
long fibular muscle	musculus peroneus longus
long flexor muscle of great toe	musculus flexor hallucis longus
long flexor muscle of thumb	musculus flexor pollicis longus
long flexor muscle of toes	musculus flexor digitorum longus
long muscle of head	musculus longus capitis
longissimus muscle	musculus longissimus
longissimus muscle of back (thorax)	musculus longissimus thoracis
longissimus muscle of head	musculus longissimus capitis

muscle	musculus (pl. musculi)
longissimus muscle of neck	musculus longissimus cervicis
longitudinal muscle of tongue, inferior	musculus longitudinalis inferior linguae
longitudinal muscle of tongue, superior	musculus longitudinalis superior linguae
long muscle of head	musculus longus capitis
long muscle of neck	musculus longus colli
long palmar muscle	musculus palmaris longus
long peroneal muscle	musculus peroneus longus
long radial extensor muscle of wrist	musculus extensor carpi radialis longus
lumbar iliocostal muscle	musculus interspinalis lumborum
lumbar interspinal muscles	musculus interspinalis lumborum
lumbar quadrate muscle	musculus quadratus lumborum
lumbar rotator muscles	musculi rotatores lumborum
lumbrical muscles of foot	musculi lumbricales pedis
lumbrical muscles of hand	musculi lumbricales manus
Marcacci's muscle	
masseter muscle	musculus masseter
medial great muscle	musculus vastus medialis
medial lumbar intertransverse muscles	musculi intertransversarii mediales lumborum
medial pterygoid muscle	musculus pterygoideus medialis
medial rectus muscle	musculus rectus medialis
medial vastus muscle	musculus vastus medialis
mentalis muscle	musculus mentalis
Merkel's muscle	musculus ceratocricoideus
mesothenar muscle	musculus adductor pollicis
middle constrictor muscle of pharynx	musculus constrictor pharyngis medius
middle scalene muscle	musculus scalenus medius
mucocutaneous muscle	
Mueller's muscle	musculus orbitalis
multifidus muscles (intermediate layer of transversospinalis muscles)	musculi multifidi
multipennate muscle	musculus multipennatus
mylohyoid muscle	musculus mylohyoideus
nasal muscle	musculus nasalis
neck, muscles of	musculi colli
nonstriated muscle (smooth muscle)	
notch of helix, muscles of	musculus incisurae helicis
oblique arytenoid muscle	musculus arytenoideus obliquus
oblique auricular muscle	musculus obliquus auriculae

muscle	musculus (pl. musculi)
oblique muscle of abdomen, external	musculus obliquus externus abdominis
oblique muscle of abdomen, internal	musculus obliquus internus abdominis
oblique muscle of head, inferior	musculus obliquus capitis inferior
oblique muscle of head, superior	musculus obliquus capitis superior
obturator muscle, external	musculus obturator externus
obturator muscle, internal	musculus obturator internus
occipitofrontal muscle	musculus occipitofrontalis
Ochsner's muscles	
ocular muscles	musculi bulbi
Oddi's muscle (sphincter)	
Oehl's muscles	
omohyoid muscle	musculus omohyoideus
opposing muscle of little finger	musculus opponens digiti minimi
opposing muscle of thumb	musculus opponens pollicis
orbicular muscle	musculus orbicularis
orbicular muscle of eye	musculus orbicularis oculi
orbicular muscle of mouth	musculus orbicularis oris
orbital muscle	musculus orbitalis
organic muscle (visceral musscle)	
palate and fauces, muscles	musculi palati et faucium
palatine muscles	musculi palati
palatoglossus muscle	musculus palatoglossus
palatopharyngeal muscle	musculus palatopharyngeus
palmar interosseous muscle	musculus interosseus palmaris
palmar muscle, short	musculus palmaris brevis
palmar muscle, long	musculus palmaris longus
papillary muscle	musculus papillaris
pectinate muscles	musculi pectinati
pectineal muscle	musculus pectineus
pectoral muscle, greater	musculus pectoralis major
pectoral muscle, smaller	musculus pectoralis minor
pectorodorsalis muscle (axillary arch)	
penniform muscle	musculus unipennatus
perineal muscles	musculi perinei
peroneal muscle, long	musculus fibularis longus
peroneal muscle, short	musculus fibularis brevis
peroneal muscle, third	musculus fibularis tertius
pharyngopalatine muscle	musculus palatopharyngeus
Phillips' muscle	

muscle	musculus (pl. musculi)
piriform muscle	musculus piriformis
plantar interosseous muscle	musculus interosseus plantaris
plantar muscle	musculus plantaris
plantar quadrate muscle	musculus quadratus plantae
platysma muscle	musculus platysma
pleuroesophageal muscle	musculus pleuroesophageus
popliteal muscle	musculus popliteus
posterior auricular muscle	musculus retrahens aurem
posterior cervical intertransverse muscles	musculi intertransversarii posteriores cervicis
posterior cricoarytenoid muscle	musculus cricoarytenoideus posterior
posterior scalene muscle	musculus scalenus posterior
posterior tibial muscle	musculus tibialis posterior
Pozzi's muscle (extensor digitorum brevis muscle of hand)	musculus extensor digitorum brevis manus
procerus muscle	musculus procerus
pronator muscle, quadrate	musculus pronator quadratus
pronator muscle, round	musculus pronator teres
psoas muscle, greater	musculus psoas major
psoas muscle, smaller	musculus psoas minor
pterygoid muscle	musculus pterygoideus
pubococcygeal muscle	musculus pubococcygeus
puboprostatic muscle	musculus puboprosticus
puborectal muscle (Braune's muscle)	musculus puborectalis
pubovaginal muscle	musculus pubovaginalis
pubovesical muscle	musculus pubovesicalis
pyloric sphincter muscle	musculus sphincter pyloricus
pyramidal auricular muscle (Jung's m.)	musculus pyramidalis auriculae
quadrate (four-sided) muscle	musculus quadratus
quadrate muscle of loins	musculus quadratus lumborum
quadrate muscle of lower lip	musculus depressor labii inferioris
quadrate muscle of sole	musculus quadratus plantae
quadrate muscle of thigh	musculus quadratus femoris
quadrate muscle of upper lip	musculus quadratus labii superioris
radial flexor muscle of wrist	musculus flexor carpi radialis
rectococcygeus muscle	musculus rectococcygeus
rectourethral muscle	musculus recto-urethralis
rectouterine muscle	musculus recto-uterinus
rectovesical muscle	musculus rectovesicalis

muscle	musculus (pl. musculi)
rectus abdominis muscle (rectus muscle of abdomen)	musculus rectus abdominis
rectus muscle of head, anterior	musculus rectus capitis anterior
rectus muscle of head, lateral	musculus rectus capitis lateralis
rectus muscle of head, greater posterior	musculus rectus capitis posterior major
rectus muscle of head, smaller posterior	musculus rectus capitis posterior minor
rectus femoris muscle (rectus muscle of thigh)	musculus rectus femoris
red muscle (slow muscle)	
Reisseisen's muscles	
rhomboid muscle, greater	musculus rhomboideus major
rhomboid muscle, lesser	musculus rhomboideus minor
ribbon muscles	musculi infrahyoidei
rider's muscles (adductor muscles of thigh)	
Riolan's muscle (cremaster muscle)	musculus cremaster
risorius muscle (Albinus' muscle, Santorini's muscle)	musculus risorius
rotator muscles	musculi rotatores
rotator muscles of neck	musculi rotatores cervicis
rotator muscles of back	musculi rotatores lumborum
rotator muscles of thorax	musculi rotatores thoracis
Rouget's muscle	
round pronator muscle	musculus pronator teres
Ruysch's muscle	
sacrococcygeal muscle	musculus sacrococcygeus
salpingopharyngeal muscle	musculus salpingopharyngeus
Santorini's muscle	musculus risorius
sartorius muscle (tailor's muscle)	musculus sartorius
scalene muscle, anterior	musculus scalenus anterior
scalene muscle, middle	musculus scalenus medius
scalene muscle, posterior	musculus scalenus posterior
scalene muscle, smallest (Albinus' m., Sibson's m.)	musculus scalenus minimus
scalp muscle (epicranius muscle)	
Sebileau's muscle	
second tibial muscle	musculus tibialis secundus
semimembranous muscle	musculus semimembranosus
semispinal muscle	musculus semispinalis
semispinal muscle of head	musculus semispinalis capitis

muscle	musculus (pl. musculi)
semispinal muscle of neck	musculus semispinalis cervicis
semispinal muscle of thorax	musculus semispinalis thoracis
semitendinous muscle	musculus semitendinosus
serratus anterior muscle	musculus serratus anterior
serratus posterior inferior muscle	musculus serratus posterior inferior
serratus posterior superior muscle	musculus serratus posterior superior
shawl muscle (trapezius muscle)	
short adductor muscle	musculus adductor brevis
short extensor musscle of great toe	musculus extensor hallucis brevis
short extensor muscle of thumb	musculus extensor pollicis brevis
short extensor muscle of toes	musculus extensor digitorum brevis
short fibular muscle	musculus peroneus brevis
short flexor muscle of great toe	musculus flexor hallucis brevis
short flexor muscle of little finger	musculus flexor digiti minimi brevis
short flexor muscle of little toe	musculus flexor digiti minimi brevis
short flexor muscle of thumb	musculus flexor pollicis brevis
short flexor muscle of toes	musculus flexor digitorum brevis
short palmar muscle	musculus palmaris brevis
short peroneal muscle	musculus peroneus brevis
short radial extensor muscle of wrist	musculus extensor carpi radialis brevis
Sibson's muscle	musculus scalenus minimus
skeletal muscles	musculi skeleti
slow muscle (red muscle)	
smaller muscle of helix	musculus helicis minor
smaller pectoral muscle	musculus pectoralis minor
smaller posterior rectus muscle of head	musculus rectus capitis posterior minor
smaller psoas muscle	musculus psoas minor
smallest scalene muscle	musculus scalenus minimus
smooth muscle (unstriated, unstriped, visceral)	
Soemmerring's muscle (levator muscle of thyroid gland)	
soleus muscle	musculus soleus
somatic muscles	musculi skeleti
sphincter muscle of anus	musculus sphincter ani
sphincter muscle of bile duct	musculus sphincter ductus choledochi
sphincter muscle of hepatopancreatic ampulla	musculus sphincter ampullae hepatopancreaticae
sphincter muscle of pupil	musculus sphincter pupillae

muscle	musculus (pl. musculi)
sphincter muscle of pylorus	musculus sphincter pyloricus
sphincter muscle of urethra	musculus sphincter urethrae
sphincter muscle of urinary bladder	musculus sphincter vesicae urinariae
spinal muscle	musculus spinalis
spinal muscle of head	musculus spinalis capitis
spinal muscle of neck	musculus spinalis cervicis
spinal muscle of thorax	musculus spinalis thoracis
spindle-shaped muscle	musculus fisiform
splenius muscle of head	musculus splenius capitis
splenius muscle of neck	musculus splenius cervicis
stapedius muscle	musculus stapedius
sternal muscle	musculus sternalis
sternochondroscapular muscle	musculus sternochondroscapularis
sternoclavicular muscle	musculus sternoclavicularis
sternocleidomastoid muscle	musculus sternocleidomastoideus
sternocostal muscle	musculus transversus thoracis
sternohyoid muscle	musculus sternohyoideus
sternomastoid muscle (sternocleidomastoid)	
sternothyroid muscle	musculus sternothyroideus
strap muscles	
striated muscle	
styloauricular muscle	musculus styloauricularis
styloglossus muscle	musculus styloglossus
stylohyoid muscle	musculus stylohyoideus
stylopharyngeal muscle	musculus stylopharyngeus
subanconeus muscle	musculus articularis cubiti
subclavian muscle	musculus subclavius
subcostal muscle	musculus subcostalis
subcrural muscle	musculus articularis genu
suboccipital muscles	musculi suboccipitales
subquadricipital muscle	musculus articularis genu
subscapular muscle	musculus subscapularis
subvertebral muscles	musculi hypaxial
superficial back muscles	
superficial flexor muscle of fingers	musculus flexor digitorum superficialis
superficial lingual muscle (of tongue)	
superficial transverse perineal muscle (Theile's muscle)	musculus transversus perinei superficialis
superior auricular muscle	musculus auricularis superior

muscle	musculus (pl. musculi)
superior constrictor muscle of pharynx	musculus constrictor pharyngis superior
superior gemellus muscle	musculus gemellus superior
superior longitudinal muscle of tongue	musculus longitudinalis superior
superior oblique muscle	musculus obliquus superior
superior oblique muscle of head	musculus obliquus capitis superior
superior posterior serratus muscle	musculus serratus posterior superior
superior rectus muscle	musculus rectus superior
superior tarsal muscle	musculus tarsalis superior
(Mueller's muscle)	
supinator muscle	musculus supinator
supraclavicular muscle	musculus supraclavicularis
suprahyoid muscles	musculi suprahyoidei
supraspinalis muscle	musculus supraspinalis
supraspinous muscle	musculus supraspinatus
suspensory muscle of duodenum	musculus suspensorius duodeni
(Treitz' ligament)	
synergic or synergistic muscles	
tailor's muscle (sartorius muscle)	
temporal muscle	musculus temporalis
temporoparietal muscle	musculus temporoparietalis
tensor muscle of fascia lata	musculus tensor fasciae latae
tensor muscle of soft palate	musculus tensor veli palati
tensor tarsi muscle	musculus orbicularis oculi
tensor muscle of tympanic membrane	musculus tensor tympani
(Toynbee's muscle)	
teres major muscle	musculus teres major
teres minor muscle	musculus teres minor
Theile's muscle (superficial transverse perineal muscle)	
third peroneal muscle	musculus peroneus tertius
thoracic interspinal muscle	musculi thoracic interspinalis
thoracic intertransverse muscles	musculi intertransversarii thoracis
thoracic longissimus muscle	musculus longissimus thoracis
thoracic rotator muscles	musculi rotatores thoracis
thorax, muscles of	musculi thoracis
thyroarytenoid muscle	musculus thyroarytenoideus
thyroepiglottic muscle	musculus thyroepiglotticus
(depressor muscle of epiglottis)	
thyrohyoid muscle	musculus thyrohyoideus

muscle	musculus (pl. musculi)
tibial muscle, anterior	musculus tibialis anterior
tibial muscle, posterior	musculus tibialis posterior
Tod's muscle (oblique auricular muscle)	
tongue, muscles of	musculi linguae
Toynbee's muscle	musculus tensor tympani
tracheal muscle	musculus trachealis
tracheloclavicular muscle	musculus tracheloclavicularis
trachelomastoid muscle	musculus longissimus capitis
tragicus muscle	musculus tragicus
(Valsalva's muscle)	
transverse arytenoid muscle	musculus arytenoideus transversus
transverse muscle of abdomen	musculus transversus abdominis
transverse muscle of auricle	musculus transversus auriculae
transverse muscle of chin	musculus transversus menti
transverse muscle of nape	musculus transversus nuchae
transverse muscle of neck	musculus transversus nuchae
transverse muscle of thorax	musculus transversus thoracis
transverse muscle of tongue	musculus transversus linguae
transversospinal muscle	musculus transversospinalis
trapezius muscle	musculus trapezius
Treitz' muscle (suspensory muscle of duodenum)	
triangular muscle	musculus triangularis
triceps muscle of arm	musculus triceps brachii
triceps muscle of hip	musculus triceps coxae
triceps muscle of calf	musculus triceps surae
trigonal muscle	
true (deep) muscles of back	musculi dorsi
two-bellied muscle (digastric muscle)	musculus digastricus
ulnar extensor muscle of wrist	musculus extensor carpi ulnaris
ulnar flexor muscle of wrist	musculus flexor carpi ulnaris
unipennate muscle	musculus unipennatus
unstriated muscle, unstriped muscle (smooth muscle)	
urogenital diaphragm, muscles of	musculi diaphragmatis urogenitalis
uvula, muscle of	musculus uvulae
Valsalva's muscle	
vastus intermedius muscle (intermediate great muscle)	musculus vastus intermedius

muscle	musculus (pl. musculi)
vastus lateralis muscle (lateral great muscle)	musculus vastus lateralis
vastus medialis muscle (medial great muscle)	musculus vastus medialis
ventral sacrococcygeal muscle	musculus sacrococcygeus ventralis
vertical muscle of tongue	musculus verticalis linguae
visceral muscle (smooth)	
vocal muscle	musculus vocalis
voluntary muscle	
white muscle (fast muscle)	
Wilson's muscle (urethral sphincter)	musculus sphincter urethrae
wrinkler muscle of eyebrow	musculus corrugator supercilii
yoked muscles	
zygomatic muscle, greater	musculus zygomaticus major
zygomatic muscle, lesser	musculus zygomaticus minor

Table of Nerves

nerve	nervus (pl. nervi)
abdominopelvic splanchnic nerves	
abducent nerve	nervus abducens
accelerator nerves	
accessory nerve	nervus accessorius
accessory nerve, vagal	ramus internus nervi accessorii
accessory phrenic nerves	nervi phrenici accessorii
acoustic nerve	
afferent nerve (centripetal; esodic)	
alveolar nerve, inferior	nervus alveolaris inferior
alveolar nerves, superior	nervi alveolares superiores
ampullar nerve, anterior	nervus ampullaris anterior
ampullar nerve, inferior	nervus ampullaris inferior
ampullar nerve, lateral	nervus ampullaris lateralis
ampullar nerve, superior	nervus ampullaris superior
anal nerves, inferior	nervi rectales inferiores
Andersch's nerve (tympanic)	
anococcygeal nerves	nervi anococcygei
anterior ampullar nerve	nervus ampullaris anterior
anterior antebrachial nerve (anterior interosseous nerve)	
anterior auricular nerves	nervi auriculares anteriores
anterior crural nerve (femoral nerve)	
anterior cutaneous nerves of abdomen (thoracoabdominal nerves)	
anterior ethmoidal nerve	nervus ethmoidalis anterior
anterior femoral cutaneous nerves	rami cutanei anteriores nervi femoralis
anterior interosseous nerve	nervus interosseous anterior
anterior labial nerves	nervi labiales anteriores
anterior scrotal nerves	nervi scrotales anteriores
anterior supraclavicular nerve (medial supraclavicular nerve)	
anterior tibial nerve (deep peroneal nerve)	

854

nerve	nervus (pl. nervi)
aortic nerve (Cyon's nerve, depressor nerve of Ludwig, Ludwig's nerve)	
Arnold's nerve	ramus auricularis nervi vagi
articular nerve	nervus articularis
auditory nerve (cochlear)	nervus vestibulocochlearis
augmentor nerves (cervical splanchnic nerves)	
auricular nerves, anterior	nervi auriculares anteriores
auricular nerve, great	nervus auricularis magnus
auricular nerve, internal	ramus posterior nervi auricularis magni
auricular nerve, posterior	nervus auricularis posterior
auricular nerve of vagus nerve	ramus auricularis nervi vagi
auriculotemporal nerve	nervus auriculotemporalis
autonomic nerve	nervus autonomicus
axillary nerve	nervus axillaris
baroreceptor nerve (pressoreceptor nerve)	
Bell's long thoracic nerve	nervus thoracicus longus
Bock's nerve	ramus pharyngeus ganglii pterygopalatini
buccal nerve	nervus buccalis
buccinator nerve (buccal nerve)	
cardiac nerve, cervical, inferior	nervus cardiacus cervicalis inferior
cardiac nerve, cervical, middle	nervus cardiacus cervicalis medius
cardiac nerve, cervical, superior	nervus cardiacus cervicalis superior
cardiac nerve, inferior	nervus cardiacus cervicalis inferior
cardiac nerve, middle	nervus cardiacus cervicalis medius
cardiac nerve, superior	nervus cardiacus cervicalis superior
cardiac nerves, supreme	rami cardiaci cervicales superiores nervi vagi
cardiac nerves, thoracic	rami cardiaci thoracici
cardiopulmonary splanchnic nerves	
caroticotympanic nerve	nervus carotidotympanicus
carotid sinus nerve (Hering's sinus)	ramus sinus carotici
cavernous nerves of clitoris	nervi cavernosi clitoridis
cavernous nerves of penis	nervi cavernosi penis
celiac nerves	rami coeliaci nervi vagi
centrifugal nerve (efferent)	
centripetal nerve (afferent)	

855

nerve	nervus (pl. nervi)
cerebral nerves	nervi craniales
cervical nerves	nervi cervicales
cervical splanchnic nerves	
(augmentor nerves)	
chorda tympani nerve	chorda tympani
ciliary nerves	nervi ciliares
circumflex nerve (axillary)	nervus axillaris
cluneal nerves	rami clunium
coccygeal nerve	nervus coccygeus
cochlear nerve	nervus cochlearis
common fibular nerve (common peroneal)	
common palmar digital nerves	nervi digitales palmares communes
common peroneal nerve	nervus fibularis communis
common plantar digital nerves	nervi digitales plantares communes
cranial nerves	nervi craniales
first (olfactory)	nervi olfactorii
second (optic)	nervus opticus
third (oculomotor)	nervus oculomotorius
fourth (trochlear)	nervus trochlearis
fifth (trigeminal)	nervus trigeminus
sixth (abducens)	nervus abducens
seventh (facial)	nervus facialis
eighth (acoustic)	nervus vestibulocochlearis
ninth (glossopharyngeal)	nervus glossopharyngeus
tenth (vagal)	nervus vagus
eleventh (accessory	nervus accessorius
twelfth (hypoglossal)	nervus hypoglossus
crural interosseous nerve	nervus interosseus cruris
cubital nerve (ulnar nerve)	nervus ulnaris
cutaneous femoral nerve, lateral	nervus cutaneus femoris lateralis
cutaneous nerve	nervus cutaneus
cutaneous nerve, femoral	nervus cutaneus femoralis
cutaneous nerve of arm, lateral, inferior	nervus cutaneus brachii lateralis inferior
cutaneous nerve of calf, medial	nervus cutaneus surae medial
cutaneous nerve of foot, dorsal, lateral	nervus cutaneus dorsalis lateralis
cutaneous nerve of forearm, medial	nervus cutaneus antebrachii medialis
cutaneous nerve of neck, anterior	nervus transversus colli
cutaneous nerve of thigh, posterior	nervus cutaneus femoralis posterior
Cyon's nerve (aortic)	

nerve	nervus (pl. nervi)
dead nerve (nonvital dental pulp)	
deep fibular nerve (deep peroneal)	
deep peroneal nerve	nervus fibularis profundus
deep petrosal nerve	nervus petrosus profundus
deep temporal nerves	nervi temporales profundi
dental nerve, inferior	nervus alveolaris inferior
depressor nerve of Ludwig (aortic)	
diaphragmatic nerve	nervus phrenicus
digastric nerve	ramus digastricus nervi facialis
digital nerves, dorsal, radial	nervi digitales dorsales nervi radialis
dorsal nerve of clitoris	nervus dorsalis clitoridis
dorsal digital nerves	
dorsal digital nerves of foot	nervi digitales dorsales pedis
dorsal digital nerves of hand	
dorsal interosseous nerve (posterior interosseous)	
dorsal lateral cutaneous nerve (lateral dorsal cutaneous)	
dorsal medial cutaneous nerve (medial dorsal cutaneous n.)	
dorsal nerve of penis	nervus dorsalis penis
dorsal nerve of scapula (dorsal scapular)	
dorsal scapular nerve	nervus dorsalis scapulae
dorsal nerves of toes	
efferent nerve (centrifugal nerve)	
eighth cranial nerve (vestibulocochlear nerve)	nervus vestibulocochlearis
eleventh cranial nerve (accessory nerve)	nervus accessorius
encephalic nerves	nervi craniales
esodic nerve (afferent nerve)	
ethmoidal nerve, anterior	nervus ethmoidalis anterior
excitor nerve	
excitoreflex nerve	
exodic nerve	
external acoustic meatus, nerve of	nervus meatus acustici externi
external carotid nerves	nervi carotici externi
external respiratory nerve of Bell (long thoracis nerve)	
external saphenous nerve (sural nerve)	

nerve	nervus (pl. nervi)
external spermatic nerve (genital branch of genitofemoral nerve)	
facial nerve	nervus facialis
femoral cutaneous nerve, intermediate	
femoral nerve	nervus femoralis
fibular nerve, superficial	nervus fibularis superficialis
fifth cranial nerve (trigeminal nerve)	nervus trigeminus
first cranial nerve (olfactory nerve)	nervus olfactorius
fourth cranial nerve (trochlear nerve)	nervus trochlearis
fourth lumbar nerve	nervus furcalis
frontal nerve	nervus frontalis
furcal nerve (fourth lumbar nerve)	
fusimotor nerves	
Galen's nerve	
gangliated nerve	
gastric nerves	truncus vagalis anterior and truncus vagalis posterior
genitocrural nerve (genitofemoral nerve)	
genitofemoral nerve	nervus genitofemoralis
glossopharyngeal nerve (ninth cranial nerve)	nervus glossopharyngeus
gluteal nerve, inferior	nervus gluteus inferior
great auricular nerve	nervus auricularis magnus
greater occipital nerve	nervus occipitalis major
greater palatine nerve	nervus palatinus major
greater petrosal nerve	
greater splanchnic nerve	nervus splanchnicus major
greater superficial petrosal nerve	nervus petrosus major
great sciatic nerve	
gustatory nerves	
hemorrhoidal nerves, inferior	nervi rectales inferiores
Hering's sinus nerve (carotid sinus)	
hypogastric nerve	nervus hypogastricus
hypoglossal nerve (twelfth cranial)	nervus hypoglossus
iliohypogastric nerve	nervus iliohypogastricus
ilioinguinal nerve	nervus ilio-inguinalis
inferior alveolar nerve	nervus alveolaris inferior
inferior cervical cardiac nerve	nervus cardiacus cervicalis inferior
inferior cluneal nerves	nervi clunium inferiores

nerve	nervus (pl. nervi)
inferior dental nerve (inferior alveolar)	
inferior gluteal nerve	nervus gluteus inferior
inferior hemorrhoidal nerves	
inferior laryngeal nerve	nervus laryngeus inferior
inferior lateral brachial cutaneous nerve	nervus cutaneus brachii lateralis inferior
inferior maxillary nerve	
inferior rectal nerves	nervi rectales inferiores
inferior vesical nerves	
infraoccipital nerve	nervus suboccipitalis
infraorbital nerve	nervus infraorbitalis
infratrochlear nerve	nervus infratrochlearis
inhibitory nerve	
intercarotid nerve	
intercostal nerves	nervi intercostales
intercostobrachial nerves	nervi intercostobrachiales
intercostohumeral nerves	
intermediary nerve	nervus intermedius
intermediate nerve	nervus intermedius
intermediate dorsal cutaneous nerve	
Jacobson's nerve (tympanic)	nervus tympanicus
jugular nerve	nervus jugularis
lacrimal nerve	nervus lacrimalis
Lancisi, nerves of	
Langley's nerves (pilomotor nerves)	
Latarjet's nerve (superior hypogastric plexus)	
laryngeal nerve, recurrent	nervus laryngealis recurrens
lateral ampullar nerve	nervus ampullaris lateralis
lateral antebrachial cutaneous nerve	nervus cutaneus antebrachii lateralis
lateral anterior thoracic nerve	
lateral cutaneous nerve of calf	
lateral cutaneous nerve of forearm	
lateral cutaneous nerve of thigh	
lateral dorsal cutaneous nerve	nervus cutaneus dorsalis lateralis
lateral femoral cutaneous nerve	nervus cutaneus femoris lateralis
lateral pectoral nerve	nervus pectoralis lateralis
lateral plantar nerve	nervus plantaris lateralis
lateral popliteal nerve	
lateral supraclavicular nerve	nervus supraclavicularis lateralis

nerve	nervus (pl. nervi)
lateral sural cutaneous nerve	nervus cutaneus surae lateralis
lesser internal cutaneous nerve	
lesser occipital nerve	nervus occipitalis minor
lesser palatine nerves	nervi palatini minores
lesser petrosal nerve	
lesser splanchnic nerve	nervus splanchnicus minor
lesser superficial petrosal nerve	nervus petrosus minor
levator ani, nerve to	
lingual nerve	nervus lingualis
long buccal nerve	
long ciliary nerve	nervus ciliaris longus
longitudinal nerves of Lancisi	
long saphenous nerve	
long subscapular nerve	
long thoracic nerve	nervus thoracicus longus
lower lateral cutaneous nerve of arm	
lowest splanchnic nerve	nervus splanchnicus imus
Ludwig's nerve (aortic nerve)	
lumbar nerves	nervi lumbales
lumbar splanchnic nerves	nervi splanchnici lumbales
lumboinguinal nerve	ramus femoralis nervi genitofemoralis
Luschka, nerve of	
mandibular nerve	nervus mandibularis
masseteric nerve	nervus massestericus
masticator nerve	
maxillary nerve	nervus maxillaris
medial antebrachial cutaneous nerve	nervus cutaneus antebrachii medialis
medial anterior thoracic nerve	
medial brachial cutaneous nerve	nervus cutaneus brachii medialis
medial cutaneous nerve of arm	
medial cutaneous nerve of forearm	
medial cutaneous nerve of leg	
medial dorsal cutaneous nerve	nervus cutaneus dorsalis medialis
medial pectoral nerve	nervus pectoralis medialis
medial plantar nerve	nervus plantaris medialis
medial popliteal nerve	
medial supraclavicular nerve	nervus supraclavicularis medialis
medial sural cutaneous nerve	nervus cutaneus surae medialis
median nerve	nervus medianus

nerve	nervus (pl. nervi)
meningeal nerve	ramus meningeus medius nervi maxillaris
mental nerve	nervus mentalis
middle cervical cardiac nerve	nervus cardiacus cervicalis medius
middle cluneal nerves	nervi clunium medii
middle meningeal nerve	
middle supraclavicular nerve	
mixed nerve	nervus mixtus
motor nerve	nervus motorius
motor nerve of tongue	nervus hypoglossus
musculocutaneous nerve	nervus musculocutaneus
musculocutaneous nerve of leg	nervus fibularis profundus
musculospiral nerve (radial)	nervus radialis
myelinated nerve	
mylohyoid nerve	nervus mylohyoideus
nasal nerve	
nasociliary nerve	nervus nasociliaris
nasopalatine nerve	nervus nasopalatinus
ninth cranial nerve (glossopharyngeal nerve)	nervus glossopharyngeus
obturator nerve	nervus obturatorius
oculomotor nerve	nervus oculomotorius
olfactory nerves	nervi olfactorii
ophthalmic nerve	nervus ophthalmicus
optic nerve (second cranial nerve)	nervus opticus
orbital nerve	
palatine nerve, anterior	nervus palatinus major
parasympathetic nerve	
parotid nerves	rami parotidei nervi auriculotemporalis
pathetic nerve	
pectoral nerve, lateral	nervus pectoralis lateralis
pelvic splanchnic nerves	nervi pelvici splanchnici
parasympathetic nerve	
perforating cutaneous nerve	
perineal nerves	nervi perineales
peroneal nerve, common	nervus fibularis communis
phrenic nerve	nervus phrenicus
pneumogastric nerve	nervus vagus
popliteal nerve, external	nervus fibularis communis

861

nerve	nervus (pl. nervi)
popliteal nerve, internal	nervus tibialis
popliteal nerve, lateral	nervus fibularis communis
popliteal nerve, medial	nervus tibialis
posterior ampullar nerve	nervus ampullaris posterior
posterior antebrachial nerve	
posterior antebrachial cutaneous nerve	nervus cutaneus antebrachii posterior
posterior auricular nerve	nervus auricularis posterior
posterior brachial cutaneous nerve	nervus cutaneus brachii posterior
posterior cutaneous nerve of arm	
posterior cutaneous nerve of forearm	
posterior cutaneous nerve of thigh	
posterior ethmoidal nerve	nervus ethmoidalis posterior
posterior femoral cutaneous nerve	nervus cutaneus femoris posterior
posterior interosseous nerve	nervus interosseus posterior
posterior labial nerves	nervi labiales posteriores
posterior scapular nerve	
posterior scrotal nerves	nervi scrotales posteriores
posterior supraclavicular nerve	
posterior thoracic nerve	
presacral nerve	plexus hypogastricus superior
pressor nerve	
pressoreceptor nerve	
proper palmar digital nerves	nervi digitales palmares proprii
proper plantar digital nerves	nervi digitales plantares proprii
pterygoid nerve	nervus pterygoideus
pterygoid canal, nerve of	nervus canalis pterygoidei
pterygopalatine nerves	nervi pterygopalatini
pudendal nerve	nervus pudendus
pudic nerve (pudendal)	nervus pudendus
quadrate muscle of thigh, nerve of	nervus musculi quadrati femoris
radial nerve	nervus radialis
recurrent nerve	nervus laryngealis recurrens
recurrent laryngeal nerve	nervus laryngeus recurrens
recurrent meningeal nerve	nervus meningeus recurrens
recurrent ophthalmic nerve	ramus tentorii nervi ophthalmici
saccular nerve	nervus saccularis
sacral nerves	nervi sacrales
sacral splanchnic nerves	nervi splanchnici sacrales
saphenous nerve	nervus saphenus

nerve	nervus (pl. nervi)
sartorius, nerve to	
Scarpa's nerve	nervus nasopalatinus
sciatic nerve	nervus ischiadicus
second cranial nerve (optic nerve)	nervus opticus
secretomotor nerve	
secretory nerve	
sensory nerve	nervus sensorius
seventh cranial nerve (facial nerve)	nervus facialis
short ciliary nerve	nervus ciliaris brevis
short saphenous nerve	nervus saphenus brevis
sinus nerve	ramus sinus carotici nervi glossopharyngei
sinus nerve of Hering	
sinuvertebral nerves	
sixth cranial nerve (abducent nerve)	nervus abducens
small deep petrosal nerve	
smallest splanchnic nerve	
small sciatic nerve	
smell, nerve of (olfactory nerve)	nervi olfactorii
somatic nerve	
space nerve	
spinal nerves	nervi spinales
spinal accessory	
splanchnic nerve	nervus splanchnicus
stapedius muscle, nerve to	nervus stapedius
statoacoustic nerve	
subclavian nerve	nervus subclavius
subcostal nerve	nervus subcostalis
sublingual nerve	nervus sublingualis
suboccipital nerve	nervus suboccipitalis
subscapular nerves	nervi subscapulares
sudomotor nerves	
superficial cervical nerve	nervus cervicalis superficialis
superficial fibular nerve	nervus fibularis superficialis
superficial peroneal nerve	nervus fibularis superficialis
superior alveolar nerves	nervi alveolares superiores
superior cervical cardiac nerve	nervus cardiacus cervicalis superior
superior cluneal nerves	nervi clunium superiores
superior dental nerves	

nerve	nervus (pl. nervi)
superior gluteal nerve	nervus gluteus superior
superior laryngeal nerve	nervus laryngeus superior
superior lateral brachial cutaneous nerve	nervus cutaneus brachii lateralis superior
superior maxillary nerve	
supraorbital nerve	nervus supraorbitalis
suprascapular nerve	nervus suprascapularis
supratrochlear nerve	nervus supratrochlearis
sural nerve	nervus suralis
sympathetic nerve	
temporomandibular nerve	
tensor tympani muscle, nerve of	nervus tensoris tympani
tensor veli palatini muscle, nerve of	nervus tensoris veli palatini
tenth cranial nerve (vagus nerve)	nervus vagus
tentorial nerve	ramus tentorii nervi ophthalmici
terminal nerves	nervi terminales
third cranial nerve (oculomotor nerve)	nervus oculomotorius
third occipital nerve	nervus occipitalis tertius
thoracic cardiac nerves	nervi cardiaci thoracici
thoracic spinal nerves	nervi thoracici
thoracic splanchnic nerve	nervus splanchnicus thoracici
thoracoabdominal nerves	nervi thoracoabdominales
thoracodorsal nerve	nervus thoracodorsalis
thyrohyoid muscle, nerve to	ramus thyrohyoideus ansae cervicalis
tibial nerve	nervus tibialis
tibial communicating nerve	
Tiedemann's nerve	
tonsillar nerves	rami tonsillares nervi glossopharyngei
transverse nerve of neck	nervus transversus colli
trifacial nerve (trigeminal nerve)	nervus trigeminus
trigeminal nerve	nervus trigeminus
trochlear nerve	nervus trochlearis
twelfth cranial nerve (hypoglossal)	nervus hypoglossus
tympanic nerve	nervus tympanicus
tympanic membrane, nerve of	
ulnar nerve	nervus ulnaris
unmyelinated nerve	
upper lateral cutaneous nerve of arm	
upper subscapular nerve	

864

nerve	nervus (pl. nervi)
upper thoracic splanchnic nerves	
utricular nerve	nervus utricularis
utriculoampullar nerve	nervus utriculoampullaris
vaginal nerves	nervi vaginales
vagus nerve	nervus vagus
Valentin's nerve	
vascular nerve	nervus vascularis
vasoconstrictor nerve	
vasodilator nerve	
vasomotor nerve	
vasosensory nerve	
vertebral nerve	nervus vertebralis
vestibular nerve	nervus vestibularis
vestibulocochlear nerve	nervus vestibulocochlearis
(eighth cranial nerve)	
vidian nerve	nervus canalis pterygoidei
visceral nerve	nervus autonomicus
volar interosseous nerve	
Willis, nerve of	nervus accessorius
Wrisberg's nerve	nervus intermedius
zygomatic nerve	nervus zygomaticus
zygomaticotemporal nerves	ramus zygomaticotemporalis nervi